foundations of massage

second edition

foundations of massage

second edition

Charles Tuchtan
Dip HSc (Remedial Therapies), Grad Cert T T & L
Head of Faculty, Remedial Therapies
Australian College of Natural Medicine
Melbourne, Australia

Vicki Tuchtan
Grad Dip TT & L, B AppSc (PhysEd), AdvDip Myotherapy, Dip Aroma
previously National Head of Teaching and Learning
Australian College of Natural Medicine
Melbourne, Australia

David Stelfox
Grad Dip Western Herbal Medicine, Dip Rem Mass, Dip Nat, Dip Herb Med
Head of Naturopathy, Clinical Studies and Research
Australian College of Natural Medicine
Melbourne, Australia

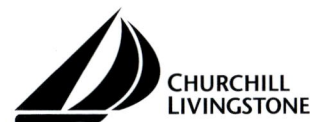

Sydney   Edinburgh   London   New York
Philadelphia   St Louis   Toronto

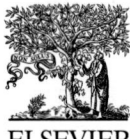

ELSEVIER

Churchill Livingstone
is an imprint of Elsevier

Elsevier Australia
30–52 Smidmore Street, Marrickville, NSW 2204

This edition © 2004 Elsevier Australia
(a division of Reed International Books Australia Pty Ltd)
ACN 001 002 357

Previously published as *Principles and Philosophies of Massage*

This publication is copyright. Except as expressly provided in the Copyright Act 1968 and the Copyright Amendment (Digital Agenda) Act 2000, no part of this publication may be reproduced, stored in any retrieval system or transmitted by any means (including electronic, mechanical, microcopying, photocopying, recording or otherwise) without prior written permission from the publisher.

National Library of Australia Cataloguing-in-Publication Data

Tuchtan, Charles C.
    Foundations of massage.

    2nd ed.
    Bibliography.
    Includes index.
    ISBN 0 7295 3734 X.

    1. Massage - Philosophy. 2. Massage - Technique. I. Tuchtan, Vicki M. II. Stelfox, David P. III. Title.

    615.822

Publisher: Vaughn Curtis
Developmental Editor: Rhiain Hull
Edited, project managed and indexed by Forsyth Publishing Services
Designed and typeset by Darben Design
Photography by Glen McCulloch Photography
Illustrations by Trina McDonald and Joe Lucia
Printed and bound in Australia by Southwood Press Pty Ltd

Foreword

Application of the hands to the human body to lend comfort, relaxation, relief of pain and improvement of function is one of the oldest and most widely used healing arts in most, if not all, cultures. This excellent text builds on this long and impressive history of service to humanity to bring massage therapy into a contemporary, scientific context without forgetting the essentials of a humanistic approach to clients.

During the last decade or so, complementary and alternative medicine (CAM) has greatly increased in acceptance and use by the community — including the importance of and acceptance of massage therapy.

This second edition of *Foundations of Massage* has been much further developed and excels the very effective first edition. In fact, it meets the aim of providing a first year text on foundations of massage with flying colours. Not only does it capture all components of the conceptual framework necessary for students to come to a full appreciation of the mosaic of what modern massage therapy represents, but it also covers the developing research basis for this important discipline.

A great deal of thinking has gone into each of the seven sections of this work that provides a methodical and logical introduction to the discipline for commencing learners.

Appropriately, it commences with a section on interesting history, demarcation of the discipline within CAM and indicating the solid foundation of massage as a credible part of mainstream medical practice and an integral part of human culture. The place of massage in an integrative, modern health care model is well presented, indicating both the responsibilities and role of massage practitioners in society.

The research evidence in favour of the benefits of massage therapy and the importance of touch is convincing and well presented.

The extensive and excellent coverage of scope of practice, principles of ethics and relevant law and the important exposition on professional boundaries issues ensures that students have all the essential information available to equip them well for professional responsibility. This is fundamental to intra-professional discipline and regulation and inter-professional cooperation in the interest of professional advancement and acceptance of massage. The discussion on massage environment recognises the importance of attention to detail and patient's rights and practice decorum.

The chapter on self-care covers this important and frequently overlooked component of practitioner training. It will guide future practitioners well in taking care of themselves in order to be able to better care for more patients for a longer period of time.

The concern for patient welfare is comprehensively addressed in the chapter on infection control — an issue that is so important as a foundation for practice.

The elegantly presented chapter on the ASTER system in practice, with case studies that nicely assist learning, provides a very solid foundation for patient assessment and management, including government requirements for clinical record keeping — all pillars of exemplary practice.

Patient safety and risk management strategies are dealt with very well in the chapter on endangerment sites and indications for the use of massage therapy, while pharmacological considerations of massage provides an excellent background for future practitioners to be able to relate effectively with medical practitioners and understand the treatment that patients on medication are undergoing.

The section on special needs serves an important purpose in providing guidance on how to serve persons with special therapeutic needs, such as the disabled.

Discussion of positioning and draping of the client covers a very important aspect of the art of practice and is clearly presented.

The chapters on body mechanics and massage, massage manipulations and massage sequence herald new initiatives and sophistication in the discipline and will add greatly to the preparation of the massage practitioner as a clinical associate to other practitioners in the field of manual medicine.

Massage during pregnancy and labour adds an important section, in the community interest, while infant massage is an important part of massage practice, and of great benefit to the sensory development of infants. Both of these aspects of the industry could benefit greatly from further research and expansion into specialty areas for the massage therapist.

The three appendices are an important, readily available, indispensable resource for the student of massage. Appendix 1, on the anatomical directional terminology and joint actions, facilitates understanding of the discipline. The anatomical plates in Appendices 2 and 3 are also a welcome ready-reference, whilst the glossary explicates commonly used terms that assist the novice in quickly mastering the language of massage.

It is a pleasure to strongly recommend this work as a comprehensive foundation textbook for therapeutic massage that not only gives an excellent introduction to the techniques of massage, but also provides a well-rounded approach to the multiple factors that play a role in clinical decision-making and client service. These include, in particular, a solid basis in patient assessment, patient safety, psychosocial, sociocultural and philosophical aspects of practice, ethics and practice management.

Andries M Kleynhans, OAM
Foundation Professor of Chiropractic
Retired Associate Dean,
Faculty of Biomedical and Health Sciences and Nursing
Retired Head of Department of
Chiropractic, Osteopathy and Complementary Medicine
RMIT University, Melbourne, Australia

Contributors

Sonya Bailey BCom, Cert Rem Mass
Lecturer
Faculty of Remedial Therapies
Australian College of Natural Medicine
Melbourne, Australia

Chris Bennett Dip Ther Mass
Lecturer
Faculty of Remedial Therapies
Australian College of Natural Medicine
Perth, Australia

Katie Callaway Dip HSc (Remedial Therapies)
Lecturer
Faculty of Remedial Therapies
Australian College of Natural Medicine
Melbourne, Australia

Lisa Casanelia BA RMT (Canada)
Lecturer
Faculty of Remedial Therapies
Australian College of Natural Medicine
Melbourne, Australia

Ellie Feeney RN, Dip HSc (Remedial Therapies)
Lecturer
Faculty of Remedial Therapies
Australian College of Natural Medicine
Melbourne, Australia

Margaret Hutchison RN, Dip FLC
Lecturer
Faculty of Remedial Therapies
Australian College of Natural Medicine
Brisbane, Australia

Dr Catherine Krejany PhD, BSc (Hons), Dip Aroma
Senior Lecturer
Faculty of Health Science
Australian College of Natural Medicine
Melbourne, Australia

Dr Heather Morrison PhD, BSc (Hons)
Head of Faculty, Health Science
Australian College of Natural Medicine
Melbourne, Australia

Dr Michael Nott PhD, BSc (Hons)
Lecturer of Pharmacology
Department of Pharmacy
La Trobe University
Bendigo, Australia

Janine Tobin BHMS, Cert Mass
Lecturer
Faculty of Health Science
Australian College of Natural Medicine
Brisbane, Australia

Sheena Worrall Dip Ther Mass, CertIV in Counselling Practice
Lecturer
Australian College of Natural Medicine
Brisbane, Australia

Contents

Foreword		v
Contributors		vii
Acknowledgments		x
Preface		xi

Section 1 Massage and Society — 1

Chapter 1	Philosophies, principles and definitions of massage and natural medicine: *David Stelfox*	3
Chapter 2	History of massage: *Katie Callaway*	15
Chapter 3	Massage and its role in an integrative health care model: *David Stelfox*	27

Section 2 Identifying the 'Legitimacy' of Massage as a Therapy — 35

Chapter 4	The evidence for massage therapy: *Vicki Tuchtan*	37
Chapter 5	The importance of touch: *Sheena Worrall*	49

Section 3 The Professional Therapist — 59

Chapter 6	Scope of practice, ethics and law in massage therapy: *Janine Tobin*	61
Chapter 7	Understanding boundaries: *Sonya Bailey and David Stelfox*	71

Section 4 Preparation for Practice — 81

Chapter 8	The massage environment: *Lisa Casanelia*	83
Chapter 9	Self-care: *Lisa Casanelia*	95
Chapter 10	Infection control in the practice of massage therapy: *Catherine Krejany, Ellie Feeney and Heather Morrison*	105

Section 5 Initial Client Contact — 117

Chapter 11	The massage process: *Charles Tuchtan*	119
Chapter 12	Endangerment sites and indications for the use of massage therapy: *Vicki Tuchtan and Charles Tuchtan*	135
Chapter 13	Pharmacological considerations for massage: *Michael Nott*	155
Chapter 14	Special needs: *Margaret Hutchison*	169

Section 6 The Massage Treatment — Hands On — 181

Chapter 15	Positioning and draping the client: *Lisa Casanelia*	183
Chapter 16	Body mechanics and massage: *Chris Bennett*	195
Chapter 17	Massage manipulations: *Charles Tuchtan*	201
Chapter 18	Putting massage into practice — the massage sequence: *Lisa Casanelia and Charles Tuchtan*	225

Section 7 Pregnancy, the Infant and Massage — 291

Chapter 19	Massage during pregnancy and labour: *Vicki Tuchtan*	293
Chapter 20	Infant massage: *Vicki Tuchtan*	301

Appendix 1	Anatomical terminology	305
Appendix 2	The human skeleton	307
Appendix 3	Overview of the muscular system	309
Glossary		311
Index		315

Acknowledgments

We are indebted to and thank all of the contributors to this book for sharing our vision for the project and working tirelessly with us to produce this book. We thank Vaughn Curtis, Helena Klijn, Amanda McGee, and Rhiain Hull from Elsevier Australia, who have all worked so diligently to ensure this text was polished and completed on schedule. A special mention to Amanda McGee who, when we were struggling to meet deadlines, kept our spirits high.

We extend our heartfelt thanks to the model clinicians and clients, who worked professionally and patiently to model for our images, namely; Lisa Casanelia, Jarrod Matthews, Anna Tuchtan and Tony Birrell. A special thank you to Lisa Casanelia who spent countless hours organising, arranging, drawing lines, checking and rechecking all of the photos and illustrations.

Charles would also like to thank the staff who took on much of his workload while he was on this special project, namely: Helena Keenan, Lisa Casanelia, Katie Callaway and Giulian Di Venuto. A special thank you is also extended to Professor Andries Kleynhans for his support and sound advice throughout this project.

Preface

One of the trends to emerge during the last decade of the twentieth century was the resurgence and growing interest in personal health and wellbeing. Combined with an increased focus on fitness and beauty, this resulted in more people in the Western world seeking natural therapies, including the pleasurable and popular experience of relaxation massage. Once viewed as an extravagance that only few could afford, these days a visit to a massage therapist is no less common than a visit to the gym or beauty therapist for many Westerners who value their health and wellbeing. In a stressed-out world, largely deprived of touch, relaxation massage provides welcome relief, and is an important therapy that may provide benefit to a wide range of people and conditions.

Much has changed over the past decades for the massage profession. In both Australia and New Zealand, national training standards aimed at establishing a benchmark for the training of massage therapists have been developed. Massage services are now easily accessible and available through local gymnasiums and health clubs, beauty salons, as well as from private health care clinics and health spas (currently the fastest growing business globally). Most new hotels incorporate a health spa as part of their facilities, and massage is one of the major services offered.

More and more workplaces are realising the benefits of massage to employees and are including a massage therapist on their payroll. Hospitals and aged-care facilities too, are involving massage therapists in their health care team. To describe massage as an 'alternative' form of therapy is no longer accurate. It has become firmly established in the 'mainstream' of health care in many Western countries.

This increased demand for massage therapy has inevitably resulted in an increased demand for competent, well-trained, professional practitioners. *Foundations of Massage* is the second edition of a broad introductory massage therapy text that covers the philosophy, principles and fundamentals of massage practice. This comprehensive text presents a uniquely Australian view of the practice of massage therapy, and includes contextual information for New Zealand also. Until now most massage training courses have relied heavily on texts from the United States of America and the United Kingdom. Those publications were written to meet the requirement for registration and regulation of massage therapists in those countries. The need for a massage text designed to meet Australian and New Zealand cultural, ethical and legal considerations was long overdue.

In this second edition, we have again brought together a group of experienced massage practitioners and educators to contribute to the writing of this book. Their expertise is drawn from both Australian and overseas training, resulting in a well-rounded perspective of massage therapy.

In essence, this edition addresses all those things you need to know about massage practice and more. We trust you will enjoy this text.

Charles Tuchtan
Vicki Tuchtan
David Stelfox

section 1

Massage and Society

chapter 1

Philosophies, principles and definitions of massage and natural medicine

David Stelfox

Learning outcomes

- Define massage
- Describe the philosophies, principles and practice of massage therapy within the context of natural medicine
- Define and provide examples of complementary and alternative health care therapies
- Compare and contrast the principles and practices of chiropractic, osteopathy, physiotherapy and massage therapy

INTRODUCTION

To be a competent and successful massage therapist — or, for that matter, a health professional of any modality — a clear understanding of the nature (definition) of the discipline, as well as its guiding philosophy and principles, is essential. Without such understanding a health care practitioner cannot deliver consistent therapeutic services that lie within a clearly defined scope of practice. It's a bit like having a car without a road map to help you find where you're going.

Massage therapy is generally classified as an 'alternative' or 'complementary' form of health care and therefore comes under the category of 'Natural Medicine' (House of Lords Report, 2000). These are terms that also require definition and understanding. This chapter aims at providing the massage student with an understanding of the various philosophies, principles and definitions associated with natural medicine practice so that they may gain an orientation to the profession in which they will be practicing.

MASSAGE THERAPY — A DEFINITION

One of the difficulties of defining massage is that the term means many things to many people. The terms massage, tactile therapy, bodywork, manual therapy and manipulative therapy have different connotations and different interpretations.

Massage as a profession has evolved significantly over the last century and today many different styles, techniques and approaches are embraced by the term 'massage'. There are now so many different techniques and approaches to soft tissue manipulation that it is difficult to classify them clearly under meaningful categories. Many have tried, but confusion has often resulted, as there will always be techniques that don't fit neatly under the proposed categories. For the purpose of this text, the more commonly known methods are classified under three broad headings —the 'subtle energy' practices, the relaxation methods, and the remedial approaches (see Table 1.1).

For the purpose of defining massage, the historical roots of the word 'massage', and their individual meanings, will be examined. 'Massage' means to touch, softly press, squeeze, rub, handle or knead with the hands. The English word 'massage' first appeared in American and European literature around 1875. It was popularised in the USA by Douglas Graham from Massachusetts (who wrote a history of the art) and in Europe by an influential Dutchman, Dr Johann Mezger.

The Greek word *masso* or *massein* means to touch, handle, knead or squeeze. *Massa* is the Latin root coming directly from the Greek, and is reflected in the Portuguese verb *amassar*, to knead. The Arabic root *mass'h*, or *mass*, is very similar and means to press softly, as does the Sanskrit *makeh*. Ancient Jewish culture held the power of touch for ritual benefit in such high esteem that the root word for anointing and rubbing with oils and for the Messiah is the same (Māshiāh).

Massage is usually applied to the skin, fascia, muscles, tendons and ligaments (the soft tissues) of the body. Since most massage has the effect of bringing about some sort of change (for the better) in the individual, then its action may be said to be therapeutic (giving physical, emotional, psychological or spiritual benefits). Therefore, the term

Table 1.1 Categories of massage therapy

SUBTLE ENERGY PRACTICES	RELAXATION METHODS	REMEDIAL APPROACHES
Reiki	Swedish massage	Manual lymphatic drainage
Therapeutic touch	Esalen massage	Neuromuscular technique
Polarity therapy		Myofascial release
Pranic healing		Aromatherapy
Aura balancing		Reflexology
Chakra balancing		Tui na (Chinese massage)
Jin shin do		Shiatsu
Zero balancing		Muscle energy technique
		Rolfing
		Postural integration
		Bowen technique
		Orthobionomy
		Cranio-sacral therapy
		Trager therapy
		Sports massage

'therapeutic massage' applies to all methods and forms of massage, since they all provide therapeutic benefit to the receiver. Reduction of muscular tension, improvement of vascular and lymphatic circulation, regulation of the nervous system and normalisation of pulmonary function are some of the claimed therapeutic physiological benefits of massage therapy (Turchaninov, 2001).

Massage therapy, then, may be defined as the use of (predominantly) the hands to physically manipulate the body's soft tissues for the purpose of effecting a desirable change in the individual. While anatomical and physiological changes are generally the focus (and may involve body systems other than the musculoskeletal system), the emotional, mental and spiritual aspects of the individual may also be affected, either objectively or subjectively due to their interrelatedness. Typical fundamental massage techniques involve (but are not necessarily restricted to) basic contact (touch), stroking (effleurage), rubbing (friction), kneading (pétrissage), percussion (tapôtement), vibration and compression. Usually a lubricant (oil or powder) is used. Hot or cold applications (thermotherapy), essential (aromatic) oils or water (hydrotherapy) may be utilised as adjuncts to massage treatment where they are considered appropriate to providing the desired therapeutic effect.

Relaxation massage seeks to relax the client, improve general wellbeing and reduce mental stress and general body tension. Techniques employed aim to soothe and loosen the body. The speed of delivery is slow and the pressure is light to moderate. An environment is created which may include soft lighting to soothe the eyes, pictures and props to create further visual pleasure, and aromatic oils dispersed in the air to satisfy the mood and emotions. Music may be played to relax the mind and enhance the spirit, and the massage table is draped for comfort and warmth (see Chapter 8 for further discussion on the massage environment).

Remedial massage is the application of more advanced techniques of treatment and assessment for neuro-musculoskeletal dysfunctions. The primary aim of remedial massage is to restore or promote motion and to reduce or prevent pain. To achieve this a variety of techniques may be employed. These may include thermotherapy, myofascial release techniques, neuromuscular techniques (trigger-point therapy), joint mobilisation, positional release techniques, post-isometric stretching and corrective exercise prescription.

NATURAL MEDICINE PHILOSOPHY AND PRINCIPLES

The philosophical basis of massage therapy draws from the philosophy and principles of natural medicine in general. The field of natural medicine embraces many different individual modalities of natural therapies (massage, homoeopathy, aromatherapy, osteopathy, colour therapy) as well as complete systems of natural healing (traditional Chinese medicine, ayurveda, naturopathy) (House of Lords Report, 2000). What draws these many different approaches together under the one umbrella is the philosophy that provides guidelines to their practice.

Natural medicine is most simply defined as *any form of health care that acknowledges and relies upon the body's natural ability to heal itself*. This principle has been a feature of traditional medicine practices for thousands of years (traditional medicine is a term used to describe any system of health care that has ancient roots, trained healers, cultural bonds and a theoretical construct; for example, traditional Chinese medicine, ayurveda, herbal medicine) (Segen, 1998). It acknowledges nature's ability to heal *(vis medicatrix naturae — the healing power of nature)*. Given the right circumstances (rest, nurturing, living according to nature's laws) a sick or injured individual can return naturally to a state of optimum health. This can be easily illustrated by the example of a fractured bone. Over a period of time the bone will heal (become whole again) of its own accord. It requires no intervention, although immobilisation may assist the bone to return to its original shape. *The body heals itself*, and nature provides the body with this ability. Any form of therapy, whether massage, nutrition, acupuncture, herbs or surgery, works simply by assisting nature's own ability to heal.

Apart from this core principle of the body's ability to heal itself, there are a number of other principles which feature commonly in natural medicine modalities and these are discussed below.

Treat the whole person

Optimum health and wellbeing is a complex interrelationship between the physical, mental, emotional and spiritual aspects of an individual (see Chapter 3). When imbalance occurs on any of these levels it eventually results in disease. For example, long-term emotional stress will eventually affect the physical body via the nervous and endocrine systems. It can then manifest physically as muscle tension, neck and back pain, headache and physical fatigue. On the physical level, natural medicine acknowledges and addresses the interrelationship between every cell, tissue, organ and system of the body. Injury or illness is never seen to be affecting just an isolated part of the body. A change to one part results in change to every part. Since illness can be the result of an imbalance in any, or a combination, of these aspects then healing must address each of them. Tactile therapy, including massage, has the potential to impact upon every aspect of the individual and so it treats the whole person.

First do no harm

Natural medicine uses therapies which are as close as possible to their natural state (e.g. human touch, herbs, food and nutrition) and that are unlikely to produce harmful side effects. Practitioners of natural medicine, including massage therapists, learn to assess the health of clients and determine whether they can effectively treat them, or if referral to another health care practitioner is more appropriate.

Prevention is better than cure

Wherever possible, the practitioner of natural medicine will promote a strategy that helps to prevent illness from eventuating, or at least from becoming worse (in the case of existing ailments). This is achieved via a combination of treatments and by involving clients in the process (e.g. regular exercise, adequate rest, balanced diet). Regular massage can serve the purpose of relaxing the nervous system, toning or relaxing muscles and regulating circulation of body fluids, thereby promoting optimum health and reducing the risk of illness or injury.

The doctor (practitioner) is a teacher

The original meaning of the word 'doctor' was 'teacher'. To achieve the best treatment outcome, to prevent the onset of illness or injury and to maintain optimum health and wellbeing, the natural medicine practitioner must educate her/his clients to take responsibility for their wellness and to get involved with creating their own health. Only by encouraging clients to live a more balanced lifestyle according to nature's laws, including healthy dietary choices, regular exercise or activity, and adequate rest, can the practitioner hope to assist. By teaching, motivating and supporting clients the practitioner–client relationship is empowered. This relationship in itself contributes significantly to the process of healing (Pizzorno and Murray, 1999).

The World Health Organization (WHO) estimates that 80 per cent of the world's population utilises natural medicine as its primary source of health care (World Health Organization, 1998). In Australia, more than 60 per cent of the population uses natural medicine of some kind. These Australians are more likely to be female, aged 30–50 years, have tertiary qualifications, earn more than $50 000 per year and be employed in a professional or managerial position. They choose natural medicine because they are dissatisfied with other approaches to health care, and because they see it as a natural, safe alternative (Therapeutic Goods Administration, 2001). In view of these facts then, natural medicine can hardly be seen as a radical, alternative healing approach on the fringe of the mainstream biomedical model of health care. With well over half of the population relying upon it to achieve a desired level of health, it is not unreasonable to view natural medicine as part of 'mainstream medicine'.

COMPLEMENTARY AND ALTERNATIVE MEDICINE

Natural medicine is sometimes referred to as 'Complementary and Alternative Medicine' (CAM). Alternative medicine is a term that was used more commonly during the 1980s and early 1990s. *The New England Journal of Medicine* (1992, p. 61) defined alternative medicine as:

> ... a heterogeneous set of practices that are offered as an alternative to conventional medicine, for the preservation of health and the diagnosis and treatment of health-related problems; its practitioners are often called healers.

At the time, this explanation reflected the fact that a minority of the population of the Western world used natural therapies as an alternative to mainstream Western biomedicine. 'Alternative' suggests an either/or choice, and provides no suggestion that Western biomedicine and natural medicine could possibly work together for the ultimate benefit of clients. Alternative medicine, then, is something which is used as an alternative to (i.e. to the exclusion of) conventional mainstream medicine approaches. These days, the natural medicine profession generally rejects the term 'alternative', as it prefers to view itself as part of an integrated approach to health care (see Chapter 3).

By definition, the term 'complementary' means to form a satisfactory or balanced whole (*Collins Concise Dictionary*, 1989). When used to describe natural medicine, 'complementary' suggests that in conjunction with the Western biomedical approach to health care, the two form a satisfactory and balanced holistic health care model (i.e. an integrated approach). However, it is taken by some to suggest that natural medicine plays only a secondary role to the biomedical model, providing merely a supplementary approach where appropriate, and cannot provide a stand-alone option to the management of health. In this respect, the term 'complementary' is an unsatisfactory description of natural medicine.

Another perspective is that complementary medicine is something which may be used to enhance, but not to replace, a conventional mainstream approach to the treatment of a health condition.

SCOPE OF PRACTICE OF NATURAL MEDICINE MODALITIES

The philosophy and principles of natural medicine define and guide the practice of the many therapies that comprise this approach to health care. Most have unique knowledge bases (i.e. the theory and skills that define how the therapy is administered), although there is some overlap (e.g. Chinese massage and acupuncture). As a result, the scope of practice (see Chapter 6) of these natural medicine modalities often overlaps, and is not always clear. It is important for massage therapists to have a basic understanding of other natural medicine modalities and their scopes of practice. The following is a brief outline of some of the more common natural medicine modalities.

Acupuncture and traditional Chinese medicine

Acupuncture involves the insertion of fine needles, and the application of a burning herb material (moxa), to very specific points or areas on the body. It is a therapy practised as part of the traditional Chinese medicine (TCM) system, which is based on the Chinese philosophical concept of health and disease. This philosophy states that health is promoted and maintained via the unobstructed flow of vital energy (Qi) through subtle channels that run throughout the body. Illness occurs when the flow of Qi becomes obstructed. Diagnosis is achieved via thorough case taking, and pulse and tongue analysis. Acupuncture and moxibustion (the burning of moxa) when administered to points located on these channels (meridians) restore and regulate the flow of Qi. The TCM system also incorporates Chinese massage (An Mo Tui Na), Chinese herbal medicine, diet and food therapy and exercise therapy (e.g. Tai qi, Qi gong). While some practitioners of Chinese medicine may include all of these therapies in their practice, others may specialise in only some or even one (e.g. acupuncture or Chinese herbs).

Aromatherapy

Aromatherapy involves the administration of essential oils distilled from plants to treat and prevent illness and to promote wellbeing. The oils may be administered topically (via massage or cosmetics), via inhalation (steam, evaporation) or less commonly through internal ingestion. An extensive range of health conditions may be treated with aromatherapy. Most aromatherapists are trained in basic relaxation massage and, more often than not, also in the technique of specialised aromatherapy massage.

Ayurveda

Ayurveda is a traditional system of healing originating from the Indian subcontinent. It is thought to be the oldest existing system of medicine practiced in the world. Ayurveda has its own unique principles based primarily on the three doshas (physiology/personality types). Pulse, tongue and urine analysis form part of the method for diagnosis. Therapies used include herbal medicine, diet and nutrition, massage, colour therapy, exercise (yoga), meditation, sound therapy, lifestyle counselling and aromatherapy. In the West, ayurveda is becoming increasingly popular due largely to the writings of Indian-born endocrinologist Dr Deepak Chopra (author of *Creating Health*, *Perfect Health*, *Quantum Healing* and other texts).

Herbal medicine

Herbal medicine practitioners usually specialise in the use of plant medicines (herbs) to treat any of a wide variety of health conditions. While naturopaths usually incorporate herbs as part of their treatment strategy, along with nutrition, massage, flower essences and perhaps homoeopathy, the herbalist will generally prescribe only herbal remedies. Phytotherapy and botanical medicine are terms also used as alternatives to 'herbal medicine'. Herbal remedies were one of the earliest forms of medication used by humankind, and most traditional healing systems include them as part of their treatment of ill health.

Homoeopathy

By comparison with ayurveda, traditional Chinese medicine and even naturopathy, homoeopathy is a relative newcomer to the field of natural medicine. It originated in Germany in the 1830s as the result of investigation by Dr Samuel Hahnemann. Based on the principle of 'like cures like' (*similia similibus curantur*), the concept of homoeopathy is that a substance that can cause illness could also cure that same illness when administered in greatly diluted doses (e.g. arsenic). Despite numerous controlled trials indicating benefits for the treatment of a wide number of health problems, homoeopathy defies explanation in terms of its mechanism of cure.

Scientists have failed to provide an explanation of how something that contains virtually no physical substance apart from water can demonstrate an efficacy comparable with, and even better than, that of pharmaceutical drugs.

Classical homoeopaths seek to establish the single best homoeopathic remedy to suit clients' presenting signs and symptoms, and prescribe no other form of therapy or remedy. However, many naturopaths incorporate homoeopathic remedies in their treatment strategy for clients when they consider them to be appropriate.

Naturopathy

The term 'naturopathy' was first used in 1899, in the USA. It was an approach to health care based on the principles of Nature Cure from Europe (Nature Cure being a general term used throughout Europe during the nineteenth century to describe the use of natural principles and therapies to prevent and treat disease). However, naturopathy's roots go back to ancient Greece and the 'Father of Medicine', Hippocrates, who believed that 'nature is the healer of all disease'. Disease is viewed as a result of violation of nature's laws, and fresh air, pure water, whole foods, sunlight, exercise and adequate rest and relaxation are seen as the cornerstones of healthy living.

In addition to promoting these healthy lifestyle measures, naturopathic practice integrates a number of modalities, principally nutrition, herbal medicine and tactile therapy. Other modalities (e.g. homoeopathy, aromatherapy, colour therapy, applied kinesiology, hydrotherapy) may also be incorporated. These modalities are applied on the basis of specific principles, and within the context of a healing environment, which endeavours to empower the individual, and motivate and educate them in order to restore, maintain and optimise wellbeing. By way of in-depth consultations, naturopaths decide upon strategies of treatment that will incorporate the most appropriate remedy/remedies to suit clients and their individual health condition. The health assessment may also be aided by iris, tongue and fingernail analysis (naturopathic diagnostic methods) and also by physical examination and pathology tests.

Nutrition therapy

Nutrition therapy, or clinical nutrition as it is also known, incorporates dietary counselling (i.e. recommending appropriate changes to clients' diets) and nutrient supplementation to treat any of a wide variety of health conditions. Supplementation with vitamins, minerals or other micronutrients is prescribed, not just where there may be deficiencies, but where an illness or injury has caused an increased demand for certain nutrients by the body. Clinical nutritionists are generally also trained in sports nutrition, an area that focuses on improving sporting performance and recovery via an optimum diet and nutrient supplementation where necessary. Treatment and management of allergies is another area in which nutrition therapists are usually trained. Where naturopaths usually incorporate diet and nutrition therapy as one of their therapeutic tools (along with herbs, massage, lifestyle counselling and sometimes homoeopathy), clinical nutritionists generally treat health problems exclusively with diet and nutrition therapy.

Tactile therapies

The field of tactile therapy includes an ever-increasing range of therapies that involve tactile manipulation (i.e. the use of touch). It is sometimes referred to as bodywork or physical therapy. While some forms of tactile therapy mainly promote beneficial changes to the anatomy and physiology of the physical body (e.g. relaxation, tonification, or stimulation of muscles, tendons, ligaments, nerves and circulation), others exert their effects mainly on the subtle anatomy/subtle energy of individuals. Reiki, therapeutic touch, aura massage and pranic healing are examples of tactile therapies that focus on changing the subtle energy/subtle body of clients. Although therapies such as Swedish massage, Chinese massage (tui na), chiropractic, osteopathy, sports massage and rolfing exert their effects mainly on the physical body, it is insisted by some that they also have an effect on the subtle energy of clients (Tappan, 1988; Chaitow, 1996).

Because there are so many approaches to tactile therapy, it is inevitable that there are many similarities between them (both similarity of technique and similarity in what they can achieve). What they share in common exceeds how they differ. For this reason there is a lot of crossover when it comes to mapping the scope of practice of these different tactile therapy approaches. While most practitioners of tactile therapy are specialists in this particular area of natural medicine, others may incorporate tactile therapy as part of their overall approach to health care (e.g. with nutrition, acupuncture, herbal medicine, flower essences). Naturopaths are an example of this.

Eastern/Asian massage therapies

Oriental bodywork techniques are based on a different set of principles and philosophy than the Western approaches to massage. The various Eastern approaches (see Box 1.1) to bodywork use different techniques and approaches, but their purpose is similar. Basically all these approaches to bodywork aim to restore, balance or maintain the flow of Qi (vital force) throughout the body (see the sections on acupuncture and traditional Chinese medicine earlier in this chapter). It is the uninterrupted and harmonious flow of Qi that is responsible for maintaining physical, mental, emotional and spiritual health. When Qi is blocked, discomfort may be experienced spiritually, emotionally, mentally or physically. If this blockage persists over time, the imbalance develops in its complexity and eventually chronic and degenerative health conditions will result.

> **Box 1.1 Eastern/Asiatic bodywork approaches**
>
> - Acupressure
> - Tui na (Chinese massage)
> - Shiatsu (Japanese bodywork)
> - Thai massage
> - Balinese massage

MANIPULATIVE THERAPIES

These days the term 'manipulative therapy' is used mainly to describe the practices of chiropractic, osteopathy and physiotherapy. The goal of manipulative therapy has been defined as '*to restore maximal, pain-free movement of the musculoskeletal system in postural balance*' (Dvorak, Dvorak and Schneider, 1985). This somewhat comprehensive definition was determined by 35 experts in the field of manipulative therapy at a workshop in Switzerland in 1983. By this widely accepted definition, massage therapy also qualifies as a form of manipulative therapy, but there are similarities and differences between them.

Manipulation therapy, like massage and other forms of tactile therapy, has been a part of the art and science of healing for thousands of years. Nearly every culture has had practitioners who specialised in bonesetting, vertebral adjustment and manipulation of tendons, fascia, ligaments and muscles (for example ancient Egypt, Greece, Africa, North and South America, India and Asia). Bonesetters practised the art of precise hand thrusts to align the spinal vertebrae and also set and promote the healing of fractured bones. They have always been popular in rural areas, where farmers and manual labourers have sought their services.

History records camel drivers in Arabia who practised manipulation on each other, English peasant women who relieved others of back pain, young girls who were taught to walk on backs, and families of bonesetters who travelled from village to village practising their special art (often a special gift handed down from generation to generation) (Kaptchuk and Croucher, 1986). During the Middle Ages the clicking of a spinal joint that resulted from a physical manipulation was thought to be the expulsion of demons or spirits from the body. The presence of manipulative therapy has always been of recognised importance in society, even though at times its popularity has declined, usually as a result of criticism or discouragement by religious bodies or biomedical practitioners. One such decline corresponded to (Greenman, 1996, p. 3):

> *the approximate time of the split of physicians and barber-surgeons. As physicians became less involved in patient contact and as direct hands-on patient care became the province of the barber-surgeons, the role of manual medicine in the healing art seems to have declined.*

However, manipulative therapy has always risen again out of such declines. The most recent renaissance took place in the late nineteenth century, a period of turmoil and conflicting views in the field of medicine. At about the same time two gifted Americans, Andrew Taylor Still (1828–1917) and Daniel David Palmer (1845–1913) originated the systems of osteopathy and chiropractic respectively.

Osteopathy

Andrew Taylor Still developed osteopathy as an alternative to the existing practice of medicine of the time. Disenchanted with the heroic approach to medicine which included blood-letting, purging and heavy-handed prescribing of laxatives, calomel (mercury), narcotics and other drugs, Still developed his new 'osteopathic medicine' on a philosophy of traditional (i.e. longstanding) healing principles combined with a contemporary understanding of the functioning of the body. He began offering his new approach to the public in 1874. Manipulation therapy was added to his approach by 1879. Today manipulative therapy is the core of osteopathic practice. For some osteopaths, manipulation is the only therapy practised.

The philosophy of osteopathy is based on five key principles as follows:

1. The body is a unit — the body does not function as separate parts. All parts (cells, tissues, organs, body systems) relate to each other and function as an integrated unit. There is no hierarchy of parts (i.e. no structure of the body is of greater importance than another). For optimum health to exist, all aspects of the body must function optimally and harmoniously.
2. The healing power of nature — the body has an innate capacity to heal and maintain health. The therapist's role is to support this capacity.

3. Structure and function are interrelated — when the structure of any body part is negatively affected, the function of that part (and other parts as well) will eventually be affected too. Conversely, if function is disturbed (e.g. through a nutrient deficiency), sooner or later the structure of the cells, tissues, organs or body systems will also be altered in some way.

4. When normal adaptability is disrupted, or when environmental changes overcome the body's capacity for self-maintenance, ill-health may follow — apart from the obvious, this also implies that the therapist must always look for the cause/s of illness and address them appropriately. It is never enough simply to treat the illness or its signs and symptoms.

5. Rational treatment is based on all of the previous principles — in any dysfunction, any illness, the function and/or structure (eventually both) will be affected. The body attempts to self-correct via its inherent self-healing mechanism. If or when the body's capacity for self-maintenance and adaptation is overcome, signs and symptoms will manifest. The role of a good therapist is not just to relieve the symptoms, but to recognise the cause/s and how the body is attempting to cope with the situation. Having established this, the appropriate treatment is one which supports, promotes and enhances the body's potential for self-healing.

It is worth noting that these osteopathic principles outlined above are in keeping with those that form the basis of natural medicine philosophy as described earlier in this chapter.

In the USA, its country of origin, osteopathy has always been a total medical approach. Students of osteopathy in that country learn surgery and how to prescribe pharmaceutical drugs, along with structural assessment and diagnosis, and manipulative therapy skills. Taught within a framework of the philosophic principles established by Still, osteopathy may be said to offer total patient care and is a licensed health care profession throughout the US. However, in Australia, New Zealand and the United Kingdom, osteopathic training and practice is restricted to the skills and practice of physical manipulation, although Still's philosophy and principles are usually espoused as guidelines to osteopathic practice.

Techniques of osteopathic manipulation

Osteopathic manipulations are applied to both the soft tissues of the body (muscles, ligaments, tendons, fascia) and also to the bones and joints (but not only the spine). The aim of osteopathic manipulation is to achieve improved physiological movement, relief of pain or discomfort, relaxation of tissues, and to support the body's self-healing capacity. It is possible to classify osteopathic manipulative techniques into two broad categories — direct and indirect. Direct technique is that which confronts any restriction of movement by applying force to the body part in the direction of the restriction. With indirect technique the body part is manipulated in the direction of ease of motion. The physiological effects of a manipulation include changes to muscular tone, central, peripheral or autonomic nervous system tone and circulatory system (lymphatic, vascular) response changes (Gallagher and Humphrey, 2001).

Osteopaths may incorporate a variety of different specific techniques. Some of these include high velocity, low amplitude (HVLA) thrusting; articulatory technique; soft tissue therapy (similar to massage); craniosacral technique; muscle energy technique; myofascial release; visceral stretching and balancing technique; and counter-strain technique.

An osteopathic treatment commences with the taking of a client's history, a physical examination of either the whole body or the region where the problem is located, possibly evaluation of X-rays, and the treatment itself. During the physical examination the osteopath seeks to identify the area/s of dysfunction in the musculoskeletal system. Having identified the problem and evaluated the cause/s, the therapist then determines the most appropriate manipulative technique and the degree of force required to achieve the desired result. Osteopaths generally use the least amount of force necessary. Follow-up treatments are determined on the basis of the client's response to the initial manipulation.

Chiropractic

Daniel David Palmer, the originator of chiropractic, was a magnetic healer and self-taught manipulative therapist from the US mid west. Palmer developed the system of chiropractic ('done by hand') manipulative therapy in the 1890s (around the same time that Still developed osteopathy). While Palmer was chiropractic's originator, it was his son, Bartlett Joshua Palmer, who promoted the practice of this therapy to a professional status with a devoted following.

Chiropractic is based on four main principles:

1. The nervous system plays an important role in health and disease — the nervous system in human beings is highly developed and influences all other systems of the body, and their organs, tissues and cells.

2. The human body has the innate capacity to heal itself (*vis medicatrix naturae*) — chiropractic is based on the vitalistic theory which states that all

living things are pervaded by a vital force, which maintains, promotes and restores health.

3. Any disease is caused by alteration of normal neural function — normal neural function can be altered as a result of misalignments of the spinal vertebrae (subluxations). These subluxations disturb the spinal nerves in their mediation of mind and body and inhibit the vital force in its attempt to maintain health.

4. 'One cause, one cure' — since sickness and disease are a result of disturbed neural function, and subluxated vertebrae are the major cause of such disturbance, then elimination of spinal subluxations via chiropractic manipulation will restore health by restoring neural function and promoting the body's capacity for self-healing.

These principles are not too dissimilar to osteopathic principles. Both chiropractic and osteopathy share the view that the body's various 'parts' (i.e. organs, tissues, cells) are interrelated and that health is dependent on this relationship. They both recognise the interdependence of structure and function, and both approaches acknowledge the importance of the body's self-healing capacity (i.e. vital force) in maintaining and restoring health.

Chiropractic manipulative techniques

Most chiropractors today restrict their manipulations to the spinal column and pelvis. Some chiropractors perform adjustments to the bones of the skull. Some also manipulate or adjust the joints of the body's extremities. Chiropractic manipulative technique consists mainly of high velocity, low amplitude (HVLA) thrusting adjustments. The aim of these adjustments is to increase mobility of the spinal joints and eliminate spasms in the associated muscles, thereby enabling the spinal nerves to function effectively. Box 1.2 outlines the most commonly used chiropractic techniques. However, it should be noted that members of the profession use numerous other adjustment techniques.

A chiropractic consultation and treatment involves the taking of a thorough case history, followed by a physical examination of the spine. X-rays of the spine are often requested to assist in the formulation of a diagnosis and treatment plan. Then follows the chiropractic treatment. Sometimes hot packs or massage are used to help relax muscles prior to the adjustment. Chiropractors may also recommend exercise therapy or offer lifestyle management advice to their clients (Kleynhans, Sweaney and Hunt, 2003).

While in the past practitioners of chiropractic fully believed that all illness was the result of subluxation and could therefore be effectively

> **Box 1.2** Chiropractic treatment techniques
>
> - Receptor-tonus method (Nimmo technique) — improves muscle function and postural balance via techniques that eliminate trigger points
> - Diversified — delivered to individual or groups of vertebral segments
> - Gonstead — direct thrust in the direction opposite to that of the motion restriction (i.e. similar to osteopathic indirect technique)
> - Activator — use of a spring-loaded gun-like device to deliver very high velocity force to vertebrae and sometimes soft tissues such as muscles or ligaments
> - Thompson Terminal Point — HVLA adjustment to the spine, especially the pelvis, using a specialised treatment table
> - Logan basic — fascial release technique to the sacrotuberous ligament for the purpose of correcting subluxation of the sacrum
> - Flexion distraction — traction-mobilisation for treatment of intervertebral disc problems
> - Hole-in-one technique — focuses on manipulation of the first two cervical vertebrae since these were seen to be crucial to the alignment of all other spinal vertebrae
> - Sacro-occipital technique — aims to achieve balance and alignment between the pelvis and the spine, thus enhancing the flow of cerebro-spinal fluid to optimise nerve function
> - Applied kinesiology — based on the concept that vertebral subluxations create specific muscle weaknesses; used to diagnose vertebral misalignment and to correct associated muscle weakness

treated with chiropractic adjustment, this view has changed. Most chiropractors today view their profession as a form of complementary therapy, which assists in the prevention, and treatment, of ill-health.

Physiotherapy

Physiotherapy began to develop as a profession in Australia after 1939 with the establishment of the Australian Physiotherapy Association (formerly the Australian Massage Association). From that time physiotherapy developed a strong reputation and a growing popularity in Australia and massage went into something of a decline during that period (see Chapter 2). Probably the main difference between the two professions was that physiotherapy focused more on rehabilitation from injury. This was largely due to the increased demand for rehabilitation services and skills as a result of World War II casualties.

Although massage techniques formed the foundation of physiotherapy practice, exercise therapy, thermotherapy, hydrotherapy and electrotherapy began to play an increasing part. Spinal manipulations also began to feature more frequently, especially where neck and back pain was concerned. Since that time physiotherapy has continued to develop as a profession, with government registration in all Australian states, university degree education programs and WorkCover recognition of its services. Geoff Maitland, a prominent South Australian physiotherapist, has been an influential figure in the development of manipulative physiotherapy in Australia. His techniques and approach to manipulative therapy have had a significant influence on orthopaedic manipulative therapy worldwide.

Health promotion and disease prevention with physiotherapy

Physiotherapy's main focus is the restoration of physical function, and an understanding of the musculoskeletal system is the therapist's key area of expertise. Manipulative therapy, prescription of therapeutic exercise and electrophysical therapy (e.g. ultrasound) are used as the primary tools for minimising physical dysfunction, restoring normal function and relieving pain. While a recent trend in manipulative therapies has seen a reduction in the use of HVLA thrusting adjustments, these still form a significant part of physiotherapy. However, a greater emphasis on rehabilitative exercise therapy is evident in most physiotherapy practices.

These days, physiotherapy training incorporates such specialty areas as neurological, cardiothoracic, paediatric, gerontological and of course, musculoskeletal physiotherapy. With health assessment there is now greater emphasis on identifying the dysfunction, its source and also the causes of the source of dysfunction, and factors contributing to it, rather than simply determining the pathophysiology. Health evaluation has become more client-centred, and the bio-psychological perspective of the dysfunction has overshadowed a patho-biological understanding. Patho-biological diagnosis serves mainly to identify precautions and contraindications to the treatment and management of the problem (Maitland, 2001). Clients are encouraged to participate in the process of rehabilitation as much as possible (by complying with the prescribed exercise regime).

Physiotherapy manipulative techniques

Manipulative physiotherapy techniques may be broadly categorised into two types, gentle pain-modulating methods and stronger mobilising techniques. The stronger mobilising techniques are similar to the HVLA methods used by chiropractors and osteopaths. They force a movement beyond its limited range of motion via a sudden thrust. The gentler methods coax a movement by passive rhythmical oscillations performed within or at the limit of the range of motion. Most areas of the body's skeleton may be treated (i.e. not just the spine). Wherever possible the gentler methods are preferred because the client has greater control, being able to resist the mobilisation if they experience too much pain, whereas the sudden HVLA manipulation prohibits any control by the client. Manipulation of the body's soft tissues also takes place where appropriate. Massage technique is rarely used these days by physiotherapists, although techniques such as trigger-point therapy, myofascial release and muscle energy technique are being used increasingly by some therapists. Physiotherapists stress that the manipulative techniques they employ are based on scientific knowledge and research. They have not been determined empirically.

A typical physiotherapy session begins with a detailed assessment that will incorporate the taking of a case history and extensive physical examination. As previously mentioned, a client-centred approach to assessment has evolved. The physiotherapist is particularly interested in the client's expression of their signs and symptoms, and how their specific dysfunction limits and affects their activities. Diagnosis of the pathology is not the 'be all and end all'. In many cases of musculoskeletal dysfunction the pathology will not be known for certain and therefore the treatment strategy will be determined largely from the information provided by the client and the signs and symptoms he/she is presenting. Evaluation of the client's full range of motion, gait, posture and strength is usually undertaken. X-rays and CT scans may assist the therapist in determining the most appropriate treatment strategy. The treatment plan will inevitably involve stretching and exercise prescription, perhaps ultrasound or other electrophysical application, thermotherapy, and possibly manipulative therapy. Some physiotherapists include musculoskeletal acupuncture (needling or laser) to the trigger points of affected areas.

Remedial massage therapy

Manipulation of the musculoskeletal system of the body is an integral part of remedial massage. While this manipulation applies mainly to the body's soft tissues, mobilisation of joints can be part of the scope of practice of the massage therapist where adequate training in the appropriate techniques has been undertaken, and where state/territory law permits (see Chapter 6).

Therapeutic massage generally does not incorporate HVLA manipulations of the spine, however vertebral subluxations may be addressed by applying massage and other soft tissue techniques (for example, trigger-point, post-isometric relaxation technique) to the soft tissues that support and surround the spine. Once these muscles or ligaments have been satisfactorily relaxed or returned to a balanced state, stretching and/or gentle mobilisation of the affected joints may correct the alignment of the vertebrae.

MASSAGE TRAINING

Training of massage practitioners has up until recently been a somewhat haphazard process (see Chapter 2). Standards and qualifications have varied enormously and control of the quality of training has been loose. However, the Australian National Training Authority (ANTA), a Federal Government department whose role it is to promote and regulate consistency of professional training standards nationally, has recently introduced national training standards for the massage profession in the Vocational Education and Training (VET) sector of education. Under ANTA's Health Training Package (Complementary and Alternative Health Care), there are several bodywork qualifications:

- Certificate IV in Massage;
- Certificate IV in Shiatsu;
- Certificate IV in Traditional Chinese Remedial Massage (An Mo Tui Na);
- Diploma of Remedial Massage;
- Diploma of Traditional Chinese Remedial Massage (An Mo Tui Na).

ANTA's Sport and Recreation Training Package includes two other massage qualifications:

- Certificate III in Sports Massage;
- Diploma of Sports Massage.

These training packages aim to ensure that all Australian massage professionals in the industry will at least have a minimum and consistent standard of training. This should result in a more consistent standard of service to Australian consumers of bodywork therapy, increased acceptance of massage and the other bodywork methods as effective health care modalities, and an even greater confidence in natural medicine generally.

CONCLUSION

As massage therapy continues to evolve as a profession and also as a therapy, it seems likely that training programs in massage, especially therapeutic massage, will incorporate more advanced assessment methods and techniques of manipulation (both of soft tissues and bony structures). When this occurs, massage as a healing method will have come full circle, in that the bodywork therapists from past civilisations and from other systems of medicine always integrated the art of bonesetting with the gentle skills of soft tissue massage, corrective exercise and posture technique.

Questions and activities

1. You are designing a promotional flyer for use in your clinic.
   (a) Write a definition of massage for inclusion that makes reference to some of the original meanings of the word.
   (b) Write a paragraph that outlines the major principles underpinning the practice of natural medicine.
2. A client has asked you for a referral for their gastric reflux. They are not sure whether to visit a traditional Chinese medicine (TCM) practitioner, ayurvedic practitioner or a naturopath. Describe what you would tell them in relation to these different modalities, including any aspects of their practice that are common.
3. A client asks you what the difference is between herbal medicine, homoeopathy and nutrition therapy. What would you say?
4. Prepare a statement that could be provided to clients that describes and outlines the benefits of each of the following modalities:
   (a) osteopathy;
   (b) chiropractic;
   (c) physiotherapy;
   (d) remedial massage therapy.

Recommended reading

Grossinger, R. (1995) *Planet Medicine: Modalities* (6th edn). North Atlantic Books, New York.

Micozzi, M. S. (ed.) (2001) *Fundamentals of Complementary and Alternative Medicine*. Churchill Livingstone, New York.

Novey, D. W. (2000) *Clinician's Complete Reference to Complementary and Alternative Medicine*. Mosby, St Louis.

Robson, T. (ed.) (2004) *An Introduction to Complementary Medicine*. Allen & Unwin, Sydney.

Ward, R. C. (ed.) (2003) *Foundations for Osteopathic Medicine* (2nd edn). Lippincott Williams & Wilkins, Philadelphia.

REFERENCES

Chaitow, L. (1996) *Muscle Energy Techniques*. Churchill Livingstone, Edinburgh.

Chopra, D. (1987) *Creating Health*. Houghton Mifflin, Boston.

—— (1989) *Quantum Healing*. Bantam Books, New York.

—— (1990) *Perfect Health*. Harmony Books, New York.

Collins Concise Dictionary (1989) Australian edition, Collins, London.

Dvorak, J., Dvorak, V. and Schneider, W. (eds) (1985) *Manual Medicine 1984*, Springer-Verlag, Heidelberg, Germany.

Gallagher, R. M. and Humphrey, F. J. (2001) *Osteopathic Medicine: A Reformation in Progress*. Churchill Livingstone, Philadelphia.

Greenman, P. E. (1996) *Principles of Manual Medicine*. Lippincott Williams & Wilkins, Philadelphia.

House of Lords — Science and Technology — Sixth Report. (2000) *Complementary and Alternative Medicine*. UK Parliament.

Kaptchuk, T. and Croucher, M. (1986) *The Healing Arts: A Journey Through the Faces of Medicine*. British Broadcasting Corporation, London.

Kleynhans, A. M., Sweaney, J. D. and Hunt, R. G. (2003) 'Chiropractic', in I. Freckelton and H. Selby (eds) *Expert Evidence*. Thomson Lawbook Co. Section 4-901–1083.

Maitland, G. D. (2001) *Maitland's Vertebral Manipulation* (6th edn). Butterworth–Heinemann, Oxford.

New England Journal of Medicine (1992), 326:61.

Pizzorno, J. E. and Murray, M. T. (1999) *Textbook of Natural Medicine* (2nd edn). Churchill Livingstone, London.

Segen, J. C. (1998) *Dictionary of Alternative Medicine*. Appleton & Lange, Stamford, Connecticut.

Tappan, F. (1988) *Healing Massage Techniques: Holistic, Classic and Emerging Methods* (2nd edn). Appleton & Lange, Norwalk.

Therapeutic Goods Administration, February (2001) Online: *www.health.gov.au/tga/docs/html/facts.pdf*

Turchaninov, R. (2001) *Therapeutic Massage — A Scientific Approach*. Aesculapius Books, Phoenix, Arizona.

World Health Organization (1998) *Traditional Medicine*. WHO Publications, Geneva, Switzerland.

chapter 2

History of massage

Katie Callaway

Learning outcomes

- Summarise the origins and history of massage
- Identify how historical events have led to current philosophies
- Develop an understanding of the importance of historical factors in the theory and practice of massage today

INTRODUCTION

The oldest written reference to what is now called massage is thousands of years old. As such, today's practitioners are quite possibly using skills that have been developed and refined over some 5000 years.

Knowledge of the history of massage will assist students to recognise their place in the profession and in forming their own beliefs and philosophies about how massage fits into society.

This chapter will discuss the development and growth of massage from its most primitive days to modern times. From its starting point in ancient history, this chapter moves through the 'Dark Ages' to modern times and includes contributions that early massage therapists made to the profession in Australia.

ANCIENT TIMES (3000 BC – AD 400)

There is evidence that massage was widely used in ancient times. The first recorded evidence dates back to around 2350 BC in Babylon (today's Iraq) where cuneiform text inscribed on clay tablets implied that massage was used.

Historians generally believe that Egyptians and Chinese cultures developed at around the same time, however dating of early Chinese texts is complicated because of the tendency at the time for Chinese writers to credit their work to a previous emperor as an expression of honour.

In Egypt, foot and hand massage was documented as a form of treatment. This is evidenced by a wall painting (c. 2330 BC) in the tomb of Ankhmahor depicting a physician massaging the hands and feet of a patient. The wall painting suggests that techniques used in this form of massage were thumb and finger pressures, as well as squeezing and pressing with the fingertips. Today such techniques might be referred to as reflexology, which is a form of pressure point massage applied to the hands, feet and ears.

The Jews gained knowledge of using aromatic oils from the Egyptian embalming process, and developed anointing and rubbing rituals to cleanse and purify the body and mind.

Archaeological discoveries in China have contributed to our knowledge of the origins of massage. A text written by Unschuld (2000) makes reference to an archaeological site that discovered a funerary complex from 168 BC known as Mawangdui, near the city of Changsha in the central Chinese province of Hunan. This site uncovered 14 medical manuscripts that document medical developments during the end of the Zhou Dynasty (1122–221 BC), during the Qin dynasty (221–207 BC) and at the beginning of the Han dynasty (206–220 AD). These manuscripts, believed to constitute the oldest medical text written in China, mention many methods of healing including what is now called massage.

Another ancient text is *The Yellow Emperor's Classic of Internal Medicine* (Nei Ching). Claimed by some to be written around 2500 BC, it was more probably written around 200 BC or even later. The translation (Veith, 1972) shows that massage was considered one of the five treatments of that era. It describes the treatment of paralysis, chills and fever and states that 'these diseases are most fittingly treated with breathing exercises, massage of the skin and flesh, and exercises of the hands and feet' (p. 168).

In ancient times, the Chinese referred to their system of massage as *amma*, which involved techniques such as rubbing and finger pressure along the meridians of the body. These ancient hand techniques are still employed, along with additional techniques such as pulling of limbs and pushing of the soft tissues. Today's Chinese system of massage is referred to as *An Mo Tui Na*, or traditional Chinese medicine remedial massage.

The trade routes are believed to have resulted in a spread of massage techniques to India where it is surmised that massage was integrated with yoga to form a system of exercise and massage to promote and maintain health, spirituality and vitality. During 1800 BC, four 'books of wisdom' were written in India, based on sacred Hindu teachings known as the Vedas. Many authors believe that massage was written about in the Ayur-Veda volume. Kleen (1918, p.1) states that '.... Professor Pagel of Berlin [could not find] anything on these subjects in the Ayur-Veda'. Later on however, in 300 BC, the *Laws of Man* mentioned massage as a duty of everyday life. Techniques such as kneading, tapôtement, frictions and cracking are listed (Beck, 1999, p. 6).

In Japan, the Chinese *amma* philosophy of working with the body's meridians lead to the development of shiatsu therapy in the seventeenth century. This therapy, which is popular today in both Eastern and Western countries, uses thumb and finger pressure on *tsubo* points (energy points along the meridians) as the fundamental technique.

Meanwhile in Ancient Greece Asclepius (Asclepiades), a practitioner of medicine, became regarded as a god due to his healing arts. Kellogg (1895) writes:

> Asclepiades ... held the practice of this art in such esteem that he abandoned the use of medicines of all sorts, relying exclusively upon massage, which he claimed effects a cure by restoring to the nutritive fluids their natural, free movements. It was this physician who made the discovery that sleep may be induced by gentle stroking.

Another legacy from Asclepius is the symbol of the medical staff with two serpents twisting around it, *cadeucus*, which is widely recognised as a symbol of medical and pharmaceutical practices.

Hippocrates of Cos (c. 460–377 BC) was a follower of Asclepius' work and was taught by Herodicus, the founder of medical gymnastics. Hippocrates became so famous he was given the title 'father of medicine'. He believed that medicine should be practised as an art inspired by the love of man. He chose surgery only as a last resort and preferred to use natural medicines and hands-on techniques as a primary cure or preventative. Hippocrates referred to his hands-on methods as *anatripsis* (rub). One of his most famous quotes relating to massage is (Beard, 1964, p. 3):

> the physician must be acquainted with many things and assuredly with anatripsis [rubbing], for things that have the same name have not the same effects. For rubbing can bind a joint that is too loose or loosen a joint that is too hard.

Claudius Galen (AD 130–199) followed Hippocrates' work and become the second most prominent physician of this time. As physician to the gladiators he used massage techniques to treat injuries. Galen's experience with the gladiators confirmed his belief in the validity of massage as a treatment. In Rome he lectured and gave physical demonstrations on the theory and practice of medicine. He also wrote over 400 books on medical practices, including massage and gymnastics (Chandler, 1980).

At much the same time in Rome, the physician Aulus Celsus (AD 129–199) published his *De Medicina*, in which rubbing and exercises are strongly favoured as a form of therapeutic relief.

Bathing culture in Greece and Rome

The bathing culture, as used by the Greeks and Romans, highlights one way in which massage was employed during ancient times. Around 400 BC large gymnasiums (known as 'Esclapeion') were built close to town or by the seashore and they were dedicated to healing, education and public discourse. In the centre of these palatial gymnasiums was the young men's hall where athletes and citizens discussed the tactics of sport and politics and would rest and massage each other (Calvert, 2002).

The Roman baths were as important as the Greek gymnasiums and followed similar themes. By the last century BC, they 'took on an importance unparalleled in human history' (Calvert, 2002). The following is a testimony to the value the Romans placed on massage (cited in Calvert, 2002, p. 60).

> The wise and able Emperor Hadrian, 76–138 AD, who will be so well remembered as having built the wall from the Solway Firth to the Tyne, and whose reign was distinguished by peace and beneficent energy, one day saw a veteran soldier rubbing himself against the marble at the public baths, and asked him why he did so. The veteran answered, 'I have no slave to rub me,' where upon the emperor gave him two slaves and gold sufficient to maintain them. Another day several old men rubbed themselves against the wall in the emperor's presence, hoping for similar good fortune, when the shrewd Hadrian, perceiving their object, directed them to rub one another!

THE DARK AGES/MIDDLE AGES (AD 400–1450)

The early Middle Ages are often referred to as the Dark Ages because of the low level of learning or 'enlightenment'. During this time information was lost, new material was not written and, in most of Europe, Christianity had a huge hold over the beliefs of men and women.

By the end of the fifth century the Roman Empire was overrun by warring tribes. As a result of such invasions, works like *De Medicina* that Celsus wrote were 'lost'. Christianity gradually became a permeating influence and knowledge that was considered to be heretical or non-Christian was suppressed. Christians did use touching as a part of their beliefs and it was referred to as 'the laying on of hands', however the use of the body for pleasure was discouraged and sickness was viewed as the invasion of an evil spirit or evil thoughts. The art of massage and its benefits were ignored by Christian leaders and followers. Folk healers may have been the only people who practised massage during this time, but due to the beliefs about sinful behaviour being against Christian doctrine, they were dubbed as witches who did Satan's work and were often punished for their actions.

While Christianity was being established in the West, a new religion and way of life which is now known as Islam was founded in Arabia, by the prophet Mohammad (c. 570–632). Around 750 the art of making paper reached the Islamic world from China, thus allowing new and rediscovered works to be transcribed. In time this learning reached Western Europe via Spain, where Islam had become established.

As a result of this, the lost work of Hippocrates, Galen and Celsus was revived and spread throughout Europe.

During the ninth and tenth centuries new medical texts were written. Some of the work of the Islamic–Persian philosopher/physician Rhazes, or Razi, (860–932) was based on the work of

Hippocrates and Galen. Razi wrote an encyclopaedia in which he praised and promoted massage, as well as exercise and diet, to maintain health and wellbeing. Another great Persian philosopher/physician, Avicenna (980–1037) wrote the *Canon of Medicine*, basing his beliefs about medicine on Galen's work and promoting the use of massage and exercise.

In about 1450 Johannes Gutenberg and his colleagues brought together the elements of modern printing for the first time. It was this creation of the Gutenberg press that allowed works such as *De Medicina* by Celsus to be circulated through the greater world once again.

THE MODERN ERA (1450–2000)

About 100 years later, well into the Renaissance, French physician Ambrois Paré (c. 1510–1590) wrote about the use of massage as a treatment. Paré was mainly interested in the effects of massage on broken joints or after orthopaedic surgery. He referred to the speeds and depths with which frictions were applied to the body, plus mobilisation of the joints (Palmer, 1912). Today these techniques are constantly employed by massage therapists.

In 1569, Girolamo Mercuriale (1530–1606) wrote *De Arte Gymnastica*, following the theme that massage and exercise were a partnership to be used during the same session.

Records show that a physician named Hoffman (1660–1742) used massage and exercise as part of his medical practice in Germany. Along with exercise, he used massage in the way that Hippocrates, Galen and Celsus advocated. Hoffman's work contributed to the medical practices in Germany, France and England and paved the way for the public to become aware of the benefits of massage and exercise.

Per Henrik Ling (1776–1839) was born in Sweden and, with two French associates, set the wheels in motion to produce *Svenska Gymnastikens* (Swedish Exercise), which today is known as Swedish massage. In 1804 Ling began lecturing at the Lunds Universitet on the art of fencing and gymnastics. He studied anatomy and physiology and further developed his knowledge of how the human body moves. While teaching fencing to his students, Ling noted that some students could not physically perform the moves he wanted them to. He learnt through teaching gymnastics to his students that posture could be re-educated to produce greater efficiency of movement.

Ling opened the Swedish Royal Central Institute of Gymnastics in 1813, where he continued the development of his ideas. Salvo (1999, p. 10) quotes Ling as saying: '[we] try by means of influencing movements to alleviate or overcome sufferings that have arisen through abnormal conditions'. Ling began to classify his gymnastic movements into *active* (performed by the client alone), *passive* (movements of the client's limbs performed by the therapist) and *duplicated* (performed by the client with assistance from the therapist). Ling's 'passive movement' incorporated massage techniques such as friction, hacking, pinching, squeezing and kneading.

By 1851, Ling's teachings had spread to 38 schools throughout Europe. However, Ling's name was exploited to market Swedish gymnastics and this brought his developments to the attention of the medical fraternity, who ridiculed his work on the basis that his education in anatomy and physiology was not extensive. Despite this, Ling's work did receive a favourable reception in parts of Europe.

In Holland, Dr Johann Mezger (1839–1909) and an English physician, Mathias Roth, have been credited for bringing Ling's work to the scientific community. Mezger introduced the terminology still used today, such as effleurage, pétrissage, tapôtement (including beating and clapping) and massage (Beard and Wood, 1964). Mezger spread massage into Germany and Austria, through his extensive practice of this art and his ability to competently display its benefits to others in the medical profession.

The French physician Just Marie Marcellin Lucas-Championnière claimed, in about 1880, that 'in fractures, the soft tissue union as well as the bony union should be considered from the start' (Tappan, 1988, p. 7). Lucas-Championnière's ideas impressed Sir William Bennett who began using massage to treat patients at St Georges Hospital in England during the late nineteenth century. The validation of massage by Bennett and Roth influenced British opinion as to its worth. Menell later writes 'those who have once seen the treatment first devised by Lucas-Championnière applied to a recent fracture cannot but admit that they have witnessed the result of a profound reflex' (1920, p. 6).

Interest in massage was not limited to Europe. In the United States in 1856, two brothers, Charles and George Taylor, introduced Ling's work. They learned the techniques from Roth and were the driving force behind Americans' belief in the benefits of massage. By 1880, medical research had begun in New York on the benefits of massage in the management of anaemia.

Back in London, specifically during 1894, the British Medical Association (BMA) made a special inquiry into the education and practice of massage practitioners. This inquiry, which fuelled the 'Massage Scandals of 1894', found that many schools of massage were using questionable tactics to enrol students. Graduates of these schools were usually unskilled and in debt and were offered employment by their schools. However, it was not unknown for this employment to include prostitution. Thus the longstanding association between massage and prostitution was reinforced. The term 'massage parlour' as a euphemism for brothels was popularised by this scandal. In addition, the BMA's inquiry found that qualifications had been forged, leading to public mistrust.

A group of women started the first massage association in London, named the Society of Trained Masseuses. They hoped to gain acceptance of massage as a legitimate field of study and an emerging career option and profession. The women used the medical model to shape their society, making high academic standards a part of the compulsory entrance requirements. Training was only done at selected schools, and these schools were monitored regularly to maintain the society's standards.

Over the next hundred years, many types of massage and bodywork developed. In 1917 Dr James Menell divided massage effects into two categories — mechanical actions and reflex actions. Menell showed that massaging a patient produced mechanical actions such as moving venous blood and lymph, and also stretched connective tissue affecting tendons and scar tissue. Menell noted that when stimulating the tactile skin receptors, reflex action occurring to soft tissue such as muscle caused it to relax or contract, depending on the type of stroke used. About 15 years later a Danish physiologist, Emil Vodder, along with his wife Estris, developed *manual lymphatic drainage*, which uses very light circular motion on the skin to work directly with the lymphatic system. Their work spread worldwide and a number of practitioners in Australia are specially trained in this technique today.

Soft tissue manipulations were also popularised at this time. In England an orthopaedic surgeon, James Cyriax, developed *transverse friction massage*. He published the *Textbook of Orthopedic Medicine: Volume 2* (11th edn, 1984), and this laid the foundation for soft-tissue manipulations.

MASSAGE IN AUSTRALIA

The Aboriginal connection

The healing methods used by the early Aboriginal people were, and still are, based on mind, body, spirit, socio-community, and environment. Approaches to healing among the Aborigines appear to vary according to region. When interviewed on 4 March 2003 Ann Warren, an Aboriginal elder from the Dtjilmamidtung region, states that 'the healings that take place cannot be compartmentalised into any one modality'. What this means is that the Aborigines do not recognise the word massage, however they do recognise the practice of touch. Warren also describes the healings as 'wholistic', whereby every part of the being is considered and the person is treated as a whole. Warren describes a method of using touch as a healing instrument in the Dtjilmamidtung region as follows (2003):

You may have a group of women in a circle exchanging words and sharing experiences. In this group there would be children sitting across laps or lying in between two people. Everyone who makes the circle would be touching in some way. Their knees may be touching the person on either side of them or they may be holding hands. As the exchange and sharing progresses, one woman may get a feeling about another woman that something is up for her. This woman would then rub, touch and soothe the other woman with a great respect for personal boundaries, and the energy of the group, and would then ask if everything was OK. This in itself is how a healing may take place. The intention of the touch is to project healing rather than to specific ally manipulate the body's soft tissue. The touch and concern of the first woman transfers into the second woman and the whole circle would be affected by this movement, the children would also be affected and then they learn how to intuit that something is up for someone, usually for their mothers and use this touch to transmit healing energy.

The period 1870–1920

By the 1870s massage therapists were known to be practising in Melbourne and Sydney. There were different ways of obtaining a massage, including referral to private rooms by medical practitioners where massage was performed by therapists who had gained credible reputations.

According to Dunstan and Bentley (2000), in 1880 an Australian doctor, Louis Henry, placed massage as 'a third branch of medical practice on equal footing with surgery and medicine'. This statement helped to pave the way for massage to be accepted as a mainstream therapy. Practitioners such as Teepoo Hall (1860–1909) became well regarded as massage therapists. Hall worked with the surgeon Thomas Fitzgerald (1838–1908) and his clients included several dignitaries. He practised at what is now the Austin and Repatriation Medical Centre (Austin Hospital) and became one of the first clinical teachers of massage, rising to the position of senior masseur and demonstrator at the Melbourne Hospital.

Likewise, Alfred Peters (1871–1944), who emigrated to Australia from England, started working as a masseur in Melbourne hospitals. He treated many sportsmen and also the Russian ballerina, Anna Pavlova. When Peters emigrated to Australia he advocated the benefits of massage and the medical profession could not ignore his claims. In his book, *Massage: Its History, Its Curative Uses and Its Practical Results* (1890), Peters refers to massage as 'one of the simplest, most rational, most efficacious and most valuable of curative agencies' (p. 3).

Figure 2.1 depicts massage in Australia before 1905.

Around 1912 a masseur by the name of Joseph Fay wrote a text titled *Scientific Massage for Athletes*. The title page heralded him as 'The Australian Authority On Massage For Athletes' and this text may well have been the first sports massage text written in Australia. Fay described what distinguishes an average massage therapist from a practical massage therapist, namely 'the former one merely pats or plays with the hide [skin], while the latter works with the meat, or muscle, between the hide and the bone so that it is in its highest state for exercise'. Fay classified three main massage movements as friction, kneading and vibration. In his text he described a method to massage the whole body such that it is done in a systemic and organised fashion (Fay c. 1912).

Australia at war

When World War I began, members of the AMA made applications to serve as massage therapists, but were turned down by the Australian Imperial Forces. Their spirit remained steady and strong and as Butler (1943, p. 595) states '...the practitioners of massage were enthusiastic and, there can be no doubt, convinced believers in the value of their art and of the importance of its proper application'.

After several further unsuccessful attempts, approval was finally given in 1915, due largely to the constant pressure from the AMA. As recorded by Butler (1943, p. 597):

The dispatch of a party or section of masseurs in the proportion of 1 male to 2 females, males to have pay and privileges of staff-sergeants, females pay and privileges of staff nurses. Under these conditions they must be prepared to serve for the term of war, and wear a uniform as directed for which allowance will be made.

One staff member alone would treat 15 cases a day. A report made by Colonel McWhae to General Howse states the following (Butler 1943, p. 613):

All soldiers with stiffness of joints, contractures of muscles or tendons and similar lesions will receive remedial gymnastic treatment, providing no acute inflammation, oedema or unhealed wounds (except in special selected cases of the latter) are present. e.g. Stiffness of the shoulder, elbow or wrist, limitation of extension of the elbow, limitation of supination and pronation of the forearm, stiffness of the wrist, hand or fingers with contractures and loss of handgrip, stiffness of the knee whether accompanied or not by a flexion, contracture, stiffness or limited mobility of the ankle, contracture of the calf muscle with resultant foot drop deformities of the foot, etc.

The AMA fought a huge battle of their own during WWI, striving for recognition. Eventually their efforts were noticed but ironically they underwent the same challenges in WWII. Butler (1943, p. 625) wrote:

This much at least is certain: whatever be the future of the Australian Service of Massage, its members can be assured that their art and technique will rest now on a scientific basis of clinical and experimental research. And for this they, and medical science in general, owe a tribute to the pioneers of the war of 1914–1918.

Modern times in Australia

In 1939 the AMA changed its name to the Australian Physiotherapy Association. Massage courses became less available during the next two decades. Physiotherapy was growing in popularity and the two fields began to separate. There are different theories about why this separation occurred. One theory is that of time management.

Figure 2.1 Massage in Australia before 1905

By 1905, massage societies were in existence in New South Wales, Victoria and South Australia. In 1906 a meeting chaired by Dr John Springthorpe resulted in the formation of the national Australasian Massage Association (AMA) and Peters was an integral influence in this association. By 25 April 1907 membership totals for the AMA stood at 302: New South Wales 112; Victoria 141; South Australia 15; Queensland 12; Western Australia 3; Tasmania 12 and New Zealand 7. Also there was a total of 196 honorary medical members on the books. Although today each state has its own massage association, a comparison has been made to indicate the membership growth of the professional massage associations: New South Wales 1200; Victoria and Tasmania 1616; South Australia and Northern Territory 650; Queensland 1100; Western Australia 200; and New Zealand 460.

To conduct a massage can take 15 to 90 minutes, resulting in fewer patients being seen in one day, whereas a physical therapy session is quicker and more patients can be treated per day. Another theory is that the use of machines may be far less invasive for some people than to have another human touch their body.

In Melbourne in the 1960s many people were treated by Bill Mitchell, who was a trainer at the South Melbourne Football Club. No appointments were available, so patients would arrive at the clubrooms and wait in turn, then be called in and treated. Mitchell would watch a client walk towards him and by the time that client reached him he would have a fair idea of what the problem was. Payment was made by placing a donation in a tin that sat on a shelf near the exit door. Mitchell was known only through word of mouth, but his reputation was huge. One reason that Mitchell was so popular was that he treated just about every size, shape, age and type of person. He treated football players, grandmothers, adolescents and business folk, but he had a hidden talent that made him a legend in Victoria, and that was charm. Mitchell, after watching patients walk across the floor, would greet patients with a handshake, look them right in the eye and through a smiling face say 'I can fix that for yah!'. This was not always the case, but people did not seem to mind as he had more successful treatments than unsuccessful.

At the St Kilda Football Club the head trainer Jim Clancy used some of the methods that the Romans used when treating their athletes in Ancient Rome. One method Jim employed was using a strigil on the players. This device was shaped liked a spoon and could remove the dust and sweat from the players before the massage was administered.

During the early 1960s two brothers, Harry and Arthur King, from Collingwood Football Club, established a trainer's college that taught students the art of massage, training the players and assessment of player injuries. This training school is still operating from Hawthorn Football Club today.

Keith Cleaver was also in the football trade and worked for Richmond Football Club from 1955 until the 1990s. Keith learned some of his skills from Mitchell. In 1977 Cleaver became head trainer for the club. He made several suggestions to the club that a freezer be installed in the clubrooms so they could have ice on hand to treat their player's injuries. Finally, in the 1980s, the club agreed to this and that put an end to the trainers rushing out on footy morning to purchase a dozen bags of ice to have on hand for the match (confirmed by Keith Cleaver, personal communication, 17 April 2003).

Events during the 1970s were absolutely vital for the survival of massage therapy. The Esalen Institute in California was established and influenced thousands of people in America, Australia, Europe and elsewhere about awareness of body, mind and spirit. Touch was integral to the Esalen philosophy and therefore massage fitted in with it perfectly. The Esalen Institute became a public platform for many people to introduce their work, including that of bodywork greats such as Ida Rolf and Moshe Feldenkrais.

MASSAGE IN NEW ZEALAND

The approach to health and wellness adopted by Maori people is very much intertwined with their way of life. Traditionally, massage (mirimiri), herbal medicine (rongoa) and spiritual healing (wairua) formed the cornerstones of holistic Maori health care. Today, mirimiri or massage is still widely practised in Maori circles by Maori healers.

According to Riley (1994), the use of mirimiri by Maori people dates back centuries. Herbal or animal oils were often used as lubricants in the application of the three main types of massage — roromi, toto and takahi. Roromi (or romiromi), usually administered by older women, was practised daily on the adults and involved squeezing and pinching strokes, whilst toto was a form of infant massage, often used to 'correct' or alter the infant structurally. For example, it was common practice to bend the thumb of female infants backwards so that when older, they may be better able to weave flax. It was a belief that the best person to perform takahi massage was someone who entered the world via a breach birth. Such people, born 'feet first', were thought destined to practise takahi massage, which involved walking on parts that were sore or injured to relieve muscular stiffness (Riley, 1994). Such forms of massage have been passed down the generations, and are used today by many Maori health networks. Parallelling the use of this traditional form of massage was the development in the early twentieth century of modern massage practices.

The development of modern massage in New Zealand followed similar lines to that of Australia. According to Anderson (1977) there were over three hundred massage therapists established in New Zealand by the early 1900s. Some of these therapists held formal massage qualifications obtained through studies overseas, whilst others had trained in New Zealand under the guidance of self-appointed massage teachers. In addition, some therapists received training in massage whilst nursing at the Auckland Hospital. Many of these massage therapists had their own practices and it was not uncommon for husbands and wives to work together.

By 1913 a massage department had been established in the Dunedin Hospital. A Mr Booth acted as Honorary Masseur within this department and later became a massage instructor to students when the department formed a school of massage. At this time an increasing number of the medical profession were becoming aware of the use and need for massage, and the importance of adequate massage training was apparent. The New Zealand branch of the British Medical Association (BMA) addressed this concern by establishing the School of Massage in Dunedin in conjunction with the Dunedin Hospital, under the auspices of the University of Otago. After administration difficulties, full responsibility of the School was transferred to the Otago Hospital Board. This board conducted examinations and issued certificates in massage, as well as medical gymnastics and the use of medical electricity (Anderson, 1977).

The government of the time was aware of these activities, and considered legal registration for all practising massage therapists. This consideration was postponed due to the great war and was acted upon shortly after when the *Masseurs Registration Act* of 1920 came into force (Sanford, 2003). In 1949 this Act was modified to the *Physiotherapy Act* (which is still in existence today) and massage therapy fell under the umbrella of physiotherapy. Those who wanted to practise massage and become registered had to adhere to the *Physiotherapy Act* and were required to undertake 600 hours of training.

Decades passed until, in 1985, a man by the name of Bill Wareham called all massage therapists in the Auckland area to a meeting. The intention Wareham had was to form an institute of massage therapists. This first meeting was fruitful and the Massage Institute of New Zealand Incorporated (MINZI) became an entity. Wareham was a massage educator during this time and he would offer his students the opportunity to become members of the institute. In 1987 Wareham travelled to Wellington where he conducted some massage education and it was during his stay that the Wellington branch of MINZI was established and Auckland became head office. MINZI has focused their efforts on the education of massage therapists and the standards of massage teachers throughout New Zealand. They have more massage teachers on the books than massage therapists but consider all types of members to be equal. The MINZI supports and assists members to obtain higher education and qualifications. The MINZI run annual conferences over a three-day period where massage therapists can attend a wide range of workshops to develop and maintain their skills (Tall, 2003, personnel communication).

In the late eighties a massage therapist named Jim Sandford invited fellow practitioners from around the country to a meeting to convey his perceived need for a professional body for therapeutic massage therapists. This initial meeting led some time later to the formation of the New Zealand Association of Therapeutic Massage Practitioners (NZATMP), a national professional body established to service the therapeutic massage profession in New Zealand.

Thus the newly formed association was up and running and set about addressing such concerns as education and training of therapeutic massage therapists, standards of professionalism amongst practitioners and recognition of the profession of therapeutic massage in New Zealand. The NZATMP duly became an incorporated society in September 1989 and has since grown from strength to strength. Perhaps the most notable achievements of the NZATMP have been in the area of developing, establishing and implementing a comprehensive programme of education for individuals interested in pursuing training in therapeutic massage. Today the association has grown to include members nationwide and has recently changed its name to the Therapeutic Massage Association (TMA). The TMA's main function today is to keep a register of massage therapists who have the National Diploma of Therapeutic Massage and to foster the ongoing training, development and mentoring of massage therapists (Vautier, 2003, personnel communication).

FUTURE OF MASSAGE

In the UK, the House of Lords Science and Technology Committee is starting to develop ways of monitoring the use of complementary and alternative medicine (CAM). Due to the large use of CAM, issues have arisen about:

- what structures and regulations are in place with practitioners of CAM to protect the public;
- whether the practitioners' level of training is adequate;
- whether evidence has been accumulated and what research is being carried out;
- whether there are adequate information sources on the subject; and
- whether the National Health Service will provide for these treatments.

Some of these issues are also on the minds of Australian legislators.

At this time in order to be considered for registration, massage would need to pose a significant health risk, and the industry would need to present a unified lobbying position. Government regulation might also follow if massage gained suitable scientific credibility, which could be achieved through conducting research programs.

However, the most common way that research is achieved is when courses are at a certain academic standard. In Australia massage is, at highest, a diploma qualification. Many people believe it needs to be lifted to a bachelor degree level before research can be seriously conducted.

Developments in England and Canada are addressing the need for higher education and it will only be a matter of time before Australia has higher academic awards, and when that occurs research will be conducted and massage will have more of a chance of being regulated and treated on a par with other professions.

In America massage research commenced around 1880. Since then the Institute of Touch has been developed at the Miami Medical School, where research is conducted to validate the benefits of massage. This research, sponsored by Johnson and Johnson, aims to look at the value of massage when used with infants, for postnatal depression, with premature babies and during pregnancy.

CONCLUSION

An appreciation of the history of massage provides the therapist with the ability to place current knowledge into an historical and developmental context, enabling the therapist to tell people briefly about its 5000 year lineage — how it survived even through the Dark Ages, the main figures in its history and the scandals that occurred along the way. The therapist can explain the fight that massage had to undertake to serve injured men during World War I, and how beneficial the massage service was in that time. See Figure 2.2 for a massage history time line.

Despite the growth of competing forms of treatment through the ages, massage has survived. Though the art of massage has sometimes faced extinction, somewhere, sometime throughout these threats, someone believed in it enough to speak highly of it and thereby influence the views of the public and medical fraternity. Current massage students represent the future of massage. In time, their work will become the history for new practitioners. As inheritors of the traditions of Hippocrates, Galen, Celsus, Avicenna, Ling, Mezger and Peters, students can think about the future of massage, what it means to them, what impact they will have on this 5000 year-old art and what direction the profession will take.

Questions and activities

1. You have been asked to present a talk to the local Rotary group on the benefits of massage. One Rotarian inquires about the development of modern massage. Detail your response to this question, making reference to the contributions of Ling.
2. Prepare a one-page visual handout that could be used for a short presentation on massage, which illustrates a timeline of significant historical events in the development of massage therapy.
3. Describe what prompted you to be drawn to the practice of massage, and define your own personal philosophies of massage.
4. It is a fact that as recently as the eighteenth and nineteenth centuries, medical physicians used massage therapy as a form of treatment. Despite the acceptance of massage then, today massage therapists are being required to scientifically validate the use of massage as a form of therapy. Why do you think this is the case?

Recommended reading

Butler, A. G. (1943) *The Official History of the Australian Army Medical Services in the War of 1914–1918*, vol. 3. Special Problems and Services, Australian War Memorial, Canberra.

Calvert, R. N. (2002) *The History of Massage: An Illustrated Survey From Around the World*. Healing Arts Press, Rochester.

Kakkib li' Dthia Warrawee'a (2002) *There Was Once a Tree Called Deru*. HarperCollins Publishers, Sydney.

Peters, A. (1890) *Massage: Its History, Its Curative Uses, and Its Practical Results*. Public Library, Melbourne.

Veith, I. (1972) Huang Ti Nei Ching Su Wen: The Yellow Emperor's Classic of Internal Medicine (new edn). University of California, California.

REFERENCES

Anderson, E. M. (1977) *The Golden Jubilee History 1923–1973: The New Zealand Association of Physiotherapists Inc.* The New Zealand Association of Physiotherapists Inc, Wellington.

Beard, G. and Wood, E. C. (1964) *Massage Principles and Techniques*. W. B. Saunders, Philadelphia.

Beck, M. F. (1999) *Milady's Theory and Practice of Therapeutic Massage* (3rd edn). Milady, Albany.

Bennett, C. (2003) email, received 24 March, admin@acnm.edu.au

Butler, Colonel A. G. (1943) *The Official History of the Australian Army Medical Services in the War of*

Figure 2.2 Time line of historical events

The arrows indicate the highs and lows of massage as a progressive healing method

10,000BC Prehistoric — Possibility massage was used to relieve tired limbs after hunting

2350BC — Babylon clay tablets discovered that depicted massage as a form of healing

2330BC — Egyptian tomb of Ankhamor shows wall painting of foot massage; Developments in healing and health made in China

1800BC Ancient Greece — Developments in healing and health made in India. Four books of wisdom (Veda's) were written

Asclepius uses massage above all other healing methods

400BC — 'Father of medicine' Hippocrates used massage as a form of healing in conjunction with herbs

300BC — Indian text The Laws of Man was written mentioning massage

200BC — The chinese text the Nei Ching was written and it documents massage as a practised healing method

160AD — Galen used massage on the gladiators and wrote over 400 text in medicine where he documented the benefits of massage

170AD — Aulus Celsus writes De Medicina and massage is documented as a method of healing

Indigenous tribes use touch as a form of healing throughout the entire world

500AD — Rome falls to waring tribes, a low level of learning occurred and many previous text were lost, stolen or ruined

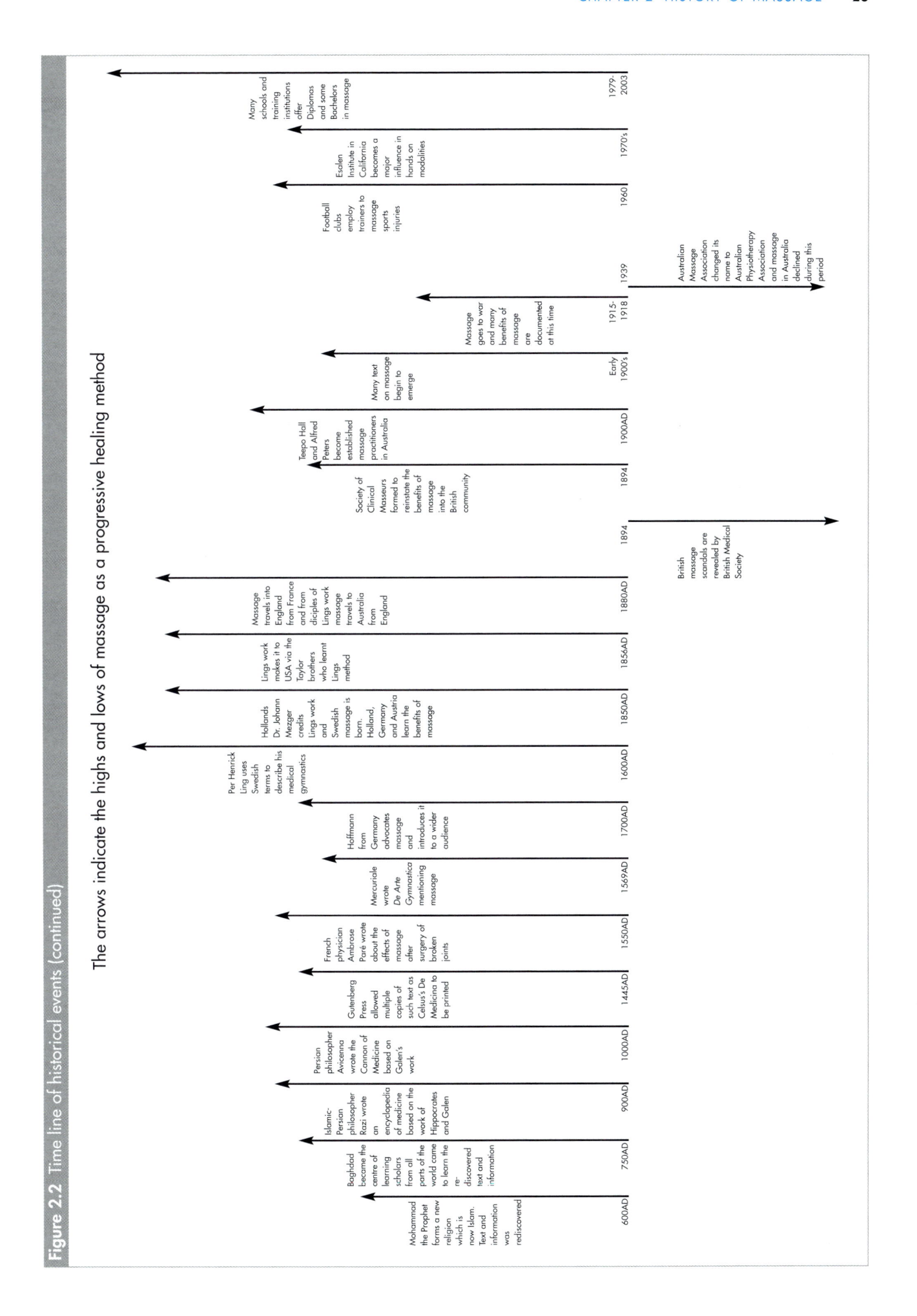

CHAPTER 2 HISTORY OF MASSAGE 25

Figure 2.2 Time line of historical events (continued)

The arrows indicate the highs and lows of massage as a progressive healing method

600AD	Mohammed the Prophet forms a new religion which is now Islam. Text and information was rediscovered
750AD	Baghdad became the centre of learning scholars from all parts of the world come to learn the re-discovered text and information
900AD	Islamic-Persian philosopher Razi wrote an encyclopedia of medicine based on the work of Hippocrates and Galen
1000AD	Persian philosopher Avicenna wrote the Cannon of Medicine based on Galen's work
1445AD	Gutenberg Press allowed multiple copies of such text as Celsus's De Medicina to be printed
1550AD	French physician Ambrose Paré wrote about the effects of massage after surgery of broken joints
1569AD	Mercuriale wrote De Arte Gymnastica mentioning massage
1700AD	Hoffmann from Germany advocates massage and introduces it to a wider audience
1600AD	Per Henrick Ling uses Swedish terms to describe his medical gymnastics
1850AD	Hollands Dr. Johann Mezger credits Lings work and Swedish massage is born. Holland, Germany and Austria learn the benefits of massage
1856AD	Lings work makes it to USA via the Taylor brothers who learnt Lings method
1880AD	Massage travels into England from France and from diciples of Lings work massage travels to Australia from England
1894	British massage scandals are revealed by British Medical Society
1894	Society of Clinical Masseurs formed to reinstate the benefits of massage into the British community
1900AD	Teepo Hall and Alfred Peters become established massage practitioners in Australia
Early 1900's	Many text on massage begin to emerge
1915-1918	Massage goes to war and many benefits of massage are documented at this time
1939	Australian Massage Association changed its name to Australian Physiotherapy Association and massage in Australia declined during this period
1960	Football clubs employ trainers to massage sports injuries
1970's	Esalen Institute in California becomes a major influence in hands on modalities
1979-2003	Many schools and training institutions offer Diplomas and some Bachelors in massage

1914–1918 vol. 3. Special Problems and Services, Australian War Memorial, Canberra.

Calvert, R. N. (2002) *The History of Massage – An Illustrated Survey From Around the World*. Healing Arts Press, Rochester, Vermont.

Chandler, C. A. (1980) 'Galen', in *The World Book Encyclopedia* vol. 8. World Book-Childcraft International Inc., Chicago.

Cyriax, J. H. (1984) *Textbook of Orthopaedic Medicine: Volume 2* (11th edn). Bailliere Tindall, London.

Dunstan, D. and Bentley, P. (unpub.) (2000) *The Australian Physiotherapy Association Draft History*.

Fay, H. J. C. (1912) *Scientific Massage for Athletes*. Ewart, Seymour & Co. Ltd, Windsor House, Kingsway, London.

Kellogg, J. H. (1895) *The Art of Massage: Its Physiological Effects and Therapeutic Applications*. Modern Medicine Publishing, Battle Creek, Michigan.

Kleen, E. A. G. (1918) *Massage and Medical Gymnastics*. J. & A. Churchill, London.

Martyr, P. (2002) *Paradise of Quacks, An Alternative History of Medicine in Australia*. Macleay Press, Sydney.

McKay, E. (2002) *Touchline Magazine*. Queensland Association of Massage Therapists (QAMT).

Menell, J. B. (1920) *Massage, Its Principles and Practice*. J. & A. Churchill, London.

Palmer, M. D. (1912) *Lessons on Massage* (4th edn). Baillière, Tindall and Cox, London.

Peters, A. (1890) *Massage: Its History, Its Curative Uses, and Its Practical Results*. Public Library, Melbourne.

Riley, M. (1994) *Maori Healing and Herbal*. Viking Sevenseas NZ Ltd, Paraparaumu.

Rowley, D. (1997) *High Profiles* vol. 8, no. 3.

Salvo, S. G. (1999) *Massage Therapy Principles and Practice*. W. B. Saunders, Philadelphia.

Sanford, J. (2003) Personal correspondence by email.

Smith, C. (1996) *ARM Massage Newsletter*, Association of Remedial Masseurs Incorporated (ARM).

Tall, N. (2003) Personnel communication, 1 May.

Tappan, F. (1988) *Healing Massage Techniques – Holistic, Classic and Emerging Methods* (2nd edn). Appleton & Lange, Connecticut.

Unschuld, P. U. (2000) *Medicine in China – Historical Artifacts and Images*. Prestel Verlag, Munich.

Vautier, B. (2003) Personnel correspondence by email, May.

Veith, I. (1972) *Huang Ti Nei Ching Su Wen: The Yellow Emperor's Classic of Internal Medicine* (new edn). University of California, California.

Warren, Ann (2003) Author's interview with Aboriginal elder from the Dtjilmamidtung region.

Watkins, K. (2003) email to author, April, *Kevin@massage.net.au*

chapter 3

Massage and its role in an integrative health care model

David Stelfox

Learning outcomes

- Define holistic health care
- Define integrative medicine
- Describe the benefits of massage therapy within an integrative approach to health care

INTRODUCTION

The art and practice of manually manipulating the body's musculoskeletal system for the purpose of promoting and restoring optimum health and wellbeing is as old as the art and science of healing itself. The majority of the cultures on this planet have incorporated bodywork, massage or manipulative therapy (i.e. physical manipulation of the body's muscles, ligaments, tendons and bones) within their traditional system of healing in some way. As outlined in Chapter 2, the earliest records of the use of massage date back over 3000 years and come from the East (Thailand and China). Other evidence suggests that over the centuries India, Tibet, Egypt, Polynesia, Indonesia, North and South America, Europe and Australia all have a history of the use of various forms of tactile therapy/bodywork within their healing traditions.

Each of these traditions recognised the benefits, indeed the necessity, of tactile therapy within its overall approach to health care. Furthermore, the indigenous healers from these cultures understood the importance of the health of mind, emotions, spirit and body, and their interrelatedness in regard to overall wellbeing. The therapies comprising these traditional healing systems were ones that aimed at specifically addressing each of these aspects of the health of a person — the mind, body, emotions and spirit.

While the techniques used or philosophies adopted may vary slightly from one culture to another, the modalities of therapy are indeed similar. Typically they include diet and nutrition therapy, the use of plant medicines (herbs), counselling (both psychological and spiritual), exercise therapy (e.g. yoga, tai qi, qi gong) and, of course, some form of tactile therapy/bodywork. Among indigenous people, massage or manipulative therapy was employed to exorcise evil spirits, to correct a person's physical structure or simply to make a person feel good. Ritual, prayer, devotion and often shamanic practice were also common features. Such practices have been passed down the generations of indigenous people, and continue to be used by many indigenous groups today.

WHAT IS HOLISTIC/ INTEGRATIVE MEDICINE?

The word 'health' originally stems from the Germanic and Old English word hœlan meaning 'whole' (*Australian Concise Oxford Dictionary*, 1995). The act of healing literally means the act of making whole, or restoring to a state of wholeness. Traditional medicine systems address each and every aspect of one's being, and as such are seen as 'holistic' or 'integrative' approaches. (W)Holistic medicine (the spelling differs for this word but the meaning is the same in either form) is an approach to health care that recognises the interconnectedness between the body, mind, emotions and spirit (i.e. it addresses the 'whole person').

The World Health Organization (WHO), a division of the United Nations, has defined holistic health care as (WHO, 1998):

that of viewing man in his totality within a wide ecological spectrum, and of emphasising the view that ill health or disease is brought about by an imbalance or disequilibrium of man in his total ecological system and not only by the causative agent and pathogenic evolution.

Furthermore, the WHO views traditional systems of health care as (WHO, 1998):

one of the surest means to achieve total health care coverage of the world's population, using safe and economically feasible methods.

'Integrative' medicine may be considered from two perspectives. The first perspective, similar to 'holistic' medicine, emphasises the unity of mind, body, spirit and emotions in a healthy, balanced individual, and the use of appropriate therapies for attending to them. However, integrative medicine goes further than this, suggesting that the practitioners of these different therapies need to work cooperatively and in consultation with each other, as well as the client, so that health/wholeness and wellbeing can be optimally achieved and maintained. In this sense the various individual therapies within a medical system, and the practitioners of them, determine which therapies will be of greatest benefit to the patient/client at the time. Since they all work within the philosophical framework of that particular health system, and the principles that define it, then they have an understanding and appreciation of each of the therapies which comprise that system and recognise the value and importance of referral to specialist practitioners where necessary. The system of healing is therefore 'integrative' from this perspective.

Integrative therapies are sometimes administered by a single therapist who is skilled in the practice and theory of all of them. Sometimes it may be that a number of practitioners, each trained and skilled in a specialty area of treatment (e.g. bodywork/herbal medicine/counselling/exercise therapy/diet or nutrition) may work within an overall guiding philosophy of a particular healing system (e.g. traditional Chinese medicine/naturopathy/ayurveda).

The second perspective of integrative health care is a more contemporary one. It is a term coined within the last five years by a new breed of general medical practitioner, one who recognises the value of integrating 'mainstream' biomedical health care with complementary/alternative/natural healing approaches. While this is an admirable view, it is often the case that such doctors (i.e. biomedical practitioners) have little understanding of the guiding philosophy/ies of the complementary healing approaches and the system of medicine they represent. It is perhaps a sad reflection of the current mainstream system of medicine that most of its practitioners are only prescribers of medicines. The integrative medicine approach, then, while appearing to integrate the best of both worlds, simply applies either 'mainstream' or 'alternative' medical approaches within the context of the Western biomedical model of health care. In such a model, natural medicine therapies are usually administered without regard to the philosophy or principles that define them (see Chapter 1), largely as alternatives to pharmaceutical drug therapy or, less commonly, surgery.

This approach is ultimately doomed to failure since it overlooks or simply dismisses the most beneficial features of the natural medicine health care model; that is, its guiding principles — one of which is the concept of the doctor as teacher (*docere*). This principle stipulates that therapists should educate their clients and encourage self-responsibility for their health. It also recognises and promotes the therapeutic potential of the practitioner–client relationship. Any health care practitioner, whether of natural or orthodox medicine, who simply prescribes medications (natural or pharmaceutical) does the art of healing a great disservice.

INTEGRATIVE MEDICINE — THE HEALTH CARE MODEL FOR THE TWENTY-FIRST CENTURY

This chapter now examines the first perspective of integrative medicine (the one that considers the importance of body, mind, emotions and spirit for maintaining and restoring optimum health) and the role that massage therapy can play in delivering this unified approach to health care in the twenty-first century.

With the conscious recognition of the complexity of modern society there has emerged an awareness of the contributions of environment, lifestyle, stress, emotional disturbance, psychosocial and cultural factors and chronic 'unwellness' to the process of disease. As a result of this recognition, health care has begun to take a turn toward self-care, mind-body therapy, personal and spiritual development and wellness enhancement to counterbalance the excesses and limitations of the biomedical model (Dacher, 2001). This turnaround is leading to a desire for a person-centred, wellness approach to health care rather than the disease-centred orientation that has characterised the Western biomedical model. The twenty-first century consumer of health care demands to be seen as an individual whose experiences constitute a dynamic unity. Today's consumer holds a certain distrust or suspicion of most things perceived as 'scientific' (Siahpush, 1998). The consumer demands an understanding of their existing health condition, and a desire to be actively involved in the process of improving that condition (Siahpush, 1998). The appropriate health care model for this century must therefore cater to these consumer demands and provide choices based on patients' preferences, respect for other therapeutic approaches and acknowledgment of the specialised skills and expertise of practitioners of other therapies.

In other sections of this book, the value, indeed the importance, of touch in maintaining and promoting health has been discussed at length. Massage, or any form of manual therapy that involves touch, inevitably impacts more than just the physical level of one's health. The idea of the body being touched in a deliberate way to achieve specific results is well documented and readily accepted, yet the ability of touch to evoke the powerful emotional responses and shifts in mental attitudes or spiritual perspective that often accompany most physical manipulations or tactile experiences is usually overlooked or ignored. Clearly, any integrative approach to healing must include massage or some other form of manipulative or tactile therapy. Let's now examine this claim in more detail.

MASSAGE AS COMPLEMENTARY THERAPY

The benefits of massage as an effective therapy in its own right must never be underestimated. However, this chapter will focus here on the valuable contribution that massage has to make as a complement or adjunct to other approaches to healing — in other words, how it can augment the therapeutic value of other healing modalities.

Massage and naturopathy

Naturopathy incorporates an eclectic blend of therapies in its attempt to promote the body's ability to heal itself. Historically, manipulative therapy or massage has always been one of the healing modalities incorporated as part of this system of holistic health care (others include diet and nutrition therapy, herbal medicines, flower essences, homoeopathy, exercise, lifestyle counselling) (Lindlahr, 1975). The main reason for the inclusion of massage or manipulative therapy is its ability to restore structural balance to the body while also helping to relieve stress and promote emotional, mental and spiritual wellbeing.

In Australia, 50 per cent of practicing naturopaths incorporate remedial massage in their practice (Hale, 2002). This percentage is probably similar in New Zealand. The inclusion of massage therapy as part of the naturopathic therapeutic strategy for a client can play a major role in helping to develop rapport between the practitioner and the client, and thereby enhance the healing potential of the client–practitioner relationship. The omission of massage from training courses in naturopathy has the potential to contribute to a trend towards 'prescription-pad medicine' (i.e. the prescribing of herbs, nutritional supplements and homoeopathic remedies). The danger this presents is that the client is no longer the focus of attention. The client's symptoms and signs, and the disease, become the focus for treatment rather than the individual. This is something for which mainstream medical practitioners have been frequently criticised over the last 50 years.

In a world deprived of the benefits of touch, massage can provide nurturing and comfort to many people (Johnson, 1985; see also Chapter 5). When so many of the health problems experienced today stem from the stress and emotional confusion associated with twenty-first century living, tactile therapy provides a means by which unexpressed or suppressed emotions such as grief, sadness, anger and frustration might be safely released. It is well known that emotions such as these are a common part of the experience of most physical illness (even having the effect of further compounding and complicating the disease picture). Therefore massage is clearly an important part of the naturopath's treatment strategy as a holistic practitioner.

Part of the process for delivering a massage or tactile therapy treatment requires provision of a suitable environment — that is, a healing environment. A healing environment is one that cocoons the client, and the therapist, from the outside world. It provides security, comfort, serenity and a feeling of nurturing. In such an environment the client feels safe to contemplate the nature of their disease, to ponder the causes or contributing factors. It is a healing space: something hard to find in the often chaotic world of today. In such a space, it is possible that the individual can discover what may be required of them to obtain a satisfactory improvement of, if not a resolution to, their health problems. The naturopath must be aware of this potential and seek to provide her/his clients with this opportunity whenever appropriate.

On the physiological level, one of the many benefits of massage therapy is to improve circulation throughout the tissues of the body. This circulation is not only restricted to the blood, but also includes lymph, interstitial and intracellular fluids. It may also extend to the circulation of energy or vital force. In many healing traditions massage and soft-tissue manipulation were employed primarily to remove obstacles and promote the unimpeded flow of life energy (for example, Qi or Prana) via the subtle energy channels or meridians.

Nutrients, oxygen, hormones, antibodies and other immunisers, and of course water, must be delivered to every single cell continually if it is to survive and respond the way it should, and all kinds of toxic wastes must be borne away. There is no tissue that cannot be weakened and ultimately destroyed by chronic interruptions of these various circulations (Juhan, 1998).

Kaptchuk and Croucher in their book *The Healing Arts – A Journey Through the Faces of Medicine* (1986) make the following comment (p. 38) concerning the omission of tactile therapy from the practice of medicine:

> *Perhaps the greatest loss that medicine has suffered over the course of the centuries is that of personal contact. Sophisticated doctors throughout the world tend to avoid the healing power of the human hand. The only form of contact that seems to have survived worldwide is the elevated art of surgery — perhaps because it can be practised in the most detached and impersonal setting. Other types of physical contact are dispersed into secondary, often disparaged categories, which are left to vie among themselves for some badge of accomplishment: osteopathy, chiropractic, acupuncture, bonesetting and manipulation and massage in its many forms.*
>
> *Far from being able to exude a feeling of fellowship and warmth, in many societies, doctors, especially men, have assumed the mantle of an unapproachable priesthood. Worse, the profession condemns some, and discourages many, of the therapies of touch that have helped millions of people physically as well as psychologically. From the perspective of other cultures and other times such attitudes could politely be described as provincial.*

Naturopaths must be careful that they do not make this same mistake and view massage as a form of second-rate manual labour, discarding it from their therapeutic repertoire in favour of the glamour and appeal of 'prescription-pad medicine'. Without the inclusion of massage as a therapy, naturopathy would struggle to address emotional, mental and spiritual aspects of health and perhaps fail in its effort to provide true holistic, integrative health care.

Massage and acupuncture

The same can be said of acupuncture, or traditional Chinese medicine, as has been stated for naturopathy. Without the inclusion of tactile therapy, acupuncture is a therapeutic modality, not a holistic system of health care. Thankfully, the practice of acupuncture involves making physical contact, but this contact may be brief, and may be administered with clinical efficiency rather than in a way that is comforting and nurturing. Similarly, the inclusion of tui na (traditional Chinese massage) in the traditional Chinese medicine (TCM) system (of which acupuncture is a part) focuses largely on achieving a therapeutic result, and the techniques employed are often strong, forceful and dynamic. While the Western approach to massage therapy (e.g. Swedish style) was derived originally from the Chinese tui na, it is generally less forceful, as pain is considered undesirable in the Western world.

The inclusion of a more gentle approach to massage in a TCM or acupuncture practice may offer many benefits to the Western client. This is certainly not suggesting that Chinese massage therapy is in any way less effective — simply that the Western mind/psyche may respond more readily to an approach that is perceived as gentler, more soothing, more comforting and more relaxing. The impact of such an approach on the emotional, mental and spiritual wellbeing of a client may be more successful than a more forceful one, and from this perspective is certainly worth considering as an adjunct to acupuncture and TCM.

Massage and homoeopathy

A typical homoeopathic consultation involves extensive case-taking on the part of the practitioner. The client undergoes a thorough interview process during which many details concerning the individual's health, symptoms and signs, personality and likes and dislikes are determined so that the most appropriate homoeopathic remedy can be determined and prescribed according to the indications. While the process is most extensive, and calls upon the client to consider issues that are physical, emotional, mental and spiritual, the interview process may be seen as very much a cerebral exercise.

The incorporation of massage as part of the treatment package for homoeopathy can certainly add another dimension to the treatment experience. As previously discussed, the benefits of tactile therapy in contributing to the client–practitioner relationship, and the contribution of that relationship to the healing process, are quite significant. The contribution of the client–practitioner relationship to the process of healing has been estimated to be at least 40 per cent. Thirty-five per cent of the process of healing is attributed to 'self-healing' and 25 per cent is attributed to the actual therapy employed (Miller, 1998). The positive experience of a massage treatment when combined with a homoeopathic prescription can only produce a therapeutic outcome with more impact for the client.

Massage and osteopathy, chiropractic and physiotherapy

It is becoming increasingly commonplace for massage therapists to work together with other manipulative therapists (i.e. osteopaths, chiropractors and physiotherapists) for the purpose of achieving optimum results with musculoskeletal health problems. While there has been a significant movement away from high velocity low amplitude (HVLA) thrusting adjustments (Chaitow, 2001) resulting in a number of chiropractors, osteopaths and physiotherapists adopting much gentler manipulations of the soft tissues of the body, a large number of these practitioners still focus predominantly on spinal adjustments. Massage complements this type of work, especially when it is administered prior to a high-speed manipulative treatment, by relaxing the muscles and nervous system, and improving circulation to the problem areas. In achieving this, the client is effectively prepared for the treatment that will follow.

Often, as a result of tight or hypertonic muscles, it may be difficult for a manipulative therapist to achieve a satisfactory result for a client, without some preliminary soft-tissue work being performed. Furthermore, regular appropriate massage may be beneficial as ongoing therapy, both to maintain the results of the manipulative therapy and also to possibly reduce the need for excessive follow-up treatment. As massage therapists and practitioners of the other various manipulative therapies see the positive results of working together cooperatively in an integrated practice, they feel more confident and comfortable with such an arrangement and their clientele spreads word of their satisfaction. Trust and effective communication are no doubt key factors to a successful integrative practice.

Massage and fitness therapy, personal training and sports coaching

While the benefit of massage therapy to sporting performance is well established, its application to fitness therapy and personal training is perhaps a little less obvious.

For decades coaches of all sports have called upon the massage therapist to prepare their sportsmen and women for optimum performance, to help them recover from the trauma of the event and from physical injury. Massage therapists now accompany most professional sporting teams and the number of massage therapists who provide their services at the Olympic games has increased significantly every four years. With the ever-increasing commercialisation of sport and the associated pressure on sportsmen and women to succeed, the inclusion of the massage therapist as a crucial member of the team is obviously essential. It seems certain that the demand for well-trained, competent massage therapists who specialise in sports massage will continue to increase.

Personal trainers and fitness therapists primarily focus on improving the level of fitness, strength and flexibility of their clients. Demand for the services of these professionals has increased markedly as a result of the trend towards improved physical health and wellbeing, and the desire to look and feel vital and youthful. These professionals work as consultants, providing advice and direction, and prescribing exercise regimens to achieve the desired result for the client. Some assist in the prevention of, and recovery from, injury. It makes perfect sense then for these trainers/therapists to offer the services of massage therapy to their clients to augment the training programs they recommend. Regular massage will speed the process of recovery from rigorous training sessions and promote optimum musculoskeletal function so that clients will get more out of their exercise schedules.

MASSAGE AND THE BIOMEDICAL MODEL OF HEALTH CARE

It seems strange when every other culture on the planet has included massage therapy in its traditional system of medicine that Western society chose in the past to abandon, and even discourage, the use of it for healing. A brief look at the history of Western medicine seems to indicate that the exclusion of massage therapy from that system had more to do with tradition than with reason.

Dr Johann Mezger, the Dutch physician (see Chapter 2), established massage as a credible part of mainstream medical practice in the mid-nineteenth century. Its use then spread throughout Europe with such famous physicians as Lucas-Championnière and Charcot, in France, promoting its use. Lucas-Championnière published the textbook *Massage and Mobilisation in the Treatment of Fractures* for the use of fellow physicians (Lucas-Championnière, 1895). But by the late 1800s, doctors in Britain were already expressing an unwillingness to administer such a manual procedure themselves, and were advocating the training of nurses (female) to deliver massage treatments, under their close supervision, in the hospitals.

It seems that this led to an increase in the popularity and demand for massage and women other than nurses undertook private training in the art of massage. Seeing such unsupervised practice as a threat to their own livelihood and status as healers, British doctors issued a warning, via *The British Medical Journal* (1894), against young women training in massage as a career. The article stated (p. 88) that there was no demand for masseuses and also warned against the unsavoury nature of massage as practised in some so-called massage establishments in London. Surgery's significant rise in status had a lot to do with the decline in use of massage and manipulative therapy by physicians. Relegated to the lowly status of barbers during the Middle Ages, surgeons were previously regarded as relatively unskilled and their 'art' was seen as a last-resort approach.

'Surgery' derives from the Greek word meaning 'hand work'. Physicians were once seen as superior to surgeons in terms of their training, knowledge and skills, and were therefore given the title of 'Doctor' (teacher) to reflect their elevated status. Surgeons, on the other hand, were manual, hands-on practitioners who were also trained as barbers (barber–surgeons). They held the title of 'Mister' which reflected their lower status. These titles are maintained today, although the status attached to each is a reversal of the previous.

While the use of massage in hospitals continued at a low level throughout the Western world during the early twentieth century (mainly due to the efforts of nurses who saw the benefits it offered to patients), its popularity within the Western system of medicine dwindled as a direct result of distrust and dissuasion of its use by doctors (Martyr, 2002).

The development of the pharmaceutical industry and the associated fascination with the potential of the 'magic bullet' (miracle drugs) was another factor. It wasn't until the 1960s when physiotherapy became a registered profession, that massage or manipulative therapy regained any sort of approval from the orthodox medical profession.

The 1970s saw the recognition of massage's value as part of a holistic approach to health care. Its increase in popularity outside of the orthodox health system brought about greater general interest and enquiry. Early research explored its potential for enhancing health. With more research, and greater awareness of its many benefits, renewed interest in the inclusion of massage in mainstream health care is occurring. Nursing homes and a few private hospitals have introduced massage therapy as a form of complementary care. While there is still considerable resistance from some doctors and hospital administrators, support for massage therapy's inclusion in the mainstream medical system is substantial. It seems certain that before long the doors will open and tactile therapies, including massage, will be seen as another branch of orthodox medical care.

In the USA, therapeutic touch (a subtle energy approach to healing) is widely administered by nurses to patients in hospital settings. Therapeutic touch, developed by nurses for nurses, stemmed from the realisation that hospital patients were usually touch deprived and that their recovery could be significantly enhanced through some form of tactile therapy. Nurses are ideally suited to delivering tactile therapy to patients in hospital wards, as they are familiar with the patient's health condition, his or her personal likes and dislikes, and have (in most cases) gained the patient's trust and acceptance.

At a time when hospital budgets are severely restricted and nurses struggle to deliver even the basic services to patients due to time and staffing constraints, it seems unlikely that tactile therapy in any form (e.g. relaxation massage, reiki, touch for health, remedial massage) will become commonplace in public hospitals. However, some hospitals have introduced massage services to patients, and experience suggests that the outcomes (in terms of patient wellbeing and recovery) are positive. More research (in particular, clinical trials) is needed to explore the potential benefits of massage or other tactile therapy in the hospital wards. It is only as a result of positive research findings that authorities may be willing to examine the possibility of providing massage therapy (whether for relaxation or remedial purposes) to hospital patients.

The prospect of massage therapy being performed prior to and after surgery, as an adjunct to the process of recovery, is an inspiring one. However, it is not an original notion. In the fourteenth century the esteemed French physician Guy de Chauliac published a book on surgical procedure. It became a standard text throughout Europe for the next 200 years. The book described the administration of various methods of massage and manipulation to augment surgical procedures.

With advances in scientific understanding, and as more is learnt about how the human organism functions, massage and manipulation therapy is once again emerging as a legitimate and desirable (perhaps essential) health care modality. Its inclusion in the mainstream biomedical health care model is inevitable. How long this will take is perhaps the only uncertainty.

Recent surveys suggest that Australians are no longer satisfied with the system of health care they have been offered to date (Siahpush, 1998). To satisfy the demands of the Australian public it is clear that an integrative model of health care is necessary.

CONCLUSION

An integrative model is one that provides choice in the range of therapeutic options it can offer. It also provides an approach that views the human being as a unity of body, mind, emotions and spirit, and appreciates the need for addressing each of these aspects as a means of promoting, restoring and maintaining optimum health.

Massage therapy has a vital role to play as part of an integrative model of health care. It complements the benefits of other therapeutic modalities and in itself has positive benefits to each of the four aspects of health (i.e. body, mind, emotions and spirit). These benefits have been established empirically due to the inclusion of massage therapy in the majority of traditional systems of healing as practised by the indigenous people of the planet's many cultures.

An integrative system of medicine also requires that the practitioners of the various therapies that comprise it are broad-minded and tolerant of each other's principles and philosophies. Furthermore, they must also have a general understanding and appreciation of how other therapies work and what they are attempting to achieve. Massage therapists therefore must be prepared to study the basic principles of other healing modalities — those that comprise what is currently described as the Western biomedical or mainstream approach to medicine, as well as those that comprise the natural therapies approach. A willingness to work cooperatively with therapists of other modalities, to refer when necessary, and to always place the interests of the client first — these are the other requirements of an integrative approach to healing.

Questions and activities

1. Briefly describe your experiences of mainstream health care and holistic health care, and identify if you have a personal preference for one over the other in any situations.

2. A client has recently read a newspaper article on the emergence of integrative medicine and asks

you to explain what it is. How would you respond?
3. You are seeking employment as a massage therapist in a clinic. You approach four different clinicians seeking work at their clinic: an acupuncturist, an osteopath, a chiropractor and a physiotherapist. Describe what you would say to each therapist about the way in which massage therapy may be integrated with his or her practice.
4. You are enjoying an academic debate with a medical practitioner at a dinner party about the value of massage. The medical practitioner agrees with you that massage therapy has a role to play in the country's healthcare system, but is not sure how it could occur. Prepare a response to this query, describing what you believe to be important for the re-inclusion of massage therapy into the Western biomedical health care system.

Recommended reading

Grossinger, R. (1995) *Planet Medicine: Modalities* (6th edn). North Atlantic Books, New York.

Leskowitz, E. (2003) *Complementary and Alternative Medicine in Rehabilitation*. Churchill Livingstone, New York.

Micozzi, M. S. (ed.) (2001) *Fundamentals of Complementary and Alternative Medicine*. Churchill Livingstone, New York.

Novey, D. W. (2000) *Clinician's Complete Reference to Complementary and Alternative Medicine*. Mosby, St Louis.

Peters, D., Chaitow, L., Harris, G. and Morrison, S. (2002) *Integrating Complementary Therapies in Primary Care: A Practical Guide for Health Professionals*. Churchill Livingstone, London.

Robson, T. (ed.) (2004) *An Introduction to Complimentary Medicine*. Allen & Unwin, Sydney.

REFERENCES

Allen, R. E. (1995) *The Australian Concise Oxford Dictionary* (8th edn). Oxford University Press, South Melbourne.

British Medical Journal (1894), p. 88.

Chaitow, L. (2001) *Muscle Energy Techniques*. Churchill Livingstone, London.

Dacher, E. (2001) 'The development of an integrated medical model', in *Fundamentals of Complementary and Alternative Medicine*, M. S. Micozzi (ed.), Churchill Livingstone, Philadelphia.

Hale, A. (2002) *Survey Data of the Australian Traditional Medicine Society as Part of the Uniform National Registration Systems Project for Suitably Qualified Practitioners in Naturopathy, Herbal Medicine and Acupuncture*. University of Sydney, Sydney.

Johnson, D. (1985) *Touch Starvation in America*. Rayid Publications, Santa Barbara.

Juhan, D. (1998) *Job's Body: A Handbook for Bodywork*. Station Hill Publishers, Barrytown, New York.

Kaptchuk, T. and Croucher, M. (1986) *The Healing Arts – A Journey Through the Faces of Medicine*. British Broadcasting Corporation, London.

Lindlahr, H. (1975) *Philosophy of Natural Therapeutics* (edited and revised edition). Maidstone Osteopathic Clinic, Kent.

Lucas-Championnière, J. (1895) *Massage and Mobilisation in the Treatment of Fractures*. Paris.

Martyr, P. (2002) *Paradise of Quacks, an Alternative History of Medicine in Australia*. Macleay Press, Sydney.

Miller, S. (1998) 'Essential Aspects of Brief Therapy', in *Brief Therapy: Lasting Impressions*. Conference, Milton H. Erikson Foundation, New York.

Siahpush, M. (1998) 'Postmodern values, dissatisfaction with conventional medicine and popularity of alternative therapies', *Journal of Sociology*, vol. 34, no. 1, Longman Publishers, New South Wales.

World Health Organization (1998) *Traditional Medicine*. WHO Publications, Geneva, Switzerland.

section 2

Identifying the 'Legitimacy' of Massage as a Therapy

chapter 4

The evidence for massage therapy

Vicki Tuchtan

Learning outcomes

- Describe the major effects of massage therapy
- Outline the research validating the effects of massage therapy on circulatory function
- Outline the research validating the effects of massage therapy on muscle tone
- Outline the research validating the effects of massage therapy on pain
- Outline the research validating the effects of massage therapy on emotional states
- Describe the benefits of massage therapy to a client
- Justify the use of massage as a therapy

INTRODUCTION

Many people can attest to the calming and pleasant sensations experienced when receiving a relaxation massage. After a massage the way in which a person feels and the effect that the therapy has had on them will vary depending upon the duration of the treatment and the combination of strokes employed by the therapist throughout the routine. Immediately after receiving a massage a client may feel relaxed or invigorated, enlivened or grounded, or maybe even a little dreamy or sleepy.

Such anecdotal reports about the effects of massage are varied. There are many claims made throughout the literature about the effects of massage therapy yet few have been substantiated through rigorous investigation. It has been said that massage reduces pain (Cassar, 1999; De Domenico and Wood, 1997; Fritz, 2000; Tappan and Benjamin, 1998), increases metabolism and promotes the circulation of blood and lymph (Cassar, 1999; Beck, 1988). According to Tappan and Benjamin (1998), massage can induce relaxation, reduce oedema, improve joint range of motion and enhance the confidence of the recipient. Other authors claim that massage is useful for stress management (Field, 2000) and can soften scar tissue and loosen adhesions (De Domenico and Wood, 1997).

Evidence exists to suggest that massage may be useful for pain management, and may also reduce depression and anxiety, and enhance immune function (Diego et al., 2001; Field et al., 1993, 1996, 2003). Researchers have been driven to determine the effectiveness of massage therapy as a treatment so that its use may be validated for a wide range of situations and conditions. Currently, more researchers are answering the call and putting massage therapy to the test by performing controlled, scientific studies that aim to determine the efficacy of massage therapy. Only when massage therapy is subjected to repeated and vigorous investigation will the benefits and mechanisms of massage therapy become evident, and massage can take its place alongside other complementary forms of therapy as a conventional and mainstream treatment in today's health care system.

SCIENTIFIC LITERATURE ON THE BENEFITS OF MASSAGE THERAPY

The intent of any massage therapy treatment is to produce an effect or a change in the person receiving the massage. Such an effect of treatment, as first described by Mennell (c. 1917), may be classified as either a reflex or a mechanical effect. A reflex is also referred to as an involuntary response; an indirect effect of the massage treatment. An example of an indirect effect of massage therapy would be the downward shift of blood pressure that is brought about by dilation of blood vessels with the application of deep effleurage movements (Salvo, 1999). Such indirect or reflex effects commonly result in neural and endocrine changes. An example of a reflex effect following massage therapy would be changes in cortisol levels (a stress hormone), which may be indicative of effects on the sympathetic nervous system. Indirect or reflex effects are thought to be an important factor in the overall benefits of massage therapy.

On the other hand, mechanical effects may be described as direct effects. A direct effect implies that a mechanical response has occurred via the application of direct force or pressure when administering massage. Such a direct effect may include the resolution of oedema via the application of effleurage that promotes lymph and venous return (De Domenico and Wood, 1997). Another mechanical effect would be the influence massage therapy has on the soft tissues of the body. For example, massage may alter the resting length of a muscle or the tonicity of a muscle. Such mechanical effects may also influence the fluid environments of the body such as the blood circulation and affect the motility of the intestines and their contents (Mennell, c. 1917; Cassar, 1999; Fritz, 2000).

Many authors of today describe the effects of massage therapy as direct or indirect. When discussing these effects, it is important to remember that they are not independent of each other. As such, it might be said that to describe these effects in isolation is limiting, due to the fact that in the larger scheme of things these actions are interrelated and interdependent when it comes to the overall effect of the massage therapy treatment. As such, the direct and indirect effects of massage should not be thought of as isolated entities. To fully appreciate the effects of massage, it is worth examining the current research that exists on the topic. This chapter presents a discussion of some of the research that supports the use of massage therapy.

THE EFFECTS OF MASSAGE THERAPY ON CIRCULATORY FUNCTION

When a massage therapist applies massage techniques to the body one of the immediate effects of massage is reddening of the skin. When they place a hand over the area an increase in temperature is also evident. Through such clinical observations massage therapists infer that local circulation is enhanced through the application of massage. The extent of such an effect and the mechanism underlying it are not fully understood, yet research-based evidence exists to validate the use of massage to improve circulation, aid the resolution of oedema and assist in controlling high blood pressure.

An early study into the effect of massage on blood flow in skeletal muscle compared the techniques of pétrissage and tapôtement in nine healthy subjects (Hovind and Nielsen, 1974). The study investigated hyperaemia, a physiological phenomenon that occurs when excess blood moves into an area, such as a skeletal muscle, when the body is preparing for exercise. The findings of this study showed that massage produced hyperaemia consistent with that which occurs with the onset of activity, which suggested that massage increased local blood flow. It is worth noting that tapôtement produced a greater effect on skeletal muscle blood flow than pétrissage.

Ernst et al. (1987) investigated the effects of whole body massage on blood fluidity (or composition) in 22 patients — 12 healthy and 10 diagnosed with ankylosing spondylitis (a chronic inflammatory condition affecting the spine and pelvis). The results of this study showed that 20 minutes of massage produced both acute and long-term declines in haematocrit, which is the percentage of blood composed of red blood cells. Declines in blood and plasma viscosities (thickness or stickiness of solution) were also observed. The investigators concluded that such changes were the result of increased fluid movement or perfusion of fluid from surrounding tissues into blood, indicative of enhanced circulation post-massage, suggesting massage to be of benefit for muscular disorders such as ankylosing spondylitis.

In addition to assisting with muscular disorders, massage may be useful for recovery from some types of surgery. Mastectomy is a surgical procedure to remove one or both breasts, usually because of a malignant tumour in the breast tissue. Such a procedure may involve removal of lymph nodes also, which can adversely affect circulation, resulting in oedema for several days or even weeks post-surgery (referred to as lymphoedema). Over a 10-year period 655 patients, primarily experiencing post-mastectomy oedema, were recruited for participation in a longitudinal study investigating massage for oedema (Yamazaki et al., 1988). Each participant received a series of pneumatic (mechanical) massage treatments for peripheral lymphoedema (oedema of the arm). Findings suggest that massage applied with undulatory (changing) pressure may be beneficial in improving lymphatic and blood flow. Yamazaki et al. (1988) concluded that such massage is useful to relieve peripheral lymphoedema as it encourages venous and lymphatic return.

Another aspect of circulatory function that massage may influence is the pressure of the blood. Research suggests that massage may be useful for reducing high blood pressure (referred to as hypertension) and related symptoms of anxiety, stress, hostility and depression. A study conducted by Hernandez-Reif et al. (2000) investigated the effects of a course of ten 30-minute massage sessions over a five-week period in 30 hypertensive subjects (21 females, 9 males). Participants were randomly assigned to either an experimental group (n = 15) that received massage or a control group (n = 15) that received instruction on progressive muscle relaxation. Decreases in both sitting and reclining blood pressure (diastolic) measurements were recorded in the massage group. Despite both the experimental and control groups reporting less anxiety, only the experimental group (which received massage) reported reductions in hostility and depression. Measurements of salivary and urinary cortisol were also reduced in the massage group, indicating a reduction in stress.

The benefits of massage therapy on skeletal muscle blood flow are evident to every practitioner, and massage has other effects on circulatory function as outlined above. The extent to which such findings can be applied to the clinical domain is not yet clear. What is clear though is that massage professionals are practising massage to assist with oedema, encourage circulation in patients who may be immobile, and enhance blood flow to remove metabolic waste products from muscles, and with promising results.

THE EFFECTS OF MASSAGE THERAPY ON MUSCLE TONE

The tone of a muscle may be described as its tension, or its resistance to passive stretch. At times muscles may be subjected to extremes of nervous stimulation resulting in hypertonicity, or put simply, muscle cramp or spasm. The over-stimulation of a muscle leads to a hyperexcitable motoneuron pool in the muscle. Such hypertonicity can produce extreme pain. One traditional technique used to relieve a hyperexcitable motoneuron pool or spasm/cramp is passive muscle stretching. In the clinical setting, when pain or limitation of joint movement does not permit for a passive muscle stretch, the application of massage may be used to relieve a cramp or a spasm.

A study by Morrelli et al. (1990) aimed to investigate the effect of massage on neuromuscular excitability. Measurements of the Hoffmann reflex (H-reflex) were obtained from nine healthy subjects to determine the degree of excitability of the spinal reflex pathway. Investigators applied pétrissage massage techniques to the triceps surae muscle group for a short period of time. The findings of this study showed that massage decreased H-reflex amplitude during the treatment, indicating that massage is effective for the relief of spasm or cramp. Further investigation into the effects of massage on motoneuron excitability confirmed these results (Sullivan et al. 1991; Goldberg et al. 1992), whilst a study conducted by Goldberg et al. (1992) showed that deep massage had a greater effect in decreasing H-reflex amplitude than light massage.

Goldberg et al. (1994) reported similar findings in a population of subjects with spinal cord injury. Ten subjects (9 males and 1 female) with traumatic spinal cord injury received pétrissage massage for three minutes. The results of this study were consistent with previous work, as a decrease in H-reflex amplitude was observed. It is worth noting that the decrease, although significant, was not as dramatic as in previous studies performed with healthy subjects. The authors noted that, when compared to healthy subjects, people with spinal cord injury do not exhibit uniform nerve stimulation. Another important finding of this study was that in more than half of the subjects, a carry-over effect was observed. Such a carry-over effect of depression of motoneuron excitability had not previously been observed in any other study prior to this one.

Abnormal muscle tone associated with excessive neuromuscular excitability may be observed in conditions such as multiple sclerosis and in people with paralysis resulting from a cerebrovascular accident or stroke. As a cost effective and safe treatment, firm massage techniques such as pétrissage may prove useful in such instances in providing immediate relief from muscle spasm or cramp.

THE EFFECTS OF MASSAGE THERAPY ON PAIN

It is not uncommon for people to seek out massage therapy treatment for the relief of pain. Whether it be a sore neck, a dull ache associated with arthritis, low back pain or pelvic pain associated with the menstrual cycle, many people find massage therapy useful in easing their suffering and taking their mind off the pain they are feeling.

Pain is a subjective experience involving both sensation and emotion. Clinically, pain may be classified as either acute or chronic, whereby each classification of pain is illustrated by its own characteristic features and is determined by differing influential factors. The reduction of pain is a physiological benefit of massage therapy described by many authors (De Domenico and Wood, 1997; Tappan and Benjamin, 1998; Trevelyan, 1993) yet little is known about the exact mechanism behind the analgesic (pain-relieving) action of this therapy. Is the perception of pain altered through purely physiological pathways, or can massage positively affect the emotional state of the recipient, thereby psychologically blocking the pain experience?

According to the gate-control theory of pain established by Melzack and Wall in 1965, sensory input of pain is transmitted to the spinal cord and the brain. Once nerve cells (referred to as neurons) in these areas are sufficiently excited, a theoretic gate opens and allows transmission of pain signals to the brain, where they are processed. A person's thoughts and emotions can directly influence the pain experience. The brain is able to close the gate and alter pain perception through psychological input such as feelings of wellness. Thus, if a person's mood is positive, the pain signals to the brain may be blocked. Another way to alter pain perception is to confuse the input of sensory information arriving at the lower centres of the central nervous system by application of a different stimulus such as the application of massage.

The way in which a person's emotional state influences their pain experience is not yet fully understood. According to a report released by the National Health & Medical Research Council (1989, p. vii):

> *pain is one of Australia's costliest health problems in terms of suffering as well as financial cost, affecting home and family life, work, recreation, and overall quality of life for many people of all ages.*

At present, the most common conventional treatment for pain consists of prescription analgesic medication. This is of concern, as long-term usage may result in dependence or iatrogenic illness.

In the clinical domain Davis, Cortez and Rubin (1990) investigated the pain management techniques tried by 82 people with rheumatic disease. Subjects were divided into two groups according to their age — young adult (n = 51) and old adult (n = 31). Fifty-nine per cent of young adults and 25 per cent of old adults had used massage as a technique to manage their pain. Both groups found massage more helpful in managing pain than non-prescription medicine and electrical stimulation. Old adults found massage more beneficial than relaxation techniques, exercise, bracing and conversation for pain management. It is interesting to note that the percentage of massage users was significantly greater in the young adults than the old adults — perhaps this is consistent with the current resurgence in complementary therapies such as massage and the awareness amongst young adults of such avenues of health management.

Using a visual analogue scale (VAS), a type of rating instrument common in many research studies involving therapeutic interventions, Weinrich and Weinrich (1990) investigated the effects of massage on pain perception in cancer patients. The study involved 28 subjects — 14 experimental (who received a relaxation back massage for 10 minutes) and 14 control (who were visited for 10 minutes). Immediately post-massage, male subjects in the experimental group showed a significant reduction in pain perception, as measured by the VAS. The results showed no significant difference between pain reports prior to massage, and one and two hours post-massage, thus investigators concluded that massage was effective for short-term pain relief.

Another investigation of massage for cancer patients was conducted in a hospital environment. Ferrell-Torry and Glick (1993) administered 30-minute massage therapy treatments over two consecutive days to male cancer patients experiencing pain (n = 9). To determine the effects of massage therapy on pain perception, anxiety and relaxation, measurements of pain (using a VAS) and anxiety levels, as well as physiological functioning (heart rate, respiratory rate and blood pressure) were recorded prior to, immediately after, and 10-minutes after massage treatment. The findings of Ferrell-Torry and Glick were consistent with those of Weinrich and Weinrich (1990), as the researchers found that massage significantly reduced patients' pain perceptions short-term. The results also showed a significant reduction in anxiety levels, and reported a relaxation effect of massage, as indicated by a decrease in all physiological measures from baseline.

Another condition associated with pain in which people may experience feelings of anxiety is fibromyalgia. A study by Field, Delage and Hernandez-Reif (2003) investigated the effects of combined massage and movement therapy for the reduction of pain associated with fibromyalgia. Forty subjects diagnosed with fibromyalgia were randomly assigned to either a control group (n = 20) to undergo relaxation via the use of progressive muscle relaxation or a massage/movement group (n = 20). All relaxation and massage/movement sessions were 50 minutes in duration, and were administered twice a week over a three-week period. Data was collected using the State Trait Anxiety Index (STAI), Profile of Mood States (POMS) and the regional pain scale. The authors noted that both the control and the massage/movement groups showed a decrease in anxiety and pain after the first and/or last sessions. However, results for the massage/movement group also showed improvements in mood, a reduction in anxiety and lower levels of pain across the three-week study period. Further investigations are required to determine the longer lasting effects of massage/movement for chronic pain conditions such as fibromyalgia.

Hernandez-Reif et al. (2001) investigated the effects of massage on pain and range of motion in 24 subjects with chronic low back pain. Subjects were randomly assigned to one of two groups — massage or control. Subjects in the massage group received a 30 minute massage twice a week over a five-week period, whilst those in the control group underwent 30 minutes of progressive muscle relaxation twice a week for five weeks. Numerous instruments were used to collect data, including the POMS, STAI, McGill Short Form pain questionnaire and VAS. At the end of the five-week period, subjects in the massage group reported less pain. Results also showed that those who received massage treatment were less depressed and anxious, exhibited positively enhanced mood and better sleep, and had greater range of trunk flexion when compared to the control group. Biochemical results for the massage group showed increased levels of dopamine and serotonin. The authors noted that the increased dopamine may have resulted from improved mood, whilst massage may have elevated serotonin levels, which become depleted in people suffering from chronic pain.

Rheumatoid arthritis is an autoimmune condition associated with chronic pain. Over a 30-day period, Field, et al. (1997) investigated the effects of daily massage on anxiety, pain and functional ability in children aged 4–16 years with mild to moderate juvenile rheumatoid arthritis. Fourteen girls and six boys were randomly assigned to either the massage group, which received a 15-minute full body massage, or the control group, which consisted of 15 minutes of progressive muscular relaxation. Parents, trained by the investigators, administered both treatments. A variety of data collection options were used to assess pain, including a VAS. The children's stress levels were monitored through measurement of salivary cortisol. Analysis of functional ability was made via parental observations. Although not statistically significant, the results of this study show a reduction in anxiety, in both the children receiving the massage and the parent performing the massage. Salivary cortisol levels were reduced post-massage and the level of pain, as measured through self-report, parental and physician assessment, was also lowered. Despite a small number of participants, the researchers recommended further investigation in the area of pain, anxiety and functional ability in rheumatoid arthritis populations, stating that 'massage seems to be a cost-effective therapy' (p. 617).

When compared to prescription medications, massage therapy may appear a more cost-effective option for the management of pain. Nixon et al. (1997) investigated the effect of relaxation massage on pain perception and usage of analgesia medication after abdominal surgery. Thirty-nine subjects were allocated to either the massage (n = 19) or control (n = 20) group. Nurses trained in relaxation massage administered massage therapy daily and data for pain perception was collected with a VAS. Patients who received massage postoperatively perceived less pain than in the control group yet did not exhibit a reduction in analgesia. One incidental finding of the study was that massage therapy intervention was particularly effective for pain reduction in the older patients.

The body can naturally modulate the pain experience through the release of endorphins; powerful analgesic substances that bind to opiate receptors in the brain dulling pain. Kaada and Torsteinbo (1989) reported a moderate elevation in plasma β-endorphin levels following connective tissue massage. Twelve subjects who experienced pain associated with myalgia and other syndromes were given a 30-minute massage. Eleven subjects reported feelings of relaxation and warmth post-intervention. The investigators concluded that feelings of relaxation and the elevation of pain thresholds were due to increased concentration of opioid (or narcotic analgesic substances). This study was flawed due to the lack of a control (or non-experimental) group, the small number of participants and the fact that subjects did not necessarily suffer from the same condition.

Dubrovskii et al. (1992) investigated the effects of massage on 69 subjects with soft tissue injury or capsular-ligament damage. It was stated that massage helped to reduce pain and swelling, and increase joint mobility. The authors found massage helpful to 'accelerate the microcirculation and to reduce histamine and muscle tone' (p. 71). This study involved a large sample size, yet there was no control group, and subjects suffered from a broad range of injuries.

It is clear from these findings that massage therapy has a significant role to play in the management of pain. A person's pain experience is a unique one, which manifests itself in a combination of physiological and psychological symptoms. Whether it be in the management of acute or chronic pain, in conditions such as cancer, rheumatoid arthritis or fibromyalgia, massage therapy is a useful treatment that may reduce pain perceptions, improve functional ability and elevate endorphin levels.

THE EFFECTS OF MASSAGE THERAPY ON EMOTIONAL STATES

One of the major reasons why people visit a massage therapist is to enhance their mood. When receiving a nurturing treatment like massage in an environment that is free from distractions and conducive to relaxation, many people find they can take time out from their busy lives; they are free to indulge their senses in a treatment that will leave them feeling calm, clear-headed, more confident and less anxious, and will assist in controlling their stress levels in addition to boosting their immune function.

Much of the research investigating the efficacy of massage therapy centres around its effects on the emotional states. What follows are summaries of research that illustrate the worth of massage for positively enhancing mood, controlling anxiety and stress, and aiding depression.

In a non-randomised investigation into the effects of massage on mood, Weinberg, Jackson and Kolodny (1988) recruited 183 university students to determine the relationship between massage, exercise and positive mood enhancement. Subjects were required to perform 30 minutes of moderate exercise (n = 87), receive a 30-minute full body relaxation massage (n = 40) or rest/read for 30 minutes (n = 56). Subjects were required to complete a series of psychological tests prior to and immediately after participation. The investigators concluded that in terms of positive mood enhancement the only groups to consistently benefit were those that received massage or performed running for exercise. This study suggests that massage may be useful in elevating mood and may elicit a 'high' similar to that experienced after moderate intensity exercise like running.

Another study reporting feelings of wellbeing investigated the effects of pre-performance massage on stride frequency in sprinters (Harmer, 1991). Although no significant increase in stride frequency was noted, subjects did report positive feelings about massage, stating they felt relaxed and refreshed post-massage treatment. Some subjects stated a carry-over effect, believing that massage allowed them to perform better in their training sessions up to five days post-massage, suggesting that enhancement of mood elevates performance.

Despite subjects reporting feelings of wellbeing post-massage, it is difficult to quantify the psychological benefits of massage. A study by Fraser and Kerr (1993) investigated the effects of massage on anxiety. The study involved 21 elderly subjects in care, assigned to one of three groups — a five-minute massage with conversation, conversation only and no intervention. Results were obtained pre- and post-test, and involved a questionnaire and quantitative measures of electromyography, heart rate and blood pressure. Although physiological improvements consistent with reduced anxiety were observed, these were not statistically significant. It should be noted that subjective qualitative data collected supported the use of massage for relaxation.

Ensuring that patients are in a relaxed state prior to undergoing surgical procedures is important for patient comfort. A study conducted by Kim et al. (2001) investigated the effects of hand massage on anxiety prior to cataract surgery. Over a two month period, 59 subjects were assigned to either a massage group (n = 29) or a control group (n = 30). Subjects in the massage group received a five-minute hand massage immediately prior to undergoing cataract surgery using local anaesthesia. Data was collected immediately prior to and post-treatment for both groups. A VAS was used to collect data on anxiety, whilst additional data was collected via blood samples and measures of blood pressure and pulse rate. The findings of the massage group indicated a significant reduction in anxiety post-massage when compared to pre-massage. Blood samples showed that epinephrine, norepinephrine and cortisol levels (all stress hormones) were reduced in the massage group, and elevated in the control group, indicating reduced anxiety amongst the massage group. The authors concluded that a hand massage administered immediately prior to surgery was a good intervention to increase patient comfort and relieve anxiety over the surgical procedure.

Patients may also become distressed or anxious also when receiving treatment regimes for conditions such as cancer. Lafreniere et al. (1999) conducted a pilot study using therapeutic touch (an energetic healing technique) as a means of investigating a possible intervention to assist breast cancer patients to cope with the side effects of chemotherapy treatment. Forty-one healthy females were randomly assigned to either an experimental group (n = 22) or a control group (n = 19). Each month, over a three-month period, the experimental group received a therapeutic touch session and then completed a series of mood questionnaires post-intervention, whilst the control group received no therapeutic touch and simply completed the same questionnaires. Results showed that mood disturbances in the experimental group reduced significantly throughout the study, whilst mood disturbances were increased over time in participants who did not receive therapeutic touch (the control group). The findings from this study suggested that therapeutic touch may be a viable intervention for patients in distress receiving chemotherapy, and recommended further study with a population of breast cancer patients.

Another study investigated the effects of massage on mood in children and adolescents. This study, conducted in 1993, investigated the effects of massage on behaviours and physiology of children and adolescent psychiatric patients (Field et al., 1993). The study involved 72 children and adolescents (32 females, 40 males) hospitalised with either depression or adjustment disorder. Using a random stratification procedure, the subjects were assigned to either a massage or control group. The subjects in the massage group (n = 52, 36 depressed and 36 adjustment disorder) received a 30 minute back massage whilst the control group (n = 20, 10 depressed and 10 adjustment disorder) viewed relaxing videos for the same time duration as the massage group. These sessions were repeated daily over a period of five days. Data was collected via STAI (for children STAIC), POMS, self-reports of anxiety and depression, behavioural observation, nursing staff observations, actometer readings for activity levels, heart rate, salivary cortisol, urinary cortisol and catecholamines and a night-time sleep video recording. Collectively, the results from the self-reports, behavioural observations and cortisol levels suggested a reduction in anxiety in both the short and long-terms for the depressed children and adolescents in the massage group. The nursing observations suggested that massage therapy may have a positive effect on children and adolescents hospitalised with either depression or adjustment disorder, whilst results from the sleep video suggested improved sleep over the five-day period. Despite having a control group, a limitation of this study was that massage therapy was not compared to another form of relaxation therapy.

Field et al. (1996) conducted a study to compare the effects of massage and relaxation therapies on anxiety and depression in a group of depressed adolescent mothers, recruited from a hospital maternity ward. Thirty-two mothers were randomly assigned to either a massage group (n = 16) or a relaxation therapy group (n = 16) that consisted of yoga exercise and progressive muscle relaxation. All treatments lasted for 30 minutes, and were administered twice a week over a five-week period. During the investigation, data was collected using the POMS, STAIC, behaviour observation scales and pulse rates. The researchers also analysed saliva and urine samples for cortisol levels. The results of this study showed that anxiety reduced on the first day for both groups, and on the last day of treatment for the massage group. The massage group also exhibited lower POMS depression scores on the first and last days of treatment and less anxiety after their sessions. It is important to note that only the massage group experienced a reduction in stress levels, as measured by a decrease in the levels of cortisol in the urine across the course of the treatment. The findings from this study are consistent with those of Field et al. (1993), and the authors note that additional research is to be done before conclusions may be drawn that massage therapy leads to longer lasting effects for depression in adolescent mothers than relaxation therapy.

A recent study investigated the effects of massage therapy on depression, anxiety and immune function in adolescents diagnosed with HIV (Diego et al., 2001). Twenty-four seropositive patients (22 females) were randomly assigned to either a massage therapy group (n = 12) or a relaxation therapy group (n = 12) which undertook progressive muscle relaxation and acted as a control.

Whilst remaining fully clothed, the massage group received a 20 minute seated massage of the back, arms, hands and neck. The investigators also randomly allocated the therapist to the patient in the massage group. All sessions were conducted twice a week for a period of 12 weeks, and results were collected using immune assay and STAI. Subjects also completed a demographic questionnaire. After treatment on the first and last days, both groups showed an immediate reduction in anxiety post-treatment, whilst only the massage group reported a reduction in depression. During the test period, cell mediated immunity was enhanced in the massage group, and after the three-month period of receiving massage therapy, the massage group was less depressed and exhibited an improved immune function. The authors postulated that stress and anxiety might result in overactivity of the hypothalamic-pituitary axis. Such overactivity may further suppress immune function, further lowering the number of killer cells. The authors believe the positive effects of massage therapy on cell mediated immunity and cytotoxicity may be explained by the ability of massage therapy to reduce stress and anxiety, which in turn may lower cortisol levels and lead to improved immune function. The findings of this study are promising, and suggest future studies be undertaken to examine the effects of massage therapy on individuals with a less compromised immune system.

Many people seek out massage therapy treatment to assist with their emotional states. It is evident from the research presented that massage therapy is of great value in such instances. A treatment that is cost-effective and non-addictive, massage therapy can reduce anxiety, aid depression and positively enhance mood. Massage may also assist with stress management and improve immune function.

THE EFFECTS OF MASSAGE THERAPY ON SLEEP

Aside from reporting feelings of emotional wellbeing, many recipients of massage report improved sleep patterns post-massage. Field et al. (1997) state that an increase in sleep may be a factor in pain reduction, hence intervention in this study was administered prior to retiring for the night. Emotional stress can be a factor in the pain experience, so targeting stress through relaxation techniques may also contribute to a decrease in the intensity and frequency of pain.

A 1998 study investigated the effect of back massage and relaxation intervention on sleep in critically ill patients (Richards, 1998). The author noted that sleep disturbances might stem from a number of factors in the critically ill patient, including psychological stress, noise, painful procedures, and physical complications associated with bed rest. The study used a polysomnograph to measure one nights sleep in 69 hospitalised male subjects with cardiovascular illness, aged 55–79 years. Patients were randomly assigned to one of three groups — massage, relaxation or control. The massage group (n = 24) received a six minute back massage prior to sleep. The relaxation group (n = 28) undertook a teaching session in relaxation and listened to an audiotape that guided them through progressive muscle relaxation prior to sleep. The control group (n = 17) received routine nursing care and six minutes of rest prior to sleep. A limitation of this study was the number of participants. Despite initial results suggesting an improved quality of sleep amongst the back massage group, when reanalysed with the groups numbers consistent (n = 17) there was no significant difference amongst the groups. Further investigation is required with a larger sample size to determine the effect of massage therapy on sleep in critically ill patients.

Many clients of massage claim that the treatment improves their sleep, yet little research exists to validate their anecdotal reports. It is anticipated that in the future, researchers will devote time to investigating the effects of massage therapy on sleep patterns.

CONCLUSION

For centuries people have instinctively used their hands to apply pressure over their painful joints without thinking about the exact mechanism behind the resultant positive emotional outcome and perceived reduction in pain. This very primitive manipulation could well be described as a form of massage therapy, a treatment that today is non-addictive, readily available and pleasurable. The details of several studies have been described throughout this chapter, and their findings are summarised in Table 4.1. Whether massage acts directly or indirectly to affect the physiological functioning of the body or to bring about a change in a person's psychological state is yet to be fully understood. One thing that is certain about massage is that it is effective for a wide range of situations and conditions. Just how effective massage can really be is yet to be tested.

Despite the current literature that exists on the effects of massage, it is clear that more controlled research studies involving large numbers of participants are required to show the benefits of the use of massage therapy for a range of conditions. With the current resurgence in complementary therapies many are discovering the benefits that

Table 4.1 Summary of study findings

YEAR	AUTHORS	FINDINGS
1974	Hovind and Nielson	Tapôtement and pétrissage techniques increase local skeletal muscle blood flow.
1987	Ernst et al.	Massage reduces haematocrit, blood viscosity and plasma viscosity.
1988	Weinberg et al.	Massage elevates mood and produces a 'high' similar to that experienced after exercise.
—	Yamazaki et al.	Undulating pneumatic massage improves lymphatic and blood flow.
1989	Kaada and Torsteinbo	Connective tissue massage elevates endorphin levels.
1990	Davis et al.	People with rheumatic disease seek complementary therapies such as massage for pain management.
—	Morrelli et al.	Pétrissage technique decreases H-reflex amplitude, with deep massage having a greater effect than light massage.
—	Weinrich and Weinrich	Massage is effective for short-term pain relief from cancer.
1991	Harmer	Massage elevates mood of sprinters.
—	Sullivan et al.	Pétrissage technique decreases H-reflex amplitude.
1992	Dubrovskii et al.	Massage aids recovery from soft tissue injury.
—	Goldberg et al.	Pétrissage technique decreases H-reflex amplitude.
1993	Ferrell-Tory and Glick	Massage is effective for short-term pain relief from cancer and relieves anxiety and induces relaxation.
—	Field et al.	Massage reduces anxiety in both the short- and long-term in children and adolescents hospitalised with depression or adjustment disorder.
—	Fraser and Kerr	Massage aids relaxation in elderly people in care.
1994	Goldberg et al.	Pétrissage technique decreases H-reflex amplitude in subjects with spinal cord injury, and has carry-over effect.
1996	Field et al.	Massage reduces stress, anxiety and depression in depressed adolescent mothers.
1997	Field et al.	Massage reduces pain and anxiety, and improves sleep in children with juvenile rheumatoid arthritis.
—	Nixon et al.	Massage reduces perceptions of pain post-operatively.
1998	Richards	Massage improves quality of sleep in some critically ill patients.
1999	Lafreniere et al.	Therapeutic touch reduces mood disturbances in patients undergoing chemotherapy treatment.
2000	Hernandez-Reif et al.	Massage reduces diastolic blood pressure, stress and feelings of anxiety, hostility and depression.
2001	Diego et al.	Massage reduces depression and improves immune function in adolescents diagnosed with HIV.
—	Hernandez-Reif et al.	Massage reduces pain in people with lower back pain, and improves range of movement, aids depression, relieves anxiety, improves mood and assists with sleep.
—	Kim et al.	Hand massage assists with patient comfort and relieves anxiety prior to surgery.
2003	Field et al.	A combination of massage and movement reduces anxiety and pain and improves mood.

massage therapy can offer. Such consumer interest has and will continue to spur researchers to test the validity of therapies such as massage for a wide range of complaints. The outcomes of such academic enquires can only add weight to the body of knowledge already established on the effects of massage therapy.

Questions and activities

1. You are giving a conference presentation on the benefits of massage when one delegate asks you to clarify the difference between the direct and indirect effects of massage therapy. What would you say?
2. As an evidence-based practitioner, you are composing a newsletter to mail out to clients. Based on research findings, write a 100 word piece describing the types of conditions that may benefit from massage therapy.
3. You are keen to commence a trial into the use of massage therapy in a hospital ward, and are asked to present your proposal to the medical board of the hospital. Your trial primarily focuses on the use of massage for the management of pain. Citing research findings, what would you say to convince these practitioners of the worth of your proposed trial?

Recommended reading

Andrade, C. and Clifford, P. (2001) *Outcome-Based Massage*. Lippincott Williams & Wilkins, Baltimore.

Field, T. (2000) *Touch Therapy*. Churchill Livingstone, London.

Field, T. M. (1998) 'Massage therapy effects', *American Psychologist*, 53(12), pp. 1270–81.

Lederman, E. (1997) *Fundamentals of Manual Therapy: Physiology, Neurology and Psychology*. Churchill Livingstone, New York.

Rich, G. J. (2002) *Massage Therapy: The Evidence for Practice*. Mosby, London.

REFERENCES

Beck, M. (1988) *The Theory & Practice of Therapeutic Massage*. Milady Publishing Co., New York.

Cassar, M. (1999) *Handbook of Massage Therapy: A Complete Guide for the Student and Professional Massage Therapist*. Butterworth–Heinemann, Oxford.

Davis, G. C., Cortez, C. and Rubin, B. R. (1990) 'Pain management in the older adult with rheumatoid arthritis or osteoarthritis', *Arthritis Care and Research*, 3(3), pp. 127–31.

De Domenico, G. and Wood, E. C. (1997) *Beard's Massage* (4th edn). W. B. Saunders, Philadelphia.

Diego, M. A., Field, T., Hernandez-Reif, M., Shaw, K., Friedman, L. and Ironson, G. (2001) 'HIV adolescents show improved immune function following massage therapy', *Intern J Neuroscience*, 106, pp. 35–45.

Dubrovskii, I., Sverdlik, Y. A., Luchshev, A. I. and Proshchalykin, A. I. (1992) 'The effect of massage on micro-circulation in athletes' musculoskeletal injuries', *Fitness and Sports Review International*, 27(2), p. 71.

Ernst, E., Matrai, A., Magyarosy, I., Liebermeister, R., Eck, M. and Breu, M. (1987) 'Massages cause changes in blood fluidity', *Physiotherapy*, 73(1), pp. 43–5.

Ferrell-Torry, A. T. and Glick, O. J. (1993) 'The use of therapeutic massage as a nursing intervention to modify anxiety and the perception of cancer pain', *Cancer Nursing*, 16(2), pp. 93–101.

Field, T. (2000) *Touch Therapy*. Churchill Livingstone, London.

Field, T., Delage, J. and Hernandez-Reif, M. (2003) 'Movement and massage therapy reduce fibromyalgia pain', *J of Bodywork and Movement Therapies*, Jan, pp. 49–52.

Field, T., Grizzle, N., Scafidi, F. and Schanberg, S. (1996) 'Massage and relaxation therapies' effects on depressed adolescent mothers', *Adolescence*, 31 (124), pp. 903–11.

Field, T., Hernandez-Reif, M., Seligman, S., Krasnegor, J. and Sunshine, W. (1997) 'Juvenile rheumatoid arthritis: benefits from massage therapy', *J of Pediatric Psychology*, 22(5), pp. 607–17.

Field, T., Morrow, C., Valdeon, C., Larson, S., Kuhn, C. and Schanberg, S. (1993) 'Massage reduces anxiety in children and adolescent psychiatric patients', *Intern J Alternative and Complementary Medicine*, July, pp. 22–7.

Fraser, J. and Kerr, J. (1993) 'Psychophysiological effects of back massage on elderly institutionalized patients', *J of Advanced Nursing*, 18, pp. 238–45.

Fritz, S. (2000) *Mosby's Fundamentals of Therapeutic Massage* (2nd edn). Mosby, St Louis.

Goldberg, J., Seaborne, D. E., Sullivan, S. J. and Leduc, B. E. (1994) 'The effect of therapeutic massage on H-reflex amplitude in persons with a spinal cord injury', *Physical Therapy*, 74(8), pp. 728–37.

Goldberg, J., Sullivan, S. J. and Seaborne, D. E. (1992) 'The effect of two intensities of massage on H-reflex amplitude', *Physical Therapy*, 72(6), pp. 449–57.

Harmer, P. A. (1991) 'The effect of pre-performance massage on stride frequency in sprinters', *Athletic Training*, 26(1), pp. 55–9.

Hernandez-Reif, M., Field, T., Krasnegor, J. and Theakston, H. (2001) 'Lower back pain is reduced and range of motion increased after massage therapy', *Intern J Neuroscience*, 106, pp. 131–45.

Hernandez-Reif, M., Field, T., Krasnegor, J., Theakston, H., Hossain, Z. and Burman, I. (2000) 'High blood pressure and associated symptoms were reduced by massage therapy', *J of Bodywork and Movement Therapies*, 4(1), pp. 31–8.

Hovind, H. and Nielsen, S. L. (1974) 'Effect of massage on blood flow in skeletal muscle', *Scand J Rehab Med*, 6, pp. 74–7.

Kaada, B. and Torsteinbo, O. (1989) 'Increase of plasma b-endorphins in connective tissue massage', *Gen Pharmac*, 20(4), pp. 487–9.

Kim, M. S., Cho, K. S., Woo, H. and Kim, J. H. (2001) 'Effects of hand massage on anxiety in cataract surgery using local anesthesia', *J Cataract Refract Surg*, 27, pp. 884–90.

Lafreniere, K. D., Mutus, B., Cameron, S., Tannous, M., Giannotti, M., Abu-Zahra, H. and Laukkanen, E. (1999) 'Effects of therapeutic touch on biochemical and mood indicators in women', *J of Alternative and Complementary Medicine*, 5(4), pp. 367–70.

Melzack, R. and Wall, P. D. (1965) 'Pain mechanisms: a new theory', *Science*, 150, p. 971.

Mennell, J. B. (c. 1917) *Massage, its Principles and Practice*. J. & A. Churchill, London.

Morrelli, M., Seaborne, D. E. and Sullivan, S. J. (1990) 'Changes in H-reflex amplitude during massage of triceps surae in healthy subjects', *JOSPT*, 12(2), pp. 55–9.

National Health and Medical Research Council (1989) *Management of Severe Pain: Report of the Working Party on Management of Severe Pain*. NH&MRC, Canberra.

Nixon, M., Teschendorff, J., Finney, J. and Karnilowicz, W. (1997) 'Expanding the nursing repertoire — the effect of massage on post operative pain', *Aust J of Advanced Nursing*, 14(3), pp. 21–6.

Richards, K. C. (1998) 'The effect of a back massage and relaxation therapy on sleep', article J of *Critical Care* 7(4), 288–99.

Salvo, S. G. (1999) *Massage Therapy: Principles and Practice*. W. B. Saunders, Philadelphia.

Sullivan, S. J., Williams, L. R. T., Seaborne, D. E. and Morrelli, M. (1991) 'Effects of massage on alpha motoneuron excitability', *Physical Therapy*, 71(8), pp. 555–60.

Tappan, F. M. and Benjamin, P. J. (1998) *Tappan's handbook of Healing Massage Techniques: Classic, Holistic, and Emerging Methods* (3rd edn). Appleton & Lange, Connecticut.

Trevelyan, J. (1993) 'Massage', *Nursing Times*, 89(19), pp. 45–7.

Weinberg, R., Jackson, A. and Kolodny, K. (1988) 'The relationship of massage and exercise to mood enhancement', *The Sport Psychologist*, 2, pp. 202–11.

Weinrich, S. P. and Weinrich, M. C. (1990) 'The effect of massage on pain in cancer patients', *Applied Nursing Research*, 3(4), pp. 140–5.

Yamazaki, Z., Idezuki, Y., Nemoto, T. and Togawa, T. (1988) 'Clinical experiences using pneumatic massage therapy for edematous limbs over the last 10 years', *Angiology – The J of Vascular Diseases*, February, pp. 154–63.

chapter 5

The importance of touch

Sheena Worrall

Learning outcomes

- Explain why touch is important for human beings
- Identify how research supports the importance of touch
- Outline the ways in which people experience touch and how it affects their self-concept and emotions
- Demonstrate an understanding of critical factors in effective touch therapy
- Develop an understanding of the mechanisms of healing energy transmission through touch

INTRODUCTION

Most people love to touch and be touched. This is evident in how often individuals touch one another, their children, their pets and themselves. Touch can communicate emotion and caring in ways that make words seem clumsy in comparison. The fact that so many people are now actively seeking out touch in the form of massage therapy is a clear indication that this is an important need that seeks to be fulfilled. In addition, the use of touch in therapy is increasingly being recognised by mainstream medicine as a powerful healing tool.

The importance of touch is evident in the way people use touch and skin references in their day-to-day language. When people talk about emotions, such as joy, happiness, sadness, anger or depression, they refer to them as 'feelings'. A deeply felt experience is one that 'touches' us. When people want to be close to other humans they get 'in touch' or 'in contact' with them. People talk about 'handling' certain people with care. Someone who is not communicating well might be said to be 'out of touch'. If they are struggling they are said to have 'lost their grip'. A person with no compassion might be described as 'unfeeling'.

Increasingly in this low-touch society, people are turning to massage and other 'hands-on' therapies to meet this need for comfort, as well as for healing. The profession of massage is a caring one. Massage therapy addresses the need for positive sensory experience and comfort. Physical contact through positive touch may foster a powerful sense of connection and caring. This sense of connection with the environment and other people may be an important source of strength and comfort for humans. Massage therapy can help with this. Whilst this may be the case, it is important for the therapist to note that not all people respond to or interpret touch in the same way, and with the same feelings (Dossey et al., 2000, p. 112).

Physiotherapy educator Gjertrud Roxendal claims that massage *is* communication. She believes that the therapist, in caring for the client, is sending messages via the skin, especially the question: 'How are you?' The client receives the care and in turn answers via changes to breathing, muscle tension and skin reactions. Roxendal also believes that massage confirms the receiver through the body. The fact that the therapist is prepared to touch the client confers on them acceptance and validation as a person (Roxendal, 1990). The purpose of this chapter is to explore the notion of touch, and to discus the benefits of touch as a form of therapy.

SKIN AND OUR TACTILE SENSE

Touch is the most extensive, important and yet neglected of our senses. People can survive without eyes, ears, or a sense of taste or smell, but without a sense of touch they are in constant physical and psychological danger. Touch stimulation is essential to people at all stages of life and touch deprivation leads to reduced levels of the neuroendocrine substances necessary for health and wellbeing (Field, 2000; Montagu, 1986).

The entire human body is covered with skin, which even turns inward and lines the gastrointestinal tract. When in the womb, the skin is the first sensory organ to be developed. Even at six weeks, when the human embryo is only about three centimetres long, gentle stimulation of the new skin on the upper lip or wings of the nose will cause the embryo to bend away from the source of stimulation (Montagu, 1986, p. 4). This occurs long before the embryo develops eyes and ears.

Through the skin people receive signals about touch, pressure, pain and heat, from the environment and the people in it. This information is conveyed to the nervous system. As an extension of the brain and nervous system, skin is very rich in nerve endings. An adult male has about 19 000 square centimetres of skin, which contains some five million sensory cells, each relaying important information to the nervous system. About half a million of these nerve receptor cells send information back to the spinal cord and brain via individual nerve pathways, providing information about texture, shape, tension, heat, vibration, and pressure. A staggering 30 per cent or more of these are located in the skin covering our hands. Fingertips have more than 160 nerve endings per square centimetre (Fritz et al., 1999).

Skin has 20 other known functions ranging from protection from trauma, foreign organisms and the elements, to regulation of body temperature and blood pressure, regeneration of tissue, excretion of waste, synthesis of vitamin D and other important compounds. Awareness of these functions is important as it helps therapists to appreciate how touching the skin (or not touching it) can produce remarkable physiological changes in humans and other species.

TOUCH AND HUMAN DEVELOPMENT

Dr Tiffany Field of the Touch Research Institute (TRI) in the United States, has conducted numerous studies concerning the importance of touch to the healthy development of babies. Her studies have shown that premature babies who received 15 minutes of massage, three times a day gained 47 per cent more weight and were discharged an average of six days earlier than babies who were only touched when they were fed or had their nappy changed (Hoffman, Sherrick and Warm, 1998).

As well as benefiting digestion, positive touch can also benefit the nervous system. A recent study on the effect of maternal contact on babies suggests that the rate at which brain cells degenerate and die is doubled when infants are neglected, thus greatly impeding their development. Curiously, the area of the brain most affected by neglect is the hippocampal region, the part of the brain where many of our emotions are evaluated (Staerker, 1999). Further studies are currently being undertaken to determine the effects of this nerve cell death (through neglect) on later adult physical and social development. Because touch stimulates the nervous system it consequently enhances general wellbeing in body systems affected by the nervous system.

Studies undertaken by the TRI suggest that tactile-kinaesthetic stimulation in the form of massage benefits newborn babies by contributing to (Field, 2000):

- greater weight gain;
- increased motor activity;
- improved alertness;
- better organised sleep patterns;
- less fussiness and more positive emotional response;
- more mature motor performance on the Brazelton scale;
- fewer postnatal complications;
- reduction of stress behaviours and levels of stress hormones;
- enhanced response to social stimulation;
- enhanced general wellbeing and reduced stress in cocaine-exposed infants;
- reduced deterioration in HIV exposed infants.

PSYCHOSOCIAL DEVELOPMENT AND TOUCH

The bond formed between parents and their child in the early months of life forms the foundation for the child's subsequent emotional and social development. A person's experiences in these early months of life help shape their beliefs about life, love and self. If all their needs are met they grow up confident that they are lovable, that they will be able to cope in life and that the world is a pleasurable place to be.

According to chiropractor Paul Staerker, touching or 'stroking' is the fundamental act of recognition for the young child (Staerker, 1999). Through it humans learn the physical outline and shape of their body, and whether they are loved and cared for. Capable, confident, mentally healthy adults develop from babies who have been given plenty of positive experience of touch. Massage is a powerful and gentle way of providing this positive touch.

Endorphins are neuropeptides that tell the cell to 'feel' blissful. Oxytocin is a neuropeptide that not only tells uterine cells to contract in childbirth but also has a strong role to play in bonding and fostering positive maternal behaviour, and cementing other kinds of relationships in both males and females. Clinical trials where blood samples were taken before and after massage therapy have shown that serum levels of both endorphins and oxytocin increase after massage (Fritz, 2000). This research sheds light on why massage not only gives people a natural 'high' but also makes them feel emotionally warmer and more connected to those around them. According to Fritz, massage also has a distinct effect on serum levels of other neuropeptides such as growth hormone, dopamine, serotonin, adrenalin and cortisol, depending on the type of technique applied and the duration.

Because positive touch in the form of massage therapy has been shown to release 'feel good' and 'feel close' neuropeptides, it is not hard to see that either an insufficient or negative experience of touch might lead to abnormal emotional and social behaviours. Developmental neuropsychologist James Prescott believes that violence has its roots in deprivation of pleasurable touch during childhood. In the 1960s Prescott and his associates discovered that lack of affectionate, intimate contact and bonding between mothers and their babies during the most sensitive periods of brain development could result in permanent brain abnormalities, particularly in the pleasure systems of the brain. These abnormalities were found to be associated with juvenile and adult patterns of aggression and violence, depression, substance abuse and eating disorders (Mendizza, 2003). Cultural anthropologists support this view too, with a study of 49 tribal cultures revealing that societies which give their babies the greatest amount of physical affection have the lowest levels of theft, killing, torture and mutilation (Prescott, 1975).

Further support for the importance of touch comes from the work of University of Wisconsin researchers Harry and Margaret Harlow. The Harlows found that female baby rhesus monkeys who were separated from their mothers at birth were neglectful and, in many cases, violently abusive towards their own young (Harlow and Harlow,

1969). Drs Steel and Pollock of the University of Colorado found that human parents who abused their children also had frequently been deprived of physical affection as children themselves (Montagu, 1986).

More recent studies conducted by researchers at Harvard University medical school's McLean Hospital clearly demonstrate that childhood neglect and maltreatment may produce permanent changes in both the structure and function of the brain. The McLean research team found that neglect and trauma led to a number of changes in the brain — brainwave abnormalities, arrested development of the left hemisphere, a reduction in the size of the corpus callosum and increased cerebellar vermis activity (which can result in dramatic mood and personality swings) (McLean Hospital, 2000).

Under the direction of developmental biopsychiatrist Martin Teicher, researchers also examined animal studies that showed that neglect and trauma increased production of cortisol and decreased production of thyroid hormone. According to Teicher, this effect on hormones and neurotransmitters resulted in brain remoulding so that the individual's nervous system was 'wired' to respond with fear, anxiety and stress. He proposes that this finding is likely to be true of people too (McLean Hospital, 2000).

These, and other recent discoveries in developmental neuroscience, clearly support Prescott's findings; that is, insufficient early positive touch may result in the kinds of brain abnormalities that are associated with juvenile and adult patterns of depression, substance abuse, aggression and violence (Prescott, 1975; Mendizza, n.d.). High levels of cortisol, resulting from neglect, and in particular a lack of touch, have also been linked to impaired development and psychological disturbance in infants. In her studies of institutionalised children in Romania, neuroscientist Mary Carlson (a former student of touch researcher Harry Harlow) found abnormally high stress levels in these children on an ongoing basis, with associated developmental retardation and autistic behaviours. Carlson claims that the lack of touching and attention the children received, due to seriously inadequate institutional care, had actually stunted the children's growth and adversely affected their behaviour (Cromie, 1998; Carlson, 1997).

In his preface to *Touching: The Human Significance of the Skin*, Ashley Montagu observed that humans have become a race of 'untouchables', avoiding all forms of 'unnecessary' physical contact, and becoming increasingly lonely and afraid of intimacy (Montagu, 1986). A number of factors have contributed to this, including 'no touch' policies in schools, institutional care settings and the workplace. Technological advances are also playing their part in contributing to low levels of touch in society as people increasingly interact with machines rather than other people. Because people have trouble touching one another, literally and figuratively, they have come to rely heavily on verbal and written communication and their non-verbal communication has suffered. This is causing a consequent impoverishment of experience and feeling.

TOUCH FOR PSYCHOLOGICAL DISORDERS

The positive effects of massage therapy are not confined to physical systems in the body. The positive impact of healing methods of touch on psychological conditions is gaining increasing attention from psychiatrists, psychologists and counsellors. Although this field is relatively new, benefits of safe, caring touch therapy are being identified for clients suffering the effects of depression, anxiety, anorexia, post-traumatic stress disorder, physical and sexual abuse, and a number of other conditions.

Studies produced at the TRI have shown that massage therapy is beneficial in a variety of psychological disorders. The TRI studies lend strong support to the use of touch therapies to decrease depression and anxiety, and lower stress hormone levels in the body. Electroencephalograph (EEG) activity following massage in depressed adolescent mothers revealed that the shifts into more positive mood states following massage were accompanied by shifts from activation of the right–front sections of the brain (normally associated with feeling sad emotionally) to activation of the left–front sections of the brain (normally associated with happy feelings). A 20 minute massage served to shift the brain activation (as revealed by the EEG) into a more symmetrical (and therefore balanced) pattern, thereby reducing feelings of depression (Jones et al., 1997).

Autism is a condition that appears to respond well to massage touch therapy. Autistic children and adults are generally described as disliking physical touch and being extremely sensitive to touch stimulus. However the TRI has found that autistic preschool children show little aversion to being massaged. Field suggests that this may be because massage is predictable, unlike some social forms of stimulation. The TRI studies show that the children who receive massage decrease their off-task behaviour in the classroom and increasingly interact socially with teachers (Hoffman et al., 1998). Similar results have been observed in TRI studies with children exhibiting attention deficit hyperactivity disorder (ADHD).

Some TRI studies have focused on the treatment of anorexia and bulimia, two eating disorders considered to be psychological in origin. After five weeks of twice-weekly massage therapy treatments administered for 30 minutes at a time, anorexia sufferers reported less body dissatisfaction on the Eating Disorder Inventory. Urine analysis revealed higher levels of dopamine and lower levels of stress hormones, and this corresponded with reports of lower anxiety and improved mood in the massaged women (Field, 2000). The TRI studies of bulimia produced similar results and the eating habits of massaged bulimic adolescents improved, along with their self-concept. Kirsty Davison, physiotherapist at the Mental Health Unit in Coney Hill Hospital, Gloucester, uses massage in the treatment of patients with anorexia. She claims that it can be used to encourage the patient with a distorted body image to feel 'in touch' with themself (Trevelyan and Booth, 1994).

Finding and creating a sense of self is an important part of developing a sense of identity, which people need in order to operate in the physical, psychological, spiritual and social worlds (Libster, 2001). Much of a person's self-concept and self-consciousness is determined by sensations felt in the body. In infancy there is no sense of separation between the self and the surrounding world. A baby's ability to differentiate him or herself from the surrounding environment or another person develops largely as a result of acting with, and feeling sensation in, his or her body. Therefore, the sense of self initially relies on the information systems provided by both the skin and the proprioceptors, which tell people what their body feels like from the inside.

In explaining how people create their own body image, psychologists Bermudez, Marcel and Eilan (1995) indicate that the sense of touch or inner feeling leads to:

- one's conscious experience of the body at a particular time;
- a changing non-conscious record of the momentary relative disposition of, and space occupied by, one's body parts; and
- emotional attitudes towards one's body, some of which are tacit and socially determined.

It seems that people define themselves, to a large extent, by the sensations experienced in their bodies or their memory of them. So if their experience of being in a body is pleasurable and positive then it is to be expected that they will feel good about themselves. This perhaps may help them to understand why massage might be of benefit in assisting to normalise the self-concept of a person with an eating disorder such as bulimia or anorexia.

Massage therapists and other bodywork specialists have long claimed that the body can resolve emotional traumas and shocks if it is assisted, through touch therapies, to release its patterns of chronic tension and blocked emotional energy. Such eminent psychotherapists and bodyworkers as Wilhelm Reich, Ida Rolf and Gerda Boyensen have developed a number of massage systems. Their methods appear to release repressed emotions and related patterns of muscle tension as well. Body tension may also develop as a defence against undesirable touch and this may result in 'body armour', as Reich termed it (Kellerman, 1985). Massage can help to release the long-held patterns of physical tension that arise from repressed emotion and painful or undesirable touch.

Traumatic experiences of the 'wrong' kind of touch (such as abuse or torture) can be healed in a particularly powerful way by the sensitive and careful application of the 'right' kind of touch. According to Ford (1989, p. 12), a chiropractor who specialises in healing emotional trauma through touch:

touch also creates a powerful therapeutic alliance, so vital to the healing process. Reaching out to touch someone is a lasting symbol of what it means to be human, and a universal sign of healing.

However, experiences of the 'wrong' kind of touch frequently lead to touch aversion, thereby making it difficult for a therapist to make physical contact in the first place. In these cases the client must be approached with particular care. Informed consent must be emphasised and 'safe' areas of the body for touching must be established in consultation with the client. The client must have a strong sense of being able to control what happens and feel he or she can stop it at any time. By giving the client control of the proceedings, a sense of safety and confidence in the therapist develops. For example, in the first session the client's hands or feet may be the only parts of the body touched. Later the lower leg or arm might be included, when the client feels ready. Progressively more and more areas of the body may be touched, at first with clothing on and later, possibly, without. Great care must be taken to be sensitive to the client's experience and anxiety levels (see Chapter 7 for further discussion on client boundaries).

A lot of the psychological benefits of massage therapy seem to relate to the establishment of a close and trusting relationship between client and therapist. Positive touch engenders a sense of confidence in the therapist (De Domenico and Wood, 1997) and demonstrates caring and concern. Massage can evoke feelings of acceptance and respect for the body and psyche of the person being touched (McCabe, 2001). It is therefore easy to understand how people with an altered body image, lowered self-esteem or those who are dependent, anxious or dying would benefit from positive messages coming in the form of touch. Elderly clients experiencing physical and social isolation and sensory impairments are one group, which appears to benefit greatly from the caring effect of massage (Vortherms, 1991).

TOUCH AS ENERGY HEALING

In nearly every culture and medical tradition on earth there is some form of hands-on healing that involves sending energy into the body, balancing existing energies, or drawing excessive or undesirable energies out of the body. Anecdotal reports indicate that many massage therapists experience sensations of energy movement when they massage clients. Some even report being able to feel energies in and around the body when they pass their hands over the body without actually touching it. Those who practice these methods claim that there is more to who and what people are than just a physical body. They believe that there are subtle bodies of finer, higher vibrational matter which interpenetrate an individual's physical body. These subtle energy aspects of humans are believed to relate to their emotions, mental functioning and spiritual experience (Gerber, 1996).

Often associated with religious and spiritual traditions, hands-on healing has been described in the Bible and other religious texts. The 'laying on of hands' healing method, practised by Jesus and continued by the early Christian church, has its modern-day adherents in some churches and cathedrals. Other versions of these methods may be found in practices such as reiki, polarity therapy, qigong therapy and some aspects of applied kinesiology. Therapeutic touch and healing touch are two systems employing energy healing principles and methods, which are taught in many nursing schools and hospitals (Quinn, 1984; Kreiger, 1975; Quinn and Strelkauskas, 1993).

Over the last 400 years a bitter controversy about subtle energies has raged between vitalists and mechanists. Vitalists believe that there is some kind of mysterious and invisible life-force energy in all things. Mechanists maintain that a phenomenon cannot be real unless it complies with basic laws of physics and chemistry and is measurable with current technologies.

With recent discoveries of the electrical and magnetic energy fields that surround the body, scientific exploration of bioenergy fields has become an important and expanding branch of biomedical research (Gerber, 1996). Biomedical researchers are increasingly investigating practitioners of traditional energy therapies. Dr John Zimmerman of the University of Colorado School of Medicine, for example, has found that some healing energy therapists emanate exceptionally strong, large biomagnetic energy fields from their hands, especially when relaxed and in a meditative frame of mind. In a recent study conducted by Zimmerman it was recorded that therapeutic touch practitioners emitted a signal, which ranged from 0.3 Hz to 30 Hz, with most of the activity in the range of 7–8 Hz. The signal appears to 'sweep' or 'scan' through a range of frequencies (Oschman, 2000). In Zimmerman's studies, non-practitioners were unable to produce these pulses. Further information on this research can be found in James Oschman's book, *Energy Medicine: The Scientific Basis* (2000) and Richard Gerber's *Vibrational Medicine* (1996).

ENSURING A POSITIVE EXPERIENCE OF TOUCH FOR CLIENTS

The practice of massage therapy is all about touching another person, and as such it is vital that therapists consider not only the physical/mechanical impact they are having on their clients, but also the mental/emotional effects. This means therapists have to take care that their clients' first experience of the therapist's touch is positive in every way.

The best time for the therapist to prepare themself and their client for this first physical contact is well before the event. Careful planning and preparation will have an enormous positive influence on the outcome of the first contact. Even before clients arrive for their appointment, they will feel much more confident and safe if they think the therapist has their best interests at heart and will treat them with courtesy, respect and gentleness. Because of this, all care should be taken, even during phone conversations, to convey an image of caring and respect for each client.

Simple strategies like shaking hands with the client at the first meeting, or a light touch on the hand or forearm to make contact in a safe way, will invoke confidence if combined with good eye contact and a friendly demeanour. If the therapist is unsure how soon they can initiate contact with their client, they should try to establish what physical distance is comfortable for the client when they meet for the first time or are taking a case history. People will naturally position themselves at a comfortable distance from others while they establish how safe they are. This individual personal distance is often an arm's length, but this distance may be greater or smaller depending on that person's family background, cultural background, life experience and other factors.

When the client's case history is taken, questions should be asked that will clearly indicate what experience of massage the client has had, and what did and did not feel comfortable for the client on these occasions. At this time clear consent must be obtained from the client for the therapist to uncover any areas of skin and touch the client's body, either directly on the skin or through clothing.

Because some individuals will involuntarily interpret any touch as threatening, regardless of their intention to receive massage, it is important for the therapist to be on the lookout for warning signs in the form of adverse body language. If a client shrinks from touch, the therapist should advise the person that they noticed them moving away when touched and ask why. The therapist should never suppose that they know the reason for any reaction from the client. It may simply be that the therapist's hands are cold, that there is pain in the area, or that the client didn't hear the therapist come into the room, or was falling asleep and was surprised by the therapist's touch.

WAYS OF TOUCHING

Different types of touch are identified by different receptors on the client's skin which relay this information to the nervous system. The client will unconsciously be registering the therapist's touch and evaluating it. The amount of pressure applied in light touch is sensed by different receptors to those that detect deep pressure and each evokes a different emotional response.

Slow, light touch is often interpreted as communicating compassion or intimacy. Slow, deep touch evokes feelings of confidence, and as such is usually associated with safety and relaxation (Fritz et al., 1999). Touch can be pleasurable, uncomfortable or even painful. If it is pleasurable people usually seek to prolong the experience. If it causes physical or psychological discomfort, distress or pain, people will withdraw from it as quickly as they can.

Massage therapists need to understand that any touch, or even the breaking of skin contact with the client, will trigger the release of neurochemicals that control various functions in the different systems of the body via the nervous system. The way in which a therapist touches their clients has a great power to influence how the client feels on virtually all levels and this means therapists must always touch with the greatest of integrity and care.

CONCLUSION

It is clear that from the moment of birth people need positive experiences of touch if they are to develop and maintain high levels of health and wellbeing throughout their lives. As the body, thoughts and emotions are intimately interconnected, the pleasurable tactile stimulus of massage therapy can enhance self-esteem and reduce feelings of anxiety, depression and social isolation. For a person to feel lonely, pessimistic, agitated or violent when their body is awash with pleasurable sensations is difficult indeed.

Therefore it is not unreasonable to expect that not only individuals can be healed of a variety of physical and psychological maladies with massage therapy, but that perhaps society as a whole may benefit. It is likely, given the profound importance of touch to emotional experience and behaviour, that therapists may begin to solve some of the huge social problems besetting the world at present if we could disseminate this information more widely (Prescott, 1975; Harlow and Harlow, 1969; McLean Hospital, 2000; Carlson, 1997). Each individual has a part to play in creating a better world, and massage therapists can do much to educate their community about the importance of touch in shaping healthy, happy individuals.

Whilst the studies discussed in this and other chapters clearly indicate a broad range of positive touch benefits, there is still much that is not known about the healing power of touch. Whether some form of healing energy is transmitted or exchanged when one person touches another person with positive intent is something that still cannot be proved or disproved at present. However, this area of research is growing very quickly in today's 'natural therapies-friendly' climate. Staying up to date with current and future research concerning the human bioenergy field will be important for massage therapists wishing to validate their experiences of this energy.

For the benefits of touch therapy to be enjoyed by clients, therapists must remain mindful and respectful of individual differences. This means handling clients with sensitivity and complying with informed consent procedures (see Chapter 6). When this is done, a high degree of trust and confidence in the therapist will develop and maximum benefits will be achieved. To be sure that therapists are part of the solution and not the problem, they must look deep into their own psyches to understand their own experiences and attitudes concerning touch. By healing themselves and getting their own touch needs met, therapists can be far more effective and sensitive in caring for others and helping them to heal.

Questions and activities

1. You have recently opened a clinic and have been fortunate enough to secure an interview on the local community radio station. The presenter of the program recalls that as a small child they loved to have their scalp massaged by their parent when they were having difficulty getting

to sleep or when they were sick. Detail how you would respond to this recollection, and convey to listeners the importance of touch to humans, and the significance of touch to the development of infants.

2. It has been claimed that massage can positively affect emotional states and people's self-perceptions. Describe the types of clients who may present for massage and benefit from such effects.

3. For a professional massage therapist it is paramount that the intent of their touch is appropriately conveyed to the client. How would you ensure that this is true of your touch in clinical practice?

4. A client makes comment one day that they feel you have a healing touch. For a massage therapist, what is the impact of healing energy on touch therapy?

Recommended reading

Field, T. (2000) *Touch Therapy*. Churchill Livingstone, London.

Montagu, A. (1986) *Touching: The Human Significance of the Skin* (3rd edn). HarperCollins, New York.

Nathan, B. (1999) *Touch and Emotion in Manual Therapy*. Churchill Livingstone, London.

Oschman, J. L. (2000) *Energy Medicine: The Scientific Basis*. Churchill Livingstone, London.

Sayre-Adams, J. and Wright, S. G. (2001) *Therapeutic Touch: Theory and Practice* (2nd edn). Churchill Livingstone, London.

REFERENCES

Bermudez, J. L., Marcel, A. and Eilan, N. (eds) (1995) *The Body and the Self*. Bradford, Cambridge.

Carlson, M. (1997) 'Understand the "Mother's Touch" on the brain', Harvard Mahoney Neuroscience Institute letter, Fall 1997/Winter 1998, vol. 7, no. 1. Online: *http://www.med.harvard.edu/ publications/on_The_Brain/volume7/number1/ commentary.html* Accessed 10 July 2003.

Cromie, W. J. (1998) 'Of hugs and hormones', *The Harvard University Gazette*, 11 June 1998. Online: *http://www.news.harvard.edu/gazette/1998/06.11/of HugsandHormones.html* Accessed 10 July 2003.

De Domenico, G. and Wood, E. (1997) *Beard's Massage* (4th edn). W. B. Saunders, Philadelphia.

Dossey, B. M., Keegan, L. and Guzzetta, C. E. (2000) *Holistic Nursing* (3rd edn). Aspen Publishers, Gaithersburg, Maryland.

Field, T. (2000) *Touch Therapy*. Churchill Livingstone, London.

Ford, C. (1989) *Where Healing Waters Meet: Touching Mind and Emotions Through the Body*. Station Hill Press, New York.

Fritz, S. (2000) *Fundamentals of Therapeutic Massage* (2nd edn). Mosby, St Louis.

Fritz, S., Paholsky, K. M. and Grosenbach, M. J. (1999) *Basic Science for Soft Tissue and Movement Therapists*. Mosby, St Louis.

Gerber, R. (1996) *Vibrational Medicine*. Bear & Co., Santa Fe, New Mexico.

Harlow, H. F. and Harlow, M. K. (1969) 'Effects of various mother–infant relationships on rhesus monkey behaviour', *Determinants of Infant Behaviour*, 4, B. M. Foss (ed.), Methuen, London, pp. 15–36.

Hoffman, R., Sherrick, M. and Warm, J. (eds) (1998) *Viewing Psychology as a Whole*. American Psychological Association, Washington.

Jones, N. A., Field, T., Fox, N., Davalos, M. and Pickens, J. (1997) 'EEG stability in infants/children of depressed mothers', *Child Psychiatry and Human Development*, 28(2), pp. 38–42.

Kellerman, S. (1985) *Emotional Anatomy*. Centre Press. Berkeley, California.

Kreiger, D. (1975) 'Therapeutic touch: the imprimatur of nursing', *American Journal of Nursing*, vol. 5, pp. 784–7.

Libster, M. (2001) *Demonstrating Care: The Art of Integrative Nursing*. Delmar Thomson Learning, New York.

McCabe, P. (ed.) (2001) *Complementary Therapies in Nursing and Midwifery*. Ausmed, Melbourne.

McLean Hospital (2000), 'McLean Researchers Document Brain Damage Linked to Child Abuse and Neglect', McLean Hospital press release, 14 December, Belmont MA, Harvard University. Online: *http://mclean.harvard.edu/Public Affairs/ 20001214_child_abuse.htm* Accessed 10 July 2003.

Mendizza, M. (nd) 'Bonding and Violence', *Touch the Future* Web article, online: *http://www.touchthefuture.org/services/bonding/main .htm* Accessed 10 July 2003.

—— (2003) *Touch The Future: Bonding and Violence*. Online: *http://www.touchthefuture.org/services/ bonding/publications.htm* Accessed 24 February 2003.

Montagu, A. (1986) *Touching: The Human Significance of the Skin* (3rd edn). Harper & Row, New York.

Oschman, J. L. (2000) *Energy Medicine: The Scientific Basis*. Churchill Livingstone, London.

Prescott, J. H. (1975) 'Body pleasure and the origins of violence', *The Futurist*, April, pp. 64–5.

Quinn, J. F. (1984) 'Therapeutic touch as energy exchange: testing the theory', *Advances in Nursing Science*, 6:42–9.

Quinn, J. F. and Strelkausaks, A. J. (1993) 'Psychoimmunologic effects of therapeutic touch on practitioners and recently bereaved recipients: a pilot study', *Advances in Nursing Science*, 15(4) pp. 13–26.

Roxendal, G. (1990) 'Physiotherapy as an approach in psychiatric care with emphasis on body awareness therapy', *Psychological and Psychosomatic Problems*, T. Hegna and M. Sveram (eds), Churchill Livingstone, Edinburgh, pp. 94–5.

Staerker, P. (1999) *Tender Touch: Massaging Your Baby to Health and Happiness*. Media Masters, Singapore.

Trevelyan, J. and Booth, B. (1994) *Complementary Medicine for Nurses, Midwives and Health Visitors*. Macmillan, Houndmills, Hampshire.

Vortherms, R. C. (1991) 'Clinically improving communication through touch', *Journal of Gerontological Nursing*, 17(5), pp. 6–10.

section 3

The Professional Therapist

chapter 6

Scope of practice, ethics and law in massage therapy

Janine Tobin

Learning outcomes

- Define the massage therapist's scope of practice
- Describe the massage therapist's limits of practice
- Know when it is appropriate to refer a client to another health care professional
- Explain why ethics are important to massage practice
- Discuss the principles of autonomy, beneficence, non-maleficence and justice
- Explain the four main principles of a negligence action
- Explain the elements of informed consent
- Decide if a client can provide informed consent for a massage

INTRODUCTION

Over the years the role of the massage therapist has continuously evolved. As described in Chapters 2 and 3, massage once formed a critical part of the mainstream medical and nursing professions, and was also the basis of the practice of physiotherapy. Massage therapy is incorporated today in many practices including naturopathy and osteopathy. This in itself raises the question as to what role massage therapy plays in today's health care system and who determines this role.

The qualified massage therapist who is a member of a professional massage association largely drives the modern day practice of massage. Such practitioners should have knowledge and understanding of their scope of practice as well as the ethics and the law that informs the legal aspects of a clinical practice. This chapter examines the scope of practice for massage therapists and discusses registration of therapists, limits of practice for a massage therapist and the referral of clients to other members of the health care team. Also discussed are the ethical principles that guide a therapist throughout their professional life. In addition, the importance of common law, torts and negligence are described for massage therapists. The importance of consent before any massage therapy commences is also discussed. Once understood, such topics provide the massage therapist with a general working knowledge of the legal and ethical issues related to the practice of massage therapy.

'Scope of practice' defines the type of professional service that the law and professional regulations entitle a massage therapist to provide in their professional capacity. The scope of practice is limited by legislation that regulates other health professions and in doing so limits the procedures a massage therapist may perform. The level of education attained by a massage therapist also defines their scope of practice. Each state and territory in Australia and New Zealand possesses their own massage associations that provide guidelines for practice. This chapter will identify the scope of practice of a massage therapist, including the relationships between massage therapists and other health care professionals. It will also explore the limits of practice and discuss the right time to refer clients to other health care professionals.

Ethics relate to determining what in a moral sense is professionally right and wrong and how people should act in a particular circumstance (van Hooft et al., 1997). Ethics encompass the application of moral principles in guiding professional relationships between the massage therapist, the client, the client's family, other health professionals and the general public (Anderson et al., 1998). This chapter will introduce the fundamental ethical principles of autonomy, beneficence, non-maleficence and justice. When applied correctly these principles can help guide the therapist in resolving ethical dilemmas that arise in professional practice.

Having a working knowledge of the relevant principles of law as they pertain to massage practice is essential to guide a therapist in their legal aspects of practice. This chapter will discuss the two principal sources of law: case law and legislation. It will also address the two distinct areas of criminal and civil law. One of the most important areas of civil law for the massage therapist is known as the law of civil wrongs, or law of torts. The aspect of the law of torts that is most often the source of potential legal action for all health care professionals is negligence (Staunton and Chiarella, 2003). The four main principles of a negligence action — duty of care, standard of care, breach of that standard of care causing damage or injury and that the risk of injury is foreseeable — will be discussed (Staunton and Chiarella, 2003).

A massage therapist would seek consent to perform therapy from the client before commencing massage therapy. Such consent provides protection for the client and the massage therapist. This chapter will address the legal importance of gaining valid consent from the client. Valid consent consists of the following three elements: that any consent from a client is given freely and voluntarily; that any consent given is informed; and that the client giving consent has the legal capacity to give such consent (Staunton and Chiarella, 2003).

As a massage therapist, the elements of scope of practice, professional ethics, and codes of practice and duty of care to the client should guide professional conduct. Adherence to these elements at all times is of utmost importance for any professional health care provider.

SCOPE OF PRACTICE

Scope of practice — the types of services that may be provided by a profession.

The scope of practice defines the type of professional service that can or cannot be provided by a massage therapist. How is the scope of practice regulated? In Australia and New Zealand many health care professions are governed by specific state and territory legislation. Legislation takes the form of an Act or Statute made by parliament. In New Zealand and each of the states and territories of Australia, the relevant Acts provide for the registration of many health care professionals. In those professions where registration is required (refer to Box 6.1) it is often an offence to practice or perform specified acts (i.e. manipulate the spine) without registration (Forrester and Griffiths, 2001).

Each state and territory is unique in its legislation and therapists should refer to their local Statute (or professional association) to determine what applies in their state or territory. Massage therapists in Australia and New Zealand (refer to Box 6.2) are not required by law to be registered to practice. New Zealand and all states and territories in Australia have massage associations that provide guidelines for practice. These guidelines are often known as a 'code of practice' (refer to Box 6.3).

> **Box 6.1** Health professionals with registration status in Australia
>
> - acupuncturists (Vic only) • chiropractors • dentists • dental technicians • Chinese herbal dispensers (Vic only) • medical practitioners • nurses • opticians • occupational therapists • optometrists • osteopaths • pharmacists • physiotherapists • podiatrists • psychologists • radiographers • dieticians • speech pathologists • traditional Chinese medicine practitioners (Vic only)
>
> (adapted from Breen, Plueckhahn and Cordner (1997), p. 147 and Forrester and Griffiths (2001) p. 304)

> **Box 6.2** Legislative requirements in New Zealand
>
> Qualified massage therapists in New Zealand may become members of one of two major professional massage associations. These major professional bodies are the Massage Institute of New Zealand Inc (MINZI) (www.minzi.org.nz) and the Therapeutic Massage Association (TMA) (www.tmanz.org.nz). Like any other professional association both of these bodies have established constitutions, a code of ethics for members and fair and equitable grievance procedures.
>
> There are numerous pieces of legislation that impact upon the practice of massage in New Zealand. These include (but are not limited to) the following:
>
> - *Massage Parlours Act 1978;*
> - *The Physiotherapy Act 1949;*
> - *Privacy Act 1993;*
> - *Medical Practitioners Act 1995;*
> - *The Health and Disability Commissioner Act 1994;*
> - *Health and Safety Employment Act 1992;* and
> - *Consumer Guarantees Act 1993.*
>
> In addition to these Acts of Parliament, The Health Practitioners Competence Assurance Bill, before Parliament in 2003, was proposed to protect the health and safety of the public by establishing mechanisms by which assurance could be given to the public that health practitioners were fit and competent to practice as health professionals. It is advised that anyone wanting to practice as a massage therapist research how such Acts impact upon the massage industry.

> **Box 6.3** Associations for massage therapists and their codes of practice
>
> Codes of practice vary amongst associations and between states and territories. The code of practice of the Australian Traditional Medicine Society (ATMS) (2001) highlights a therapist's:
>
> - duty of care;
> - professional conduct;
> - confidentiality of patient information;
> - management of patient records;
> - guidelines for advertising;
> - code of ethics; and
> - disciplinary action in cases of breaches of the code.

Guidelines for scope of practice

The Australian National Training Authority (ANTA) that oversees vocational education in Australia sets guidelines for registered training organisations that offer massage courses within the endorsed health training package for complementary and alternative health care (2000). The package outlines, amongst other things, the knowledge and skills as well as the legislative responsibilities necessary to work legally, safely and effectively as a massage therapist. The guidelines include knowledge about:

- the codes of practice of relevant national, state and territory associations;
- relevant national, state, territory and local government regulations and guidelines;
- workplace health and safety;
- duty of care;
- informed consent;
- legal aspects of documentation;
- ethical professional care considering clients' cultural, social and religious needs;
- principles of confidentiality;
- professional boundaries;
- methods of therapy including effleurage, pétrissage, passive joint movement and neuromuscular techniques;

- other techniques in which the massage therapist is trained;
- referral to other complementary therapy and allopathic professionals; and
- contraindications for massage therapy.

This list does not include all of ANTA's guidelines, but it shows how massage courses provide the knowledge required for therapists to work responsibly within their scope of practice. A similar body exists in New Zealand (see Box 6.4).

> **Box 6.4** New Zealand
>
> A regulatory body that is similar to ANTA in New Zealand is the New Zealand Qualifications Authority (NZQA). The NZQA oversees the accreditation of tertiary education awards. In 2002, through consultation with the massage industry, the NZQA registered two national qualifications for massage therapists — the National Certificate in Massage (Relaxation Massage) (Level 4) and the National Diploma in Massage (Therapeutic Massage) (Level 6). Registered training organisations may register to deliver these nationally recognised awards, or provide training in their own accredited programs.

Limits for the scope of practice

Under the law, the scope of practice of a massage therapist is determined by statutory limitations, yet within the profession the level of education obtained and the recognition provided by a professional association also determines the scope of practice. It is important for therapists to keep abreast of any new state or territory legislation regarding regulation for massage therapists and their scope of practice. Also important is the need to keep up with changes in legislation relevant to other health professionals (i.e. medical practitioners, physiotherapists, osteopaths and chiropractors). The legislative scope of practice of these health professions can impact on the scope of practice of massage therapists. It is the responsibility of the therapist to ensure the client is made aware of the scope of practice and types of services offered by the therapist and to refer the client as necessary to other health care providers.

According to Weir (2000), depending on local statutes and regulations the effect of the scope of practice of registered health professionals may exclude massage therapists from:

- diagnosis of illness or injury;
- prescribing or advising the use of medications, vitamins, minerals or herbs;
- spinal or joint manipulations;
- treatment or cure of a wide variety of illnesses; and
- counselling clients.

A massage therapist should ensure their clients understand their scope of practice and what professional service they offer. In some cases, the expertise of a number of health care professionals, in a multidisciplinary approach, may be required to provide the best quality holistic care for the client. The multidisciplinary team may consist of the naturopath, osteopath, physiotherapist, counsellor, medical practitioner and others. In the multidisciplinary environment it is important to be able to communicate effectively with other professionals with whom the therapist works or to whom the therapist refers clients. The massage therapist needs to be familiar with medical terminology to be able to communicate professionally about client care. This is part of the reason why the therapist will find that reputable training institutions also teach Western health science as part of the underpinning knowledge that supports particular massage techniques and practices. In addition to the massage therapist's professional boundaries, their ethical boundaries are also important in their scope of practice.

ETHICS

Ethics — the moral principles by which our actions are guided.

For a massage therapist ethics will guide the making of right and wrong decisions within their professional life. Therapists are in a unique position to provide care and give advice to clients, the client's family, other health professionals and the general public. A therapist has ethical obligations to these people and is accountable for them, and will need to make ethically sensitive decisions that are acceptable to all concerned (van Hooft et al., 1997). The ethical principles of autonomy (the obligation to respect the decision making capacities of individuals), beneficence (doing good), non-maleficence (refraining from doing harm) and justice (the obligation of fairness in the distribution of benefits and risks) when applied correctly will guide a therapist in making decisions for clients (Mathes, 2000; Wiley, 1994).

Autonomy

Autonomy — the personal freedom to make moral decisions and act upon them.

The everyday meaning of 'autonomy' is that a person has the right to make his or her own decisions and to act independently. As applied to clinical practice this means that a therapist should respect their client's entitlement to make their own decisions about their health care. Autonomy implies that clients have a right to decide on the type of treatment they receive, and have a right to consent to or refuse treatment (Hawley, 1997).

In multicultural societies like Australia and New Zealand, it is especially important for the massage therapist to consider therapy from the client's unique cultural perspective (see Chapter 7). A client's personal values and beliefs will influence the decisions they make in regard to the type of therapy and massage they wish to receive. Cultural values will influence approaches to many aspects of health care, spirituality or sex roles (Lee, 1999). Similarly the therapist will have his or her own beliefs, expectations, and personal feelings dependent on cultural background, education and life experience (Geldard, 1993). As Parsons (1990, p. 130) states:

> Some health professionals feel discomfort at what they regard as an uncaring attitude, or an excessive emotional display, without realising it is simply their own cultural expectations that generate the discomfort.

Remember both the client and the massage therapist will bring their worlds into the clinical practice. The therapist must respect a client's autonomy by respecting their decisions and encouraging them to make their own decisions.

Beneficence

Beneficence — a good or charitable act aimed at proving a beneficial outcome.

The ethical principle of beneficence implies that the therapy provided is aimed at what is appropriate for the wellbeing of the client; the delivery of therapy or interventions that have a beneficial outcome (Hawley, 1997). The massage therapist has an ethical obligation to do everything within his or her scope of practice and professional ability to enhance a client's health and wellbeing.

Non-maleficence

Non-maleficence — to do no harm.

The ethical principle of non-maleficence means, above all, do no harm. Non-maleficence not only involves a duty of care to avoid actual harm to a client but also to avoid the risk of harm (Hawley, 1997). Therefore, the massage therapist shall not knowingly perform any therapy that could adversely affect the health of a client. In addition to physical harm, non-maleficence applies to financial exploitation and emotional harm (Weir, 2000).

Justice

Justice — the fair and reasonable manner in which people are treated or decisions regarding them are made.

Justice refers to society's expectations of what is fair and right in the clinical setting. It would suggest the need to provide the appropriate massage therapy for all clients, regardless of socio-economic status, race, sex or religion (Hawley, 1997). It is not possible to provide equal health care to all clients, but it is possible to view massage as a service that everyone in the community should have equal access to, in accordance with their needs. For example, 'massage therapists should avoid making professional decisions based on discriminatory grounds, or for personal reasons of convenience or financial advantage' (Weir, 2000, p. 14).

LAW

In Australia and New Zealand there are two sources of the law. The first is legislation and the second is common (or case) law (Chisholm and Nettheim, 1992). According to Forrester and Griffiths (2001) 'common law is the accumulated body of law made by judges as a result of decisions in cases that come before the courts' (p. 7). As such, common law results from rules of law created by the courts rather than by legislation enacted by parliament (Chisholm and Nettheim, 1992). Law is divided into either criminal law or civil law.

Criminal versus civil law

Criminal law provides the rules of behaviour that govern our community. Criminal law deals with criminal sanctions for taking another person's property, assault or breaches of the road traffic regulations. Criminal law prosecution is initiated by the state or territory, in the form of the police or the public prosecutor, against a private citizen or other entity such as a company. The prosecution needs to prove that the accused is guilty beyond reasonable doubt (Staunton and Chiarella, 2003).

Civil law on the other hand has nothing to do with the police force and punishment. It relates to those legal proceedings between private citizens or private and public bodies. An example of this would be a client bringing legal proceedings against a massage therapist. Civil law will often involve an action to recover compensation for wrongs done (Dimond, 1998; Forrester and Griffiths, 2001). Civil wrongs are categorised as 'torts' and include negligence, trespass, assault, nuisance and defamation.

It should be noted that one incident could give rise to both civil and criminal law proceedings. For example, to assault a person would be a criminal act as well as trespass to the person (Dimond, 1998).

Law of torts

Negligence is the civil wrong of greatest significance as a source of potential legal action for health professionals (Staunton and Chiarella, 2003). Clinical situations that may lead to a negligence action include a client falling on a slippery floor, a client falling off a massage table that has collapsed due to faulty manufacturing or a client receiving injury as a result of incorrect application of massage techniques. See Box 6.5 for a case study.

> **Box 6.5** Case study 1
>
> *A therapist in a remedial massage therapy practice charges $50 for an hour-long session involving massage, aromatherapy and stretching. For clients who are pensioners a charge of $35 is applied. A client who arrives in a BMW would appear more affluent, therefore is charged $80 for the same therapy.*
>
> Question — is this an ethical practice?
>
> Answer — no this practice is not ethical. It does not show ethical practice in regard to the fairness of its approach (justice) and the potential for exploitation (non-maleficence). It may also be a breach of statutory provisions about false and misleading practices (Salvo, 1999). However, state and territory laws do not require massage therapists to charge a fee for a given service or to charge every client equally — assuming the pricing is not on discriminatory grounds (i.e. race; religion). The therapist is free to offer discounts to pensioners, children or financially disadvantaged individuals.

Negligence action

Clients or (in the case of a death occurring) relatives of clients are entitled to seek financial compensation for a negligent act that has caused or will continue to cause personal injury, pain and financial loss (Forrester and Griffiths, 2001; Staunton and Chiarella, 2003). For the massage therapist to be found negligent, the plaintiff must prove four things:

1. that the therapist owed a duty of care to the client;
2. that the therapist failed to adhere to appropriate standards of care;
3. as a consequence of the therapist's breach of the appropriate standards of care, the client suffered injury;
4. that the risk of injury was reasonably foreseeable by the therapist.

If the client is unable to demonstrate that all of these conditions existed, then the negligence action will not succeed (Showers, 2000; Staunton and Chiarella, 2003). (See Box 6.6 regarding safeguarding against negligence.)

Duty of care

A duty of care is a duty that exists when one person can reasonably foresee that their actions or omissions could cause harm to another person. In other words, liability can arise as much from failure to do an act as it can from doing it and doing it incorrectly (Staunton and Chiarella, 2003). A duty of care always exists between a massage therapist

> **Box 6.6** Tips for safeguarding against negligence
>
> Maintain your competency through continuing education (CE): read journals, attend educational seminars and earn CE points normally offered through the professional association.
>
> Know your clinic's policies on adverse incidents, know your responsibilities and meet them.
>
> Learn about other health professionals who are part of your multidisciplinary team; for example, physiotherapists, occupational therapists, diabetes counsellors, breast cancer nurses and chiropractors, and utilise their services when appropriate.
>
> Know where drug, herb, vitamin and mineral references and other resources are located and keep them up to date. Purchase your own references if necessary.
>
> If you don't understand a condition, consult other appropriate health professionals. Ask for help.
>
> Treat each client as you would like to be treated — show respect for your clients, involve them in decisions, educate them and answer their questions. Clear and open communication is vital to a sound client–therapist relationship.
>
> Report to your clinic manager any problems that may endanger your client. Failure to do so may lead to negligence actions.
>
> If an incident occurs, follow your clinic's procedures for reporting, and document any incident correctly.
>
> When you document, be factual, accurate, complete and timely.
>
> Maintain a hygienic clinic, with well-maintained equipment.
>
> (adapted from Showers, 2000)

and a client. The duty commences at the point a referral is accepted or there is an agreement between the therapist and the client for provision of services. In addition, the client/therapist is not the only relationship where a duty of care exists, as the massage therapist owes a professional duty of care to the following people also:

- any person who enters the premises;
- any person to whom advice is given;
- any person to whom instruction is provided (including over the telephone, the internet or in printed form);
- any person treated;
- any persons related to a client;
- any employees.

This list is by no means exhaustive. As can clearly be seen, the massage therapist owes a duty of care to a great deal of people (Dimond, 1998; Forrester and Griffiths, 2001).

Standard of care

We have established that a duty of care exists between a massage therapist and a client and sometimes other people concerned with that client. In court, to establish what standard of care should be provided, evidence would be sought from experts. Professional massage therapists would be consulted as to what they consider should establish a standard of care in the same or similar circumstances to the case in question. These people would be respected members of the profession, such as the president of the massage association or a scholar from an academic institution. In such instances, the court would ask 'what should the ordinary reasonable massage therapist do in this situation?' (Dimond, 1998; Staunton and Chiarella, 2003).

Breach of the standard of care

Once the court has established the standards by which to evaluate the massage therapist, the prosecutor then needs to demonstrate that the therapist breached those standards (Showers, 2000). A therapist would breach a duty of care by falling below that reasonable standard of care. Examples of a breach of duty may be:

- failure to maintain all equipment to a safe standard;
- use of oil that the client was allergic to;
- failure to maintain the clinic to a safe standard, such as allowing slippery floors or loose rugs on which to trip;
- failure to act on a contraindication to treatment;

> **Box 6.7** Case study 2
>
> *Following a manual handling incident Todd was referred to a remedial massage therapist by his general practitioner. After several months of attendance, an orthopaedic surgeon has told Todd that the remedial massage was not an appropriate treatment for the injury sustained and the massage has caused additional permanent damage.*
>
> Question — can Todd claim compensation?
>
> Answer — the general practitioner that referred Todd to the inappropriate massage therapy might possibly be jointly liable for the referral for inappropriate treatment. If it could be shown that a reasonably competent massage therapist would not have provided the type of massage given and would have referred back to the doctor because of the risk of further injury (or would have applied other techniques) then liability for negligence could be found against the massage therapist. Liability would only accrue if it could be demonstrated that treatment was the cause of further injury. If Todd had suffered harm, over and above the original injury, he may claim damages for:
>
> - medical costs;
> - pain and suffering;
> - present and future economic loss; and
> - special damages; for example, items such as medication or special transportation.
>
> These damages can be quite expensive. In some cases settlements made for injuries have amounted to very substantial sums.
>
> (adapted from Dimond, 1998)

- failure to maintain the client's confidentiality; and
- failure to maintain adequate hygiene.

See Box 6.7 for a case study.

Foreseeability

There is a duty of care owed to a person if it can be reasonably foreseen that the person might be injured by negligent actions. For example, when driving a motor vehicle, the driver is responsible for driving with due care, and if they fail to observe certain rules it can be reasonably foreseen that somebody may get hurt (Staunton and Chiarella, 2003). A massage therapist may fail to ask a client about sensitivities to lubricants, which is expected of a reasonably competent practitioner. If the client subsequently develops an allergic reaction to a lubricant used and the therapist should have reasonably foreseen that an allergic reaction could occur, then the therapist may be considered liable in negligence for that omission.

CONSENT

Valid consent

Consent to massage therapy should be obtained from the client before the therapist commences massage. Valid consent consists of three elements:

1. consent is given freely and voluntarily;
2. consent given is informed; and
3. the client giving consent has the legal capacity to give such consent.

Informed consent is supported by the ethical principle of autonomy and the legal principle that people have the right to determine what shall be done to their bodies (Hawley, 1997; Staunton and Chiarella, 2003).

Consent can be given in three ways:

1. implied;
2. verbally;
3. in writing.

Implied consent occurs where a client undresses and lies on the massage table as instructed in readiness for a massage to begin, but no words of consent are spoken. The client's compliance with the request would probably imply consent to begin massage. Verbal consent occurs when the client is on the massage table in readiness for the massage to begin and the therapist asks if it is okay to begin, to which the client verbally agrees. Consent provided in writing, as occurs when a client signs a consent form prior to treatment, serves as documentary evidence of what the client has verbally given consent for.

There is no legal requirement that consent forms must exist, but a written consent form is documentary evidence that consent was given should a controversy arise over that point (Staunton and Chiarella, 2003). One should not assume that the signing of a consent form means consent cannot be a matter of controversy, as a client may not have read the consent form nor understood its terms. This may nullify the protection this document provides. Note that consent for one therapist to do a massage does not assume that another therapist may perform the massage (Forrester and Griffiths, 2001). The three elements of consent are now detailed below.

Free and voluntary consent

This is consent given by a client without any undue pressure from the massage therapist or other staff. The therapist must respect the autonomy of the client in regard to their choice of massage therapy. If it can be established that any undue persuasion or influence was brought to bear on a client to obtain consent, that consent will be invalid (Staunton and Chiarella, 2003).

Informed consent

Informed consent requires that the client have sufficient information to determine if they want to receive a particular massage or therapy (see Box 6.8). The massage therapist needs to explain the massage procedure, how long it will last, what is expected of the client, other options available, the proposed benefits, the common side effects or risks of treatment, who will provide the massage, that confidentiality is assured and the costs for the massage including any ongoing costs. Time should be provided for the client to ask questions (Fritz, 2000; Staunton and Chiarella, 2003).

> **Box 6.8 Providing information for informed consent**
>
> - Discuss the massage procedure.
> - Discuss the proposed benefits.
> - Discuss the common side effects or risks.
> - Discuss that confidentiality is assured.
> - Discuss who will provide the massage, their expertise and qualifications.
> - Discuss the time involved.
> - Discuss the costs involved.
> - Discuss other options available for treatment if necessary.
> - Answer all questions asked by the client.
> - Draw diagrams and give written information where appropriate.
>
> (adapted from Staunton and Whyburn, 2003)

Legal capacity to give consent

Legally, any person 18 years and over can give and withhold consent to massage therapy. The client must also have the cognitive capacity to understand the nature and consequences of the proposed therapy. Generally though, a child over the age of 16 years is usually considered capable of giving valid consent. It is possible but problematic to obtain consent from a child under 16 years, as age cut-off points vary between states and territories in Australia. In New Zealand a child is a person under 16 years of age, or less than 20 years of age in cases of diminished capacity to provide consent to undergo treatment (Geer, 2000). Accordingly, caution suggests the need to obtain consent from the parent or guardian of a child under 16 years (Breen et al., 1997; Staunton and Chiarella, 2003).

An adult with an intellectual disability who is able to comprehend the nature and consequences of the massage therapy is legally able to give consent. Where the individual is unable to comprehend the nature and consequences of massage therapy, consent will need to be obtained from the parent or legal guardian on behalf of that person. It is necessary for a client to give a valid consent (that includes all the principles discussed) to treatment otherwise a civil action in assault may arise (Staunton and Chiarella, 2003). It is advisable for any health professional to consult with the relevant legislation in their state or territory.

Remember litigation concerning informed consent should never occur because failure to obtain consent before an examination and massage is professional negligence and constitutes substandard care. Clearly gaining a valid consent is essential before the therapist commences massage.

CONCLUSION

As part of their routine practice a massage therapist makes countless decisions regarding client care every day. Such decisions are informed by the therapist's knowledge and understanding of the various legal requirements and ethical principles that affect the way in which they practice. With an understanding of their legal and ethical responsibilities, a therapist may adhere to simple procedures and safeguards to avoid common legal and ethical pitfalls.

An understanding of a therapist's scope of practice, ethics and law will assist in guiding the therapist through the legal aspects of a massage practice. Therapists should be aware of their scope of practice, including professional regulation for massage therapists, limits of practice and referral of clients to other members of the health care team. Consideration of the ethical principles will also assist in guiding a therapist throughout their professional life.

Ongoing professional education, competent skills and sound procedures should prevent any client suffering or experiencing loss. Should it occur, a demonstrable adherence to proper lawful requirements is essential to prevent a potential negligence action. All health care professionals should have a thorough understanding of the law and regulations, and be sure to obtain consent before any treatment. Before establishing a massage practice it is essential to obtain legal advice so as to provide lawful and ethically principled health care.

Questions and activities

1. Describe the scope of practice of a massage therapist, taking into consideration specific state and territory legislation and professional association guidelines.
2. Define non-maleficence and describe how it relates to duty of care as a massage therapist.
3. Describe how a negligence action might arise from a massage practice.
4. Discuss how the ethical principle of 'autonomy' relates to a therapist's personal decisions in regard to how they communicate with a client. Think about your personal values and beliefs and how they will influence you.
5. A person who is 15 years old makes an appointment for a massage. Discuss the responsibilities of the therapist with regard to consent for massage, taking into consideration any state or territory legislation.

Recommended reading

Breen, K., Plueckhahn, V. and Cordner, S. (1997) *Ethics, Law and Medical Practice*. Allen & Unwin, St Leonards, NSW.

Dimond, B. (1998) *The Legal Aspects of Complementary Therapy Practice: A Guide for Health Care Professionals*. Churchill Livingstone, London.

Forrester, K. and Griffiths, D. (2001) *Essentials of Law for Health Professionals*. Harcourt, Sydney.

Weir, M. (2000) *Complementary Medicine: Ethics and Law*. Prometheus, Brisbane.

REFERENCES

Anderson, K., Anderson, L. and Glanze, W. (eds) (1998) *Mosby's Medical, Nursing and Allied Health Dictionary* (5th edn). Mosby, St Louis.

Australian National Training Authority (2002) *Health Training Package for Complementary & Alternative Health Care*. Australian National Training Authority, Brisbane.

Australian Traditional Medicine Society (2001) *Code of Practice*. Australian Traditional Medicine Society (ATMS), NSW.

Breen, K., Plueckhahn, V. and Cordner, S. (1997) *Ethics, Law and Medical Practice*. Allen & Unwin, St Leonards, NSW.

Chisholm, R. and Nettheim, G. (1992) *Understanding Law* (4th edn). Butterworths, Sydney.

Dimond, B. (1998) *The Legal Aspects of Complementary Therapy Practice: A Guide for Health Care Professionals.* Churchill Livingstone, London.

Forrester, K. and Griffiths, D. (2001) *Essentials of Law for Health Professionals.* Harcourt, Sydney.

Fritz, S. (2000) *Mosby's Fundamentals of Therapeutic Massage.* Mosby, St Louis.

Geer, B. (2000) 'Legal Implications in nursing Practice', New Zealand Supplement, Chapter 21 in Potter, P. and Perry, A. *Fundamentals of Nursing*, J. Crisp and C. Taylor (eds), Mosby, Sydney.

Geldard, D. (1993) *Basic Personal Counselling* (2nd edn). Prentice Hall, Australia.

Hawley, G. (1997) 'Ethical issues, principles and theories', Chapter 2 in *Ethics Workbook for Nurses*, G. Hawley (ed.), Social Science Press, Sydney, pp. 24–38.

Lee, W. (1999) *An Introduction to Multicultural Counselling.* Taylor & Francis, USA.

Mathes, M. (2000) 'Ethical Challenges and Nursing', *MedSurg nursing*, 9(1), p. 44.

Parsons, C. (1990) 'Cross-cultural issues in health care', in *The Health of Immigrant Australia: A Social Perspective*, J. Reid and P. Trompf (eds), Harcourt Brace, Sydney, pp. 108–53.

Salvo, S. (1999) *Massage Therapy: Principles and Practice.* W. B. Saunders, Philadelphia.

Showers, J. (2000) 'What you need to know about negligence lawsuits', *Nursing*, 30(2), pp. 45–50.

Staunton, P. and Chiarella, M. (2003) *Nursing and the Law* (5th edn). Churchill Livingstone, NSW.

van Hooft, S. Gillam, L. and Byrnes, M. (1997) *Facts and Values, An Introduction to Critical Thinking for Nurses.* MacLennan & Petty, Sydney.

Weir, M. (2000) *Complementary Medicine: Ethics and Law.* Prometheus, Brisbane.

Wiley, E. (1994) 'Principles of health care ethics', BMJ, 308, pp. 988–9.

chapter 7

Understanding boundaries

Sonya Bailey and David Stelfox

Learning outcomes

- Identify physical and emotional boundaries that relate to massage practice
- Establish and maintain professional boundaries with clients
- Deal effectively and respectfully with people of differing cultures
- Describe the importance of professionalism in providing a safe environment
- Demonstrate sensitivity and respect for a client's physical and emotional boundaries

INTRODUCTION

Society is regulated not just by laws but also by a general adherence to more voluntary codes or standards of behaviour. People draw from their culture, their life experiences and their upbringing, to determine what they think is acceptable behaviour — and beyond the boundary of that lies behaviour that they personally find puzzling, distressing or offensive.

Although there may be general societal norms regarding 'being polite', due to the personal nature of the boundaries people set, there is plenty of scope for misinterpretation of anyone else's actions. For example, while one person on a train might think it polite to mind their own business, the passenger in the seat next to them might feel rudely ignored if attempts at conversation are not reciprocated.

In fact people are often not aware that a boundary exists until it has been challenged or trespassed. An interaction may occur after which emotions flare and the mood changes. Sometimes a person's reaction can be as subtle as coughing to clear their throats in response to a somewhat personal question. Alternatively, the person may perceive the question as a more serious violation and respond by becoming defensive, confused or even aggressive. Box 7.1 defines boundaries.

> **Box 7.1** Defining boundaries
>
> In general terms, a boundary may be defined as a line, or a set of parameters, which indicates the limits of an area or territory. Boundaries can be personal or professional.
>
> Personal boundaries are self-created limits for the purpose of establishing and maintaining a healthy sense of separateness from others. These boundaries offer protection, recognition and a sound sense of self.
>
> Professional boundaries are limits established for the purpose of promoting and maintaining integrity in professional relationships. A professional therapeutic relationship is where there is a balance between safety and objectivity, and between care and distance (Salvo, 1999).

An awareness of the boundaries of others is vital for all health care therapists. It is particularly relevant in massage therapy, which necessitates the therapist invading the client's 'personal space' or transgressing what is normally perceived as 'intimate distance'. In this regard, Northouse and Northouse write (1998, p. 144):

> *Due to the types of interventions and activities carried out in health care settings, clinicians often need to enter the patient's intimate distance zone ... Some people will accept and appreciate clinicians' willingness to provide needed care within these close distances. However, those situations in which the clinician enters the intimate distance zone by accident or with little attentiveness to the patient may produce discomfort.*

Massage may bring to the surface very personal emotions and feelings for either the client or the therapist, which are outside the client–therapist relationship. Given the characteristically unconscious or unarticulated nature of boundaries and their fickle, often unpredictable and fluctuating state, it is easy to see how confusion and misunderstanding can occur.

> **Box 7.2** Activity 1
>
> Consider the different types of relationships you have with people: friends, acquaintances, work associates, family. How does your interaction with them differ? Observe the type and style of conversation — is it feeling-based or thought-based? Does your body language alter depending on the type of relationship you have with a person? Check the distance between you and the person you are interacting with: public distance is usually defined as 3.6 to 7.6 metres (lecture, public presentation); social distance is usually 1.2 to 3.6 metres (casual or workplace settings); personal distance is defined as 0.45 to 0.75 metres (conversations with close friends); 0.45 metres or less defines what is known as intimate distance (reserved for very close friends, partners, lovers, children).

As a health professional, it is up to the massage therapist to create clear, healthy boundaries with their clients. In fact it is their professional duty. Well-located boundaries provide a safe, supportive and sustainable environment for therapist and client alike. Because of the fluid and individualistic nature of the participants' boundaries, the therapeutic relationship is dynamic. As such it requires constant reassessment and attentiveness on the part of the therapist (Taylor and Ziegler, 1999).

PERSONAL AND PROFESSIONAL BOUNDARIES

Boundaries can be divided into two broad categories, professional and personal. Professional boundaries are dictated by the relevant professional associations, which dictate guidelines for scope of practice, code of conduct, ethical responsibilities and standards of practice. Personal boundaries relate more to the experience of living, a person's identity and perception of the world and themselves. They are determined by beliefs, prejudices, personal experiences, family upbringing, culture and customs.

Personal boundaries tend to be subjective in nature. For the purpose of this chapter the term *subjective* refers to an individual's personal, emotional experiences — 'belonging to the individual consciousness or perception'. Objective on the other hand is 'dealing with outward things or exhibiting facts uncoloured by feelings or opinions' (*The Australian Concise Oxford Dictionary*, 1995). For example, an objective assessment of a client may refer to their age, sex and medical history, whereas a subjective assessment may engender feelings. A therapist may feel uncomfortable about massaging a client because they remind the therapist of a former associate or partner.

> **Box 7.3 Activity 2**
>
> Take a separate piece of paper and quickly write down the personality traits and mannerisms you like in people, and those that you don't like. Try to avoid rational thought or political correctness; write down whatever occurs to you spontaneously. Your responses to this exercise can serve to illustrate how personal perceptions and prejudices (that is, subjective experiences) can determine your personal boundaries, and therefore the parameters of your client–therapist relationships.

Understanding his or her own personal boundaries may help the therapist to define the parameters of their client–therapist relationship so that they can confidently give a massage to a stranger without feeling threatened, uncomfortable or unsafe. It may also assist in developing appreciation and empathy for the client's boundaries, allowing the therapist to be sensitive to the client's vulnerabilities, fears and insecurities. By observing their responses to other people, the therapist's own boundaries may become clearer. If someone speaks to a therapist in a harsh tone, how do they respond? Responses may vary from aggression, assertiveness, fear or confusion. The therapist may even remain neutral — that is, not experience any emotional response. How the therapist responds will be dependant on a number of variables — such as the therapist's physical and personal wellbeing, mood and time of day — as well as the parameters of the therapist's own personal boundaries.

SELF-DISCLOSURE

In order to gain as much information as possible about a client before formulating an understanding of their condition of health and determining a treatment plan, it is important to encourage them to openly and honestly disclose details of their current situation pertaining to their health. Self-disclosure may be defined as the act of verbally or non-verbally communicating to others some degree of personal information.

This can be an issue from both the client's perspective and the therapist's perspective. As a therapist, it is important to be objective in choosing the questions to ask a client. It is a good idea for the therapist to always ask themself, 'Is this question of therapeutic significance or am I just being curious?' In this regard it is important to be familiar with the *Privacy Act 1988* and *The Privacy Amendment (Private Sector) Act 2000* and the conditions contained therein. One way of assisting the client to feel at ease with a line of questioning is to provide them with an explanation of how the information sought may contribute to a better treatment outcome. It is important to assure the client that the questioning is relevant to the consultation.

The client will possibly feel obliged to answer regardless of whether or not they are comfortable with the degree of disclosure. Some clients may ask personal questions of the therapist and even place the therapist in a difficult position ethically. It is best for the therapist to stay honest with the client if this occurs and tell them that they are not comfortable with the direction of the conversation. By doing this in a positive and friendly manner the therapist will allow the client to do the same if they are not comfortable with any aspect of the therapist's case-taking practices.

> **Box 7.4 Activity 3**
>
> What topics of conversation would you not be comfortable to talk to a client about? The answer to this question may help you empathise with your client. If you are not comfortable, consider whether your question may result in the same response for your client.

RIGHT TO REFUSE

Both the client and the therapist have the right to refuse the treatment (that is, receiving and giving). If the therapist finds that they are unable to express positive regard for a prospective client because of their personal boundaries or because they do not feel that the client can respect their professional boundaries, then they have the right to refuse service. However the therapist should be able to justify their decision to the client. If the therapist explains to the client their right, as a client, to refuse any or all aspects of the treatment at any time, then the client's sense of empowerment and safety can be enhanced and the therapist–client relationship can flourish (Fritz, 2000).

DUAL ROLES

Dual roles can occur where the therapist has more than one type of relationship with their client. In each relationship there is likely to be a different set of expectations and responses. The most common dual roles/relationships that can occur involve:

- family;
- social;
- friendship;
- dating;
- sexual;
- employee/employer; and
- client/therapist.

Stepping into the role of therapist with a friend, partner, parent, co-worker or sibling can be a challenging transition. The main issue arising in dual relationships revolves around shifts in which one player holds the greater power or knowledge according to their role at the time. When a power differential exists (that is, one person holds more power or knowledge than the other), there are two considerations: firstly, how will the person in power use the power advantage that they have at this time and, secondly, how will the person in a situation of less power respond to the situation?

When dealing with dual role situations as a therapist, the therapist must always remember that the power advantage they hold in that role must never be abused regardless of whether the client is a stranger, friend, family member, employer or acquaintance. One of the therapist's primary roles is to support and nurture the client. Intimate sexual relationships between therapist and client should be avoided. Most professional codes of ethics prohibit such relationships and, should one develop between the therapist and the client, it is wise to terminate the professional relationship without hesitation.

In dual role situations it is important to establish clear professional boundaries such as the duration of the consultation, the fee for service (see Box 7.5) and the treatment plan. Such clear professional boundaries will assist in avoiding any misunderstandings or unclear expectations regarding the service.

PHYSICAL BOUNDARIES

In a professional environment the physical space between people is generally arm's length. In fact this would generally hold true of any non-intimate relationship, as people need a certain amount of physical space between themselves and the next person. In elevators people are not able to get this physical space so they tend to compensate by avoiding eye contact and focusing their attention on the door. Although this response may be quite unconscious, its purpose is to reduce the intimacy of the experience.

A massage therapist will be asking their clients to undress, and the therapist will be touching their skin, palpating their muscles and providing a certain degree of nurturing and soothing that is generally only provided or exchanged by intimates (Taylor and Ziegler, 1999). In order for this not to be a boundary violation for either the therapist or the client, certain protocols can be put in place to help draw the experience into the professional realm. Such protocols include:

- creating a treatment plan with the client so that the purpose and sequence of events are well mapped before treatment begins;
- providing the client with every opportunity to speak up if there is something they are not comfortable with;
- providing the client with very clear instructions about what clothing they need to remove and what they may leave on, as confusion about the degree of undress can be very disconcerting for the client;
- leaving the room when the client undresses and instructing them to cover themselves with draping that has been provided;
- draping body parts that are not being massaged (see Chapter 15); and
- avoiding massaging or touching erogenous zones (these are parts of the body that are particularly sensitive to sexual stimulation and include the genitals, anus and breasts).

> **Box 7.5** Pricing in dual role situations
>
> When considering discount pricing policies or 'mates rates' it is important to take into account the following:
> - Does this pricing structure support your value and skill-base as a professional therapist?
> - What is an equitable exchange for your time and energy?
> - Is the discount sustainable with respect to your ability to make a living?

INTIMACY

The word intimate comes from the Latin *intimus*, meaning inmost (*The Australian Concise Oxford Dictionary*, 1995). What that actually means to an individual appears to range between a sense of closeness and unity with all things, including inanimate objects and plants, to hosting an intimate dinner for a select few, or to having sexual relations with someone. Intimacy appears to move across planes from spiritual to social to sexual but what is consistent is the element of connection with an 'other'.

> **Box 7.6** Activity 4
>
> Consider the forms or ways that intimacy manifests in your life. Who do you feel close to and why?

EMOTIONAL BOUNDARIES

Emotional boundaries are fluid and can change with each client and from session to session with the same client. The degree of intimacy is usually an unspoken contract between two people. There are some obvious limits within the professional relationship, in that sexual intimacy is not an option, yet the degree of connection the therapist has with the client is reflective of the boundaries of both client and therapist.

So what happens when that contract cannot be agreed upon? Much of how people interact or respond with other people can occur on an unconscious level. For example, the therapist may remind their client of their daughter and interact with them on that level. The therapist may become a party to this contract without realising it and take on the role of daughter unknowingly. What is occurring here is that the client is projecting a personal relationship onto the therapist (transference) and the therapist is responding to that projection (counter-transference). The therapist needs an objective basis upon which to relate to the client to avoid responding to the transference of the client. That objectivity may come in the form of reassessing the goals of the session; the therapist checking in with his or her self and asking the question 'Is this conversation or behaviour in the best interest of the client for the purpose of achieving the desired therapeutic outcome?' In this way the therapist can step outside of the immediate relationship and redirect it to a healthier arena (Salvo, 1999).

SEXUAL BOUNDARIES

A boundary issue that arises frequently for the practising massage therapist as well as their clients is the issue of sexuality. Massage may be a very intimate and personal experience so it is not surprising that it may evoke sexual feelings or responses. This becomes a problem if either party feels unsafe, uncomfortable or violated in some way. Confusion can also arise when massage therapists advertise their services as some people still associate massage with the sex industry (Howard, 1999). The term *massage therapist* is used throughout this book in preference to the term 'masseur' since it conveys the fact that the practitioner is indeed a therapist, and it is less likely to convey connotations of a sexual nature. All graduates of massage training courses are encouraged to use this term when referring to their profession and when advertising and promoting the services they offer.

Confusion relating to sexual boundaries may arise in massage therapy for three main reasons. The first reason is that massage may be, for some, a very intimate and physical experience; two attributes that are usually present in sexual relations. For the client this may be mistaken for or translated as a sexual experience. This connection tends to be more evident in today's culture, where there are limited outlets for touch and intimacy outside of sexual relations (Jordan, 2000).

The second reason relates to the associations attached to the word 'massage'. 'Massage' has sometimes been used as a cover for the illegal sex industry and although it has diminished considerably since the legalisation of prostitution, the association is sometimes still apparent. This confusion is constantly being reduced by such factors as increased public awareness and education about therapeutic massage, state legislation regarding use of the term 'massage' in advertising, greater acceptance and referrals by the medical profession, and increased scientific validation of the benefits of massage (Howard, 1999).

The third reason is the parasympathetic nervous system's response to massage. As Polseno (2000) explains, this response occurs when mind and body are quietened and all of a person's fears, pressures, stresses and 'shoulds' are put to one side; a more fundamental or essential nature emerges and the experience of massage may in fact awaken sexual feeling. The peripheral nervous system can be categorised into sympathetic and parasympathetic.

> **Box 7.7** Activity 5
>
> A client is having problems in their relationship with their teenage son and asks for your advice. What role are they projecting onto you? How do you respond?

> **Box 7.8** Suggestions for promoting clear sexual boundaries
>
> - Assume a professional phone manner. Provide a clear description of the service you provide as a massage therapist.
> - Dress professionally. Consider the image you wish to project to your client with respect to dress.
> - Ensure your workplace is professional in its appearance and function.
> - Clearly explain the procedure you wish to implement in delivering the treatment, including which parts of the body you intend to massage. Gain the client's consent before proceeding.
> - Give clear instructions to the client about what clothing, if any, needs to be removed prior to treatment.
> - Drape the client appropriately. Only undrape that specific part of the body you are currently working on.
> - Make your touch deliberate and purposeful.
> - Some parts of the body are more sexually charged than others, so if one part elicits a sexual response, attend to another part of the body.
> - By explaining the parasympathetic response to male clients it may prevent embarrassment, or concerns they have about becoming aroused during a massage.
>
> (Association of Massage Therapists Australia, 2001)

The sympathetic nervous system is often referred to as the 'flight/fight' response, which is a high-stress state that suppresses non-essential functions of the body — one of those functions being sex drive. The parasympathetic system 're-normalises' the body and returns homeostasis or balance. Massage encourages the relaxation response and sometimes that includes the reawakening of sexual desire. It is the process of massage as opposed to the massage therapist that may kindle this reawakening (Polseno, 2000). See Box 7.8 for suggestions for promoting clear sexual boundaries.

CULTURAL CONSIDERATIONS

Massage therapy is practised in many forms throughout the world, each with its own style, customs and techniques. Australia as a multicultural nation offers the massage therapist the potential to work with clients from a variety of cultural backgrounds, with each bringing an experience and expectation of massage that may differ from the therapists. It is important to be aware of cultural differences and to adapt the treatment accordingly.

Probably the most obvious issue relating to the cultural background of a client in a massage setting may be a concern of body boundaries. People of some ethnic groups and associated religious beliefs (e.g. Islam, Hindu) may have different perceptions of their physical body. To some the body may be considered sacred. To others it may be held as very private, something that cannot be revealed readily to others. In addition, beliefs about the shape and size of the body can differ significantly from one culture to another.

Disrobing for a massage, then, may be cause for concern to both female and male clients. It may seem logical that unless a person feels comfortable with disrobing then they are unlikely to make an appointment for a massage in the first place, though this is not necessarily the case. Massage is an acceptable and most desirable approach to the treatment of many health conditions in some cultures. Furthermore, a client may be of the belief that the massage can be delivered without the need for removal of clothing.

People from countries where civil unrest and political violence have occurred (for example, Central and South American countries) may have been victims of brutality and torture. They may still carry the physical and emotional scars of these experiences with them. Such clients should be dealt with sensitively. While it is natural for the therapist to express strong concern at the sight of disfigurements such as scarring and malformations due to fractures, it must be realised that the client is usually self-conscious of them, and too much attention may lead to further distress. The massage therapist should also be aware that body mutilations or alterations, such as scarification, body piercing or tattooing, are culturally sanctioned in many ethnic groups. In such cases the therapist need not show concern and, in fact, should be careful not to express shock or surprise in the client's presence.

A complexity of emotions and troubled thoughts may exist below the surface and massage therapy can beneficially unlock and release these. However, the massage therapist must work with sensitivity, developing the client's faith and trust so that they feel comfortable to release the physical and emotional tension that the body has held within it. It is possible that in some cases this may result in the need for referral to a qualified counsellor, psychotherapist or psychologist. Competence in counselling is generally outside the scope of practice of a massage therapist so the benefit of referral for counselling needs to be considered.

Disrobing and draping are dealt with in Chapter 15 and the guidelines provided there apply for every client. A key consideration is the gaining of informed consent from the client before beginning any massage or physical assessment. This must include the provision of information to the client about the need to disrobe, clarification of what is required where necessary, and non-pressured consent from the client (see Chapter 6). Where language may be a problem for a client of a different cultural background it may be necessary to have someone present who is able to translate.

Menstruation may have certain cultural beliefs associated with it and a woman may not feel comfortable receiving a massage treatment at such time. (Regardless of cultural beliefs, any female may feel uncomfortable with the prospect of massage during menstruation.) It should also be realised that the sex of the client, and the therapist, may prove an issue for consideration. People of many ethnic groups (e.g. people of Islamic faith, orthodox Jews, and even people of Anglo-Saxon culture) have preference for a therapist of the same sex as themselves. This should be acknowledged and respected.

Different areas of the body can have cultural beliefs associated with them. As such some individuals may not feel comfortable having those parts massaged or even touched. For example, in some cultures a person's soul is believed to be attached to their head and touching, massaging or manipulating it may cause the soul to escape, eventually resulting in death or in the person going mad (Waxler-Morrison et al., 1990). Once again, if informed consent is gained for the intended areas of the body to be worked on then no issue should arise.

In some cultures, high value is placed on stoicism, especially by males (e.g. South-East Asian ethnic groups), and the client may not complain about pain — either pre-existing pain or pain that is experienced during a massage treatment. This should be taken into consideration so that the treatment plan is adjusted accordingly and the need for possible referral to another health care therapist is determined. The massage therapist should look for indications that the client may be experiencing pain or discomfort. Such indicators may be flinching, body armouring (tensing up in certain areas), facial contortions or perspiration.

People of some Middle-Eastern cultures, for example, may not respond well to the suggestion of exercise or stretching as part of their treatment. If a therapist wishes to propose such a strategy, careful and thorough explanation of the benefits of exercise to the client's health condition may help. Such an issue should never be pushed too vehemently though.

Guidelines for dealing with clients of a different cultural or ethnic background

Establish the possible influence of the client's ethnicity and culture on the proposed treatment

There are many cultural factors that contribute to an individual's perception of their health and how they feel their health condition is best treated. People from different cultures explain the causes of ill-health differently (e.g. to some it is the intrusion of an evil spirit or the result of living outside of the laws of their society or nature). Different ethnic groups have faith in different types of treatments and may turn to therapists of quite different health care approaches when confronted with illness.

This may seem strange and even inappropriate to some people in Western society. For example, Western biomedicine (its pharmaceutical drugs and surgical procedures) is perceived by many cultures (e.g. South Asian, Chinese, South American) as too strong. The Chinese and Vietnamese believe that it is too 'hot' or 'yang'. When ill, these people often turn to massage or other traditional healing approaches as an alternative to the Western biomedical approach. While this may seem fine, it is always important for the therapist to evaluate the appropriateness of massage to the treatment of the client's problem. For example, in Trinidad and other islands of the West Indies, conditions such as cancer, mental illness and even oedema of the legs are seen as the result of an evil spirit that has entered the body. Massage therapy is viewed as a legitimate means of expelling or exorcising this spirit and thereby restoring health.

As a guiding principle, always gather as much information as possible about the client, their ethnic background, their beliefs about health, illness and treatment, and their expectations of the treatment. Most of this information can be gained during the early 'ice-breaking stage' of the consultation. The therapist should be aware that it may be appropriate to recommend that the client seek the services of another health care provider whom the therapist considers may be better suited to treating their condition.

Encourage the client to ask questions and express themselves freely during the case-taking and massage treatment

People of some cultures (e.g. Chinese, Nepalese, Japanese and South-East Asian) seldom ask questions of a health therapist because they consider it impolite. Clear and open communication is the best means of avoiding dissatisfaction and achieving positive results. Encourage the client to provide input and feedback at all stages of the massage session.

Accommodate the client's perspective of their illness when determining the best treatment approach

As mentioned previously, some cultures have entirely different perceptions of health, illness and health care. These perceptions should be acknowledged, respected and accommodated. For example, people from some regions in the north of India have a cultural belief (ārdha-angani = 'half-body') where the left half of a married woman's body belongs to her husband and his family (Waxler-Morrison et al., 1990). This has obvious implications where massage or physical examination of this half of the body is considered necessary. Another consideration is that any marital problems may be seen to manifest as muscular tension, pain or paralysis to the left side of the body.

Refer where appropriate to other health therapists

People from many ethnic groups (for example, from rural India, Vietnam, Sri Lanka, Nepal) and older people from countries such as Greece, Turkey, Italy and Cyprus turn to traditional healing practices for both simple and serious health problems. These may include home remedies, folk medicine, massage or other forms of tactile therapy. Throughout South-East Asia Tiger Balm and other similar ointments and oils, which tend to be associated with the treatment of muscular aches and pains, are used internally and topically to treat a wide range of health conditions (cure-alls), including quite serious ones. A professional massage therapist must be aware of these perceptions and know when it may be necessary to encourage a client to visit a more appropriate health care provider who can best treat their health problem.

Avoid ethnic stereotyping

Usually there will be shared experiences, values and beliefs among people of a given ethnic group. However, there may also be significant intra-ethnic diversity. In Indonesia, for example, there are people of Muslim, Hindu, Christian and Buddhist faiths, so their religious beliefs can be different. In addition, social class, level of education and area of origin (urban or rural) can have a considerable influence and contribute to major differences within ethnic groups. Massage therapists should not make any assumptions. Just because someone from a particular ethnic group dresses in Western clothes and speaks perfect English doesn't mean that they

---

Box 7.9 Questions for determining the influence of culture on treatment of clients

- Place of birth — city or rural?
- Length of time in Australia and did you have any family living here before immigrating (this may determine the degree of familiarity they have of their new cultural setting)?
- Occupation in country of origin?
- Occupation in Australia?
- Describe the nature of your health problem?
- What do you think may have caused it?
- How has it affected you (at home, at work)?
- What results do you hope the treatment will achieve?

---

don't live according to strict traditional practices and beliefs. Conversely, a woman dressed in traditional ethnic clothing may be quite casual or non-observant of the traditional cultural practices of her homeland.

Clear communication, awareness of special considerations associated with particular ethnic groups and a willingness to respect and accommodate cultural differences in clients are probably the keys to effectively dealing with clients of different cultural backgrounds to the therapist.

CONCLUSION

Boundaries are an implicit and inevitable facet of all individuals. They may be attributable to someone's cultural background or simply the result of someone's upbringing and life experiences. The quality of the therapeutic relationship is greatly dependent upon the skill and sensitivity with which boundaries are acknowledged and handled.

Sound therapist protocols in the massage setting not only help to define the professional relationship, they also remove impediments to therapeutic outcomes. Client and therapist safety requirements must also be met and treatment expectations must be mutual. These various objectives can be created and maintained by the careful monitoring and maintaining of workable boundaries between therapist and client.

Some basic tools that can be put in place for avoiding most misunderstandings are:

- solid communication skills;
- a high level of professionalism;
- awareness and adherence to the professional code of ethics;

- sensitivity to the client's boundaries; and
- the therapist's awareness of their own subjective boundaries.

Although someone's boundaries may be radically different from a massage therapist's, and therefore lead to vastly different behaviours and expectations, those boundaries are not necessarily right or wrong, good or bad. The important thing is to recognise and respect the boundaries, for with consciousness and consideration they can be positively navigated to enhance relations. With recognition and respect of such boundaries comes the solid foundation for a sound and healthy working relationship between the massage therapist and client.

Questions and activities

1. Professional and personal boundaries may become blurred when treating friends or family. Differentiate between personal and professional boundaries, and describe some strategies you may adopt to ensure these boundaries are maintained, even when providing treatment to friends or family.
2. For a professional massage therapist it is important to respect a client's physical boundaries. When in clinical practice, what strategies could you adopt to avoiding violations of a client's physical boundaries?
3. When in practice, you sense that a client may be making unwanted advances towards you. Describe how you would establish and maintain clear sexual boundaries with this client.

Recommended reading

Helman, C. G. (1997) *Culture, Health and Illness* (3rd edn). Butterworth–Heinemann, Oxford.

Northouse, L. L. and Northouse, P. G. (1998) *Health Communication: Strategies for Health Professionals*. Appleton & Lange, Stamford.

Salvo, S. (2003) *Massage Therapy: Principles and Practice* (2nd edn). W. B. Saunders, Philadelphia.

Fritz, S. (2000) *Mosby's Fundamentals of Therapeutic Massage*. Mosby, St Louis.

REFERENCES

Association of Massage Therapists Australia (AMTA) (2001) 'The issue of sexuality and massage', *AMTA Journal 2001*, 12(2), pp. 6–9.

Australian Concise Oxford Dictionary (1995). Oxford University Press, Melbourne.

Fritz, S. (2000) *Mosby's Fundamentals of Therapeutic Massage*. Mosby, St Louis.

Jordan, D. (2000) 'Sexual vs compassionate touch', *Massage Therapy Journal*, Summer.

Howard, H. (1999) 'Sexual harassment survey', *AMTA Journal*, 10(5), p. 17.

Northouse, L. L. and Northouse, P. G. (1998) *Health Communication: Strategies for Health Professionals*. Appleton & Lange, Stamford, Connecticut.

Polseno, D. (2000) 'Desexualising the massage experience', *Massage Therapy Journal*, vol. 39, pp. 136–43.

Salvo, S. (1999) *Massage Therapy: Principles and Practice*. W. B. Saunders, Philadelphia.

Taylor, K. and Ziegler, K. (1999) 'Self-examination in healing relationships', *Massage Therapy Journal*, Summer, vol. 38(2). pp. 65–74.

Waxler-Morrison, N., Anderson J. and Richardson, E. (eds) (1990) *Cross-Cultural Caring: A Handbook for Health Professionals*. UBC Press, Vancouver.

section 4

Preparation for Practice

chapter 8

The massage environment

Lisa Casanelia

Learning outcomes

- Create an atmosphere and environment that is conducive to massage
- Differentiate between the varying types of massage environments
- Describe the various forms of massage equipment and their specialised use
- Identify the benefits, necessary precautions and hygienic application of the different types of oils and lubricants used for massage

INTRODUCTION

As the public image of massage therapy has developed over recent years more and more people are turning to massage as a form of preventative health care. This broadened awareness has created greater scope for the massage therapist to provide their services in many diverse settings. For example, the massage therapist may establish a practice in their home, in a clinic with a combination of different health practitioners, in a spa, in a corporate environment, at sporting clubs or events, in shopping centres, at markets or at exhibitions. They may also choose to provide treatments at nursing homes, hospitals, in private homes or hotels so as to allow the broader community to enjoy the benefits of massage therapy.

Irrespective of locality, it is important for the therapist to provide a setting for the massage that will enhance the effects of relaxation when providing a massage treatment. Factors that a therapist would take into consideration include the temperature of the room, privacy of the client, standard of hygiene, professionalism and ethical practice, use of suitable lighting, aromas and the addition of music. Such factors are important in enhancing the sensory ambience of the massage. The type of environment the therapist chooses to work from will dictate how much control the therapist has over the massage setting. The atmosphere of the massage room and the supplies required by the massage therapist, such as massage table and linen, are determined by whether the therapist is mobile, home-based, in a clinic, or providing seated massage in a work environment. This chapter describes how to prepare a setting suitable for massage and addresses some of the varying types of massage environments that a therapist may work from.

THE MASSAGE SETTING

When providing a service, the massage therapist has a professional responsibility to provide a clean and safe environment for the client. The therapist should also ensure they maintain a high standard of personal hygiene (see Chapter 10). When in practice it is essential for the massage therapist to work within the boundaries of ethical practice at all times (see Chapter 6) and maintain adequate professional indemnity insurance, in addition to maintaining proper records (see Chapter 11) and displaying their qualifications and professional association memberships. As a professional health care provider the massage therapist has the responsibility to keep their skills current and to refer clients to other health practitioners where necessary (see Chapter 6).

When providing a massage treatment the therapist should always allow adequate time for each client, and leave time to prepare for the next client to ensure clients are not kept waiting. As with any business, a client reassured by the subtle indicators of a professionally conducted business will gain the most from the service. The care taken by the therapist to ensure the massage room is kept clean and inviting will provide important cues for the client about the assiduousness the therapist has for their work and bestow vital first impressions on the client.

When preparing a massage room for treatment, there are four factors that must be considered. These factors may be referred to as the tranquillity, aroma, ambience and comfort of the treatment room. The features of these important considerations are described below. When combined, these factors make for an ideal massage setting that is sure to induce feelings of wellness, comfort, security and relaxation in any client.

Tranquillity

The massage therapist should create a peaceful, quiet space for massage that is free from external disturbances, distractions and interruptions. The external sound of telephones, traffic din, television, radio or machinery can be most disruptive to the relaxation process and can startle clients from a relaxed state. Even a ticking clock might distract some people. Certain clients may find music intrusive in the massage setting and others will find it enhances their ability to relax. Where possible, a therapist should allow the client the preference with regard to the type of music played. Conversation should be kept to a minimum and relevant to the massage setting. A therapist who uses the massage time to tell clients about their personal life and talk incessantly through a massage can be annoying and, more importantly, professionally inappropriate. Likewise, a therapist who loses contact during the massage to answer the telephone, the door or to attend to something other than the massage will be disrupting the relaxation process by breaking the flow and continuance of the massage treatment. Disruptions to the massage as well as unexpected and obtrusive noises can interfere with the client's ability to relax during a massage. As such the therapist should attempt to minimise all such annoyances to optimise the tranquillity of the massage environment.

Aroma

The massage therapist should give consideration to the smell of a massage room. A fresh, pleasant-smelling environment that is welcoming and not overpowering will enhance the surrounding ambience. Massage rooms can tend to become stuffy with the warmth of the room and all the varying odours clients bring with them. The use of a fan to stimulate circulation of air can help disperse stale smells and minimise any odours. The subtle use of essential oils in a vaporiser, or essential oil mist sprays, can assist in enhancing the mood and freshness of a massage room. Plants can also be used to cleanse the air and increase the energy in a room. As some clients may be sensitive or even allergic to certain aromas or flowers, the therapist should always check for individual sensitivities prior to treatment. When used appropriately, however, a client may find the use of subtle aromas a welcome addition to the massage treatment.

Ambience

Visually the massage room should be pleasing to the eye; uncluttered, clean and enhanced by subtle lighting. The paintwork should look fresh and be free of greasy hand marks. As certain colours are believed to enhance relaxation, the therapist may make use of such colours on the walls or on accessories to create the right effect. Shades of blue, violet and turquoise are colours that promote feelings of calm and relaxation and as such would be well suited to a massage treatment room. Red and orange on the other hand are colours that are warm and inviting but may be too stimulating to be used in the massage setting, which aims to enhance relaxation (Gimbel, 1994). A massage therapist may enhance a room further with the use of appropriate pictures on the walls and subtle lighting. Where possible, overhead lights should be operated by a dimmer switch or alternatively the room lit with a soft bulb. The addition of a lamp that is appropriately placed to provide lighting that is soft enough to create a mood of relaxation, but bright enough for the therapist to observe the client's skin for any abnormalities, may also prove useful in enhancing the massage setting. In terms of ambience in the massage setting, a tidy and uncluttered room that is pleasing to the eye will convey the impression of an organised professional therapist who takes pride in their work, thereby instilling confidence in the client about the therapist's abilities.

Comfort

Client comfort is of utmost importance to the massage therapist. The massage room should be warm, the towels soft and the massage table comfortable. Massage is all about touch, and the application of the various massage techniques will serve to stimulate different tactile skin receptors, creating a wide range of sensations and responses for the client. Comfort on the massage table is very important in encouraging the body to relax. So, to increase the clients' level of relaxation the therapist should make use of bolsters and pillows and position them to suit the individual needs, size and shape of the client.

The linens used for the massage should be soft and clean and, where possible, warmed to really encourage the body to relax into the massage. A client who is cold on the massage table will tense their muscles, making it difficult for the massage to achieve a relaxation effect. As such the massage room should be at a temperature that is comfortable for the client. A temperature in the massage room between 22 and 25 degrees Celsius is ideal, as during the treatment the client will relax and their body temperature will decrease. In addition to this, the therapist can use blankets, hot packs, electric blankets and heated towel racks (that warm the towels) to keep the client sufficiently warm throughout the massage. Creating a comfortable environment is vital during the massage, as a client who is comfortable during the treatment will benefit most from the massage.

Factors such as the tranquillity, aroma, ambience and comfort of the treatment room are important for a successful massage treatment. A massage room that beckons the client into its tranquil space and encourages a sense of relaxation simply from entering is a blessing for a therapist. A client should begin to relax simply by breathing in the beautiful surroundings and easing themselves into the soft warm towels that drape the massage table. It is to the therapist's advantage to create such a welcoming massage setting; one that will only serve to enhance the treatment provided.

The therapist should take as much care in their own presentation as they would with the presentation of the massage room. The dress of the therapist should be conservative, neat and clean and portray a professional image to the client. A massage therapist's attire should be comfortable and allow freedom of movement. The practice of massage may be inclined to attract the wrong kind of clientele at times and the therapist's attire should not lend itself to any doubt about the services that are being provided.

Box 8.1 provides a summary of a typical sequence of the massage consultation from preparing the massage room to writing the treatment record.

DIFFERENT MASSAGE ENVIRONMENTS

Massage therapists can invent their own image and style, be self-employed or work as an employee, have one job or several, and work in one field or many. As such they have a variety of wonderful

> **Box 8.1** Putting the massage into practice
>
> - Prepare the massage room.
> - Greet the client and introduce yourself.
> - Take the client's case history.
> - Explain the massage procedures.
> - Receive consent for the treatment recommended.
> - Explain preparation of the client on the massage table.
> - Leave the room while the client prepares.
> - Wash your hands and forearms.
> - Knock before re-entering the room.
> - Adjust the client draping and pillows to ensure client comfort and warmth.
> - Commence massage as discussed and consented to.
> - Check in with the client during the massage regarding depth of pressure, client comfort and warmth.
> - If treatment changes or time is running short, renegotiate treatment plan and gain consent for any changes made before proceeding.
> - At the end of the massage, allow time for the client to rest a few moments to refocus, and assist your client off the massage table if necessary.
> - Leave the room while your client gets dressed again.
> - Wash your hands and forearms.
> - Knock before entering the room, ask how the client feels and offer a drink of water.
> - Make suggestions about how to enhance the feelings of relaxation and explain what to expect after a massage, recommend any self-care or exercises to do at home and educate the client where appropriate about the correct use of posture, exercise and the benefits of regular massage.
> - Collect payment for the massage, provide a receipt and check if the client wishes to schedule another appointment.
> - Ensure the client has all their belongings and see them to the door.
> - Write up ongoing client treatment record.
> - Prepare the room for the next client, change linens, clean equipment and refresh the room.
> - Therapist should have enough time to refresh themselves, have a snack, drink some water, and stretch in preparation for their next client.
> - Repeat the cycle.

options and these options are diversifying as massage increases in popularity. An understanding of the advantages and disadvantages associated with the various options for practice may help the therapist in deciding the option that best suits them.

Home-based massage practice

The home-based massage practice, as the name implies, is a massage practice established in the therapist's home. How the therapist decides to set this up will largely be dependent on the available space in their home. Ideally in this situation the clinic room will be separated from the rest of the house, with its own bathroom and separate entrance. A therapist setting up a professional practice could not expect clients to feel comfortable entering their private home for massage treatment if it involved walking through living spaces, meeting the family members, using the bathroom, which may be an ensuite to a bedroom, or having the massage in a room that doubles as a spare bedroom or is cluttered with things that are unrelated to massage. Such an environment would appear unprofessional to the client and perhaps a little too intimate and personal for their level of comfort.

When appropriately established, a home-based massage practice can be a lovely tranquil space for massage, separated from hectic street noises of shopping centres and activity, offering a special space; a space that the therapist has more control

> **Box 8.2** Advantages and disadvantages of a home-based practice
>
> Advantages of a home-based practice include:
> - convenience of location for the therapist;
> - cost effectiveness for the therapist;
> - can combine home-duties in between clients;
> - greater control over external and internal environment;
> - access to washing machine and clothes dryer for linens;
> - flexible working hours; and
> - part of home, thus home expenses may be tax deductible.
>
> Disadvantages of a home-based practice include:
> - clients may feel more vulnerable entering a therapist's private home;
> - clients may expect the therapist to be on call at hours beyond their specified clinic hours; and
> - therapists may feel isolated in their massage practice.

over in terms of windows and fresh air, lighting, paintwork and room fittings.

Box 8.2 provides a list of advantages and disadvantages of a home-based practice.

Mobile massage practice

The mobile massage practice is where the therapist visits the client in his or her own home or hotel. The therapist transports the massage table and accessories to the clients' premises and sets the equipment up in the space provided. In such practice, the therapist will have less control over the surroundings and should encourage the client to set aside a quiet space that is free from the distractions of telephone, family, visitors, television and the like. It is possible to ask the client to provide articles such as pillows, linens, music, hot packs or other tools that will make the load the therapist has to carry less demanding. Box 8.3 provides a list of advantages and disadvantages of mobile massage practice.

> **Box 8.3** Advantages and disadvantages of a mobile massage practice
>
> Advantages of a mobile massage practice include:
> - overheads are low (petrol costs and vehicle maintenance);
> - price of treatment is usually more expensive;
> - the environment is varied throughout the day, which may add interest to the therapist's work;
> - the client may feel more at ease in their own home; and
> - the client has greater opportunity to be relaxed before and after massage.
>
> Disadvantages of a mobile massage practice include:
> - the therapist may feel vulnerable entering an environment they are unfamiliar with;
> - the therapist has little control over the massage setting;
> - the therapist is restricted by the amount of equipment they can physically carry; and
> - the distance of travel between clients may be time consuming.

Clinic-based practice

A clinic-based practice generally refers to a practice that is set up commercially. This could include a therapist working in a beauty salon, hairdressing salon, medical practice, physiotherapy, chiropractic or osteopathic practice, personal training studio, natural therapies practice or may involve the therapist working on their own or with a combination of different therapists. The therapist could be self-employed or an employee, or perhaps even an associate with other practitioners. The clinic-based therapist would be in a setting where they have greater visibility to the general public and as such may acquire more clients from passers by than any other practice set up. The clinic may have a more professional set up of facilities, have a receptionist and may have the ability to offer clients a variety of different services, attracting a range of clientele into the clinic. Box 8.4 provides a list of advantages and disadvantages of clinic-based practice.

> **Box 8.4** Advantages and disadvantages of a clinic-based practice
>
> Advantages of a clinic-based practice include:
> - greater exposure to the general public;
> - professional image;
> - shared knowledge with other practitioners and feeling less isolated in a multidisciplinary clinic;
> - shared expenses, advertising and reception duties with other practitioners;
> - the clinic can provide more varied equipment for clients;
> - client database can be shared between therapists; and
> - a diversity of practitioners may draw a wide range of clients.
>
> Disadvantages of a clinic-based practice include:
> - higher overheads; and
> - parking may be restricted.

Work-site massage practice

With today's fast paced workplaces, many employees are becoming increasingly aware of the benefits of injury and stress reduction strategies to benefit their businesses. Having employees off work due to stress or injury places a significant financial burden on companies annually; a burden that is not necessary considering workplace stress and injuries are largely preventable. Evidence suggests that massage may positively impact upon workplace stress and aid employee productivity and wellbeing (Rich, 2002). As more and more employers are turning to massage in the workplace to assist employee health and morale, the good news is that almost any type of workplace setting has the possibility for massage to be utilised regardless of the type, size or location of the business.

The work-site massage is ideally suited to provide massage to employees in their work environment. Like the mobile massage therapist, the therapist will travel with their equipment to the work site. The massage itself can be with a massage table or, more commonly in the work environment, it will be a seated, clothed massage. The seated massage is more suited to the workplace setting as it poses fewer interruptions to the work environment. The seated massage may be applied at the client's desk or in a separate space with a specialised seated massage chair. The duration of the seated massage is generally 10 to 20 minutes and the techniques are performed through the client's clothing. Regular massage using a massage table will require a private room and more time for the massage appointments, which may not be possible in some work environments. Box 8.5 provides a list of advantages and disadvantages of work-site massage based on a clothed seated massage of short duration in the work environment.

> **Box 8.5** Advantages and disadvantages of work-site massage
>
> Advantages of work-site massage include:
> - the closed environment of a workplace means that word of your services will move fast;
> - the massage is easily accessible to anyone in the office;
> - the massage is not disruptive to the client's working day as they can stay in the office;
> - the massage through the clothing and in a seated position may mean it is less intimidating for some people who would be reluctant to have massage normally;
> - if the practitioner also has a massage practice then this will become a good source of advertising and attract new clientele; and
> - overheads will be low (petrol costs and car maintenance).
>
> Disadvantages of work-site massage include:
> - the environment may be disruptive and the massage may be interrupted by work priorities;
> - the therapist is limited by brief massage time;
> - the therapist is limited by what they can physically carry to the job;
> - the seated massage techniques are usually more taxing on the therapist's hands; and
> - travelling to the office site may be time consuming.

MASSAGE EQUIPMENT

There are a few pieces of equipment needed by a therapist to perform massage. The massage therapist must feel confident about the quality and effectiveness of their equipment and should choose carefully as they have a duty of care to provide a safe environment for their clients. A massage table that is old and rackety and groans and rattles under the weight of the client will not bestow a sense of comfort or safety and will no doubt interfere with the client's ability to relax and enjoy the massage. The quality of the therapist's equipment will impart valuable impressions regarding their professional standards and the quality of care provided to the client.

The massage table is the most important piece of equipment. Not only necessary for client comfort, the massage table also determines the ease with which the therapist can provide the massage treatment. For most therapists the massage table will be the most expensive piece of equipment they will purchase. As such, investment in a massage table requires thought and thorough research on the part of the therapist.

Massage tables can be stationary, portable, electric or in the form of a chair. The type of table the therapist chooses to buy will be dependent on how they wish to set up their clinical practice. The portable massage table will of course be the most versatile option, allowing the therapist to easily store, carry and transport their practice to different locations. The therapist can choose from a wide range of massage tables at varying degrees of quality and price. A therapist may be tempted to purchase the least expensive massage table and end up with a table that is uncomfortable, unstable and prone to breaking easily. The following features of a massage table are explained to aid the therapist in the purchase of a table that best suits their needs.

Massage table features

Height

The height of the massage table is critical for assisting the therapist to maintain good body positioning and thereby place minimal strain on their body. Most massage tables permit adjustment of the height of the table, and this is a most important feature for the therapist. Table height it seems is a matter of personal preference and a general rule commonly used to determine height is to have the massage table reach the therapist's knuckles when the hands are curled loosely into a fist hanging by the therapist's side. A table that is too high will mean the therapist will resort to using upper body muscle strength as a result of being unable to use their body weight over the top of the massage strokes. As the therapist develops their skills and develops greater body awareness they will be able to determine a table height that best suits their needs. The size of the client on the massage table, the type of techniques and modalities being employed and the body areas being worked will all generate a need to vary the height of the massage table. The electric massage table offers the massage therapist the perfect solution for adjusting table height throughout a massage treatment. A standard portable or fixed massage table will range from 64 cm to 80 cm in height, with increments of 5 cm on a height adjustable table.

Width

The width of the massage table is also an important factor, especially when considering client comfort. A large adult should fit comfortably on the massage table and have enough room for their arms to be supported by the table. For the therapist's benefit, a narrow table allows for greater reach and less strain on their body. A compromise between these two is a contoured table allowing for support of the client and easy access by the therapist. The width of standard massage tables will vary between 610 mm to 700 mm with the most popular width being 680 mm.

Length

A standard massage table should be approximately 1850 mm in length. This can be further extended by approximately 335 mm with the addition of a face cradle, making it long enough to accommodate taller clients.

Table frame

The frame of the massage table provides the table with stability and strength. A steel-framed massage table is sturdiest when the legs are attached directly to the frame, providing greater stability. The addition of cables and struts to the frame provides even greater support. The table can be tested for stability, movement, comfort and squeaks by having someone lie on the massage table while the therapist applies downward force and rocking movements to the person's body.

Padding and vinyl

The comfort of the massage table is dependent on the quality and density of the foam and the quality of the vinyl. The softness of the vinyl will add to the table's level of comfort and the durability of the vinyl will extend its life. Double density foam is fairly standard for a massage table. However, the difference in the quality of the foam used will dictate its level of comfort and its lifespan. Cheaper foams will lose their cushioning effect much faster than higher-quality foams, regardless of the density.

Weight

The weight of portable massage tables will vary from approximately 12 kilograms to 18 kilograms.

Massage table accessories

The face cradle can be added to a standard massage table and it can be fixed or adjustable. The cushioning is generally much softer and more supportive than the face hole that is part of a standard massage table. In terms of client comfort this is a most important accessory for the massage table.

Armrests can be helpful for clients who are larger, with longer limbs, or for those who find it more comfortable with their arms supported in front of them when lying prone. Armrests are generally attached to the face cradle.

Bolsters are great tools for the therapist and can be acquired in different shapes and sizes for the purpose of supporting the client in various positions.

Carry cases are an essential tool for the therapist who plans to provide mobile massage services. The case provides protection for the table, keeping it clean as well as protecting the vinyl from nicks and added wear. It also permits the table to be transported with greater ease by use of a shoulder strap or wheels.

The wedge is a big wedge-shaped piece of foam covered in vinyl that is suitable for supporting a client in a seated or semi-reclined position, and is ideal for the pregnant client.

The face recess plug fills the face hole recess to support the client when they are lying face up.

Footstools are ideal for aiding clients onto and off the massage table.

Stools on wheels and fit balls are ideal for maintaining good posture when accessing awkward parts of the client's body such as the head and neck, the feet or when the client is in a side-lying position.

Caring for the massage table

Considerations of hygiene dictate the need to clean the massage table surface after coming into contact with a client. Strong disinfecting solutions tend to have an eroding effect on the vinyl and as a result manufacturers of massage tables tend to suggest the use of mild detergents with warm water to clean the surface. Oils and perspiration coming in contact with the vinyl can also harden and erode the vinyl over time. If strong disinfecting solutions are used on the massage table for cleaning, they should be followed with a wipe with a damp cloth or warm soapy water to reduce the drying-out effect on the vinyl.

To protect a table the less contact the vinyl has with these eroding factors the greater its longevity. A simple solution to reduce wear on a table is to keep the vinyl protected with fitted covers that can be removed and replaced after each client.

The massage chair

The massage chair is designed for therapists who wish to provide massage in workplace environments, markets, exhibitions or really anywhere inventive they wish to set up their service. The chair is easily transported. It either folds up or divides into two easy pieces and weighs between 10 to 12 kilograms. Such chairs are designed for the client to be comfortably supported as well as relaxed in the seated position. Some chairs can be fully adjustable to suit each client's individual needs and others will have more basic fixed attachments.

The desktop massager is another option, where a chest pad and face cradle are put together in an attachment that sits on a desk.

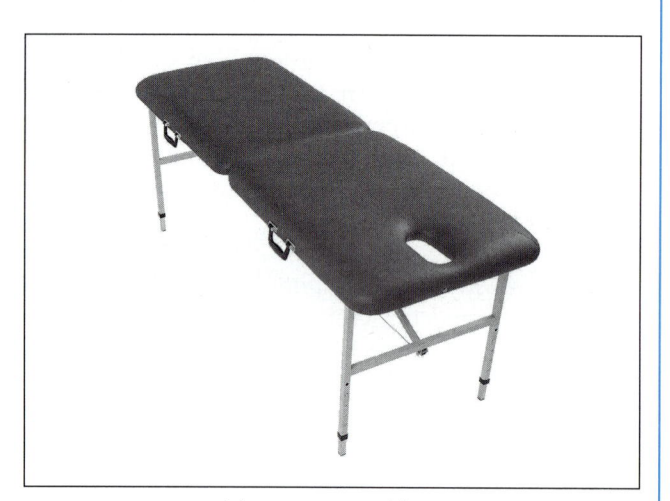

Figure 8.1a Portable massage table

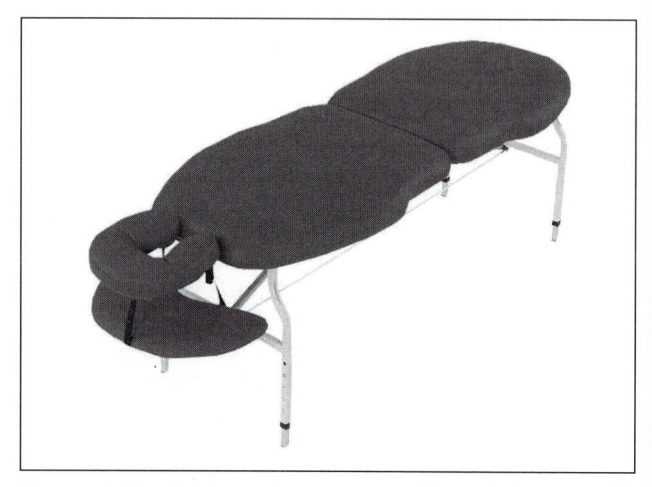

Figure 8.1b Contoured massage table with face cradle and arm rest attachments

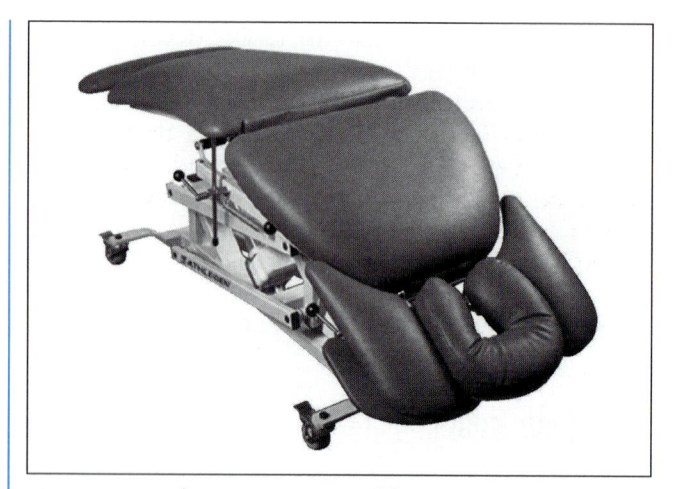

Figure 8.1c Electric massage table

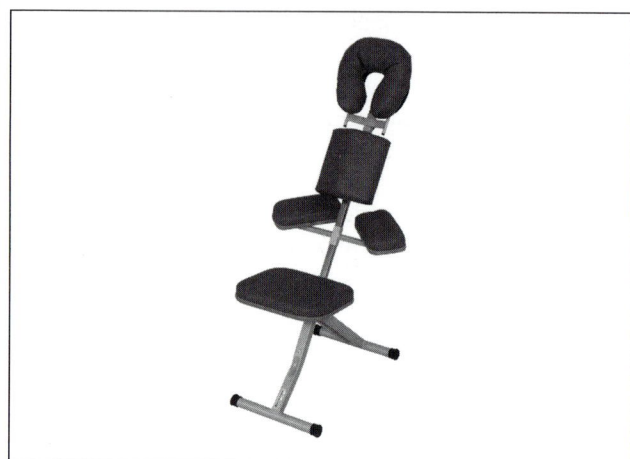

Figure 8.1d Massage chair

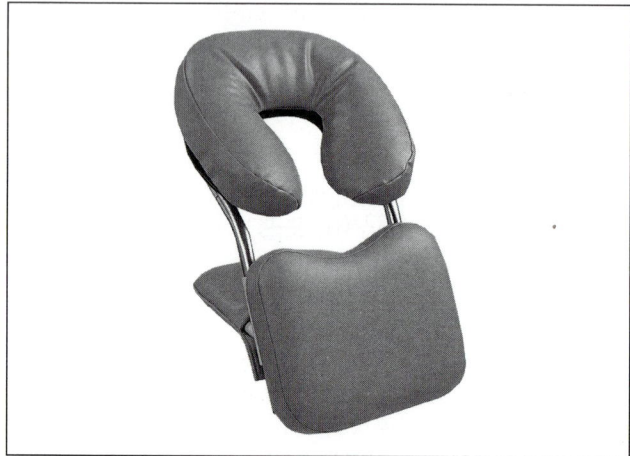

Figure 8.1e Adjustable desktop positioner

(photographs courtesy of Athlegen)

Figures 8.1a–e show a portable massage table, contoured massage table, electric massage table and massage chair.

Lubricants

For the application of Swedish massage techniques a lubricant is required to reduce drag and assist in the gliding strokes. There are many options for the therapist in choosing a type of lubricant, each providing a different texture, viscosity, odour and absorption rate.

Vegetable oils

Vegetable oils can be extracted from nuts, seeds or fruit by cold pressing or by heat extraction. Heat extraction follows a complicated refining process that uses very high temperatures to extract the oil. Refining can have a destructive effect on the vitamin and enzyme content of the oil as well as removing the natural flavour and aromas of the oil. Refining does, however, give an oil greater stability and a longer shelf life. Cold-pressed unrefined oils are more desirable to use in massage because of their nutritive qualities (Price, 1993).

Most vegetable oils are suitable for the application of massage. Figure 8.2 highlights some of the more commonly used oils, their uses in massage, and a comparative cost guide.

Vegetable oils will have a tendency to become rancid over a period of time when exposed to air, heat or light. The stability of a vegetable oil will depend on its fatty acid content. Oils high in saturated fatty acids are more stable than those high in unsaturated fatty acids. The vitamin E content of an oil will also increase stability, therefore those oils containing both saturated fatty acids and vitamin E will have a longer shelf life (Price, 1993).

Figure 8.2 Vegetable oils commonly used in massage therapy

Almond oil
- Properties: Contains vitamins A, B1, B2 and B6 and a small amount of vitamin E with mono and polyunsaturated fatty acids. It keeps reasonably well.
- Uses: Protects and nourishes the skin and is good for dry skin and eczema.
- Cost: $$

Apricot kernel oil
- Properties: Apricot kernel oil is very similar in make-up to sweet almond oil.
- Uses: Good for dry skin, especially the face.
- Cost: $$$$

Avocado oil
- Properties: Contains vitamins A, B, D and E. The unrefined oil is dark in colour and may have a cloudy appearance. Slightly pungent smell.
- Uses: Good cosmetic qualities for dry and wrinkled skin.
- Cost: $$$

Grapeseed oil
- Properties: Contains a high percentage of linoleic acid and some vitamin E, and is usually a refined oil processed by solvent extraction.
- Uses: Is popular with therapists for its light non-greasy properties.
- Cost: $

Olive oil
- Properties: The best grade to use is extra virgin. It is primarily a monounsaturated oil and has a slightly pungent smell.
- Uses: Beneficial for dehydrated, itchy or inflamed skin.
- Cost: $$

Safflower oil
- Properties: There are two types of safflower oil; a monounsaturated oil with oleic acid and a polyunsaturated fat with linoleic acid. The polyunsaturated oil will go rancid fairly quickly.
- Uses: Beneficial on painful inflamed joints, sprains and bruises.
- Cost: $

Sunflower oil
- Properties: Contains vitamins A, B, D and E and is high in unsaturated fatty acids, light in texture and has a non-greasy feel.
- Uses: Beneficial to bruises, skin diseases and leg ulcers.
- Cost: $

Sesame oil
- Properties: Is rich in vitamins and minerals and its high content of vitamin E gives it excellent stability.
- Uses: Beneficial for dry skin, eczema and psoriasis.
- Cost: $$

Key:
$ = inexpensive
$$ = average
$$$ = above average
$$$$ = expensive

(Goldberg, 2001; Wildwood, 1996; Battaglia, 1995; Price, 1993)

To increase the shelf life of vegetable oils follow these steps:

- store in amber glass;
- keep stored in a dark cool place away from direct sunlight;
- keep the lid tightly on the oil bottle when not in use;
- add vitamin E oil to extend shelf life;
- purchase in small quantities rather than stockpiling larger amounts.

Water soluble vegetable oils

These oils have been developed especially for massage therapists to ease the laundering of oil from their linens and clothing. An emulsifier has been added to the oil to make it easily dispersed in water.

Mineral oils

Mineral oils are saturated hydrocarbons extracted from petroleum. Being a foreign substance to the human body that does not nourish or penetrate the skin, mineral oil smothers the skin leading to blocking of the pores. Prolonged use may lead to dry skin conditions as a result of the mineral oil removing the skin's natural oils. Mineral oils are not recommended in skin care, despite the fact they are very common in many cosmetics and creams (Mehran, 2000). Some massage therapists choose to use mineral oil for massage because it is odourless, cheap, non-staining and doesn't go rancid.

Talcum powder

Talcum powder may be used as a lubricant for massage. It provides a surface that is less slippery than oil and would be more commonly used in sports or remedial massage, where deeper more specific techniques are applied and less glide is necessary.

Lotions and creams

Various lotions and creams may be used as an alternative to oils. They will generally be less greasy in texture and provide a less slippery surface than oil, requiring more frequent application. Some lotions and creams specially formulated for massage have a similar feel to oil and allow for easy glide.

Lotions and creams may be preferred by the therapist because they are less staining to linens and clothing and will have a longer shelf life than vegetable oils. They may be preferred by the client because they are less greasy on the skin, can be scent-free, and possibly available as a hypoallergenic lotion, which in some cases may be an important consideration.

Box 8.6 The essential pieces of equipment for massage

- Massage table or massage chair.
- A collection of pillows and bolsters of assorted sizes.
- A variety of linens and a blanket to drape the client and keep them warm.
- A suitable music collection and a means for playing the music.
- Oils and lubricants appropriate for massage.
- Client consent forms and treatment forms for record keeping.
- Cleaning and disinfectant supplies.
- Tissues.
- A chair for the client to sit on.
- A mirror.

Dispensing the lubricant

Dispensing the lubricants must be done in a contamination-proof way. This means using containers with a squeeze top or a pump top for easy and safe application. Thick creams that cannot be squeezed from a bottle will require disposable spatulas to retrieve them from the container.

The right amount of oil will depend on the dryness of the skin and the type of lubricant in use. The lubricant should be applied to the therapist's hands first rather than directly to the client. The therapist warms the lubricant in their hands by gently rubbing them together, and applies it sparingly to the area to be massaged. The lubricant is reapplied until the area is covered sufficiently — allowing for an easy glide over the surface with minimal friction but not so much that the therapist's hand is slipping off the surface. Experience will determine an appropriate amount of lubricant to use as well as determining when it is necessary to reapply.

Box 8.6 summarises the essential equipment for a massage therapist.

CONCLUSION

There are many factors that come together to make a massage therapist successful in their practice. The technical skills of massage are only a small part of the whole package that clients will seek out when looking for a therapist. The massage setting and all of the factors that comprise it, such as tranquillity, aroma, ambience and comfort contribute significantly to the client's experience of massage. Because massage requires touch, the therapist must instil a sense of security and trust in their service by ensuring that all of these factors are in place. It takes some effort to learn the skills of massage and be a good therapist, but it requires a great deal of thought and care to become an outstanding therapist. To be successful in practice a massage therapist must set themselves apart — creating a successful business by paying attention to all the small details that contribute to an enjoyable massage treatment.

Questions and activities

1. State five strategies to increase the shelf life of vegetable oils.
2. Write a proposal for a corporate client that describes the benefits of work-site massage.
3. Based on the factors that contribute to an ideal massage environment (tranquillity, aroma, ambience and comfort) describe in detail the features of your ideal massage room.
4. State the equipment required by a mobile massage therapist and describe how best they could pack and carry such equipment to create a setting in someone's home that would be suitable for massage.
5. Describe the features of a comfortable massage table set-up.

REFERENCES

Battaglia, S. (1995) *The Complete Guide to Aromatherapy*. Watson Ferguson & Co, Brisbane.

Gimbel, T. (1994) *Healing with Colour*. Simon & Schuster, Sydney.

Goldberg, L. (2001) *Massage and Aromatherapy: A Practical Approach* (2nd edn). Nelson Thornes Ltd, Cheltenham.

Mehran, D. (2000) *Nature in Cosmetics and Skin Care: A Compendium of Ingredients Used in Cosmetic and Skin Care Chemistry* (translated). Allured Publishing Corporation, Illinois.

Price, S. (1993) *Shirley Price's Aromatherapy Workbook. Understanding Essential Oils from Plant to Bottle*. Thorsons/HarperCollins, London.

Rich, G. (2002) *Massage Therapy: The Evidence for Practice*. Mosby, St Louis.

Wildwood, C. (1996) *The Bloomsbury Encyclopedia of Aromatherapy*. Bloomsbury Publishing, London.

chapter 9

Self-care

Lisa Casanelia

Learning outcomes

- Develop strength and flexibility in preparation for massage
- Perform self-massage techniques
- Develop a self-care program to minimise the strain of performing massage
- Cultivate awareness of individual strengths and weaknesses

INTRODUCTION

The human hand is a unique part of the body. Mechanical massage devices and other such apparatus can never replace the ability of the hand to mould to the contours of the human body or sensitively interpret the soft tissues of the body. The quality of the human touch and the contact it provides is far superior in therapeutic value to any machines or tools designed to replicate massage. As such the hands are appropriately designed to perform intricate patterns of touch and movement that allow massage techniques to be varied in their application. This ability combined with the dense distribution of tactile skin receptors through the fingertips make for a powerful combination of interpretation and application ability through touch.

The massage therapist is indeed fortunate and has the ability to apply unique strokes and assess the client's condition through the use of their hands. Those who have received a massage from a skilled therapist would be well aware of the types of strokes and touch that can be applied to the body with the hands. The ability to provide such touch is the primary tool of the massage therapist and a therapist working in a busy practice would perform their skill many times over in the course of a day. As in any profession, the tools of the trade, the therapist's hands, must be protected and cared for so as to prolong the working life of the therapist.

As massage is a manual therapy that is repetitive in nature it is not uncommon for massage therapists to develop overuse injuries. The thumbs, fingers, wrists and forearms are common injury sites arising from improper use and positioning of the therapist while performing massage. Prevention of injury, fatigue and muscle strain can be achieved in a number of practical ways. Just as any athlete would train to build strength and endurance, so too should the massage therapist slowly increase the number of treatments they perform to allow the body to slowly adapt to the increased demands placed upon it as a result of performing manual therapy (Greene, 1995). To avoid developing injuries when in practice the massage therapist can cultivate an awareness of how the hands and body move whilst performing massage. They may then adopt a daily exercises regime that encourages mobility and flexibility whilst strengthening the hands, forearms and body. Without such regular exercise a therapist may find that their wrists, fingers or hands start to ache after months or years of practice. Exercise strengthens the hands so they can cope with the demands of massage, minimising the possibility of repetitive injury. This chapter will introduce a self-care regimen for therapists to maintain their strength, endurance and flexibility.

A DAILY REGIME

The massage therapist should perform specific exercises designed to stretch and strengthen the thumbs, fingers, wrists and forearms on a daily basis. Such exercises will assist the therapist to perform in their clinical practice. The old adage 'you should practice what you preach' holds true for the massage therapist. As advocates of regular massage the therapist should also partake in regular massage; the use of self-massage will benefit the health of the therapist and assist in increasing the longevity of their massage career. It is very easy for the massage therapist to incorporate exercise and self-massage into their practice regime. What follows are simple recommendations for self-care of the hands and body that serve as a guide for the therapist in developing a daily self-care regime to suit their practice.

Flexibility and mobility exercises

Muscles in nature display qualities of contractility and elasticity; allowing them to contract and shorten when stimulated and relax when not stimulated. It is important for the health of muscles that their mobility is maintained as a muscle that is shortened for a prolonged period may become hypertonic or over contracted and loose its flexibility. This is not ideal as a muscle in its shortened position is a muscle that has a decreased range of movement and a compromised ability to provide maximal effort or strength. Whilst performing a massage a therapist is continually contracting and relaxing their musculature. After performing repeated massages it is not uncommon for a therapist's muscles to feel fatigued.

Day in and day out the massage therapist works and replicates the same movements; uses the same muscles. A therapist who does not stretch their muscles under such conditions, so as to elongate them back to their normal resting length, may end up with a posture that is contracted and hunched, and hands and forearms that feel weary and ache. Mobility and flexibility are very important for the massage therapist to allow for proper functioning and health of the muscles and for correct alignment and posture. As such a therapist should incorporate a daily stretching routine into their massage practice as part of their self-care.

A stretching program for the massage therapist must target specific muscles of the body. The following mobility and flexibility exercises focus on muscle groups that are commonly overworked during massage and have the potential to become contracted from overuse.

When a therapist performs these exercises the following recommendations apply:

- The feeling in the muscle should be a gentle stretch rather than an intense or painful feeling.
- Breathing should be relaxed throughout the exercise.
- The stretch should be held for a period of approximately eight to ten slow breaths.
- The exercise should be performed equally on both sides of the body.
- The exercise should be performed at the beginning and end of a working day and, where possible, in between clients.

Hand mobility exercises

Use the right hand to work on the left hand, which will remain relaxed and passive throughout. Begin by gently folding and unfolding each of the fingers in turn (3–5 repetitions per finger); start with the little finger, finish with the thumb. Gently hold the end of the little finger and take it through a large easy circle (circumduction) several times clockwise, then anticlockwise; this movement is not a stretch but rather a light and easy movement. Repeat on each of the other fingers including the thumb.

Gently hold the knuckle (metacarpophalangeal joint) of the little finger and move it back and forth (extension followed by flexion of the carpal metacarpal joint). Repeat this movement several times, then do the same for each of the fingers and the thumb.

The entire sequence should be repeated on the opposite hand.

Flexibility of the forearm flexors

Stand in front of a desk and place the palms and fingers flat on the desktop with the fingers facing back toward the body. Move the body away from the desk until a stretch is felt in the front of the forearms and wrists. If this stretch feels too strong it can be modified by allowing the fingers to curl over the edge of the desk to lessen the intensity of the stretch. (See Figure 9.1.)

Flexibility of the forearm extensors

In a similar manner to the above exercise, place the back of the hands flat on the desktop with the fingers facing back toward the body. Move the body away from the desk until a stretch is felt in the back of the forearms and wrists. (See Figure 9.2.)

Finger flexibility

Resting on a table, spread the thumb and index finger out and away from each other. Repeat the process with index finger and middle finger and so on to stretch each finger in turn. (See Figure 9.3.)

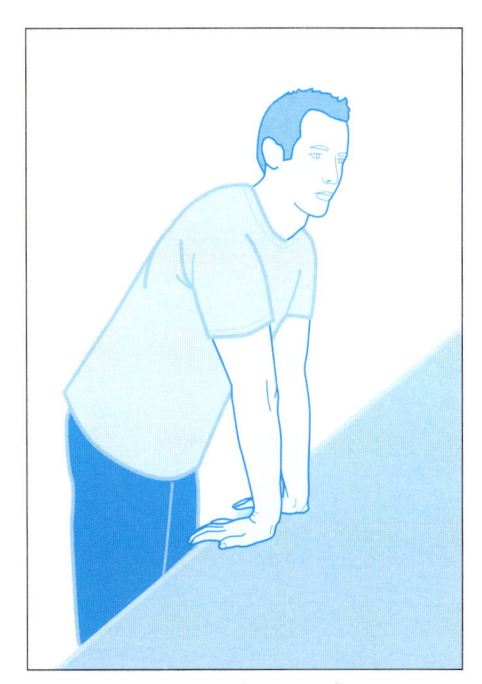

Figure 9.1 Flexibilty of the forearm flexors

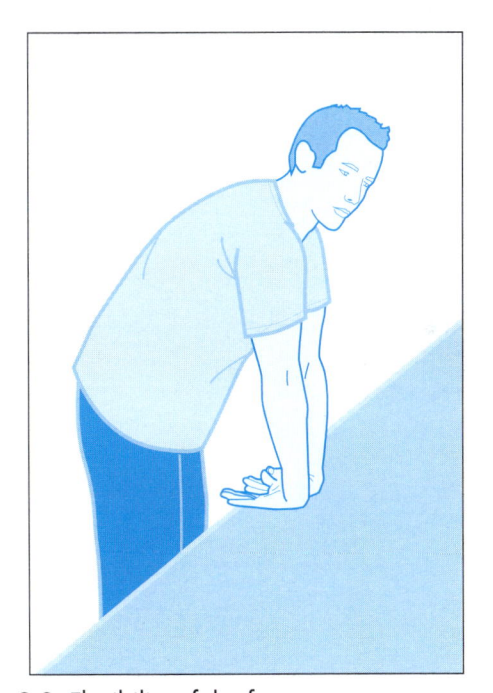

Figure 9.2 Flexibility of the forearm extensors

Flexibility of pectoralis major

Stand close to a wall or a corner with one arm out to the side at shoulder height and with the elbow bent and the hand facing forward. Rest the forearm on the wall and lunge the body forward, away from the arm. A stretch should be felt across the top of the chest and into the front of the shoulder. (See Figure 9.4.)

Flexibility of latissimus dorsi

Rest the back flat against the wall with the knees bent as if sitting in a chair. Bring the arms together in front of the chest, with the elbows bent and

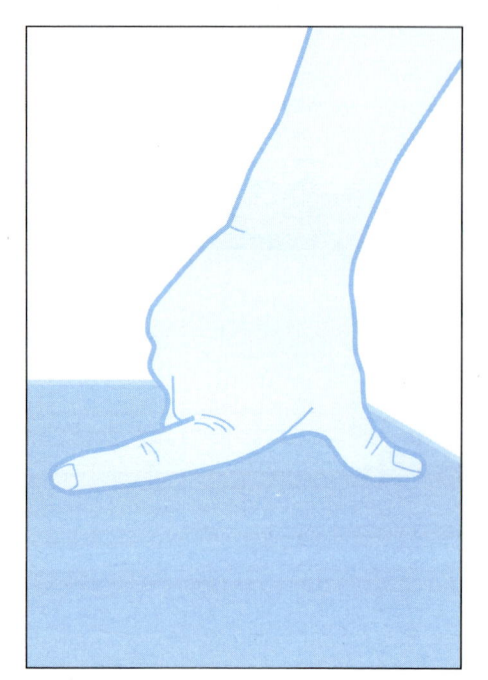

Figure 9.3 Finger flexibility

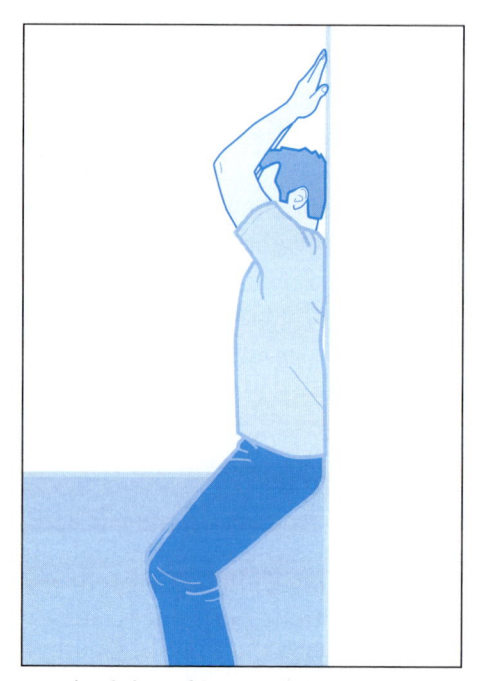

Figure 9.5 Flexibility of latissimus dorsi

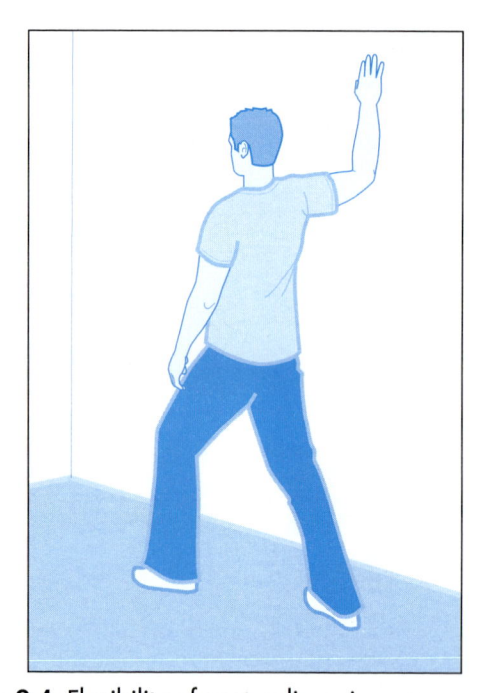

Figure 9.4 Flexibility of pectoralis major

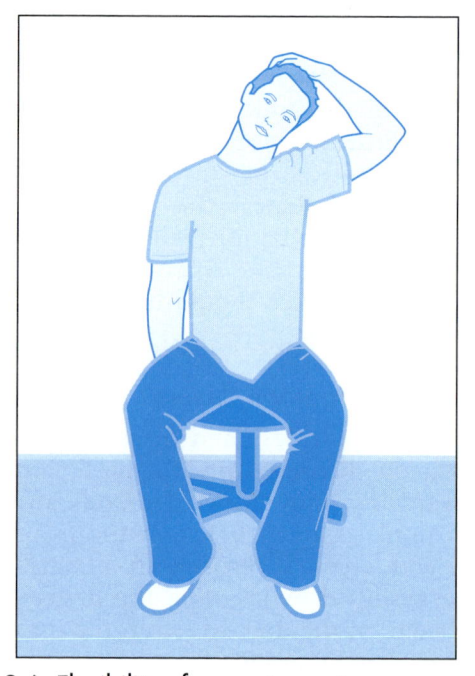

Figure 9.6 Flexibility of upper trapezius

touching each other. The palms should also be touching and facing toward the body. Take a deep breath in and on the exhale lift the arms up as a unit over the head and towards the wall. The hands should touch the wall above the head and slide up the wall as high as they can go. At the maximum stretch, hold and breathe deeply several times before releasing the position. (See Figure 9.5.)

Flexibility of upper trapezius

Sit on a chair with an upright posture and stabilise the trunk and shoulder girdle by holding onto the side of the chair with one hand. The other hand guides the head in gentle side-bending where the ear is moving toward the shoulder. (See Figure 9.6.)

Flexibility of rhomboids

Sitting in a chair, cross the arms in front of the chest and grasp the sides of the chair, drop the head forward and open up the shoulder blades by moving them away from the spine. Hold this stretch and breathe deeply several times. (See Figure 9.7.)

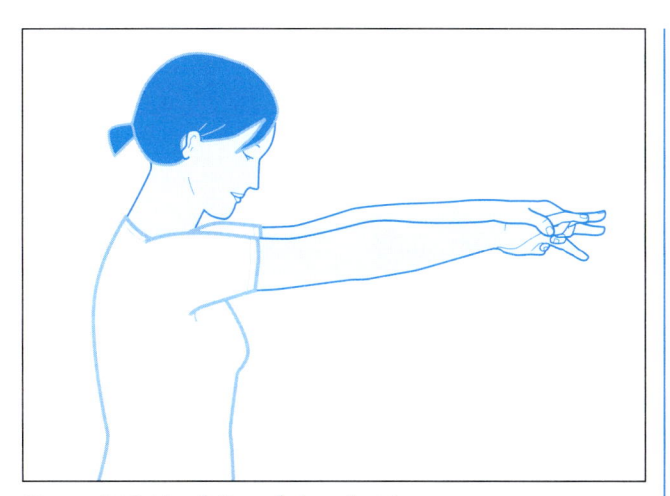

Figure 9.7 Flexibility of rhomboids

Flexibility of anterior shoulder

Kneel down next to a massage table facing away from it, clasp the hands together behind the back and lift them as a unit to rest on the massage table, and keep the chest open and body upright. To maximise the stretch lower the body so the buttocks are lowered toward the heels. Hold this stretch for a minute, rest and repeat several times. (See Figure 9.8.)

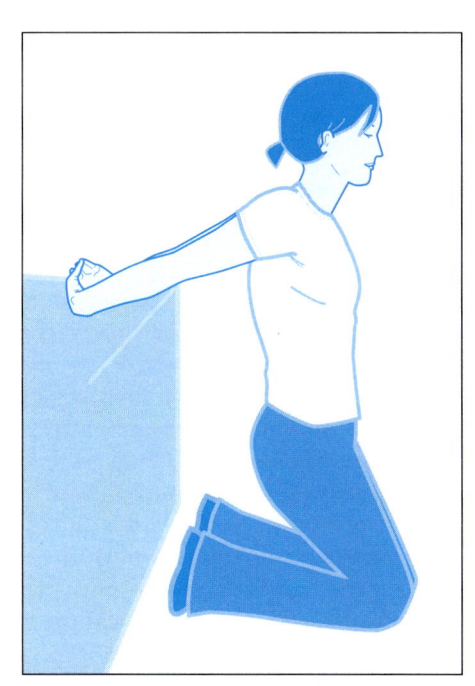

Figure 9.8 Flexibility of anterior shoulder

Flexibility of triceps brachii

Bring one arm up straight beside the head with the fingertips stretched up and the palm facing backward. Bend the arm at the elbow until the fingertips are reaching down toward the shoulder blade. The other hand reaches across toward the elbow and increases the stretch by grasping the elbow and pulling it backward. Hold this stretch as you breathe deeply several times. (See Figure 9.9.)

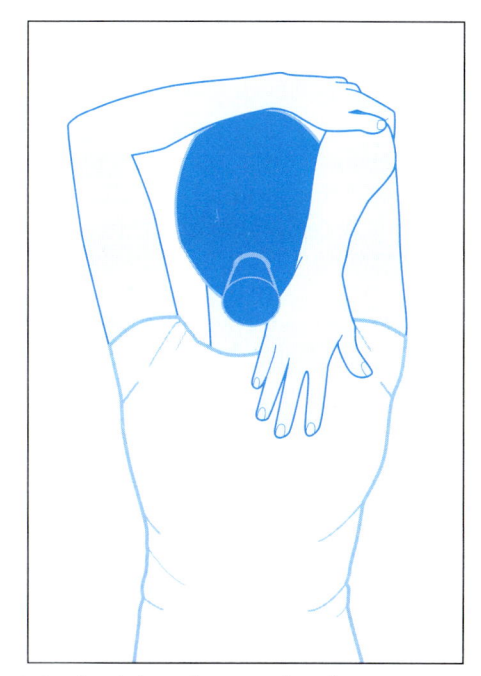

Figure 9.9 Flexibility of triceps brachii

Flexibility of thoracic spine

Lying on the floor use a bolster (or a towel rolled up to create a bolster) and place it across the spine and just below the shoulder blades. Lay over the bolster and allow the thoracic spine to extend and the chest to open up. Lay there for several minutes, breathing deeply. (See Figure 9.10.)

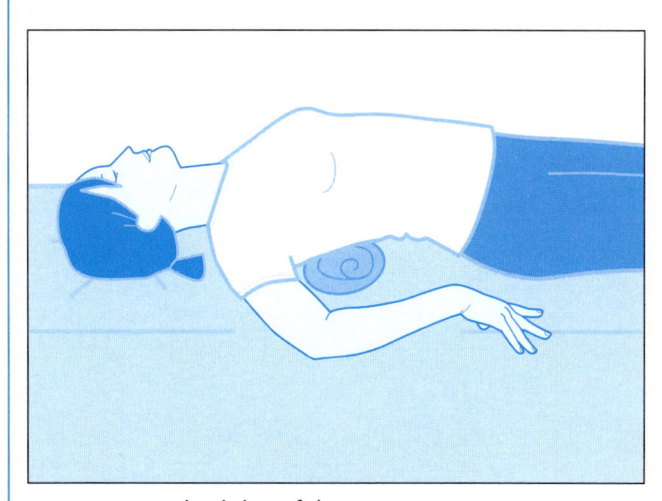

Figure 9.10 Flexibility of thoracic spine

Back loosening exercise

Lie supine on a carpeted floor or folded blanket and bend both knees so the feet are flat on the floor about hip width apart. With the knees apart and arms resting on the floor away from the body, slowly move both legs, tipping them over to the right as far as is comfortable. Slowly bring the legs back to the middle and then over to the other side. Repeat this movement several times, paying attention to the back and hips, consciously softening and relaxing these areas as they move (see Figure 9.11a). Stretch the legs out in front of the body and rest for 30 seconds.

Bend the knees again and continue the movement as before, only this time, gently roll the head in the same direction as the legs. Repeat this movement slowly and gently from side to side several times, paying attention to relaxing the back, hips and neck (see Figure 9.11b). Rest as before.

Bend the knees and resume the movement as before, this time rolling the head in the opposite direction to the legs. Repeat this several times, paying attention to areas in the body holding

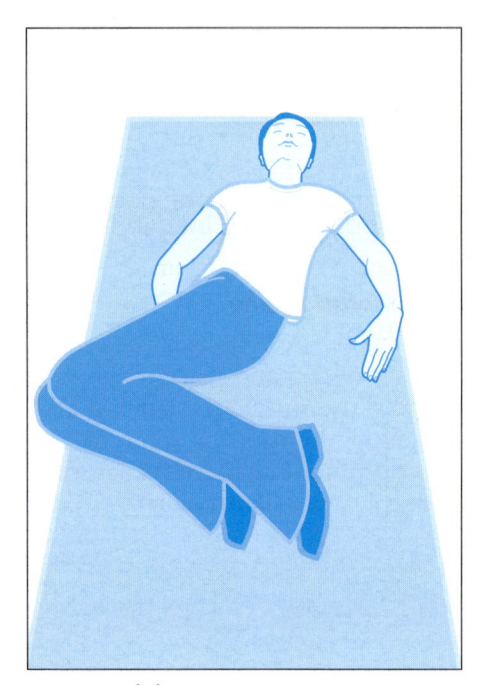

Figure 9.11a Back loosening exercise

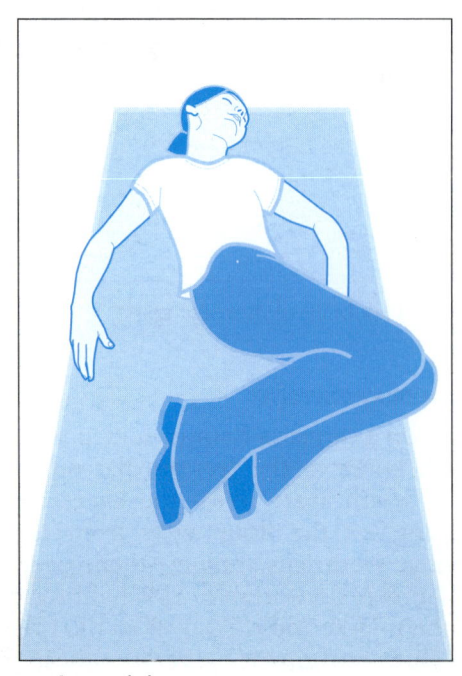

Figure 9.11b Back loosening exercise

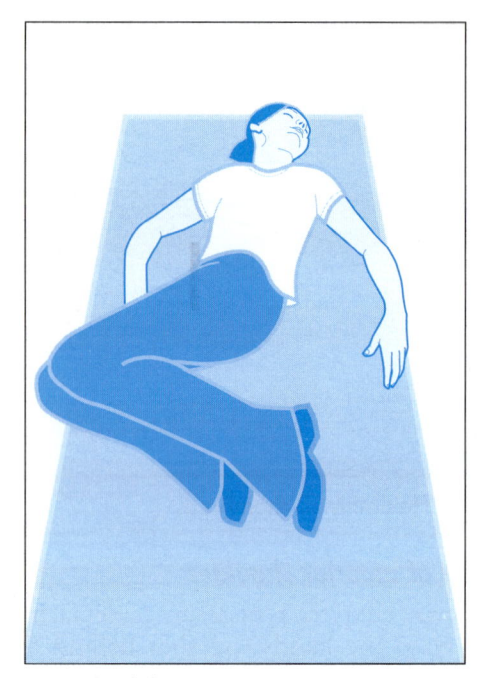

Figure 9.11c Back loosening exercise

tension and consciously let it go (see Figure 9.11c). Rest as before.

Bend the knees up and resume the original movement (i.e. only the legs tipping side to side). Notice if it feels easier and if the rest of the body automatically participates. Rest as before. Observe while resting if the body feels more comfortable and notice if the back, hips and legs feel more relaxed.

Resistance exercises

For the therapist to perform a one-hour massage with ease they require a minimum degree of strength. To perform eight massages in one day, over five working days a week, the therapist requires a much greater degree of muscle strength and endurance. The development of such strength and endurance of the musculature is imperative so that the therapist does not fatigue during their working day, thereby increasing the chance of injury.

The following resistance exercises are designed to build strength, improve function, increase muscular endurance and increase power in muscles that are commonly used whilst performing massage.

When a therapist performs these exercises the following recommendations apply:

- Start out with a minimal resistance and progress to a heavier load over time as the exercise becomes easier.
- Aim to perform up to ten repetitions of the exercise and repeat three sets of these repetitions on each side of the body.
- Perform strengthening exercises every other day.

Strengthening the forearm flexors and extensors

Hold a weight in one hand with the palm facing down, the elbow bent and the wrist in a neutral position (neither flexed nor extended). Bend the wrist upward and then release it back to the starting position, repeat 10 times. (See Figure 9.12.) Repeat this exercise with the palm facing up. (See Figure 9.13.)

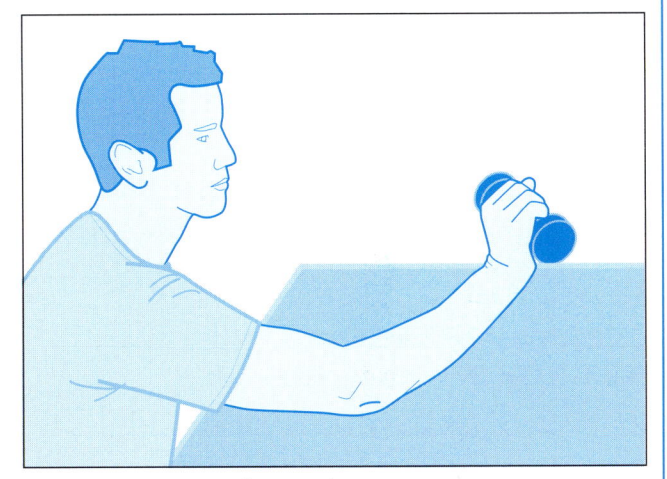

Figure 9.12 Strengthening forearm extensors

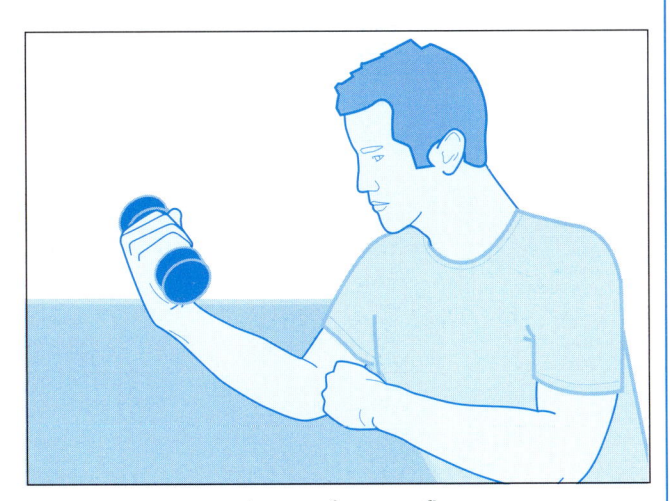

Figure 9.13 Strengthening forearm flexors

Strengthening the hand

A variety of objects can be squeezed in the palm of the hand to increase strength and avoid overusing any one set of muscles. Such objects include a tennis ball, squash ball or stress ball. Squeeze the object with moderate strength, with the wrist in a neutral position (neither flexed nor extended). Repeat 10–20 times on each hand. (See Figure 9.14.)

Strengthening the fingers

Using a peg or a butterfly clip (used to fasten papers) place the end between the thumb and index finger and squeeze the two fingers together to open the peg or clip. Repeat this several times and move on to the second digit and thumb. Continue this

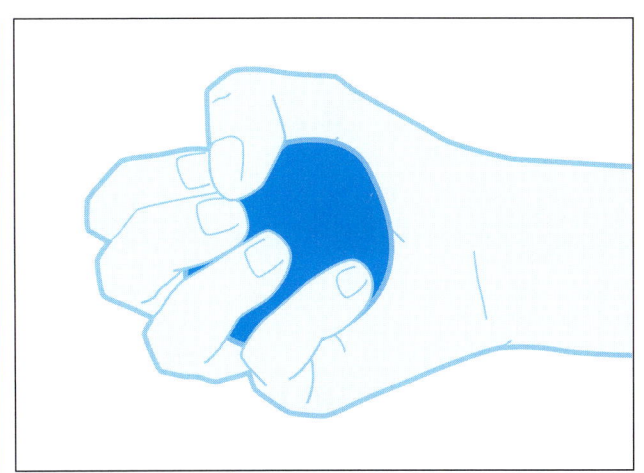

Figure 9.14 Strengthening the hand

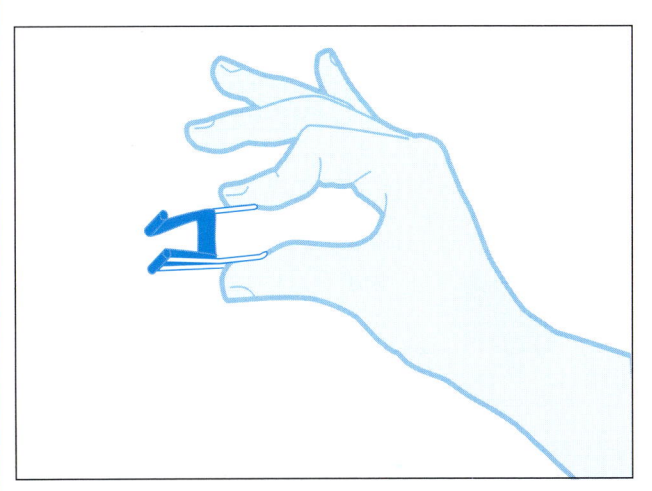

Figure 9.15 Strengthening the fingers

through the fingers, noticing the difference in strength between each finger. (See Figure 9.15.)

Strengthening serratus anterior

Lie supine on the floor with the knees bent and a folded towel placed between the floor and shoulder blades. Place weights in either hand and extend the arms up in front of the chest with the palms facing each other. Keeping the arms straight, stretch one arm up higher, extending it out from the shoulder, and then drop it back so that the shoulder blade compresses back into the towel. Repeat this on the same side 10 times and then repeat on the other side. Repeat the cycle three times. (See Figure 9.16.)

Strengthening rhomboids

Lean down over a low bench and support the body with one knee and arm resting on the bench. The free hand holds a weight and the arm hangs down by the side. Bend the elbow as you bring the hand with the weight back toward the chest. The action comes from the scapula being squeezed toward the midline. Repeat 10 times on each side and repeat the cycle three times. (See Figure 9.17.)

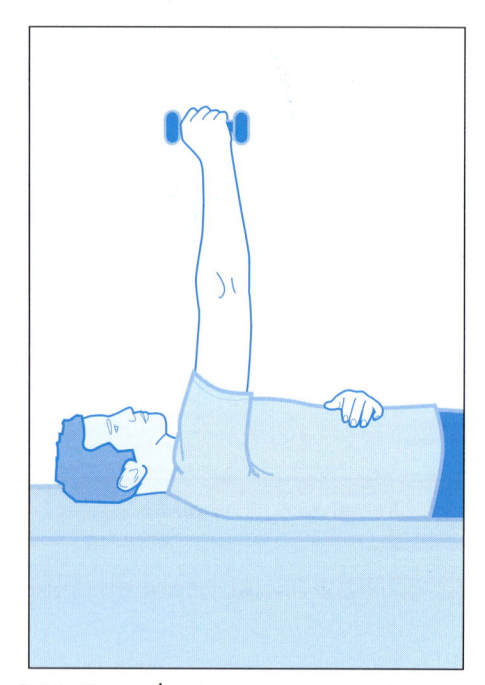

Figure 9.16 Strengthening serratus anterior

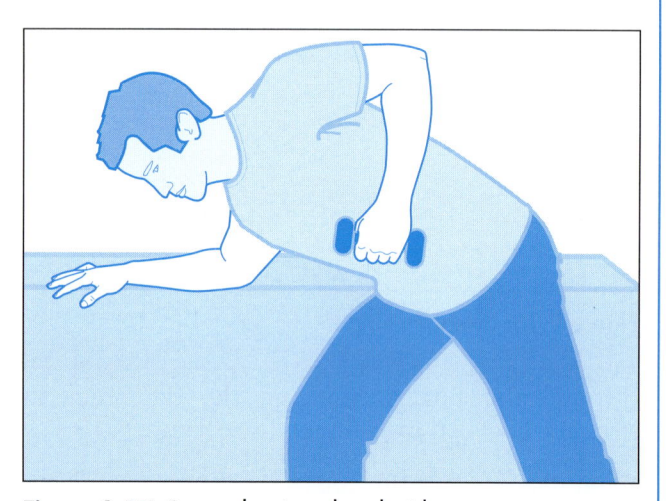

Figure 9.17 Strengthening rhomboids

Strengthening rotator cuff

Sit on the edge of a chair, holding a weight in either hand in front of your chest. The elbows are bent and together and the palms are facing each other (see Figure 9.18a). From this position bring the arms out to the sides keeping the elbows bent and parallel to the ground (see Figure 9.18b). From here lift your arms up straight over your head with the palms facing forward (see Figure 9.18c). Finally bring the arms back to the starting position by first turning the palms to face each other, then bring the elbows together as they are lowered. Repeat this cycle seven times and then reverse the order for the last three cycles. Rest in between repeating this sequence twice more.

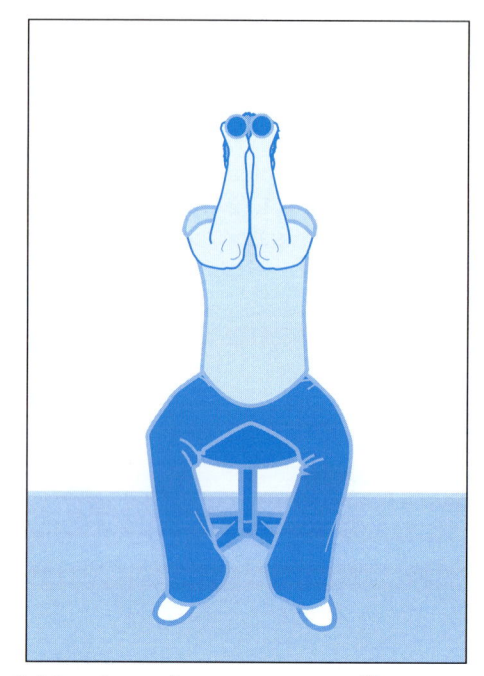

Figure 9.18a Strengthening rotator cuff

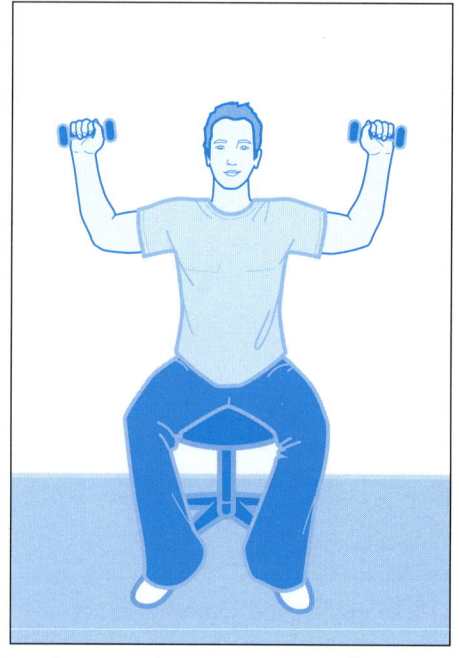

Figure 9.18b Strengthening rotator cuff

SELF-MASSAGE

All massage therapists would be aware of the benefits of massage. Massage therapy may assist in relieving tension in tight and contracted muscles and as such is of benefit to the therapist. Possessing the skills of massage application the therapist is limited only by their imagination when it comes to self-massage and it is recommended that the therapist employ a variety of techniques and gadgets to apply self-massage to their body.

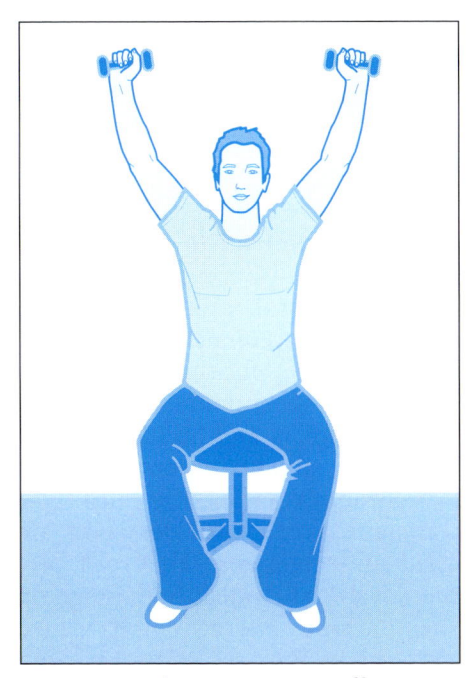

Figure 9.18c Strengthening rotator cuff

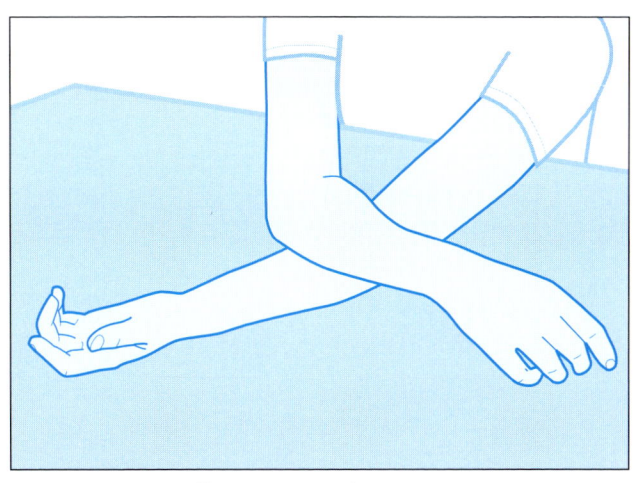

Figure 9.19b Self-massage to forearm extensors

There is a wide range of massage tools on the market that can assist the therapist in applying self-massage to areas of the body that may be difficult to access. A simple and inexpensive self-massage tool that is readily available in many households is a tennis ball or golf ball. The therapist can use a tennis ball or golf ball to assist in massaging muscles that are not easy to access by placing the ball against a wall or on the floor and using their body weight to lean into the ball and roll it around on the muscles.

The forearm flexors and extensors are muscles that are frequently overused during massage and self-massage can be applied to these muscles by using the forearm of the opposite arm to stroke along their length (see Figures 9.19a–b). Self-massage techniques should be incorporated into the therapist's daily warm-up and warm-down routines and used in between massage treatments where possible to maintain the health of the muscles and minimise the risk of injury.

CONTRAST ARM BATHS

To reduce fatigue and aid recovery after a day of massage a therapist may find relief through the use of hydrotherapy treatments. A simple hydrotherapy method to use is a contrast arm bath. Using a double sink or two small tubs about sink size, fill one with hot water (as hot as can be tolerated) and the other with cold water (ice may be added to make it extra cold). Beginning with the hot water, place the forearm and hands into the water and leave for approximately two minutes, follow directly into the cold water and leave for approximately 30 seconds. Repeat the cycle from hot to cold three times, beginning with hot and ending with cold. At the end of the sequence shake the excess water from the arms and hands and allow to air dry. The arms and hands should be tingling and feeling very much alive.

GENERAL HEALTH

As a health care provider the massage therapist has the responsibility to educate clients about how to look after themselves and maintain optimal health and wellness. It is also important that, as a practitioner, the massage therapist also adopts a lifestyle that promotes health and wellness so as to provide a role model for their clients. For instance, a therapist will generally recommend that a client receive regular massage as a form of preventative health. So too must the therapist receive regular massage. A therapist that looks after their health, receives regular massage, follows an exercise program and has a healthy diet and lifestyle will portray a positive image to the client and serve as a worthy advocate for the massage profession.

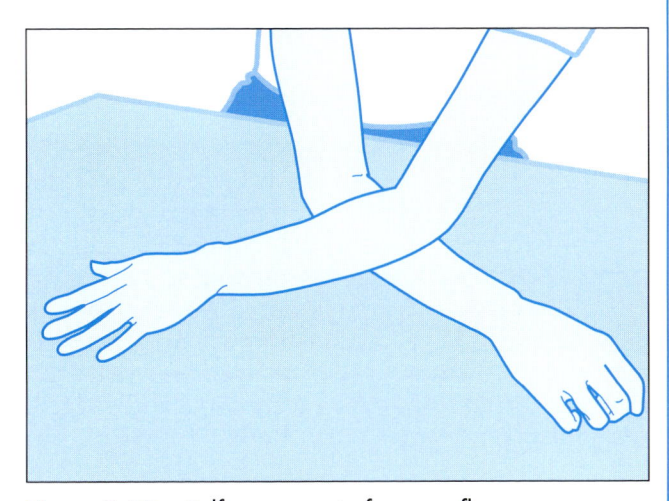

Figure 9.19a Self-massage to forearm flexors

> **Box 9.1** Suggestions for massage therapists to maintain their health
>
> - Receive regular massage.
> - Maintain the health and integrity of the skin of the hands and forearms.
> - Maintain the health and integrity of the nails.
> - Vary the part of the arm and hand used in performing massage to decrease the risk of repetitive strain injuries.
> - Adopt a healthy diet and lifestyle.
> - Maintain flexibility and mobility through regular exercise.
> - Maintain the strength and endurance of muscles required to perform massage.
> - Cultivate awareness of movement and posture by practising movement therapies such as yoga, tai chi, pilates, qi gong, Feldenkrais or martial arts.
> - Become aware of the makeup of the hand and take note of any individual weaknesses that may exist.
> - Use correct hand technique and correct body mechanics.
> - Recognise and respond to any injuries promptly.

The suggestions in Box 9.1 may assist the massage therapist in looking after their health whilst in clinical practice.

CONCLUSION

Students about to embark on careers as massage therapists must recognise the physical nature of the profession. As manual practitioners, therapists perform repetitive movements, many whilst leaning over a massage table; movements that are both physically demanding and draining on the body. The strength, flexibility and health of therapists are key factors in the ability of therapists to execute massage techniques efficiently and effectively. Massage therapists can provide good treatment when skilled at techniques. They can provide an excellent, enjoyable and effective massage treatment when they adopt correct body mechanics, strengthen their weaknesses and take care of their tools of the trade, their hands. Massage therapists who preserve the strength, flexibility and health of their hands and body will go a long way towards ensuring a healthy and rewarding career.

Questions and activities

Design a weekly health and fitness plan specifically for the practising massage therapist that takes into consideration strength and flexibility of the relevant muscle groups, providing a rational for each activity.

REFERENCES

Greene, L. (1995) *Save Your Hands! Injury Prevention for Massage Therapists.* Gilded Age Press, Colorado.

BIBLIOGRAPHY

Kisner, C. and Colby, L. (1996) *Therapeutic Exercise, Foundations and Techniques.* FA Davis Company, Philadelphia.

chapter 10

Infection control in the practice of massage therapy

Catherine Krejany, Ellie Feeney, Heather Morrison

Learning outcomes

- Demonstrate and apply the principles of infection control in the practice of massage therapy
- Describe the consequences of infection
- State the causes of infection
- Discuss the routes of transmission and methods of entry of infectious agents into the human body
- Describe the effects of infection on the human body
- Discuss the necessity for Standard and Additional Precautions in infection control
- Describe the application of Standard and Additional Precautions in the workplace
- Recognise and respond appropriately to potential infection risks

INTRODUCTION

Infectious diseases by their very nature are communicable; that is, they can be transmitted from person to person. Understanding the concepts of basic hygiene and infection control is therefore necessary to be able to implement techniques to prevent the spread of infectious diseases in the workplace. The massage therapist has both a moral and legal duty of care to protect themselves, their employees and their clients from harm.

Massage therapy is a relatively safe health care modality. There are very few reports of disease transmission as a result of massage treatments (Vickers and Zollman, 1999). However, massage by its very nature involves direct human contact and there is always the possibility that transmission of infections from clients to therapists, or therapists to clients, can occur. Not all clients encountered will have an infectious disease but everyone has the potential to spread infection. To prevent potential harm in a massage clinic environment adequate hygiene and infection control measures must be routinely practised. It is vital then that massage therapists understand and utilise best practice techniques in personal hygiene and clinic management. This chapter aims to outline the causes and consequences of infection and disease transmission and outlines the procedures and protocols that need to be employed within a massage setting to ensure a safe work environment for both massage therapists and clients.

WHAT IS INFECTION?

Before the practices of infection control can be discussed and implemented it is necessary to understand what infection is and where it comes from. Infections are caused by micro-organisms such as bacteria and viruses that replicate inside the human body and, as a result of this growth, cause disease symptoms. These micro-organisms or microbes may be a natural component of the body or may occur in the body as a result of attack and invasion. Therefore, infection is a term used to describe the symptoms of dysfunction in the body that are caused by the new growth of either a pre-existing micro-organism or one that has invaded the body.

The characteristic features of infection differ depending on the location of the infection within the body and may be due to either the action of the micro-organisms or alternatively to the action of the body's immune system that is seeking to destroy them. The next section contains an overview of the likely micro-organisms involved, where they're found and how they are transmitted from person to person.

INFECTIOUS AGENTS

History of infectious agents

Historically people had no knowledge that infectious diseases were caused by micro-organisms. This ignorance resulted in infectious diseases being regarded with much fear and superstition. Myth and misinformation was commonplace and many bizarre practices such as excessive bleeding and purging were endorsed in the hope of treating the illness and controlling the spread of such afflictions.

Infectious diseases can reach epidemic proportions in the absence of infection control measures. During the twelfth to fifteenth centuries it is estimated that tens of millions of people died in Europe in successive epidemics of the bubonic plague — a bacterial infection (Black, 2002). In fact early surgical procedures were carried out using the same instruments for all patients and hand washing was not employed, as there was still no comprehension of micro-organisms and their relationship to disease.

It was not until the first primitive microscope was produced in the seventeenth century that micro-organisms were even observed. Despite these observations these micro-organisms were not linked to the causation of infectious diseases and infections such as the bubonic plague and anthrax continued to ravage communities worldwide. It took another 200 years before the germ theory of disease was proposed and infectious diseases were proved to result from micro-organisms. Disinfection and hygiene practices were not implemented until the late 1800s when these infection control activities began to impact on the transmission of infectious agents (Lee and Bishop, 2002).

What are infectious agents?

Advancing technologies enable the observation of the amazing diversity of the microbial world. The environment in which people live is teeming with an immense variety of micro-organisms. The vast majority of such microbes live with people in harmony and are incapable of causing damage to the human body. These minute organisms are found in all aspects of the environment, from soil and water to the food people eat and the air they breathe. Many of these tiny creatures are even found on and in the human body, actually assisting in vital functions such as digestion.

Micro-organisms that exist in balance with the human body are referred to as 'normal flora'. The microbes present in normal flora are diverse and exist in harmony with each other and with the physiology of the human body. It is essential that this balance be maintained for good health as changes in the physiological condition of the body can alter the distribution of microbes, commonly resulting in the overgrowth of one species to the detriment of others. Such an overgrowth disrupts the balance of normal flora and can result in infection and disease.

The abnormal overgrowth of normal flora can be one way in which disease manifests. In addition to this, other micro-organisms which are not normally a part of the body can attempt to invade it. These microbes are referred to as pathogens, which are by definition disease causing organisms.

Pathogens are derived from four main groups of micro-organisms — viruses, bacteria, parasites and fungi. Other rare infectious agents such as prions, which are proteins, occasionally cause infectious diseases. Each of the major pathogenic groups will be discussed in turn.

Viruses

Viruses are amongst the smallest of the micro-organisms and are incapable of living outside of a host cell. They survive by infecting a normal cell and inserting their own genetic material. The viral genetic material hijacks the cellular metabolism of the host cell and forces it to manufacture viral proteins. These viral proteins are assembled into new viruses and released from the host cell. One infected cell is capable of producing hundreds of new virus particles. The newly released viral particles are then free to infect neighbouring cells and further the infection.

Bacteria

Bacteria are larger than viruses and are unicellular organisms that can survive in the environment on their own. Bacteria replicate quickly and divide and multiply to produce a bacterial colony. The colony requires specific temperatures and nutrients for replication and dies quickly if these requirements are not met. The human body by its nature is warm, moist and nutritious and provides an ideal environment for bacterial growth.

When bacteria enter the human body they replicate and are usually required to produce relatively large numbers before disease symptoms occur. Damage to the human body from bacterial infections is usually a result of either the secretion of toxic substances from the bacteria, damage to the host cells from the formation of the bacterial colony or the consequences of the body's immune response to the bacterial invasion.

Parasites

A parasite is an organism that derives its nutrients from the host. Technically all pathogens are parasitic as they derive their nutrients from the body after infecting it. It is a convention however that parasitic micro-organisms refer to a diverse group of microbes containing helminths (worms), protozoa (amoeba-primitive cells), and arthropods (insects). These organisms can be very small and microscopic such as the protozoa or large such as the tapeworm, which can grow inside human intestines to an amazing length of several metres (Haslett et al., 1999).

Generally, parasites enter the body through contaminated food and water or from direct contact with the parasite in the environment. Parasites then infect the body in various ways, creating infestations that cause tissue damage.

Fungi

A few micro-organisms that cause disease in humans are classified as fungi. Fungi are a very diverse group of organisms that range from small single-celled organisms such as yeast to large plant-like structures such as mushrooms. The majority of fungi are harmless to humans, however the few that are capable of causing infections fall into two main groups — yeasts and moulds. Although both yeast and moulds can cause infections this occurs more commonly if there are other predisposing factors in the host, such as immunosuppression from a pre-existing illness or drug therapy. Such infections are classified as opportunistic as the body usually has to be weakened in some way before a fungal infection can establish. The fungus then takes the 'opportunity' to grow into higher numbers and cause an infection.

Where are infectious agents found?

As mentioned previously, microbes can be found almost anywhere — in air, water, soil, food, and on animals, people and even the surfaces of inanimate objects. Remember that the majority of these microbes are completely harmless to humans and form a natural part of our ecosystem. However, some are pathogenic to humans and are responsible for a large variety of infectious diseases.

Box 10.1 Potential sources of microbes in the massage clinic

- Massage tables
- Oil bottles or containers
- Doors and door handles
- Light switches
- Bathroom facilities
- Linen
- Furniture and furnishings

In the massage clinic environment the sources of micro-organisms that may be pathogenic include those that have been left behind on inanimate surfaces, such as door handles, light switches, linens and massage tables, as a result of direct or indirect contact with people. In particular the deposition of bodily fluids is of great concern as these are potentially infectious to both the therapist as well as the next client unless properly managed and handled.

Transmission and entry of infectious agents

Although many pathogens have a great potential for harm to humans they can only do so if they can be transmitted and enter the human body. It is important then, for infection control, to understand the ways in which microbes can be transmitted. Mechanisms of transmission of micro-organisms may be categorised under three main headings — contact, vehicle and vector.

> **Box 10.2** Three major ways that micro-organisms can be transmitted
>
> - Through contact
> - With the use of vehicles
> - With the use of vectors

Transmission of organisms via contact

Contact transmission itself can be divided into three subgroups — direct, indirect and droplet. Direct contact transmission of micro-organisms means contact with the source of infection such as another person or animal. Indirect contact transmission means there is an intermediate between the source of infection and the newly infected person. These intermediates can be inanimate objects such as tables, computers, workbenches and writing implements; in fact just about anything that is found in a workplace or clinic. Droplet contact transmission occurs when someone sneezes or coughs on another person or within one metre of their presence. This person is not in physical contact with the person who sneezes, only their secretions.

Contact transmission is of major importance in massage therapy as an integral part of the massage treatment process involves touching the skin of clients as well as objects they have come into direct contact with. The massage therapist may take precautions to protect themselves, however unless they manage the clinic environment their next client may be exposed to infectious agents left behind by the previous client. Therefore infection control measures must take into account not just the therapist but also other employees and clients.

Transmission of organisms via vehicles

Certain components of our environment can act as vehicles of transmission that facilitate the transfer of microbes to new human hosts — air, water and food. Viruses and bacteria can both be airborne and travel on air currents. Breathing in air that contains pathogenic organisms is an efficient way for a microbe to establish an infection in the respiratory tract.

Ingestion of contaminated food products facilitates infections of the digestive tract. Water is also a vehicle for bacteria, viruses and common parasitic protozoa to enter the digestive system. Knowledge of these transmission mechanisms has obvious applications. It is essential that any food or water offered to clients meets acceptable food handling guidelines.

Transmission of organisms via vectors

As already discussed, it is not necessary to come into direct contact with the source of infection to enable transmission of infectious diseases. In addition to indirect contact and vehicle transmission it is also possible to transmit infectious agents using vectors. Vectors such as insects are carriers of disease and transmit infectious agents such as bacteria and viruses from infected sources to humans. The obvious examples of this are bites from mosquitoes, fleas and ticks. It is necessary then for a massage therapist to ensure that pests, vermin and insects cannot gain access to the treatment room and take measures to ensure that any such infestations that may arise are dealt with appropriately. Household pets such as cats and dogs should also be denied access to the treatment area as insects as well as infectious agents may be transferred from these animals into the clinic area.

How do infectious agents enter and exit the body?

For a microbe to be pathogenic it must first gain entry into the host and then multiply in sufficient numbers to cause disease. The human body is designed in such a way as to prevent or minimise this potential invasion.

The major barrier to infection is human skin. Skin is a thick impenetrable multi-layered barrier for micro-organisms and it is difficult for any microbe to cross the skin unless the barrier has been breached or damaged in some way, such as through cuts, burns or insect bites. The areas of the body where there is no skin covering are more likely portals of entry for pathogens. These areas include the:

- respiratory system: nose and mouth;
- digestive system: mouth and anus;
- urogenital system: vagina and urethra; and
- mucous membranes: conjunctiva, ears, eyes and lacrimal glands.

Different types of infectious agents use different portals of entry. For example, an airborne virus or bacteria is more likely to enter the respiratory tract than cross the skin. Knowing how infectious agents enter the body enables the application of preventative measures. However, knowing the exit routes is of equal importance as microbes that exit the body also act as sources of infection. During an infection the immune system, together with other processes of the body, acts to eradicate or remove the invading pathogen. As a result the infectious agent is shed from the body in sputum and mucosal secretions, saliva, semen and vaginal secretions, urine, faeces and blood. It is very likely that the massage therapist at some point in their practice experience will have to handle situations in which exposure to these bodily fluids occurs, either through accident, through injury or circumstances particular to individual clients. Knowledge of infection control and appropriate cleaning techniques will minimise the risks for both therapist and clients in the aftermath of being presented with these hazards.

> **Box 10.3** Potential routes of entry of micro-organisms into the body
>
> - Damaged or broken skin
> - Mucosal surfaces
> - Eyes, conjunctiva, ears
> - Respiratory tract through inhalation
> - Gastrointestinal tract through ingestion of food or water
> - Urinary tract through poor hygiene

IMPLEMENTING INFECTION CONTROL IN THE WORKPLACE

To localise the spread of micro-organisms and prevent the transmission of infectious disease in the workplace a series of work practices have been developed to ensure minimum risk of harm to workers and their clients. These work practices are known as Standard Precautions (National Health and Medical Research Council, 2002).

Standard Precautions, when adopted, offer a basic standard of infection control and apply to all patients regardless of their disease state, diagnosis or presumed infectious status. This means that broken skin and mucous membranes, blood and body fluids are treated as if they offer a potential infectious risk. When a client is known or suspected to be infectious Standard Precautions provide the therapist with further tools and procedures in the form of Additional Precautions to ensure adequate infection control.

The most common application of Additional Precautions for the massage therapist will occur during exposure to blood or body fluids that are known to be infectious. These instances should be handled appropriately to prevent the risk of infection to the therapist or other employees and clients. In the instance of known infectious material handling the basics of Standard Precautions still apply, including high standard hygiene practices and the application of personal protective equipment in cleaning and disinfection routines and situations of exposure to sources of infection. In addition to these procedures Additional Precautions can be adopted that are specific to the infectious agent involved. These work practices are designed to prevent the transmission of infection particularly when highly contagious infectious agents are involved, such as those that utilise airborne transmission, respiratory droplet transmission, direct contact with dry skin or contaminated surfaces or combinations of these infectious routes (National Health and Medical Research Council, 1996). In these instances application of face masks (for client and therapist), gloves and protective eyewear may be used during the treatment to reduce the transmission potential.

Within Standard Precautions the techniques and protocols that are adopted are divided into two main categories — aseptic techniques and clean techniques. Asepsis is the term used to describe the process of sterilisation that involves the complete removal of all micro-organisms. True asepsis cannot be achieved in the massage clinic as it involves sterilisation equipment that will not normally be accessible to a massage therapist. Instead procedures of clean techniques are adopted to minimise as much as possible the transmission of micro-organisms.

Clean techniques refer to the protocols that centre on a number of areas of action including personal hygiene, the use of barriers to reduce the transmission of infectious agents, the use of environmental controls to reduce transmission and the appropriate processing of instrumentation and equipment between clients. The application of these procedures in the massage setting will be discussed in the next section.

Application of infection control precautions

Personal hygiene

Personal hygiene is paramount to infection control. As a massage therapist, direct person to person contact is a part of every treatment regime. It is therefore essential that every aspect of personal hygiene be attended to at the highest possible standard.

Personal cleanliness should be maintained at all times. Therapists should ensure their hair is clean and tied back if long enough to contact the client in any way during the application of massage techniques. This prevents intrusion in the therapy technique as well as decreasing transmission of microbes.

Hand and nail care is of particular importance as hands represent the contact between client and therapist. The massage therapist should ensure that there is no broken skin on their hands or in the skin of the client. Any broken skin should be covered appropriately with non-absorbent covering or the application of personal protective equipment such as gloves should be employed (see next section). The therapists nails need special attention and all fingernails should be cut short and be free from all traces of dirt or foreign matter.

Jewellery on the hands and wrists is also a potential source of infection and may injure the client, so it should be removed when massaging and hand washing. The therapist may opt for more personal protection through vaccination against common transmissible diseases. This is, however, a very personal choice and all aspects of this option should be considered, such as relevance of the vaccine, cost, potential of infection and possible side effects.

One of the most vital protocols that should be adopted is the correct hand-washing routine. Hand washing is the single most effective mechanism known to prevent transmission of microbes from therapist to client. There is no substitute for a good hand-washing technique and even the use of gloves alone is not as effective (National Health and Medical Research Council, 2002). Hands must be washed before and after significant client contact of any type, after engaging in any activities likely to cause contamination and after the removal of gloves.

The procedure for correct hand washing is shown in Figures 10.1a–d. Correct hand washing begins by removing all jewellery and thoroughly wetting the hands with water. A mild detergent is then applied and a vigorous lather is built up across all aspects of the hands, incorporating the palms, back of hands, wrists, between the fingers and thumbs, under the fingernails and up the forearms to the elbows. The lather is then washed off in running water. Care must be taken at this point not to touch the tap handles with clean hands. If elbow or foot controls are not available then a paper towel should be used to turn the tap off. Hand washing should continue for a minimum of 10–15 seconds. Hands can then be patted dry with a clean paper towel or hand towel.

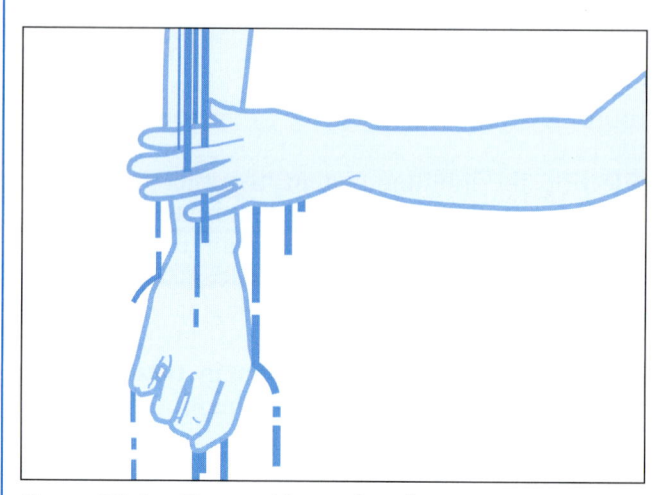

Figure 10.1a Thoroughly wet hands

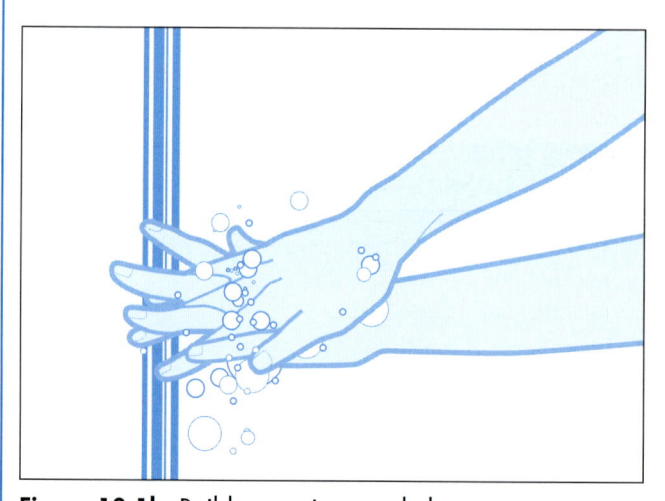

Figure 10.1b Build up a vigorous lather

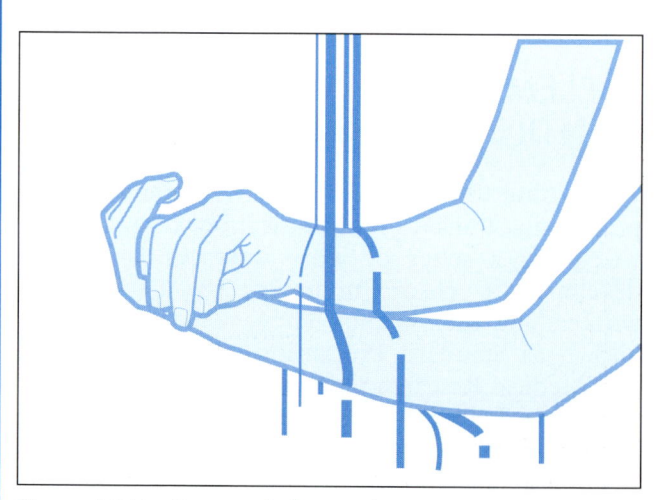

Figure 10.1c Remove lather under running water

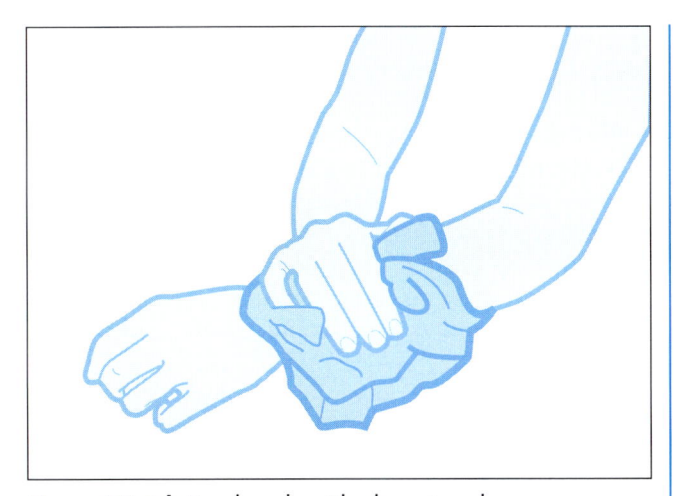

Figure 10.1d Dry hands with clean towel

Personal protective equipment

There is a range of personal protective equipment that may be of use to the massage therapist such as gloves, face masks, eye protection and appropriate footwear. Each of these items is designed to protect the therapist from infectious agents. The majority of personal protective equipment may be more useful in clean-up procedures than during client treatment.

Examination gloves

Gloves should be used when there is a risk of exposure to blood or body fluids. They must be of high standard and meet Australian guidelines for patient examination. If the therapist has damaged or broken skin on their hands or if the client has damaged or broken skin, there should not be direct contact between client and therapist and gloves should be used. Alternatively there may be a spill of blood or bodily fluid (such as urine or faeces from incontinent clients) that needs to be cleaned and in these situations gloves are also essential. There is also a particular procedure for the correct removal of the gloves after clean up or contact with the potential hazard. After contact with the bodily fluid or infected material the gloves themselves become sources of infection and must be handled appropriately. It is necessary that the therapist does not touch the outer surface of the contaminated gloves in order to remove them. Instead the therapist needs to follow the following procedure:

1. Grasp the outside of the cuff of one glove below the wrist.
2. Pull the glove down over the hand, turning the glove inside out and continue to hold that glove.
3. Insert the un-gloved fingers inside the cuff of the other glove.
4. Pull the glove downwards and over the hand and first glove, turning the glove inside out.
5. Drop the inverted gloves directly into a bin for disposal.

This procedure is illustrated in Figures 10.2a–d. If this procedure is followed correctly there will be no contact with the contaminated surface of the gloves. Gloves that have been contaminated then need to be disposed of appropriately (see section on waste disposal).

Face masks

During the clean up of an infectious hazard or in any other circumstance where there is the potential for splashing or spraying of blood or body substances or where there is the potential for

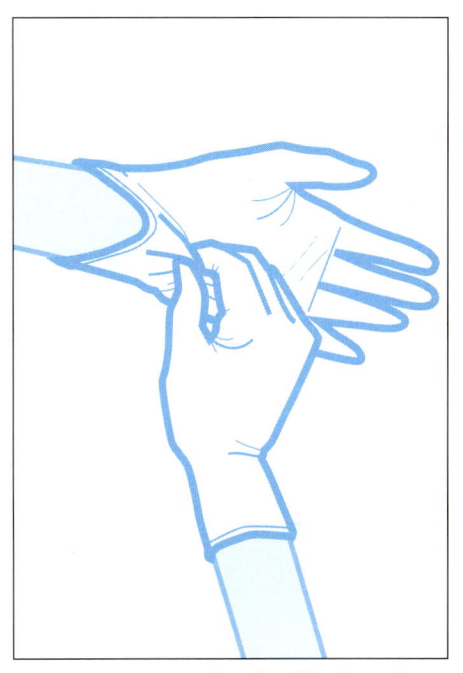

Figure 10.2a Grasp outside of cuff below the wrist

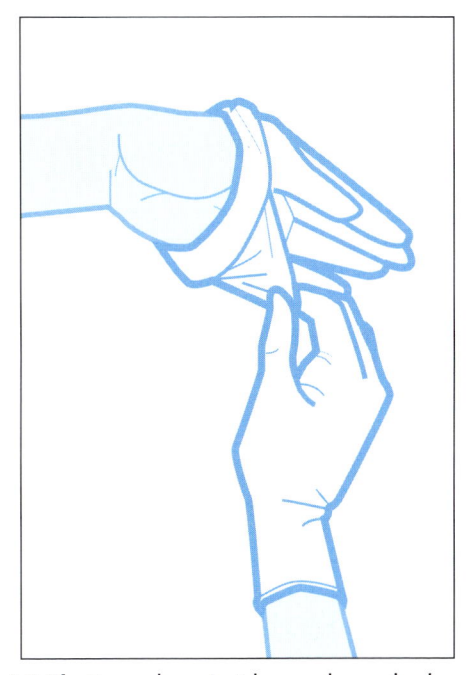

Figure 10.2b Turn glove inside out down the hand

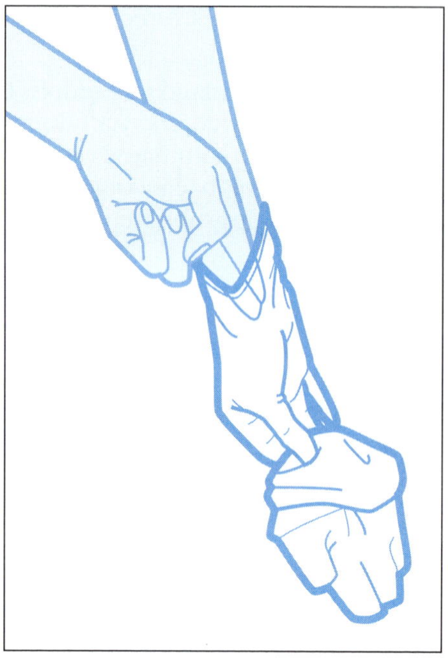

Figure 10.2c Ungloved fingers into cuff of remaining glove

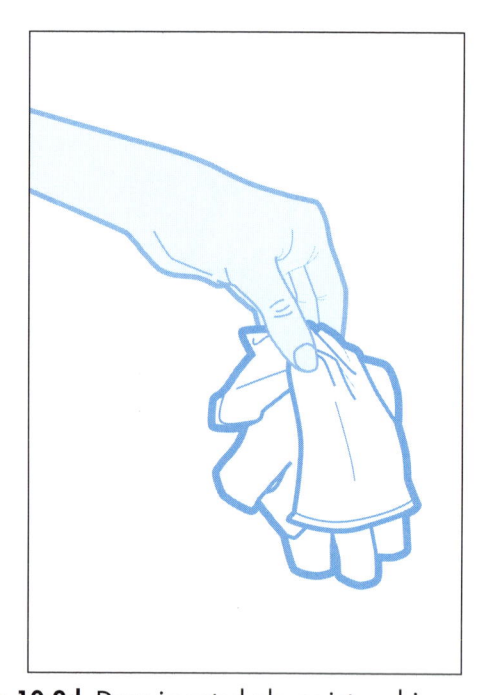

Figure 10.2d Drop inverted gloves into a bin

airborne infection, face masks should be employed. These act as barriers to infection from airborne microbes and can be used to protect the therapist and client.

For a face mask to be effective it must be fitted and worn according to manufacturers' instructions. It should not be touched by hand while being worn and needs to cover both the nose and mouth to be effective. A face mask should be removed as soon as practicable after becoming moist or visibly soiled and this needs to be carried out by touching the strings and loops only. A mask must be discarded as soon as practicable after use and if a single-use mask is employed the therapist must ensure that it is indeed used only once.

Clothing

The clothing worn during treatment of clients can also be considered protective equipment for both the therapist and client. To be protective the clothes must be kept clean and laundered regularly. If contamination with bodily fluids occurs, clothes must be changed as soon as practicable and bagged for laundering.

Footwear should also be considered. Covered footwear offers the best protection from sharp objects, heavy objects and also spills and exposure to body fluids. Shoes should also be cleaned regularly to prevent spread of infectious agents.

Eye protection

The final piece of protective equipment that may be of benefit to the massage therapist is eye protection. This is likely to be of most benefit in the cleaning of spills and liquid hazards where there is a potential for splashing of blood or body fluids or cleaning chemicals into the eyes.

If each of the pieces of personal protective equipment is employed appropriately this offers a great level of protection to the therapist (and the clients indirectly) from occupational exposure to infectious agents.

Storage, cleaning and disinfection

Personal protective equipment is of great use in infection control but is not adequate, in the absence of other infection control measures, to prevent the spread of infectious agents. The massage clinic or treatment area must be managed appropriately and cleaned effectively. Procedures have to be adopted for storage of items in the workplace and cleaning of communal areas.

The entire work environment needs to be considered for adequate infection control. This includes the walls and surfaces of the room, all furnishings, work equipment, bathroom and toilet facilities and the air supply to the work area.

Routine cleaning of work areas is important because deposits of dust, soil and microbes on surfaces can transmit infection. The regular and routine cleaning and maintenance are therefore necessary to help maintain a safe environment for therapist and clients.

Standard cleaning equipment should be readily available for routine cleaning as well as spills management. Standard equipment should include cleaning solutions, water, buckets, cleaning cloths and mop heads. It should be stored safely in a place known to all employees of the clinic. All cleaning items should be changed routinely and especially after dealing with blood or body fluid spills. For all routine and general cleaning a neutral detergent and warm water should be used. It is not necessary to use disinfectants or bleach.

Cleaning the work environment

Regular cleaning of the environment and workplace enables therapists to comply with Standard and Additional Precautions. Each massage clinic should develop written cleaning protocols, including cleaning methods and frequency of the cleaning routine. Consideration should be given to the order in which items are cleaned. Commonsense dictates this should be from cleanest to dirtiest and from top to bottom of the room to prevent the depositing of dirt on clean items.

Routine surface cleaning

Work surfaces should be cleaned and dried after each session and when soiled.

Floors should be cleaned daily and damp dusting should be used on surfaces, including window furnishings.

Wet areas

Toilets, sinks, and washbasins need to be cleaned at least daily. During this process avoid the generation of aerosols (avoid splashing and spraying).

Walls and fittings

All walls and fittings including curtains need to be cleaned regularly and when soiled. This applies particularly for those in high traffic areas such as reception rooms, children's play areas and treatment rooms.

Storage of cleaning equipment

Cleaning equipment should be cleaned and dried before storage. Mop heads (if detachable) and cloths should be laundered and buckets emptied and dried to prevent microbial growth on wet materials.

Cleaning the work equipment

The cleaning routine for work equipment will vary depending on the equipment in question and also on the exposure of that equipment to potential sources of infection. All equipment that comes into contact with the client's skin, such as massage tables, should be cleaned in between clients. Equipment that has been repeatedly used but not necessarily in direct client contact should be cleaned at the end of the day, and some equipment may require a more thorough cleaning at the end of the day. At the end of the week or month, depending on client loadings, all work equipment should be cleaned or disinfected.

Laundry

For a massage therapist one of the major pieces of work equipment that must be handled well is laundry. As linens used during massage therapy come into direct contact with the skin of the client they must be clean to begin with and dirty linen needs to be handled appropriately.

When handling dirty linen check soiled linen for foreign objects. Place soiled linen in appropriate container or bag at point of generation. Appropriate containers are able to be either laundered, washed or disposed of. Sort linen in appropriate areas; not the treatment room. Do not shake the linen out as this spreads microbes to other surfaces. Linen heavily soiled with bodily substances should be placed in an impermeable bag for transport from the treatment area.

When washing linen use detergent and hot water and wash linen as soon as practicable to reduce the time allowed for growth of microbes. After washing, clean linen should be stored appropriately. If linen is to be used within a day it can be stored on open shelves within the treatment room. If the linen is not to be used straight away it should be stored in a closed cupboard to avoid the settling of dust and dirt on the clean laundry. Be very careful to handle and store clean and dirty linens separately.

Managing waste

The majority of waste generated by a clinic will fall into the category of general or recyclable waste and should be treated as domestic or household waste. In the massage clinic there are rarely exceptions from this. However some therapists work in clinic rooms that are shared in a multi-modal setting and there are biological wastes and sharps containers used for the disposal of contaminated items, syringes or acupuncture needles for other health professionals. The key to effective waste management is in the organisation and set up of appropriate containers so that waste can be handled appropriately from its generation to its storage and safe disposal.

Collection

Use appropriate containers to ensure segregation of clinical waste from household waste at point of generation. Needles or syringes must be deposited into an approved clinical waste sharps container. Clients who are diabetic or carry medication that needs to be injected may require such a container to dispose of needles appropriately.

Sharps containers are yellow and bear a clearly marked international biohazard symbol. They must meet Australian standards and cannot be disposed of with household waste. Disposal is organised through the company that supplies the containers.

Collection of blood and body substance spills

The massage clinic should have a protocol in place for managing blood and body fluid spills. These protocols should follow Standard Precautions including the use of personal protective equipment and, where needed, Additional Precautions. The basic principles of blood and body fluid management are outlined in Box 10.4. These basic steps should be flexible enough to adapt to different circumstances such as the size of the spill, the differing surfaces that the spill is on, the nature of the spill (blood, urine, vomit, or faeces) the location of the spill, the likely pathogens involved and whether there is a likelihood of contact of the spill area with bare skin.

> **Box 10.4 The basic principles of blood and body fluid management**
>
> - Spills should be cleared before the area is cleaned, as adding cleaning solutions (detergent) to the spill increases the size of the spill to be dealt with.
> - The generation of aerosols should be avoided, so prevent vigorous scrubbing when potentially infectious fluid is present.
> - Using personal protective equipment such as gloves, masks, and eye goggles.
> - Carefully remove as much of the spill as possible with absorbent material, such as a paper towel or hand towel, and dispose of it in a plastic bag or container.
> - Clean the area with warm water and detergent.
> - If contact with bare skin is likely, disinfect the area with a diluted bleach solution with at least 1000ppm available chlorine and allow to dry.
> - Wash hands thoroughly after clean up.

Items that have been used to clean up body fluid spills should be collected using a strong sealable plastic container or a series of two plastic bags to hold these items to prevent leakage and spillage. Such items, once secured, can be placed with and disposed of with normal household rubbish.

Handling

When handling potentially infectious material use the appropriate personal protective equipment. Have a container or heavy duty plastic bag ready to dispose of gloves, paper towels and other cleaning equipment exposed to potentially infectious wastes. Do not carry contaminated cleaning products to the place of disposal through other rooms of the clinic. Instead have a sealable container ready to receive contaminated waste and seal carefully before moving the waste for disposal.

Storage

Storage of items used to clean up and disinfect must be safe and secure while awaiting disposal. If dealing with broken glass or other sharp objects ensure the container is adequately sealed to prevent further hazards with sharp objects protruding from the container. All waste containers should have a closable lid, and not be an open bin. Store waste in small bags or containers rather than large bins that take a while to fill. This prevents unnecessary waste accumulation and reduces the attraction of vermin or other pests that may spread disease.

Disposal

General rubbish should be disposed of with the local rubbish collection. Care should be taken to separate recyclable items from normal household rubbish. The therapist should also take care with paper items to ensure that any form of confidential client information is not included with household rubbish.

IDENTIFYING AND RESPONDING TO INFECTION RISKS

There is no way of describing or identifying all of the potential disease-causing organisms that a massage therapist may be exposed to within the clinical setting. This will be very dependent on the location of the clinic and the clients that frequent it. For example, if the client base is specialised to treat a large number of children the range of infectious diseases a therapist will be exposed to will be different than if the clinic's clients are predominantly elderly. Despite the differences in client demographics some commonalities will exist based on the disease prevalence within the community. Table 10.1 identifies some of the more common infectious diseases that may be encountered within a clinical environment and their corresponding modes of transmission and spread.

It is important for the massage therapist to be aware that infectious agents are a part of the working environment. Knowledge of the sources and spread of infectious diseases, as already discussed in this chapter, enables the therapist to use professional judgment in the application of personal protective equipment and disinfection and cleaning routines for the clinic to achieve the best outcome for personal and client care.

Table 10.1 Examples of some common diseases in a clinical setting and their mechanisms of transmission

ORGANISM	TYPE OF ORGANISM	TRANSMITTED BY	DISEASE
Influenza virus A Influenza virus B Influenza virus C	Virus	Respiratory droplets Water aerosols	Influenza
Rhinovirus Parainfluenza virus	Virus	Respiratory droplets Water aerosols	Common cold
Staphylococcus aureus	Bacteria	Direct contact Indirect contact (clothes, furnishings etc.)	Can infect most parts of the body including skin
Streptococcus pyogenes	Bacteria	Direct contact Airborne Cellulitis	Tonsillitis Scarlet fever
Tinea pedis (athlete's foot) *Tinea corporis* (ringworm)	Fungus	Direct skin-to-skin contact Foot baths (for Tinea pedis)	Cutaneous fungal infection
Pediculus humanus (body lice) *Pediculus capitus* (head lice)	Parasite	Direct contact Indirect contact with eggs	Dermatitis

POLICIES AND PROCEDURAL REQUIREMENTS

Many sections throughout this chapter discuss the implementation of policies and procedures for the workplace. The legal requirements of written documentation of these procedures will differ dependent on local state or territory legislation and it can be difficult in a busy clinic environment to regulate and monitor all of these practices. A well organised and safe clinic workplace should allocate time for these procedures to be proactively implemented and develop a routine quality control protocol to check that all cleaning and disinfecting tasks are completed and a safe workplace results. A simple checklist can be developed for each room to ensure that procedures are carried out and signed off. As well as the reassurance this provides for the therapist in the knowledge that they are providing a safe environment for themselves, their employees and their clients, it is also a written record that the clinic is adopting best practices. Other documentation that may be useful for the massage clinic is an incident reporting protocol. Any incidents or accidents are recorded and policies can then be set in place to prevent any further occurrences.

Further information

The topics and areas of discussion around infection control are vast and cannot be completely covered in this chapter. Therapists seeking further information on infection control measures, the epidemiology of infectious diseases in Australia and safe work practices are directed to the National Health and Medical Research Council (2002) working document on infection control and the Victorian Government *Blue Book*. Therapists in New Zealand are advised to consult their governing authority or professional massage association.

CONCLUSION

This chapter has described the importance of infection control practices for massage therapists in the clinical environment. Therapists need to be aware of the potential hazards that infectious diseases pose to themselves and others in their care. Although the risk of disease transmission is small, the implementation of Standard Precautions in the clinic environment will reduce that risk, dramatically providing a safe workplace for therapists and clients. In addition, these practices offer therapists information and techniques to safely and confidently handle accidents and incidents that may arise.

Questions and activities

1. For the professional massage therapist, cleanliness of the massage environment is of utmost importance. Describe the massage process and state all potential sources of microbes in the massage environment.
2. As a massage therapist, what would you do to ensure your personal hygiene is of a high standard for practice?
3. Discuss the factors that would need to be considered when designing policies and procedures for the control of infection in a clinical setting.

REFERENCES

Black, J. G. (2002) *Microbiology: Principles and Explorations* (5th edn). John Wiley and Sons, New York.

Haslett, C., Chilvers, E. R., Hunter, J. A. A. and Boon, N. A. (eds) (1999) *Davidson's Principles and Practice of Medicine* (18th edn). Churchill Livingstone, Edinburgh, p. 178.

Lee, G. and Bishop, P. (2002) *Microbiology and infection control for the health professions* (2nd edn). Prentice Hall Health, Australia.

National Health and Medical Research Council (1996) *Infection Control in the Health Care Setting; Guidelines for the Prevention of Transmission of Infectious Diseases*. National Health and Medical Research Council (NHMRC), Canberra.

—— (2002) *Draft Infection Control in the Health Care Setting*. National Health and Medical Research Council (NHMRC), Canberra.

Vickers, A and Zollman, C. (1999) 'Massage Therapies', *British Medical Journal*, 319, pp. 1254–7.

Victorian Government (2003) *The Blue Book: Infection Control Procedures and Practices*. Victorian Government Printing Service, Victoria.

section 5

Initial Client Contact

chapter 11

The massage process

Charles Tuchtan

Learning outcomes

- Apply the ASTER system to guide consultations
- Record appropriate information without hesitation or omission
- Describe the format and list the benefits of a health history form
- Conduct fruitful client interviews
- Follow the statutory guidelines governing data collection
- Fill in ASTER charts quickly, using an accepted system of abbreviations

INTRODUCTION

To be successful in clinical practice a massage therapist needs the ability to perform massage manipulations in a masterful fashion. In addition to this the massage therapist must also have the skills to assess the needs of the client, develop a treatment plan that is designed specifically for that client, perform the treatment, evaluate the treatment and then accurately and thoroughly record the entire consultation process.

To assist in the accomplishment of these tasks, it is common for the massage therapist to adopt a strategy or use a 'formula' to prompt them to complete each of these tasks in a thorough and precise manner. Such formulas are often abbreviated to acronyms, and one common process often adopted by experienced therapists is SOAP charting.

The acronym SOAP stands for Subjective Objective Assessment Plan. A useful tool for experienced therapists, SOAP charting requires a sound knowledge of clinical assessment skills to be able to document all the requirements of a SOAP chart. As such, this chapter introduces the concept of ASTER charting as a functional alternative that is easy to use and assist the massage therapist in practice to accomplish each of the objectives of a professional consultation.

The ASTER formula provides a consultation process and a documentation chart for the massage therapist. Through learning the ASTER formula the massage student will effectively learn to conduct a professional relaxation massage consultation and be able to employ the formula as a prompt during consultations, after they are competent and skilled in clinical practice. The ASTER system of charting is comprised of five sequential components, as follows:

A – Assess client needs
S – Select treatment plan
T – Treat
E – Evaluate
R – Record

The purpose of this chapter is to identify and explain each of the components of the ASTER charting system. Each of the components will be addressed within the context of the scope of practice of a relaxation massage therapist. For this reason discussion of the range of joint movement, orthopaedic assessment and muscle testing have been excluded from this chapter.

A – ASSESS CLIENT NEEDS

The first component of ASTER involves the assessment. Such an assessment aims to ascertain the presenting needs of the client. The assessment of a client's needs involves evaluating the client's own goals for massage therapy and establishing the client's previous medical history. The assessment would also include discussion of the presenting symptomatology, any aggravating circumstances, any changes in activity due to the complaint and the onset or initial cause of the symptoms.

The gathering and recording of such information is vital for several reasons. Firstly, such information will assist in determining the client's needs and expectations for the massage. A therapist will encounter clients who have differing previous experiences with massage; one may have received massage treatments in the past with another therapist whilst one may have never received any form of massage therapy. As such, clients may present with very clear expectations of what the experience of receiving a massage might entail. For example, some clients may prefer and expect a deep treatment, whereas others may be seeking a light touch. If the therapist gains an insight of the client's previous experiences and/or current expectations the massage can then be appropriately designed to best meet the client's needs.

A therapist also gathers information to evaluate whether massage is a suitable treatment for the client's condition. Occasionally a client may present to a massage therapist with a known disease state or symptoms that would sound an alarm bell for the therapist. Take, for example, a client presenting with acute ankle pain. Upon questioning, the therapist may learn that the client injured the ankle by twisting it while playing football one week earlier and that the pain and swelling has not yet fully subsided. The client may also explain that they experience difficulty when trying to bear weight on the affected ankle during walking and thus have been forced to rest the ankle frequently and seek relief through the application of ice several times a day. They may also admit to using non-steroidal anti-inflammatory drugs (see Chapter 13) to reduce the pain. Through questioning, the massage therapist is able to determine that the injury sustained during the football game has not yet healed and that the affected region may still be inflamed (swollen). As acute (short-term) inflammation is considered an absolute contraindication to massage the therapist would automatically refer the client with the inflamed ankle injury to an appropriate health care practitioner for further investigation. Where the therapist, through appropriate questioning during the assessment, has ruled out any serious pathology, massage may be applied as indicated (see Chapter 12).

The massage therapist would gather information to establish the indications and any precautions to the use of massage therapy. Such information allows for the implementation of a safe and effective treatment plan. To illustrate this point let's consider a client who announces during questioning that he or she experiences chronic fatigue syndrome (CFS) (see Chapter 12). This client might complain of reduced energy levels and muscular aches and pains over most areas of their body. From the client's case history the therapist could determine the most appropriate treatment plan. Prior knowledge of the medical condition would allow the therapist to deliver an appropriate treatment strategy, which may involve light soft tissue manipulations as opposed to deep techniques, and last for only a short duration thereby reducing the possibility of exhausting the client. Box 11.1 lists valid reasons for the gathering and recording of client information.

> **Box 11.1** Reasons for gathering and recording client information
>
> - To determine the client's needs and expectations for massage.
> - To evaluate whether massage is appropriate for the client's condition.
> - To consider the indications and precautions of massage therapy, to enable a safe and effective treatment strategy.
> - To prompt the client to explore their physical sensations.
> - To note changes from previous massage sessions.
> - To exclude any contraindications that may preclude massage therapy.
> - To reveal where referral to an appropriate health care professional is necessary.

The assessment component of the ASTER charting system forms a critical first step in the consultation process. During the assessment the client and therapist take time to interact and determine the individual needs of the client whilst developing a mutual understanding and respect that will underpin all future treatments. Affording a client time to focus and reflect on their needs, although a novel experience for some therapists, is a vital part of the assessment process. With society's hectic pace many people find themselves constantly on 'fast forward', leaving their mind focused on their external environments with little time to consider their own physical and emotional needs. Encouraging a client to focus on and discuss their needs and sensations, whilst integrating the body and mind, will encourage them to be active participants in their own healing process.

The consultation process will highlight the exact needs and expectations of the client. Such information is best obtained through the completion of a health history form by the client, or elicited via an interview and accurately recorded in detail on an ASTER chart by the massage therapist.

Health history form

An efficient way to assess the client's needs is to have the client fill in a questionnaire prior to the commencement of the consultation. Aside from collecting the client's personal details, indications and contraindications for massage therapy, and previous massage experience, the health history form also serves as a written consent to the massage treatment.

A good health history form will contain the following particulars and be updated yearly or whenever there is a change in the client's details, whichever is sooner.

Personal information:
- name
- address
- phone number/s
- date of birth
- emergency contact details
- occupation
- recreational activities

Massage therapy information:
- previous massage treatment
- areas to be included/excluded from massage

Health history:
- previous medical history
- current medical history
- current medications
- recent treatment (such as surgery)

Disclaimer:
- consent to massage therapy
- outline of the scope of practice of the massage therapist
- outline of the confidential nature of the consultation and related procedures
- statement that all information provided is true and correct

This form may be given to the client prior to the commencement of massage on the day of treatment or alternatively may be mailed to the client prior to their first consultation for them to complete ahead of time. All details recorded on the health history form would be discussed during the client interview, allowing the client the opportunity to elaborate on their health history, previous massage experience and expectations. A sample health history form is provided in Figure 11.1.

Client interview

Once the client's health history form has been completed, it is discussed as part of the consultation during the client interview. Lasting for a short period, the interview aims to gather the necessary information already detailed above, and also generate further details about information given on the health history form (see Figure 11.1). The client interview will only be successful in meeting its aims if a positive and trusting relationship is established between the therapist and the client. Factors that contribute to the development of such a relationship include the setting of the clinic (see Chapter 8), the therapist's appearance, the therapist's intent and interviewing skills.

Figure 11.1 Sample health history form

CONFIDENTIAL MASSAGE HEALTH HISTORY FORM

Please complete this form as best as you can and return it to the receptionist. Please print clearly.

Name: ....
Address: ....
.... Post Code: ....
Phone Home: .... Work: ....
Occupation: ....
Date of birth: ....
Recreational activities: ....
Contact telephone number in case of emergency: ....
How did you first hear about us? ....
Have you had a massage before?   Yes ❑   No ❑
Do you experience any difficulty lying on your front?   Yes ❑   No ❑
Do you experience any difficulty lying on your back?   Yes ❑   No ❑
Please tick (✓) all conditions that apply now. Put a **P** for past conditions.

___ Heart, circulatory problems   ___ Cancer/tumours   ___ Vision problems or contact lenses
___ High/low blood pressure   ___ Asthma or lung conditions   ___ Hearing problems
___ Varicose veins   ___ Hernias   ___ Fatigue
___ Blood clots   ___ Abdominal or digestive problems   ___ Depression
___ Phlebitis   ___ Arthritis   ___ Seizures
___ Infectious disease   ___ Numbness or tingling   ___ Stroke
___ Rash, athlete's foot/tinea   ___ Muscle, bone injuries   ___ Skin disorders
___ Allergies   ___ Muscle or joint pain   ___ Previous motor vehicle
___ Diabetes   ___ Chronic pain   accident/trauma
___ Pregnancy   ___ Headaches or migraines   ___ Prosthesis or dentures

Other medical conditions or injuries not listed (past and present): ....
....
....
Current medications, including aspirin, ibuprofen, herbs, vitamin, etc: ....
....
....
Recent surgeries: ....
....
....
Consent is required to massage each part of the body. Please indicate which areas you would like included:
❑ Back   ❑ Buttocks   ❑ Legs   ❑ Feet   ❑ Arms   ❑ Stomach   ❑ Chest   ❑ Face   ❑ Head
I understand that:
In accordance with the scope of practice of a massage therapist as well as adhering to regulatory and statutory requirements it is not the role of the massage therapist to diagnose injury or illness, or prescribe medication.
Signature:...Date: ....

During this information-gathering process the therapist may gain information from the client by asking simple, clear and precise questions. It is essential that the therapist possess good listening skills, including the ability to be an attentive listener. The style of the client interview may be tailored to suit the therapist's preference and the line of questioning may include open-ended or closed questions or a combination of both types of questioning. Open-ended questions allow the client to respond freely without restriction. For example, asking a client if they can describe their pain enables the client to express their feelings using their own terminology, thus avoiding the client being led to a particular response. As this type of questioning provides much freedom to the respondent it is essential that the question be precise to prevent long and irrelevant responses.

Closed questions may be phrased in a similar manner to a multiple-choice question, in that there is usually a correct or desired response. For example, a therapist may enquire as to the quality of a client's pain, asking 'is it dull and aching, sharp and localised or throbbing and intense?' Although this type of questioning is to the point, it may be limiting and lead to inaccurate responses as the client may feel they need to choose one of the options despite their situation not ideally matching any of the response choices offered. Such styles of questioning may require follow-up questions to facilitate further discussion to allow the therapist to gain a better insight into the client's condition.

As a general rule carefully structured open-ended questions should predominate during the client interview whilst closed questions are best kept to a minimum. Examples of questions that may assist the therapist to determine the appropriate treatment plan are detailed below.

Questions to evaluate the reasons for massage

- What brings you in for a massage today?
- Have you ever had a professional massage, and if so, when was the last time you had a massage?
- What are you looking for in massage?
- Which part(s) of your body become fatigued or ache?
- In which part(s) of your body do you feel stress most often (head, neck, shoulders, back, digestive tract, extremities, other)?
- Do you have a preference for music or aroma (essential oils)?
- You have indicated on you health history form that you would like the following areas included during the massage. Can I clarify these with you before we begin?

Questions to evaluate indications and contraindications

After reviewing the client's health history form the following questions may be asked:

- You have marked … on your health history form; can you tell me how this condition affects you?
- How long have you had this condition?
- What treatments, if any, are you receiving for this condition?
- Who is/are the health professional(s) providing the treatment? Do I have permission to contact them?
- Are you currently taking any medication? If so, what medications?

Questions to evaluate current symptoms

Clients often present to the massage clinic with aches and pains without having seen an appropriate health professional for a diagnosis. Many aches and pains presenting to a massage therapist could be the result of the strains of everyday life including stress, postural habits or overuse. Through gaining an awareness and understanding of the client's symptoms a massage therapist may determine whether massage therapy is in fact the most suitable form of treatment or if referral is more appropriate for the client. If massage is appropriate then a determination should be sought as to whether the massage should be modified (see Chapter 12). If the therapist is unsure of what path to take, referral to an appropriate health professional should be made prior to any treatment being performed. It should be noted that the formulation of a diagnosis is outside the scope of practice of a massage therapist (see Chapter 6).

The following questions may be asked to enable the therapist to evaluate the client's current symptoms:

- Do you have any pain, discomfort and/or stiffness today?
- Can you show me where the pain, discomfort and/or stiffness is?
- What is the pain like?
- How and when did the symptoms begin?
- What makes the pain worse?
- What relieves the pain?
- Is there any time of the day that the pain eases or is worse?
- How has this problem affected your life?
- Have you seen a health professional for this problem? If so, do you mind if I contact them in relation to your condition?

It is imperative that all relevant information obtained through questioning during the client interview is accurately recorded.

S – SELECT TREATMENT PLAN

Once the client has completed the health history form, and its contents have been discussed during a client interview, the massage therapist together with the client may determine the best course of treatment. This would involve the development of a treatment plan that the client should consent to. The therapist has a professional and ethical responsibility to liaise with the client when devising the treatment plan. Any treatment should always be designed around the client's needs. The therapist has a duty to explain the benefits and/or risks of the suggested treatment plan to the client. On occasions, based on the information gathered, the therapist may need to refuse to provide a treatment; this is referred to as the *right of refusal* (see Chapter 7). Such refusal would most likely occur when the therapist discovers an absolute contraindication to the application of massage therapy. The therapist is obliged to discuss the reasons for refusal with the client and refer them to an appropriate health professional.

Once the massage therapist has discussed the benefits and potential risks (such as residual pain following deep treatment) of the proposed treatment plan they must seek informed consent before commencing any treatment (see Chapter 6). It should be noted that the client has the right to accept, refuse or amend any proposed treatment plan in consultation with the therapist. Such procedures could be carried out verbally. However, health professionals are increasingly seeking a written consent that is signed by the client prior to administration of treatment. Along with the client's written permission for massage a consent agreement may also include the following information:

- the treatment goals;
- the areas of the body that are to be massaged and in what order;
- the duration of the massage;
- the degree of undress that is recommended and the draping procedures;
- the positions the client will adopt during the massage;
- the procedure to climb on and off the massage table;
- the obligation of the client to inform the therapist of any unusual sensation or discomfort during the treatment;
- an explanation of the potential muscle soreness that can be experienced following the massage treatment;
- the role of massage as an ancillary health aid rather than a primary medical treatment;
- the right of the client to alter any part of the treatment plan or cease the massage at any time.

If a written consent agreement is to be used its existence and the client's consent to treatment should be noted in the treatment record documents.

T – TREAT

Once all relevant information pertaining to the client has been gathered through the assessment and client interview, and the treatment plan has been selected in consultation with the client, the massage therapist should be ready to commence the treatment the client consented to during the interview.

Whilst performing the massage treatment the therapist should use palpation to assess the tissue for any problem areas. Palpation is the primary skill of the massage therapist and involves the placement of the therapist's hands on the client's tissues to assess their condition. Palpation skills are cumulative and like any skill must be practised and refined (Rattray and Ludwig, 2000). Through practice the therapist's palpation skills can be refined and improved with every treatment they perform. The greater the number of clients the therapist encounters the greater the variations in tissue quality the therapist will experience.

Rattray and Ludwig (2000) describe the four 'Ts' of palpation: temperature, texture, tenderness and tone. When the therapist palpates the client's tissues during the massage each of the four Ts provides valuable information to the therapist. Such information may lead the therapist to reconsider the treatment plan and, after discussion with the client, perform a revised treatment plan.

Placing a hand over the forehead of someone to assess their temperature is an assessment tool that has been used by the layperson as well as health professionals for centuries. A massage therapist may adapt this same crude assessment technique during treatment, as an area of tissue that feels excessively hot may indicate local inflammation, resulting from infection or even injury.

The term 'texture' is used to describe the way in which a surface feels beneath the fingertips. Whilst performing soft tissue manipulations the therapist will notice the texture of the body tissues. When massaging over healthy areas of tissue the texture will feel uniform and uninterrupted. However tissues that are injured or damaged will possess a distinctive texture, often quite different to that of healthy tissue. For example, when feeling acute oedema the texture of the tissue will be firm. When a therapist massages over a soft tissue adhesion the texture may feel quite rough and bumpy, almost like corrugated iron. During the treatment the therapist should make note of the texture of the regions they are massaging and note changes in texture over subsequent treatments.

During the massage the therapist may stroke over the soft tissues such as muscle, tendon or ligaments. Occasionally while compressing these tissues the client may indicate discomfort, tenderness or even pain. They may convey such feelings verbally by saying 'ouch' or imply them via their body language, perhaps by tensing an area of tissue or making a pained expression. Such feedback on the tenderness of tissue will assist the therapist with their treatment.

Muscle tone is defined as the tension within a muscle at rest (Tuchtan and Tuchtan, 2000). When a muscle is overused, misused or guarding an injured area, the muscle shortens, thus increasing the muscle's tension. Such an area would be referred to as a hypertonic (hyper = excess) muscle lesion. The opposite may occur when a muscle is under-utilised, such as following six weeks in a plaster cast due to a broken limb, during which time the muscle becomes small, weak and flaccid. Such areas would be known as a hypotonic (hypo = insufficient) muscle lesion. More often than not a massage therapist deals with hypertonic musculature. Such lesions are located predominantly in postural muscles, including the paraspinal muscles of the back and the superficial muscles of the neck, as well as the regions of the low back and buttocks.

The massage treatment should follow the treatment plan outlined by the therapist and agreed to by the client. If during the course of the treatment the client identifies an area of pain or discomfort not initially outlined in the health history form or discussed in the client interview, the therapist should first consult the client and gain consent for any modification to the original treatment plan. All information pertaining to temperature, texture, tenderness and tone, gathered during a treatment through the palpation skills of the therapist, should be noted in the treatment records. Such a treatment record chronicles all treatment sessions, and details the client's information and responses relating to the massage therapy in the ASTER charting system.

E – EVALUATE

From the minute the massage therapist makes first contact with the client an evaluation has already begun; this includes evaluating the suitability of the client while making an initial appointment, assessing the client's needs and a continual evaluation throughout the treatment. Evaluation is ongoing. However, the fourth component of the ASTER charting process is the formal evaluation, which establishes the success of the treatment performed. During the application of the treatment the therapist may detect changes in the texture of tissues via palpation that will serve as a form of evaluation. For example, when commencing massage of the posterior thigh and leg with a rowing stroke the therapist is able to evaluate the state of the tissue, noting the four Ts. The therapist may detect hypertonicity in the hamstring muscle group and, when appropriate, continue to perform massage manipulations over the area. In doing so, such massage may potentially create a change in the tissue texture, via a decrease in muscle tone. During any massage treatment the therapist should perform evaluations of the tissue at regular intervals, to assess any changes in condition.

During a treatment a client will also provide verbal feedback as to the effectiveness of the treatment. Gaining verbal feedback from the client plays an essential role in evaluating the success of the treatment. For example, a client may notice a change in their muscle tone during the massage, and may report a reduction in local muscle pain. Once the massage treatment has concluded the client should be encouraged to stand and gently move their joints, to notice any changes. The client may report increased freedom of movement, reduced stiffness or increased comfort, providing a vital evaluation of the success of the treatment. All verbal feedback from the client should be noted in the treatment record. If the client reports a negative response to the treatment consideration must be given as to the reason for such feedback. The massage therapist must explain the reason for this to the client, reassess the treatment plan for future sessions or refer the client to an appropriate health professional.

R – RECORD

The final stage of the ASTER process involves recording the consultation process. The client record is considered to be an accurate account of the client's related medical information, and consists of the health history form, additional information gathered during the client interview, and information regarding prior assessment, treatment or referral for the client. This process of ongoing record keeping is known as *charting*.

Medical records are an essential component of any massage consultation. The information collected and recorded assists the massage therapist to provide ongoing professional client care. The written document is a testament to the assessment, treatment plan, treatment and evaluation performed. Reasons for keeping a client record include:

- to enable the therapist to track a client's progress;
- to assist the therapist to recall previous assessment, treatment and evaluation, enabling the therapist to deliver more specific and beneficial treatment;
- to allow the therapist to communicate with other health care professionals in the same clinic who may be treating the same client;
- to form, with the client's written permission, a part of the medico-legal report;
- to provide, with the client's written permission, a record of treatment for private health insurance companies;
- to provide the therapist with accurate information of the entire consultation if the therapist is called as a witness in any legal proceeding.

As a complete document the client record consists of the client questionnaire (as discussed earlier), the ASTER chart and any other documentation collected from other health professionals. There are key features that must be documented on the ASTER chart, and these include: reasons for the treatment, presenting signs and symptoms, contraindications and precautions, treatment plan, client consent, treatment findings and the evaluation (see Box 11.2).

Guidelines for good record keeping

It is vital that the massage therapist maintain accurate, thorough and detailed client records. As no professional body, insurance agency or government department currently stipulate guidelines as to how to correctly format or document medical reports, the following recommendations are suggested to assist the therapist to maintain accurate, thorough and detailed client records.

Accurate, concise and comprehensive records

A massage therapist must ensure that the information recorded in the client record is accurate and comprehensive, yet brief. Everything that is medically relevant should be concisely included. The accuracy of the record is imperative. For example, there is a marked difference between stating the 'client has low back pain' and 'client complains of low back pain'. The first statement is definitive whereas the second statement describes the view of the client who may instead have buttock or pelvic pain and calls it low back pain. The therapist should be sure to include the client's informed consent or refusal of any part of the treatment.

The documentation must be able to withstand independent scrutiny. This is important as the record or part of the record may be passed onto other health care professionals or be subpoenaed in cases of legal action. As such the therapist should keep in mind that the written comments contained in the client's record, including those referring to the type of care given, the client's condition, their observed demeanour or perceived state of mind may be used at a later time as evidence in an action for negligence, malpractice or the like. The therapist must ensure the record is an honest and thorough account of all interactions with the client.

Objectivity

All language used within a written report should be objective and definitive. The massage therapist should ensure all words used in the report describe what was observed rather than make assumptions as to the client's condition or allude to a diagnosis. For example, 'the client appears to have suffered a stroke' would be best reported as follows:

- the client's speech is slurred;
- the client has motor and sensory impairment on the right-hand side.

Time

When a therapist works in a busy practice it may be difficult to recall accurate details of clients and any previous treatments. To assist with recall the client record may be used. Once a treatment has been performed the therapist should document all details in the client record immediately after the consultation or as soon as possible after the treatment has ceased. For accuracy of record keeping it is recommended that the recording of the client's needs and clinical presentation takes

---

Box 11.2 Recording the consultation

- Name
- Date of consultation
- Current medication
- Reasons for treatment
- Presenting signs and symptoms
- Contraindications and precautions
- Needs of referral
- Overall health
- Treatment plan
- Consent
- Finding on treatment
- Evaluation

place during the interview, and that the treatment plan be recorded prior to the application of any treatment. Once the treatment has concluded, and the client is returning to a state of dress, the treatment procedures and the evaluation should be recorded. All entries should be prefaced with the date, time and signature of the therapist.

Legibility

All contents of the client record must be legible. Records that are unable to be read or understood by others may lead to incorrect interpretation that may result in mistakes being made. If decisions impact upon illegible writing it is essential that the massage therapist checks with the source before continuing the treatment.

Medical terminology

The massage therapist should have a thorough understanding of appropriate medical terminology. Using medical terminology incorrectly may prove to be ambiguous or confusing to another health practitioner.

Abbreviations and symbols

Abbreviations and symbols are often used as a shorthand form of documenting information that is used to save time and space. The abbreviations and symbols in Table 11.1 are common abbreviations used throughout the massage profession as well as abbreviations used in medical terminology. It is important that the therapist adopt the use of such abbreviations as the use of any uncommon abbreviations may confuse other health practitioners accessing client records. To enable the massage therapist and any other health professional with approved access to client files to interpret all records it is recommended a key to abbreviated terms be available, located within proximity of the file; for example, on the front of a filing cabinet that stores records.

> **Box 11.3** Guidelines for good record keeping
>
> - Record client's name. Check spelling is correct. Date of birth can be a further identifier.
> - Write accurately, concisely and comprehensively.
> - Write objectively.
> - Record during the consultation or immediately after treatment.
> - Begin each new entry with the date, time and your signature.
> - Write legibly.
> - Use appropriate medical terminology.
> - Use only commonly accepted abbreviations, symbols and terms.
> - Use ink.
> - Cross through a mistake with a single line, and initial the change.
> - Never erase or use white-out.
> - If blank spaces exist, draw a line through it so that other information cannot be added by others who may have access to the file.
>
> (adapted from Forrester and Griffiths, 2001; Van Leuven, 2000; Staunton and Chiarella, 2003)

Errors

As client reports are legal documents they must be written in ink. If a therapist makes an error on the record a correction should be made by simply placing a single line through the incorrect information. The use of correction fluid or total obliteration of the incorrect entry may suggest to a third party that the massage therapist may have something they wish to conceal. Writing over or altering the mistaken words may cause confusion and misunderstanding and should be avoided.

Table 11.1 Common abbreviations and symbols

MASSAGE TERMS		MUSCLE ABBREVIATIONS	
XFF	cross fibre friction	QL	quadratus lumborum
MLD	manual lymph drainage	SCM	sternocleidomastoid
MET	muscle energy technique	lats	latissimus dorsi
PNF	proprioceptive neuromuscular facilitation	lev scap	levator scapulae
		trap	trapezius
STM	soft tissue manipulation	delt	deltoid
DTM	deep tissue manipulation	pec −, +	pectoralis minor, major
Ⓜ	massage	gastroc	gastrocnemius
FBM	full body massage	TFL	tensor fascia latae

Table 11.1 Common abbreviations and symbols (continued)

Sw	Swedish massage	abs	abdominals
MFR	myofascial release	bi	biceps
TPR	trigger-point release	gluts	gluteal muscle group
NMT	neuromuscular technique	quads	quadriceps femoris
CS	counter-strain	rhomb	rhomboids
PRT	positional release technique	sol	soleus
		tri	triceps

JOINT ACTIONS

flex	flexion
ext	extension
Add	adduction
Abd	abduction
rot	rotation
Ext rot	external rotation
Int rot	internal rotation
sup	supination
pron	pronation
SB	side bending
inv	inversion
evr	eversion
U/Dev	ulnar deviation
R/dev	radial deviation
protr	protraction
retr	retraction
ROM	range of motion
A, P, R-ROM	active, passive, resisted-range of motion
WNL	within normal limits

SYMBOLS

∅	none, no
ⓟ	pain
Δ	change
−	minus
+	plus
x	times
↑	increase, higher
↓	decrease, lower
→	leads to
<	less than
>	greater than
≈	approximately

ANATOMICAL LOCATIONS

C1-7	cervical vertebrae 1 through to 7
T1-12	thoracic vertebrae 1 through to 12
L1-5	lumbar vertebrae 1 through to 5
Cx	cervical spine
Tx	thoracic spine
Lx	lumbar spine
Sx	sacral spine
ft	foot or feet
lig	ligament
jt	joint
AC	acromio-clavicular
Paravert	around or attaching to the vertebrae
TVP	transverse process
SP	spinous process
ITB	ilio-tibial band
SI	sacro-iliac
LB	low back

DIRECTIONAL TERMINOLOGY

Ⓛ	left
Ⓡ	right
sup.	superior
inf.	inferior
ant.	anterior
post.	posterior
med.	medial
lat.	lateral
caud.	caudal
ceph.	cephalad
prox.	proximal
dist.	distal
int.	internal
ext.	external
SL	side lying

Table 11.1 Common abbreviations and symbols (continued)

ABD	abdomen
IVD	intervertebral disc
Z jt	zygophophyseal joint
CES	cervical erector spinae
TES	thoracic erector spinae
LES	lumbar erector spinae
Sh	shoulder

BODY SYSTEMS, ASSESSMENT FINDINGS AND MALADIES

LxP	lumbar spinal pain			
SxP	sacral spinal pain			
Loin P	loin pain			
Glut P	gluteal pain			
TxP	thoracic spinal pain			
CxP	cervical spinal pain			
GI	gastrointestinal			
GU	genitourinary			
Resp	respiration			
Circ	circulation			
HT	hypertonicity			
Adh.	adhesion			
TrP	trigger point			
AMC	abnormal muscle contraction			
Sp	spasm			
Ten^n	tension			
str.	strain			
spr.	sprain			
#	fracture			
Scol	scoliosis			
Lord	lordosis			
kyph	kyphosis			
OA	osteoarthritis			
RA	rheumatoid arthritis			
DJD	degenerative joint disease			
CA	cancer			
CVA	cerebrovascular accident, stroke			
MVA	motor vehicle accident			
H/A	headache			
CFS	chronic fatigue syndrome			
MS	multiple sclerosis			
CP	cerebral palsy			
DM	diabetes mellitus			
UTI	urinary tract infection			
URI	upper respiratory infection			
Agg	aggravate			
Rel	relieve			
NAR	no apparent reason			
NAD	nothing abnormal detected			

MEDICAL RECORD TERMS

Rx	treatment
Hx	history
Dx	diagnosis
N/A	not applicable
c/o	complains of
mm	muscle
pt	patient
cl	client
Ⓚ	constant
freq.	frequency
inter.	intermittent
hr	hour
1/7	1 day
1/52	1 week
1/12	1 month
meds	medication
OTC	over the counter
PRN	as necessary/as needed
qd	every day
bid	twice a day
qid	four times a day
qod	every other day
ac	before meals
pc	after meals
qhs	at bedtime
po	orally
pr	rectally
iv	intravenous
sc	subcutaneous
im	intramuscular
PA	postural analysis
DDx	differential diagnosis
Prog	prognosis
HW	home work

Recording using ASTER

It is unfortunate that at times a therapist may consider the recording of information to be a cumbersome and time-consuming task. To assist in making this necessary task easier the massage therapist would be wise to adopt a recording system such as the ASTER approach. Such an approach also ensures the therapist maintains accurate, thorough and detailed client records.

Three ASTER charts are illustrated in Figure 11.2. As each ASTER chart has limited space for information to be documented the therapist should adopt the abbreviation system previously described. An example of a documented case using the abbreviations described is provided in Figure 11.3.

SOAP charting

SOAP (Subjective, Objective, Assessment, Plan) charting, similar to ASTER charting, is another documentation system used widely throughout the massage profession as well as with the medical and other allied health professions. SOAP is an acronym that is broken down into four categories (Thompson, 2002):

1. *Subjective*: stores the client perceptions — current health concern, recent and past medical history.
2. *Objective*: stores the therapist's findings — observations, testing and other measurable data; intervention and client's response to treatment.
3. *Assessment*: formulates diagnosis and prognosis (the likely course and outcome of the disease).
4. *Plan*: documents the treatment plan and any take-home exercises prescribed, documents any referrals.

SOAP charting may be difficult for many massage therapists in Australia and New Zealand, who have minimal clinical assessment skills except that of history taking, and have a limited knowledge of pathology and are therefore unable to formulate a diagnosis or prognosis. The ASTER process may be an easier and more effective format for these individuals.

Government legislation and record keeping

All client records are subject to certain legal requirements. These legal requirements were formed either through government legislation or common law. Many of the recommendations under guidelines for good record keeping were based on recommendations made through common law cases. The information below is privacy and health record Acts and Codes developed in Australia and New Zealand over the last decade.

Australia

The *Privacy Act 1988* was amended in 2000 to cover comprehensive privacy law for private organisations including health service providers in Australia. This Act provides privacy protections for clients as well as providing scope for health professionals to share information. The amendment to the Act provides 10 National Privacy Principles (NPP), which establish the minimum standard for the private health care sector (see Figure 11.4).

At present Victoria and New South Wales (NSW) are the only states to have a comprehensive data protection regime. The Victorian state government passed the *Health Records Act* in 2001 and the NSW state government passed the *Health Records and Information Privacy Act* in 2002. Like the Commonwealth's *Privacy Act 2000*, the Victorian *Health Records Act 2001* and the NSW *Health Records and Information Privacy Act 2002* establishes standards for the handling of health information. This Act describes Health Privacy Principles (HPP) similar to those of the Commonwealth's *Privacy Act*. In the Victorian *Health Records Act* Principle 4 of the HPP discusses data security and data retention. It states that a health professional must keep client information for a period of no less than seven years following the last occasion on which a health service was provided to the client, or if the client was a minor (under 18 years of age) at the time of the last consultation, then all records must be kept until the child reaches 25 years of age. Similarly this is also discussed in Part 4, Division 2 of the NSW *Health Records and Information Privacy Act 2002* under Retention of Health Information.

The Australian Capital Territory passed the *Health Records (Access & Privacy) Act* in 1997. It is based on the NPP and is intended to allow patients access to their own medical records in the public and private sectors.

The Northern Territory Government is currently developing privacy legislation for use in the public sector.

The other states have issued instructions requiring broad compliance by government agencies with the NPP but appear to be moving towards separate privacy legislation covering public or private sector bodies. In regard to retention of client records it is advisable that all massage therapists follow similar requirements to those for Victoria and NSW.

CHAPTER 11 THE MASSAGE PROCESS 131

Figure 11.2 Three ASTER chart samples

Client's Name: ....

Rx Date: ....Time: ....Current Meds: ....

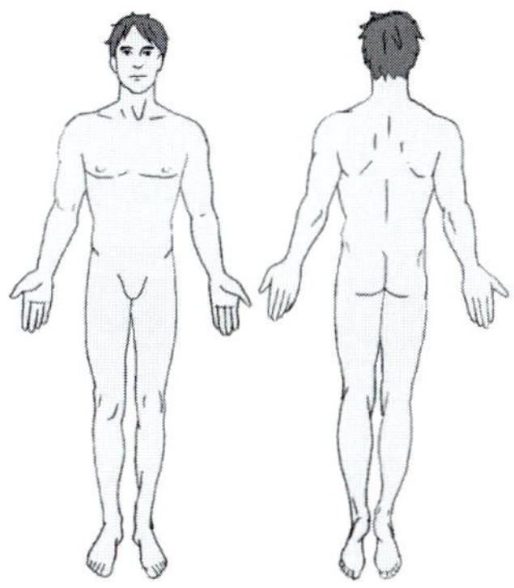

Therapist's signature: ....recording date & time: ....

Rx Date: ....Time: ....Current Meds: ....

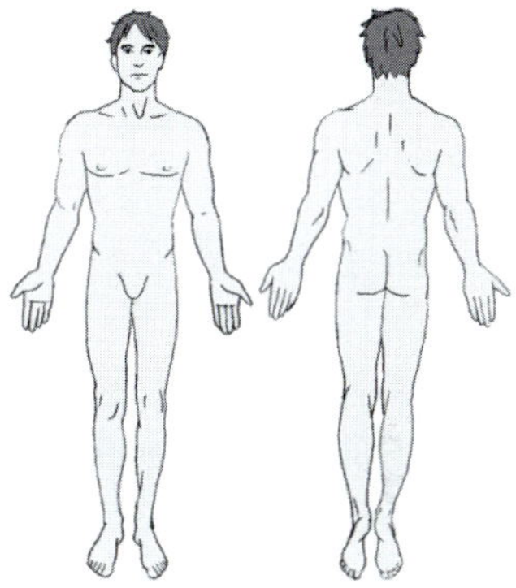

Therapist's signature: ....recording date & time: ....

Rx Date: ....Time: ....Current Meds: ....

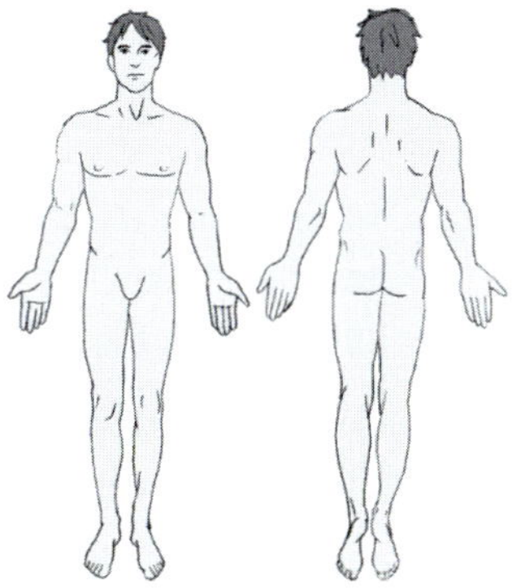

Therapist's signature: ....recording date & time: ....

Symbols for figure drawing:

X	Trp
≈	Spasm

∿	Adh
Ⓟ	Pain

≡	Hypertonicity
( )	Rotation

✱	Swelling
↗	Elevation

Figure 11.3 Case study

ASSESS NEEDS

Therapist. What can I do for you today?
Client. I'd like a relaxation massage.
T. Do you have any problem areas?
C. Yes, I fell off my bike yesterday and landed on my left hand and shoulder, grazing the whole area.
T. Have you seen your local doctor regarding this fall?
C. Yes, and he said I have just a few grazes that will clear up in a few weeks.
T. Are you on any medication at present?
C. The doctor told me to take aspirin twice a day to reduce the pain and reduce the inflammation.
T. (check contraindications list from client questionnaire)

SELECT TREATMENT PLAN

T. Today I think it would be best if we give you a full body relaxation massage with the exception of your left arm, so that it can recover. How does that sound?
C. Sounds fine.
T. A full body massage will commence with the back and neck followed by the back of the thighs, legs and feet. I will then ask you to turn over and massage the front of the legs, thighs, abdomen, chest, right arm and conclude with the face and scalp. How does that sound?
C. Sounds great.
T. Once I've left the room, could you disrobe to your underwear and lie face down on the treatment table and place your face in the hole? Here are some towels you can use to cover yourself up.
C. Okay.

TREAT

While performing a full body massage I found very tight and tender lower back muscles and buttocks. I also found a trigger point in the client's right levator scapulae muscle. I spent extra time working on these areas using deep cross-fibre friction techniques over the low back and buttocks, and trigger-point release and stretching on levator scapulae muscles. Client fell asleep during the massage.

EVALUATE

Decreased muscle tension was found throughout the lumbar erector spinae muscles and the gluteal muscle groups. The client reported a feeling of relaxation and an increased freedom of movement in his low back.

RECORD

Rx Date: 26-03-02   **Time:** 3:30 pm   **Current Meds:** Aspirin bid

A.   FBM, Reported: fell off bike and grazed Ⓛ arm & hand 1/7
S.   FBM – Ⓛ arm & hand, obtained client consent
T.   FBM, found AMC to LES & gluts used XFF over this region
     Ⓡ lev scap TrP found used TPR & STR
E.   ↓ LES & Glut AMC, ↓ TrP lev scap.
     Client reports feeling relaxed & ↑ Lx ROM

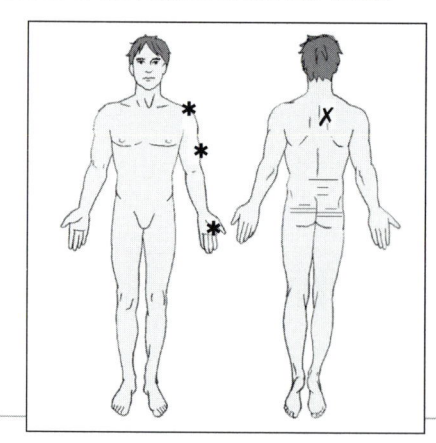

New Zealand

The New Zealand *Privacy Act 1993* applies to the handling of all personal information collected or held by government agencies and most businesses including health professionals. The legislation identifies 'personal information' as information about an identifiable living person, irrespective of whether it is on a computer or a paper file.

The legislation is based on 12 Information Privacy Principles (IPP), which are similar to the Australian NPP in the *Privacy Amendment (Private*

Sector) Act 2000. The Act allows the Privacy Commissioner to establish Codes of Practice that apply the Information Privacy Principles to specific activities and industries or to allow exemptions. In 1994 the commissioner established the *Health Information Privacy Code* which covers the Health Information Privacy Rules. For further information regarding New Zealand's Health Information Privacy Code 1994 go to *http://www.privacy.org.nz/comply/hinfopc.html#rule9*

Figure 11.4 The National Privacy Principles

1. COLLECTION

This section sets out the health professional's requirements for collecting information. Only necessary personal information can be collected by lawful and fair means. Before collecting the individual's personal information the health professional must explain the purpose for collecting information and any law that requires specific information to be collected, as well as gaining client consent before collecting the information.

2. USE AND DISCLOSURE

This section prohibits the use or disclosure of personal information about an individual for any purpose other than the primary reason for collecting the data, unless: the client has consented to it; the information is not of a sensitive nature; the information is health information and is necessary for research relevant to public health or safety; to prevent serious and imminent threat to the client's life, health or safety or to public health and safety; or if it is required or authorised by or under law.

3. DATA QUALITY

The health professional must take reasonable steps to ensure the personal information collected, used or disclosed is accurate, complete and up to date.

4. DATA SECURITY

The health professional must ensure reasonable steps are taken to protect the client's personal information from misuse and loss, or from unauthorised access, modification or disclosure.

5. OPENNESS

This section requires the health professional to be open about what client records are held, why and how they are kept, how they are collected and how they are used. This section also requires the health professional to develop a policy document on how client information is managed. This document must be made available to all who ask.

6. ACCESS AND CORRECTION

This section gives the client the right to access their personal records and a right to have the information corrected if incorrect, incomplete or out of date.

7. IDENTIFIERS

This section limits the use of identifiers (a number assigned by an organisation to identify the client, such as a Medicare number or private health insurance number) by a health professional to the purposes for which they were issued. That is, these identifiers cannot be used as client identification codes.

8. ANONYMITY

Where lawful and practicable, the client has the option of not identifying themselves when presenting at the clinic.

9. TRANSBORDER DATA FLOWS

This section sets out the terms for transferring client information out of Australia.

10. SENSITIVE INFORMATION

The health professional may collect sensitive information from the client only when the client has consented or is required to by law.

National Privacy Principles adapted from the *Privacy Amendment (Private Sector) Act 2000*

CONCLUSION

Adherence to the ASTER system can form the backbone of consistent, professional and comprehensive consultations. Good record keeping benefits both the client and the therapist. Accurate and up-to-date records help a therapist to recall quickly all relevant details of an individual client, assisting them to deliver the most appropriate treatment and to be alert to health changes over time. Useful information such as emergency contact details are always readily at hand, and during the consultation and recording process important information can be exchanged. The client is protected by statutory guidelines governing information collection and distribution, and the therapist is protected by having a signed consent form.

Questions and activities

1. Your client, Nancy, is suffering from neck pain and stiffness. The right side is mostly affected and is accompanied with restriction in movement. Headaches occur frequently for Nancy and she attributes this to stress and tension that builds up throughout her working day in front of a computer. She enjoys regular massage to ease the build up of tension in her neck and to reduce her levels of stress.

   On her health history form Nancy has noted that she has Type I diabetes and takes insulin injections to regulate her blood sugar levels.

   Nancy takes Panadol® (paracetamol) for her headaches when needed and uses a hot pack to ease the tension at the end of a working day.

   (a) Nancy is coming to you for massage for relief of tension in her neck and back. You are seeing her for the first time and wish to assess her needs thoroughly in this first meeting. What questions would you ask Nancy to gain information about her presenting complaint?

   (b) You are not familiar with the condition of diabetes and unsure about the impact massage will have. What questions will you ask Nancy to gain enough insight to perform a safe and effective massage?

   (c) Are there contraindications or precautions to this massage? If so list them.

   (d) You have gathered all the appropriate information from your client. What treatment plan would you recommend for a one-hour massage?

   (e) How would you record all this information on an ASTER form?

2. Erica is a 19 year-old girl who is undergoing psychiatric treatment for anorexia nervosa. She has never had a massage before and has been referred to you by her psychiatrist. She is currently on anti-depressant medication and feels nervous about receiving a massage.

   (a) How might massage benefit Erica?

   (b) What concerns might she have that you need to be aware of?

   (c) What modifications would you make to provide a safe and effective massage?

   (d) Complete an ASTER form using correct abbreviations to record a theoretical massage treatment you have performed on Erica.

Further reading

Forrester, K. and Griffiths, D. (2001) *Essentials of Law for Health Professionals*. Mosby, Sydney.

Fryer, G. (2001) 'Abbreviations for use in osteopathic case notes', *Journal of Osteopathic Medicine*, 4(1), pp. 21–4.

Sloane, S. B. (1997) *Medical Abbreviations and Eponyms* (2nd edn). Mosby, St Louis.

Thompson, D. L. (2002) *Hands Heal: Communication, Documentation, and Insurance Billing for Manual Therapists* (2nd edn). Lippincott Williams & Wilkins, Baltimore.

REFERENCES

Forrester, K. and Griffiths, D. (2001) *Essentials of Law for Health Professionals*. Mosby, Sydney.

Rattray, F. S. and Ludwig, L. M. (2000) *Clinical Massage Therapy: Understanding, Assessing and Treating Over 70 Conditions*. Talus Inc., Toronto.

Staunton, P. and Chiarella, B. (2003) *Nursing and the Law* (5th edn). Churchill Livingstone, Sydney.

Thompson, D. L. (2002) *Hands Heal: Communication, Documentation, and Insurance Billing for Manual Therapists* (2nd edn). Lippincott Williams & Wilkins, Baltimore.

Tuchtan, C. C. and Tuchtan, V. M. (2000) *Theory in Practice: Modern Soft Tissue Techniques*. Self-published, Melbourne.

Van Leuven, K. (2000) *Clinical Companion: Fundamentals of Nursing*. Prentice-Hall Health, New Jersey.

chapter 12

Endangerment sites and indications for the use of massage therapy

Vicki Tuchtan and Charles Tuchtan

Learning outcomes

- Recognise, locate and deal appropriately with endangerment sites
- Assess when massage treatment is contraindicated
- Recognise a large range of conditions or afflictions
- Safely treat partially contraindicated conditions to the beneficial extent available
- Know when referral to other health care professionals is necessary

INTRODUCTION

People can present to a massage therapist with a vast array of complaints, seeking outcomes ranging from temporary relief of pain or discomfort to a more curative treatment. On the whole, massage therapy may be indicated for many types of people and a multitude of bodily conditions. However, every therapist must be aware of certain regions of the body over which massage should be applied with caution. Such anatomical areas of the body are referred to as endangerment sites, and are massaged with care during the massage routine as manipulations over or around such locations may produce harm and result in temporary or permanent damage. In some circumstances, massage treatment is an unsuitable therapy to use on a person.

When massage therapy is contraindicated for use in certain situations, the symptoms responsible are referred to as absolute contraindications. A skilled massage therapist would be alerted to any absolute contraindications a client may exhibit during the initial consultation process. For clients presenting with any absolute contraindications, the application of massage therapy is likely to worsen their condition. A massage therapist would be wise to refer such clients to their primary care practitioner (such as a general practitioner, naturopath, osteopath or chiropractor) and avoid administering any massage treatment when absolute contraindications exist.

In addition to absolute contraindications this chapter outlines some common conditions with which clients may present to a massage therapist and describes the clinical features of each condition. The times when massage therapy should be used with caution or is best avoided are also discussed. By having an awareness of the typical presentation of many conditions that clients may present with, the skilled massage therapist is able to select and provide the best care and treatment for each and every individual client.

ENDANGERMENT SITES

Endangerment sites are areas of the body where bones, organs, nerves and blood vessels close to the skin are not well protected by muscles or connective tissue. Massage over these structures may damage them or cause discomfort or pain if caution is not used. The following section identifies the endangerment sites, their anatomical location and what precautions need to be applied (see Figure 12.1).

Back

Kidney region

The kidneys are located on both sides of the spine between the 12th thoracic vertebra and the 3rd lumbar vertebra, and sit in front of the posterior muscular wall. Heavy tapôtement should be avoided over the kidney region.

Neck

Anterior triangle of the neck

The anterior triangle of the neck is bordered by the sternocleidomastoid laterally, the mandible superiorly, the sternum inferiorly and the cervical midline medially. Included within these borders are the carotid artery, jugular vein, vagus nerve, larynx and thyroid gland. Deep pressure over any of these structures may be uncomfortable and dangerous, and should be avoided.

Posterior triangle of the neck

The posterior triangle of the neck is bordered inferiorly by the clavicle, anteriorly by the sternocleidomastoid and posteriorly by the anterior border of the trapezius. The superficial branches of the brachial plexus, the brachiocephalic artery, axillary artery and vein are found within the borders of the posterior triangle. Compression of these structures due to deep pressure can cause pain, paraesthesia and numbness of the upper extremity.

Anterior throat

The front of the throat consists of the larynx (the voice box) and the trachea (the windpipe). Although these structures are supported by cartilage, mild pressure over the anterior throat may cause discomfort and restriction of respiration. The application of massage should not be applied over the anterior throat.

Lymph nodes

Lymph nodes are small bean-shaped organs located along lymphatic vessels. In the neck region there are several concentrated areas of these nodes. The superficial cervical nodes lie along the external jugular vein and over the sternocleidomastoid. The occipital lymph nodes lie on the upper end of the trapezius muscle at the apex of the posterior triangle of the neck. Deep sustained pressure can inflame these lymphatic nodes, causing pain and discomfort; therefore deep pressure over these areas is best avoided.

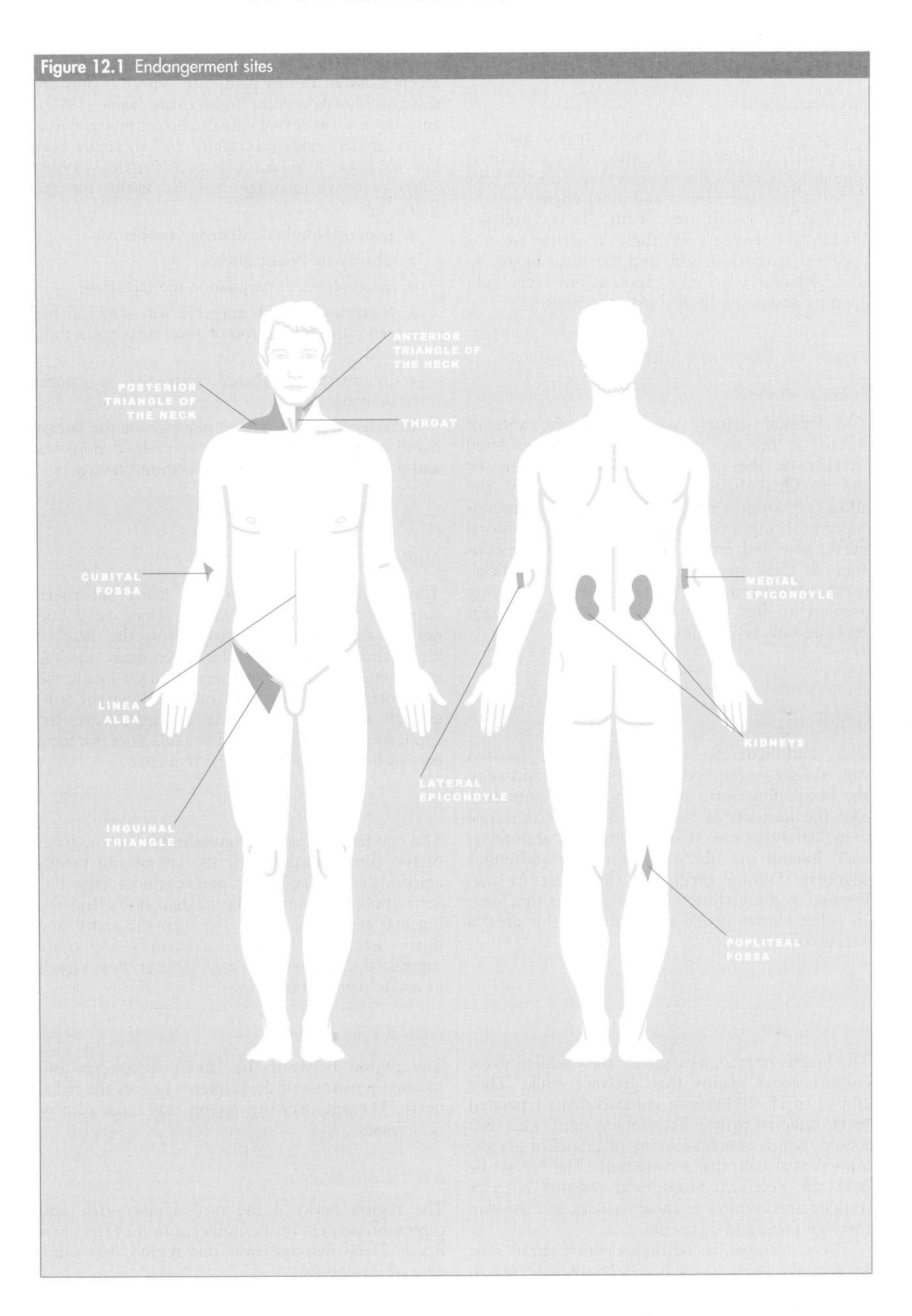

CHAPTER 12 ENDANGERMENT SITES AND INDICATIONS FOR MASSAGE THERAPY 137

Figure 12.1 Endangerment sites

- ANTERIOR TRIANGLE OF THE NECK
- POSTERIOR TRIANGLE OF THE NECK
- THROAT
- CUBITAL FOSSA
- MEDIAL EPICONDYLE
- LINEA ALBA
- KIDNEYS
- INGUINAL TRIANGLE
- LATERAL EPICONDYLE
- POPLITEAL FOSSA

Back of thighs and legs
Popliteal fossa
The popliteal fossa is a diamond-shaped space on the posterior surface of the knee. It is a relatively unguarded space as the muscles that cross the knee do so at the knee's outer and inner edges, thereby forming the boundaries of the fossa (hollow). Within the borders of these muscles are the popliteal artery and vein, and the tibial nerve. As these structures are very exposed, only very light pressure should be applied over this region.

Front of thigh and legs
Femoral triangle
The femoral triangle space is on the anterior surface at the top of the thigh. It is bordered laterally by the sartorius muscle, superiorly by the inguinal ligament and medially by the adductor longus muscle. The region contains superficial inguinal lymph nodes, the femoral nerve, vein and artery, and the great saphenous vein. As these structures are relatively superficial, great care needs to be taken when applying pressure to this region. The application of light pressure only is recommended.

Abdomen
Umbilicus area
The umbilicus is a sensitive area located superficially to the body's largest artery and vein; the descending aorta and inferior vena cava. It is also the location of the linea alba, a connective tissue band that runs centrally down the abdominal wall, joining the fibres of the rectus abdominis together. During pregnancy this structure can herniate and therefore is best avoided at this time. In other clients gentle massage over this area is permitted.

Chest
Breast tissue
The breasts or mammary glands are modified sweat (sudoriferous) glands that produce milk. They consist of 15–20 lobes or compartments separated by fat (adipose tissue). Each lobe is subdivided into lobules which contain clusters of grapelike glands, known as alveoli, that secrete milk. The breasts lie over the pectoralis major and serratus anterior muscles and connect to these muscles and the skin through fascia and ligaments.

Breast massage has become a controversial issue for several reasons. There is no scientific evidence to support the therapeutic benefits of breast massage. Deep massage causes pain, and repeated pressure can cause breakdown of breast tissue (Salvo, 1999). In today's socio-sexual climate, breast massage may create anxiety and uncertainty and therefore may fail to have a relaxing effect. Curties (1999) suggests breast massage may be useful for the following:

- general lymphatic drainage problems;
- fibrocystic breast disease;
- discomforts of pregnancy and lactation;
- following recent surgery, for symptomatic relief and promotion of good quality scarring; and
- treatment of adhered, restrictive or painful scarring.

It is recommended that massage of the breast tissue be performed only for specialised purposes and not as part of a general relaxation massage.

Arm and forearm
Axilla
The axilla or armpit contains many superficial structures including the axillary artery, veins and nerves, the brachial plexus nerves, the brachial artery and many lymph nodes. Deep tissue massage may compress these structures leading to pain and numbness (which may travel or refer down the arm) as well as inflammation. As a general rule, the application of massage over the axilla does not form part of the relaxation massage sequence.

Cubital fossa
The cubital fossa is a triangular hollow at the front of the elbow bordered by the lateral and medial epicondyles, pronator teres and brachioradialis. The fossa (hollow) contains the median nerve and the brachial artery, which divides into the radial and ulnar arteries. As these structures are quite superficial, deep massage may damage these vessels or create pain or numbness.

Lateral epicondyle
The region between the lateral epicondyle and olecranon process of the humerus houses the radial nerve. Massage over this region may cause pain or numbness.

Medial epicondyle
The region between the medial epicondyle and olecranon process of the humerus houses the ulnar nerve. Deep massage over this region may cause pain or numbness.

Face

Eyes

Light compression over and around the eye area is permissible, however, if the client is wearing contact lenses, massage is not advised.

INDICATIONS FOR THE USE OF MASSAGE THERAPY

Certain conditions or situations may render the application of massage therapy unsuitable. Such conditions or situations are referred to as absolute contraindications and are described in Box 12.1. The application of massage may be contraindicated as the condition may be life threatening (heart failure); a serious medical emergency (acute accident such as motor vehicle trauma) or contagious and pose a health threat to others (tuberculosis). In other instances the condition may be exacerbated through massage therapy (acute inflammatory conditions) or massage may in fact pose a risk of damaging the recipient when applied (embolism or haemophilia).

> **Box 12.1 Absolute contraindications**
>
> - Acute accidents and emergencies (appendicitis, bronchial asthma, cerebrovascular accident, heart failure, myocardial ischaemia, shock)
> - Acute inflammatory conditions
> - Acute psychosis
> - Aneurism
> - Embolism
> - Fever
> - Haemophilia
> - Infections (encephalitis, meningitis)
> - Infectious skin conditions
> - Kidney failure
> - Leukaemia
> - Malignant tumours
> - Tuberculosis

When taking a case history, the massage therapist should inquire as to the existence of any absolute contraindications. If any of these exist, the therapist should refer the client immediately to their primary care practitioner or nearest emergency department for treatment. If a client reveals a past history of any absolute contraindications, it is recommended to treat the client with care after first seeking a written clearance from a primary care practitioner.

Aside from medical conditions that fall under the classification of absolute contraindications, clients may present to a massage therapist with a wide range of other types of conditions or under a variety of situations. For some conditions, the application of massage is not absolutely contraindicated, but rather cautioned.

This chapter outlines some common conditions with which clients may present to a massage therapist and these are detailed on the following pages (listed alphabetically for quick reference). The systems of the body most affected by the condition are listed for easy reference. The nature of each condition is described, and the clinical signs are explained. When massage therapy is suitable as a form of therapy in a particular condition, it would be indicated for use. The indications for massage, as well as any cautions to treatment are also discussed. As the clinical features of each condition may fluctuate in the client at varying times there may be times when massage should be used with caution and times when it is best avoided. These times are flagged for easy reference using the following symbols:

⚠ = massage therapy should be used with caution

🛑 = massage therapy is best avoided

> **Box 12.2 Remember**
>
> When a client presents with any absolute contraindications, refer them to their primary care practitioner or nearest emergency department. Conditions labelled ⚠ indicate that under certain circumstances massage is used with caution, whereas those labelled 🛑 indicate that massage is best avoided.

Anorexia nervosa

(nervous system, digestive system)

An eating disorder characterised by an obsessive desire to achieve extremes of weight loss and to be thin.

Clinical features

Primarily observed in adolescent females, people with anorexia nervosa refuse to eat for prolonged periods, leading to emaciation. Symptoms include amenorrhoea, low body fat and dry and scaly skin. Considered a psychoneurotic disorder, anorexia nervosa is often associated with feelings of anger, fear and anxiety.

Indications for massage

As the condition is characterised by emotional stress or conflict, massage therapy may assist with stress management, and may contribute to improved awareness and perceptions of body image.

Caution

As those with anorexia nervosa are suffering from the effects of poor nutrition, gentle manipulations are recommended. Excessive pressure over bony areas, which may result from reclining too long in the same posture, may cause discomfort or even damage surrounding tissue. Avoid such pressure areas by padding the treatment table well, and moving the patient regularly.

Best avoided

Avoid massaging directly over bony prominences, which will appear more pronounced in a person with anorexia nervosa.

Anxiety

(nervous system)

Anxiety is a normal emotion, felt by all people at some time, in response to stress. Persistent anxiety produces feelings of inner fear, uncertainty and uneasiness. Anxiety may become problematic if the feeling is disproportionate to the apparent threat or agent of stress.

Clinical features

There exist many categories of anxiety disorders. Common features of such disorders include physical symptoms such as tension headaches, muscle tightness, fatigue, palpitations, dizziness, abdominal distress and sweating. Psychological symptoms include panic, impatience, noise sensitivity and irritability.

Indications for massage

One of the treatment modalities recommended for anxiety disorders includes relaxation techniques to calm the mind and body. Therapeutic relaxation massage may assist with stress management, and can contribute to the control of feelings of anxiety.

Asthma

(respiratory system)

A chronic inflammatory respiratory disorder characterised by episodes of wheezing caused by constriction of the bronchi. Episodes, often referred to as 'attacks', may result from irritation by an inhaled allergen, such as pollen, or triggers such as emotional distress. Asthma tends to develop between the ages of two and seven years, and may first present as a persistent cough.

Clinical features

Asthma attacks vary greatly. Episodes may involve mild wheezing and coughing, or may be more severe, characterised by total obstruction of the airways. During an attack the sufferer may panic, and their respiratory rate may increase. Stimulation of excessive bronchial secretions results in the production of thick sputum.

Indications for massage

The main focus for the management of asthma is prevention of episodes. This would involve removal of allergens or triggers. By aiding stress management, massage therapy may assist when emotional distress is the trigger of attacks. By improving circulation, massage may assist immune function and would be useful in asthmatics whose episodes are preceded by respiratory infections. Hacking manipulations may assist with mobilisation and removal of excess bronchial secretions.

Caution

To reduce the risk of triggering an asthma attack in an asthmatic client, eliminate the use of synthetic products or fragrances in the clinic, and ensure the treatment room is maintained in a clean and dust-free state, and all linen is thoroughly cleaned and aired.

Best avoided

Massage is not indicated during an asthma attack, which is considered a medical emergency.

Attention deficit hyperactivity disorder

(nervous system)

Attention deficit hyperactivity disorder (ADHD) is a condition characterised by behavioural and learning difficulties, affecting children and adolescents. Attention deficit hyperactivity disorder affects boys more than girls, and may be carried into adulthood.

Clinical features

People with ADHD exhibit overactivity and inattentiveness. They are often impulsive, irritable, moody and disorganised. Attention deficit hyperactivity disorder sufferers typically have poor coordination.

Indications for massage

As ADHD is believed to be of nervous system origin, massage therapy may be useful to relax the client and assist with stress management. Massage may assist with improving feelings of self-esteem, particularly in children with ADHD.

Caution ⚠

To avoid a learned negative association with massage in children, discontinue any treatment if the child does not wish to participate. Treatment may resume when the child is more attentive, or may require rescheduling to another day or time.

Bell's palsy

(nervous system, muscular system)

A facial paralysis caused by damage to any or all branches of the facial nerve. Such damage may be the result of trauma, infection or compression of the nerve anywhere along its course. Growths such as tumours may compress the nerve, affecting its function.

Clinical features

Due to inactivity of the nerve, the person exhibits difficulty in closing the eye or mouth on the affected side of the face. Symptoms include drooping of the face unilaterally, drooling of the mouth and slurred speech. The majority of cases experience spontaneous recovery, whilst a few are left with permanent paralysis.

Indications for massage

During the recovery period, massage therapy is useful to enhance circulation, aid muscle tone and stimulate nervous activity.

Caution ⚠

As the person may be experiencing a loss of sensation, gentle massage is recommended. Reduced sensitivity may result in the client being unable to give adequate feedback on treatment techniques being applied.

Bulimia

(nervous system, digestive system)

An eating disorder characterised by episodes of binge eating followed by self-induced vomiting, purging and periods of depression.

Clinical features

Observed most frequently in young females, bulimia is commonly seen between the ages of 17 to 25 years. This psychoneurotic disorder is associated with depression, and is characterised by fluctuations in body weight. Symptoms include irregular menstruation, hypokalaemia (low potassium levels) and tooth decay.

Indications for massage

As the condition is associated with depression, massage therapy may assist with stress management, and may assist with elevating emotional states.

Cellulitis

(integumentary system)

An inflammatory skin disorder resulting from infection of the skin. If left untreated it may develop into abscess formation and other skin destruction. Cellulitis is commonly seen in people with poor circulation, diabetes mellitus and damaged skin conditions.

Clinical features

The skin appears swollen and red, and is painful and hot to touch. Other symptoms may include headache, malaise and fever.

Indications for massage

Massage is not indicated for the treatment of this condition.

Best avoided 🛑

Avoid massaging directly over or around any areas affected by cellulitis. To reduce the risk of infection, ensure all linen is changed and thoroughly washed, and massage equipment (including table) is disinfected at all times (see Chapter 10).

Cerebrovascular accident (stroke)

(circulatory system, nervous system, muscular system)

A medical emergency leading to ischaemia (reduced blood supply) of the tissues of the brain, often the result of an embolus or haemorrhage of cerebral blood vessels.

Clinical features

The location and extent of ischaemia will determine the resultant damage of the stroke. Survivors may exhibit muscle weakness, paralysis and spasticity and possibly speech difficulties.

Indications for massage

During the rehabilitation period, massage therapy manipulations may assist with restoration of motor function. Relaxation techniques may be useful for the relief of muscular pain, and may aid stress management.

Caution ⚠

As the person may be experiencing a loss of sensation, gentle massage is recommended. Reduced sensitivity may result in the client being unable to give adequate feedback on treatment techniques being applied.

Best avoided 🛑

Massage is not indicated during a cerebrovascular attack, which is considered a medical emergency.

Chronic fatigue syndrome

(immune system, nervous system, muscular system)

An immune disorder with no clearly defined origin, chronic fatigue syndrome (CFS) is also referred to as chronic Ebstein-Barr virus, myalgic encephalomyelitis and chronic neuromuscular viral syndrome. Just as there is no clearly defined cause of CFS, there exists no diagnostic test for this syndrome. Approximately two-thirds of all patients with CFS report a preceding viral infection, yet the type of virus is inconsistent amongst sufferers. A common feature of CFS is extreme tiredness and fatigue.

Clinical features

Chronic fatigue syndrome is characterised by depression, extreme lethargy and exhaustion, aching musculature, sleep disturbances and flu-like symptoms. One of the major criteria for diagnosis of CFS is the presence of debilitating muscular fatigue that impairs daily functioning and has been present for longer than six months.

Indications for massage

Relaxation techniques may be useful for the relief of muscular pain, and may aid stress management. Massage therapy may be useful in relieving fatigue and aiding sleep, as well as enhancing emotional states to assist with feelings of depression.

Caution ⚠

Chronic fatigue syndrome sufferers often experience changes in energy levels throughout the day. By discussing with the client their energy peaks and troughs over a 24-hour period, appointments for massage therapy may be made for times during the day when they are feeling at their best, and are the least fatigued. Clients with CFS may be taking prescription analgesic or anti-inflammatory medications. Such medicines may reduce sensitivity and mask pain; thus clients may not be able to give adequate feedback on treatment techniques being applied.

Best avoided 🛑

Avoid deep manipulations as these may have a 'draining' or exhausting effect on people with CFS.

Constipation

(digestive system)

Constipation is described as difficulty in passing small, hard stools. The most common likely cause of this disorder is poor eating habits, namely insufficient fluid and dietary fibre from sources such as whole grains, fresh fruits and vegetables. Constipation may also result from disease states of the large bowel, metabolic disorders like hypothyroidism, and psychogenic conditions. Depression, anxiety, anorexia nervosa and schizophrenia are some psychogenic disorders that may manifest in constipation. Several drug classes — including analgesics and antacids — are also risk factors in the development of this condition.

Clinical features

People experiencing constipation report hard stools, a reduced frequency of defecation, a reduction in bowel sounds, increased intra-abdominal pressure and nausea. Those with constipation may be exhibiting other symptoms, including an altered appetite, back pain, headache and abdominal pain.

Indications for massage

To encourage faecal motility, gentle massage strokes may be applied over the abdomen following the direction of the large bowel. In those people where constipation has a psychogenic component, relaxation techniques may be useful to aid stress management.

Best avoided 🛑

Avoid massaging the abdomen of a person who has recently eaten a large meal. If constipation is associated with bleeding, or is of sudden onset in the middle aged and elderly, refer the person to their primary care practitioner for investigation.

Depression

(nervous system)

Depression is the mental state or emotional disorder characterised by extreme feelings of sadness, melancholy, despair and worthlessness.

Considered to be one of the more common disorders presenting for treatment to medical practitioners, depression may result from many different variables, and involves a loss of interest in life's pleasures, as well as altered mood states.

Clinical features

People with depression typically exhibit both physical and mental symptoms. Such symptoms include tiredness, fatigue, headache, constipation, tension, anger, anxiety and irritability.

Indications for massage

Massage therapy may assist symptomatically with physical symptoms such as constipation, headache, and fatigue. Relaxation techniques may be useful to aid stress management, and enhance emotional states. People with depression will benefit from the nurturing and relaxing effects of a full body relaxation massage. To assist the depressed client to gain maximum benefit from a full body relaxation massage, it is important to create a safe and relaxing massage experience. In doing so, ensure environmental stressors such as background noise and bright overhead lighting are kept to a minimum. The relaxation effect may be enhanced when the massage recipient is kept warm and adequately draped throughout the treatment.

Caution

As people with depression may have underlying pathologies, it is vital for the skilled massage therapist to extract a full case history from the client prior to commencement of any massage therapy treatment. Clients with depression may be taking prescription analgesic or anti-inflammatory medications. Such medicines may reduce sensitivity and mask pain; thus clients may not be able to give adequate feedback on treatment techniques being applied.

Best avoided

If a person presents in poor health, with major symptoms, or suicidal thoughts, refer the person to their primary care practitioner for assessment.

Diabetes mellitus

(endocrine system, circulatory system, nervous system)

There are two main types of this metabolic disorder, characterised by a lack of or inadequate secretion of insulin, or altered sensitivity of receptor cells to the presence of insulin. Type I diabetes mellitus (DM) is referred to as insulin dependent diabetes mellitus (IDDM), and is sometimes still known as juvenile onset diabetes. Those with IDDM rely on insulin — often in the form of injection — to prevent ketosis, a build up of ketones in the body as a result of excessive breakdown of fats when carbohydrates cannot be metabolised. Type II DM is known as adult onset or non-insulin dependent diabetes mellitus (NIDDM). As this type has a more insidious onset than type I, those with NIDDM may remain asymptomatic.

Clinical features

In uncontrolled DM, symptoms would include polyuria, polydipsia and hyperglycaemia. Weight loss is typically observed in type I DM. Diseased small blood vessels can result in loss of vision, poor wound healing and infections and kidney problems while effects on the nervous system may result in peripheral neuropathies.

Indications for massage

Massage may assist with circulation and metabolism, and may have a beneficial effect on insulin requirements. Therapeutic relaxation techniques may be useful to aid stress management.

Caution

Amongst the complications with DM are changes in vascular and nervous condition. People with DM may present with altered sensation, particularly in the peripheries. Such reduced sensitivity may mask any pain; thus clients may not be able to give adequate feedback on treatment techniques being applied. To reduce the risk of infection, ensure all linen is changed and thoroughly washed, and massage equipment (including table) is disinfected at all times (see Chapter 10).

Best avoided

Those with DM are prone to skin lesions and infections. Avoid massaging directly over or around any skin lesions or infections. People with DM may become hypoglycaemic, presenting with symptoms of sweating, rapid heart rate and dizziness. In such situations a source of glucose should be administered, such as sugar sweets (jelly babies or marshmallows) or fruit juice (most people with DM carry some form of glucose with them). Any treatment should be discontinued and the client referred to their primary care practitioner for further assistance.

Down syndrome

(nervous system, muscular system, respiratory system)

A congenital syndrome, resulting usually from an extra chromosome 21. It occurs in approximately one in 600 births, and has a higher incidence in children born to women over 35 years of age. Down syndrome is also referred to as Trisomy 21.

Clinical features

Children born with this syndrome display typical facial features of slanting eyes, low-set small ears and a large protruding tongue. The hands and feet are broad and short, and musculature is hypotonic. Down syndrome people exhibit mental retardation, and may develop respiratory complications.

Indications for massage

Massage therapy may be useful in enhancing muscle tone. Gentle relaxation strokes may be beneficial for stress management, and may assist in controlling extremes of mood.

Caution

To avoid a learned negative association with massage in people with mental retardation, discontinue any treatment if the Down syndrome client does not wish to participate. If the mental retardation were severe, a Down syndrome client would attend for treatment with a carer. Such carers may provide insight into patient history, and may assist with patient management if required.

Dysmenorrhoea

(genito-urinary system, endocrine system)

Dysmenorrhoea, a condition affecting most women at some stage in their reproductive life, is the pain associated with periods. Dysmenorrhoea may be classified as either primary or secondary. Primary dysmenorrhoea may commence in adolescence, and involve the pain associated with the menstrual cycle, whereas secondary dysmenorrhoea is related to another condition, such as endometriosis or pelvic inflammatory disease, and often presents around 30 years of age or older.

Clinical features

In primary dysmenorrhoea, pain commences at the onset of menses, and symptoms include abdominal pain that radiates to the low back and thighs, nausea, dizziness and vomiting. In secondary dysmenorrhoea, pain may present as a dull ache three to four days before the menses, and may increase in intensity throughout menstruation. Both forms of dysmenorrhoea may be accompanied by changes in bowel functions.

Indications for massage

Massage therapy may assist to relieve pain and cramping, when applied to the abdomen. Relaxation massage may be useful for stress management. Heat may be applied over the abdominal area to provide pain relief.

Caution

As the person may be experiencing intense abdominal pain, gentle massage is recommended. Clients with pain may be taking prescription analgesic medications. Such medicines may reduce sensitivity and mask pain; thus clients may not be able to give adequate feedback on treatment techniques being applied. A menstruating woman may be sensitive to unrobing, so adequate draping is important, both for coverage and warmth.

Best avoided

Avoid deep manipulations over pelvic organs during menstruation, as these may lead to endometrial regurgitation, a risk factor for the development of endometriosis (see below). Clients presenting with secondary dysmenorrhoea should be referred to their primary care practitioner to establish underlying organic pathology.

Endometriosis

(genito-urinary system, endocrine system)

A gynaecological condition in which endometrial tissue grows outside of the uterus. Such tissue responds cyclically to female sex hormones and haemorrhages. Although an exact cause is yet to be established, it is known that the incidence of endometriosis is increased with delayed pregnancy.

Clinical features

Symptoms are similar to those of secondary dysmenorrhoea. Other symptoms include premenstrual spotting and infertility.

Indications for massage

Massage therapy would primarily assist in controlling pain, and heat applied over the painful areas may also provide relief. The application of gentle relaxation massage may be useful for stress management.

Caution

Clients with pain may be taking prescription analgesic medications. Such medicines may reduce sensitivity and mask pain; thus clients may not be able to give adequate feedback on treatment techniques being applied. A menstruating woman may be sensitive to disrobing, so adequate draping is important, both for coverage and warmth.

Epilepsy

(nervous system)

Epilepsy is a term used to describe a group of neurological disorders of unknown origin. Such disorders are characterised by seizures resulting from abnormal firing of brain cells. Epilepsy may also involve sensory disturbances, and attacks may occur several times a day, or may appear years apart.

Clinical features

In most epileptics, an attack leads to a sudden loss of consciousness. The duration and symptoms of an attack vary depending on the type of seizure.

Indications for massage

Massage therapy is suitable for people with epilepsy. Relaxation massage may be useful for stress management.

Caution

Most epileptics will have their seizures under control through the use of prescription medication. Depending on the severity of their condition, it may be necessary to schedule massage appointments around their medication times so as to maximise treatment benefits, by performing massage when they feel at their best. Be sure to ascertain contact details for their primary care practitioner during the initial consultation, and ensure such details are current with subsequent visits, in case of medical emergency.

Best avoided

Massage is not indicated during an epileptic seizure. If a client experiences a seizure whilst under a therapist's care, the client should be protected from injury and not restrained. Their airway should be monitored to ensure breathing is not restricted or lost. Once the client regains consciousness, any treatment should be discontinued and the client referred to their primary care practitioner for further assistance. A seizure in a person who has a history of epilepsy is not considered a medical emergency if it lasts for less than five minutes, if they regain consciousness without further complications, and if there are no signs of injury. A seizure is considered a medical emergency if it lasts for longer than five minutes, is preceded by another seizure, occurs in an epileptic who is pregnant, diabetic or injured, or occurs in a person with no prior history of seizure. In such instances, emergency medical assistance should be sought immediately.

Fibromyalgia

(nervous system, muscular system)

The term fibromyalgia — literally meaning pain in the muscles — is used to describe a painful muscle syndrome of unknown cause. It should not be confused with the symptom of fibrositis, which is inflammation of the connective tissue, observed mostly in the cervical and thoracic regions. People with fibromyalgia exhibit characteristic tender points that are painful on palpation, and have a history of muscular pain. It is believed to be associated with poor sleep patterns, and affects four times as many females as males.

Clinical features

The symptoms of fibromyalgia are similar to those of chronic fatigue syndrome, namely muscular pain and fatigue, tiredness and depression. Sufferers may present with tension headaches, anxiety and digestive disturbances (such as constipation, diarrhoea, nausea and abdominal gas). Another common condition associated with fibromyalgia is temporomandibular joint dysfunction (TMJ dysfunction), in which people complain of pain and tenderness around the face and jaw. Female sufferers may also report dysmenorrhoea.

Indications for massage

Relaxation techniques may be useful for the relief of muscular pain, and may aid stress management. Massage therapy may be useful in relieving fatigue and aiding sleep, as well as enhancing emotional states to assist with feelings of depression. Gentle manipulations are advised, as deep manipulations may worsen the pain experience. It is worth noting that this chronic condition is often unresponsive to treatment, and as such a multi-faceted management approach is recommended.

Caution

People with fibromyalgia often experience changes in energy levels throughout the day. By discussing with the client their energy peaks and troughs over a 24-hour period, appointments for massage therapy may be made for times during the day when they are feeling at their best and are the least fatigued. Clients with fibromyalgia may be taking prescription analgesic or anti-inflammatory medications. Such medicines may reduce sensitivity and mask pain; thus clients may not be able to give adequate feedback on treatment techniques being applied.

Best avoided 🛑

Avoid deep manipulations as these may have a 'draining' or exhausting effect on people with fibromyalgia, and intensify the pain experience.

Folliculitis

(immune system, integumentary system)

An inflammation of the hair follicles of the skin, folliculitis is often bacterial in origin (*Staphylococcus aureus*). It may result from irritation of the follicle, such as when massage is applied without adequate lubricant, resulting in a 'pulling' of the hair follicles leading to inflammation. To avoid such irritation when applying massage, ensure adequate lubricant is used. When performing deep strokes such as pétrissage, ensure the manipulations are applied slowly and smoothly, thus reducing the pulling action of the hair.

Clinical features

Local inflammatory signs, including redness and swelling, appear around the follicle. A small pustule (round fluid-filled elevation) is evident at the base of the hair follicle. Folliculitis is commonly seen on the thighs, lower legs, arms, face and scalp.

Indications for massage

Massage is not indicated for the treatment of this condition.

Best avoided 🛑

Avoid massaging directly over or around any areas affected by folliculitis. Cover affected regions with adhesive plasters (such as bandaids) to reduce the risk of infection. Post treatment, ensure all linen is changed and thoroughly washed, and massage equipment (including table) is disinfected (see Chapter 10).

Fractures

(skeletal system)

A fracture is characterised by a break in the continuity of a bone, and may be classified as either closed or open, and complete or incomplete. In a closed fracture, the skin remains intact, whereas an open fracture involves the bone breaking through the skin or into a body cavity (making the injury more susceptible to infection). A complete fracture occurs when the bone breaks into two or more pieces. When the bone is bent or cracked, the fracture is referred to as incomplete, as the periosteum surrounding the bone remains intact. The most common cause of fracture is the sudden application of force greater than the bone can withstand, resulting in the tissue distorting or breaking. Other causes of fracture include overuse injury (including stress fractures) and pathological conditions (such as fractures occurring in bone weakened by tumour or other disease states).

Clinical features

Typical signs and symptoms of fracture include:
- pain;
- swelling;
- bruising/ skin discoloration;
- deformity;
- loss of function;
- abnormal movement; and
- crepitus (the grating sound of bony surfaces rubbing together)

Indications for massage

The conventional management of a fracture includes reduction (realignment) and immobilisation, through the use of a plaster cast. The rate at which a fracture heals is dependent on several factors, including the location and classification of the fracture, as well as the age of the person affected. As a result, immobilisation periods vary. For example, an upper limb fracture in an adult may take six weeks to heal whereas in a child healing may occur within a month. When in a cast, the aim of treatment is to preserve or maintain the functional capacity of the affected region and surrounding structures. During this immobilisation period, massage therapy may be applied around the affected region and plaster cast to assist circulation, maintain joint mobility, and reduce oedema and pain. This can be achieved by:

- elevating the affected limb, thereby reducing oedema;
- applying heat therapy to encourage circulation, and to reduce muscle spasm and pain in the surrounding musculature;
- gently moving surrounding joints to encourage venous return and reduce stiffness;
- applying relaxation massage to gross body areas (such as the back) to assist with stress management.

After successful reduction, the treatment aim shifts to restoration of function. Once immobilisation has been removed, gentle massage therapy manipulations may be applied to:

- enhance joint range of movement;
- alleviate adhesions in connective tissue;
- promote local circulation;
- reduce muscular pain.

Caution ⚠

During the immobilisation period, the massage therapist should ensure that any techniques employed during treatment do not aggravate the inflammatory process. Treatment should cease if there is any increase in swelling or pain. Once immobilisation is removed, tissues will be weakened and soft. The massage therapist must take care to avoid overstretching connective tissue during this period, which may result in tearing of the tissue, thus further delaying full rehabilitation. Deep techniques should be introduced gradually so as to avoid aggravating the weakened tissue.

Best avoided 🛑

Avoid massaging directly over the fracture site. Avoid the use of oil as a lubricant near the plaster site as it can soften the cast.

Guillain-Barré syndrome

(nervous system, immune system)

Also referred to as acute idiopathic demyelinating polyneuropathy, Guillain-Barré (pronounced Geeyan bara) syndrome (GBS) is an inflammatory condition affecting the peripheral nerves. Characterised by segmental demyelination of the nerves, it may appear several weeks after a viral infection, or even post immunisation.

Clinical features

People with GBS rapidly develop weakness of the limbs, which may result in paralysis. Other symptoms include pain in the limbs and altered sensations. GBS may lead to respiratory paralysis, which can be fatal in a small percentage of cases. In most cases though, a full recovery is observed over a period of many months, and often after hospitalisation.

Indications for massage

Gentle massage therapy may be administered to the limbs to assist with pain relief and fatigue. Massage may encourage circulation and aid stress management.

Caution ⚠

As paralysis and altered sensation are associated with GBS, clients may not be able to give adequate feedback on treatment techniques being applied; as such reduced sensitivity may mask any pain.

Best avoided 🛑

Avoid deep manipulations due to altered sensation and risk of thrombophlebitis.

Hay fever

(immune system, respiratory system)

Referred to as allergic rhinitis, hay fever is an inflammatory condition of the nasal mucosa. Also affecting the eyes, hay fever has a strong association to asthma and most commonly presents as seasonal rhinitis. Hay fever is triggered by allergens, including pollen, dust mites and animal fur. Such triggers result in an excessive amount of histamine circulation in the body, resulting in the symptoms of hay fever.

Clinical features

Symptoms include sneezing, nasal congestion, excessive nasal discharge, watery eyes and itchiness. People with hay fever may also experience pressure in the ears, sinus congestion, altered sense of smell and a dry, sore throat.

Indications for massage

Massage therapy applied to the face may assist in relieving congestion and reducing pain associated with increased pressure. Relaxation massage may also assist with stress management.

Caution ⚠

So as not to aggravate hay fever, eliminate the presence of allergens by ensuring the treatment room is maintained in a clean and dust-free state and that all linen is thoroughly cleaned and aired. Remove all flower arrangements from the treatment room prior to massaging those prone to allergic hay fever.

Best avoided 🛑

Avoid possible damage to eyes by asking clients to remove contact lenses where necessary.

Headache

(nervous system)

A headache, as the name implies, refers to any pain in the head, regardless of cause. Everyone experiences a headache at some stage in his or her life, and over a 12-month period, nearly 90 per cent of the population is likely to complain of headache. There are many different types of headache, and these are commonly classified as either primary or secondary headaches. Primary headaches are those which have no underlying pathology; for example, tension headaches, cluster headaches and migraines. Secondary headaches result from an underlying medical condition, such as tumour or infection, and account for a minority of headaches.

Clinical features

Tension headaches are very common and present as a throbbing ache on both sides of the head. Undue stress or anxiety often precipitates a tension headache, which may last for several hours, and recur each day. Tension headaches are also known as muscle contraction headaches, as sufferers may exhibit neck disorders. Cluster headaches are more common amongst males and present as intense pain over one eye. Such headaches are of sudden onset and usually last minutes to hours. Alcohol may be a trigger for cluster headaches, and attacks are said to be as regular as clockwork, characteristically appearing in the middle of the night and around the same times during the day.

A migraine headache may take many forms, and is most commonly triggered by stress. Migraines, which tend to affect more females than males, are debilitating and produce a throbbing pain on one side of the head. Symptoms of migraine include sound and light sensitivity, as well as nausea, vomiting and irritability. Many migraine headaches are preceded by an aura phase (typically involving visual disturbances), and may last for several days. Known triggers of headaches include stress, certain foods (such as caffeine), intense odours, hormonal changes, exercise, oversleeping and anxiety.

Indications for massage

Massage therapy is most beneficial for the prevention of primary headaches. As stress and emotional disturbances are common factors associated with headaches, relaxation massage administered regularly will assist with stress management and may enhance mood. As cervical dysfunction is also associated with the majority of primary headaches, deep manipulations applied to the musculature of the neck and shoulders will help to prevent headache attacks related to tight musculature. During an attack, gentle massage therapy may be of benefit. Depending on the type of headache, some clients may gain relief from a face and scalp massage, whilst others may find a foot or hand massage more relaxing. The application of cold packs to the forehead and neck may also provide relief from pain.

Caution

Avoid deep manipulations during an attack, as they may aggravate the condition. During an attack a client may be taking prescription analgesic medications. Such medicines may reduce sensitivity and mask pain; thus clients may not be able to give adequate feedback on treatment techniques being applied.

Best avoided

A client should be referred to their primary care practitioner for assessment if they:

- complain of more than three attacks per week;
- feel the need to take analgesic medication every day;
- are experiencing fever or shortness of breath;
- exhibit altered speech or paraesthesia;
- are experiencing their first-ever headache;
- are over 50 years of age and headaches have just begun;
- notice changes in the nature of their headaches.

Hepatitis

(immune system, digestive system)

Hepatitis is a term used to describe any condition resulting in inflammation (pain and swelling) of the liver. The liver is the body's largest gland, and its functions include the conversion of ammonia to urea, the production of bile, the secretion of glucose as an energy source and the production of heat. As one of the most complex and vital organs of the body, it may lead to serious illness if not functioning properly. There are several factors that may result in hepatitis. Recreational drug usage (including alcohol and illegal drugs) may lead to inflammation of the liver. Hepatitis may also result from viral or bacterial infection, or parasitic infestation. There are several forms of viral hepatitis, each referred to by a letter, such as hepatitis B. Each viral form results in similar complications, yet transmission occurs in varying ways. For example, hepatitis A virus is often spread through faecal-contaminated water or food, whereas hepatitis B virus may be contracted from contaminated blood products, syringes or equipment (such as dialysis machinery).

Clinical features

Symptoms vary for each type of hepatitis, but generally include loss of appetite, pain in the liver, jaundice, and nausea or vomiting. Depending on the cause of hepatitis, symptoms may last weeks to months. In cases that persist longer than six months, the hepatitis is termed chronic. Hepatitis B, when more serious, may lead to progressive illness or even death. Hepatitis resulting from substance abuse is not contagious. Some forms of viral hepatitis (including hepatitis B and C) may be transmitted if a contaminated person's blood comes into contact with open cuts on another person. As the virus is present in the blood of the infected person, any infected blood that enters another person's bloodstream through damaged skin such as a cut or a wound may lead to them becoming infected also. It is recommended that all health care providers be vaccinated against hepatitis B.

Indications for massage

Massage is not indicated in this condition in the acute stages. Massage therapy may assist with stress management following the acute stage.

Caution

As a therapist, ensure hands and arms are free of open lesions when administering massage to a client with viral hepatitis. Tight-fitting latex or vinyl gloves may be worn as a precautionary measure. Post treatment, ensure hands are thoroughly washed, change and thoroughly wash all linen, and disinfect all massage equipment (including table).

Best avoided

Avoid massaging directly over an inflamed liver in chronic hepatitis. In cases of viral hepatitis, avoid massaging over or around any skin that is damaged or broken.

Hypertension

(circulatory system, nervous system)

Hypertension is elevated blood pressure in excess of 140/90mmHg that is unrelated to another disorder.

Clinical features

In many cases, hypertension may be asymptomatic. Symptoms may include dizziness, headaches and palpitations. If left untreated, hypertension may result in left ventricular hypertrophy, myocardial infarction or stroke. Elevated blood pressure correlates with an increased risk of cardiovascular disease.

Indications for massage

Massage therapy may assist in controlling or normalising blood pressure, and as a relaxation therapy is useful for stress management.

Caution

Anti-hypertensive medications are often prescribed in cases of moderate to severe hypertension. A side effect of such medicines is postural (or orthostatic) hypotension, which involves a downward shift in blood pressure when one moves from a reclining to seated position, or seated to standing position. Care should be taken to assist such patients in the gradual transition to a standing posture post-massage.

Best avoided

A hypertensive crisis may occur in a person who has undiagnosed hypertension or in someone who has stopped taking prescription anti-hypertensive drugs. Such a crisis involves a rapid elevation of blood pressure to 200/120mmHg or greater. Symptoms include severe headache, bleeding from the nose, defined and distended neck veins, cardiac arrhythmia and vomiting. Massage is not indicated during a hypertensive crisis, which is considered a medical emergency.

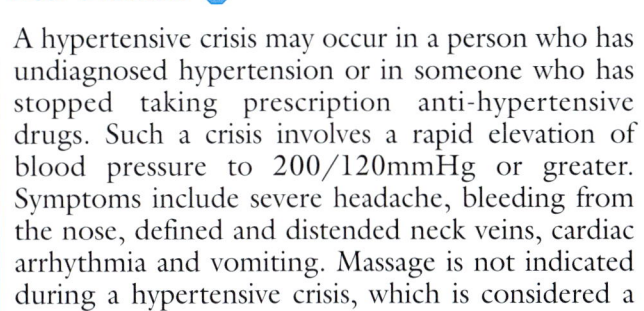

Irritable bowel syndrome

(digestive system, nervous system)

Irritable bowel syndrome (IBS) is an intestinal disorder, characterised by colicky abdominal pain and constipation, diarrhoea or both. Common in females between the ages of 20 to 40 years, diagnosis of IBS involves first excluding other pathologies, such as inflammatory bowel diseases. Irritable bowel syndrome results from irregular motility of the intestines, and is often associated with psychological disturbances, including emotional stress and anxiety.

Clinical features

The symptoms of IBS often present after meals, and include alternating diarrhoea and constipation, painful abdominal cramping (usually relieved by defecation), bloating and fatigue. Exacerbated by stress and anxiety, IBS is a condition often observed in the 'perfectionist' personality.

Indications for massage

As clearly stressful situations and emotional pressures affect IBS, massage therapy has a large part to play in the management of this disorder. Relaxation massage is beneficial when incorporated as part of the prevention of IBS. Relaxation massage administered regularly will assist with stress management and may enhance mood.

Menopause

(genito-urinary system, endocrine system)

Strictly speaking, menopause is the cessation of menstruation, or the presence of amenorrhoea for a period greater than 12 months. Menopause commonly occurs between the ages of 45 to 55 years, and is a consequence of a decline in the production of oestrogen by the ovaries.

Clinical features

The symptomatic features of menopause are varied for each woman. Hot flushes, night sweats, migraine, dizziness, and vaginal and skin dryness are some of the physical symptoms that may be present. Psychologically, altered sleep patterns, depression, tearfulness, a loss of confidence and reduced short-term memory may be noted. If symptoms are severe and greatly impact upon quality of life, drug intervention such as hormone replacement therapy (HRT) may be recommended. Menopausal women may also experience muscular and joint pain.

Indications for massage

Massage therapy may assist in controlling psychological symptoms, and can aid relaxation and stress management. When applied with care and in a supportive environment, massage may also enhance feelings of self-worth and boost self-confidence. Deep soft tissue manipulations may help relieve muscular and joint pain. The use of a good quality cold-pressed vegetable oil as a lubricant during massage will contribute to a reduction in dry skin and improve the appearance and feel of the skin. Such a visible physical change may also aid the confidence of the client.

Multiple sclerosis

(nervous system)

Multiple sclerosis (MS) is a degenerative disease of unknown cause, affecting the brain and spinal cord. Having a peak onset between the ages of 20 to 40 years, this neurological disorder appears to be more prevalent in females than in males. Characterised by a loss in both motor and sensory function, the condition involves destruction of the lipoprotein content of nerve cells, leading to the formation of zones of demyelination referred to as plaques. Symptoms depend on the size and distribution of such plaques.

Clinical features

Early symptoms may include visual disturbances, pins and needles, numbness, subtle sensory changes and fatigue. As the condition progresses the MS sufferer may exhibit obvious disabling disease affecting mobility and muscle coordination. As well as spasticity, increases in body temperature and fatigue can be severe and disabling.

Indications for massage

Massage therapy may be useful in improving circulation and muscle tone, and may stimulate nervous activity. Gentle relaxation massage may assist with stress management.

Caution ⚠

As the person may be experiencing a loss of sensation, gentle massage is recommended. Reduced sensitivity may result in the client being unable to give adequate feedback on treatment techniques being applied. Clients with MS may be taking prescription analgesic or anti-inflammatory medications. Such medicines may reduce sensitivity and mask pain, also reducing the client's ability to give adequate feedback on treatment techniques being applied.

Best avoided 🛑

Avoid deep manipulations due to altered sensation, and the risk of deep manipulations having a 'draining' or exhausting effect on people with MS.

Obesity

(nervous system)

Obesity is an increasing health concern in Western civilisations and is characterised by excessive accumulation of fat, or adipose tissue. Having a genetic link, obesity is more prevalent in females than males. Obesity is associated with a lack of physical activity, and emotional disturbances such as depression.

Clinical features

Obese people are susceptible to hypertension, infertility, type II diabetes, and vascular and mechanical disorders. There is an increased mortality amongst obese people compared with people of healthy weight. Obese people may be self-conscious, and exhibit low self-esteem and a lack of confidence.

Indications for massage

As an obese client may be feeling self-conscious, it is important to drape adequately and considerately. Massage therapy may assist with stress management, and when applied with care and in a supportive environment, may enhance feelings of self-worth and boost self-confidence. Massage may also encourage circulation and promote digestive function.

Caution ⚠

If the obese client has type II diabetes, they may present with altered sensation, particularly in the peripheries. Such reduced sensitivity may mask any pain; thus clients may not be able to give adequate feedback on treatment techniques being applied. If the obese client presents with hypertension, they may be taking anti-hypertensive medications. A side effect of such medicines is postural hypotension, which involves a downward shift in blood pressure when one moves from a reclining to seated position, or seated to standing position. Care should be taken to assist such patients in a gradual transition to a standing posture post-massage. As the obese patient may not be comfortable in a reclining position for extended periods of time, massage therapy may be more effective if administered in a seated position. So as to maximise comfort and security for the client, a purpose-built massage chair is recommended (see Chapter 8).

Best avoided

Avoid deep manipulations over excessive adipose tissue, as this may prove quite painful and could lead to vascular or connective tissue damage.

Oedema

(circulatory system)

Oedema is an excessive accumulation of fluid in the interstitial regions of the tissues. Many factors contribute to the formation of oedema, including elevated capillary blood pressure, venous or lymphatic obstruction, pressure disorders, renal failure, tissue inflammation and corticosteroid usage.

Clinical features

Symptoms of oedema include swelling, reduced functional ability and pain from increased pressure.

Indications for massage

Gentle massage therapy manipulations in the direction of venous flow may assist with resolution of oedema. Once resolved, pain will be relieved and functional ability will be restored. The wearing of compression bandages or supportive stockings may assist to control oedema between massage treatments.

Caution

Prior to commencement of any treatment, the underlying cause of oedema should be established.

Osteoarthritis

(skeletal system)

Osteoarthritis (OA) is a chronic, degenerative condition affecting the articular cartilage covering the ends of long bones. Also referred to as osteoarthrosis, it is the most common form of arthritis, affecting men and women equally, and usually appearing between the ages of 45 to 90 years. The primary function of articular cartilage is to cushion movement at the joint. As a person ages, this cartilage thins and weakens. In OA, the cartilage wears away completely, exposing the underlining bone. This results in the outward growth of the bony ends, producing osteophytes. Joints most commonly affected include the fingers, neck, knees, feet, hips and low back. Osteoarthritis is more prone to occur in joints that have been previously injured.

Clinical features

Many people with OA present with little or no symptomatology. Osteoarthritis commonly produces pain and stiffness in the affected joints. Such joints may be swollen, resulting in limitations of joint movement.

Indications for massage

The aims of treatment include:
- reduction of pain and stiffness;
- alleviation of muscle spasm;
- reduction of oedema;
- increasing joint range of movement.

As the client may be experiencing pain, heat may be applied prior to manual treatment to relax the superficial fascia and enhance local blood flow to underlying structures. Swedish massage may reduce pain, stiffness and oedema. Deep soft tissue manipulations may be used to alleviate muscle spasm. Gentle stretching may assist with improving joint movement.

Caution

Use deep manipulations with care, as they may lead to excessive pain. Clients with OA may be taking prescription analgesic or anti-inflammatory medications. Such medicines may reduce sensitivity and mask pain; thus clients may not be able to give adequate feedback on treatment techniques being applied.

Best avoided

Avoid deep soft tissue manipulations or excessive stretching in elderly patients or those with pronounced OA.

Paget's disease (osteitis deformans)

(skeletal system, endocrine system)

A common, progressive bone disease of unknown origin, Paget's disease is characterised by abnormal bone growth. Affecting middle-aged to elderly people, this condition involves an imbalance of bone destruction, resorption and re-growth, leading to bone being replaced by fibrous tissue. As a result, bone becomes thickened, spongy and may bend. Bones commonly affected include the pelvis, vertebrae and long bones such as the femur. As the disease progresses, the bones may become dense and very hard.

Clinical features

This condition is often discovered by accident on routine radiographic examination (X-ray), as the patient usually complains of no symptoms. When the condition progresses or the long bones are affected, the client may complain of pain. In more advanced cases deformity of bones may be present, most commonly at the femur, tibia or fibula where bowing may be noted. Pain, as well as an increased risk of pathological fracture, increase as the disease progresses. Paget's disease is more prevalent amongst males and is rare before the age of 40 years.

Indications

Massage may provide symptomatic relief from pain and aid in stress management.

Caution

Clients with Paget's disease may be taking prescription analgesic or anti-inflammatory medications. Such medicines may reduce sensitivity and mask pain; thus clients may not be able to give adequate feedback on treatment techniques being applied.

Best avoided

Avoid deep soft tissue manipulations as excessive pressure may lead to pathological fracture.

Premenstrual syndrome

(genito-urinary system, endocrine system)

Premenstrual syndrome (PMS) is a disorder of varying severity affecting most menstruating women at some stage in their lives. Symptoms present prior to the onset of menses, and are often relieved with the commencement of menstruation.

Clinical features

There exists a multitude of varying symptoms reported to be associated with PMS. Such symptoms include depression and fatigue, breast tenderness, fluid retention, headache, cramping or pain (see dysmenorrhoea) and weight gain.

Indications for massage

Gentle massage therapy manipulations may assist circulation and encourage the resolution of oedema. Relaxation massage is recommended for the control of psychological symptoms, and to aid stress management.

Caution

Clients experiencing headaches associated with PMS may be taking prescription analgesic medications. Such medicines may reduce sensitivity and mask pain; thus clients may not be able to give adequate feedback on treatment techniques being applied.

Psoriasis

(integumentary system, nervous system)

Psoriasis, a skin disorder of unknown origin, is not an uncommon condition. Presenting as reddened, silvery, scaly lesions, psoriasis plaques are the result of abnormally excessive skin cell development leading to thickening of the skin. The condition is frequently hereditary, and may be precipitated by emotional stress, infection and medications (including oral contraceptives).

Clinical features

Lesions commonly appear on the inside of the elbows, behind the knees, on the scalp and over the sacrum. The rash appears to worsen in winter months, and is improved by exposure to ultraviolet rays. In severe cases, psoriasis may develop into arthritis primarily affecting the small digits of the hands and the feet.

Indications for massage

As the condition can be precipitated by emotional stress, therapeutic relaxation massage may assist with stress management.

Best avoided

Avoid massaging directly over or around any areas affected by psoriasis. To reduce the risk of causing infection, ensure all linen is changed and thoroughly washed, and massage equipment (including table) is disinfected at all times (see Chapter 10).

Rheumatoid arthritis

(immune system, skeletal system)

Rheumatoid arthritis (RA) is an autoimmune disease that is characterised by an inflammatory response as the body attacks its own connective tissue. It is estimated that approximately two per cent of the Australian population experiences this condition, which is considered the most common inflammatory joint disease. Despite Rheumatoid arthritus being a debilitating disease of the immune system, the exact cause of RA is still largely unknown. Rheumatoid arthritis is referred to as a multisystem disease — although most of the inflammation and tissue destruction occurs in the joints, other body tissues are affected also. Women are three times more likely to experience the condition than men, and the onset of RA can occur between 16 to 70 years of age, but is most common between the ages of 20 to 55 years.

Clinical features

Rheumatoid arthritis places the human body under both physical and psychological stress. The major symptoms of RA include pain, stiffness and loss of joint function. Rheumatoid arthritis is characterised by periods of exacerbation ('flare-ups') and remission. The pain caused by inflammation during a flare-up may be of an acute nature, yet during periods of remission chronic pain presents from both physiological and psychological causes. The physiological causes of pain are due to weight bearing on the affected joints, and psychological causes of pain are due to the stress, anxiety and depression experienced when so-called 'normal' function is lost. The symptoms of RA are most often observed to be bilateral, and it is largely the smaller joints of the body that are involved. The joints usually affected include shoulder, hip, elbow, knee, wrist, ankle, hand and foot.

Indications for massage

Another source of pain is joint swelling (which produces stretching) and weakening of the joint capsule and surrounding ligamentous structures, leading to instability of the joint. As the joint weakens, the altered biomechanics of the musculature associated with the affected region can also produce pain. There is often pain in the surrounding muscles, with muscle weakness and atrophy occurring as the condition progresses. This results in muscle imbalance, which further exacerbates the deformity. Surrounding musculature may become taut or contracted to protect the area. Massage therapy is useful for RA during periods of remission to encourage local circulation, and aid the relaxation of muscle tissue. Massage may also assist to reduce pain and is useful for stress management.

Caution

Clients with RA may be taking prescription analgesic or anti-inflammatory medications. Such medicines may reduce sensitivity and mask pain; thus clients may not be able to give adequate feedback on treatment techniques being applied.

Best avoided

Avoid massage when joints are acutely inflamed during flare-up periods.

CONCLUSION

Massage therapy is a safe and effective form of therapy for a vast array of medical complaints, and as such is suitable for a multitude of different situations. When a person first presents for massage, a skilled therapist ascertains the client's needs, and develops a detailed profile of their current health status. Armed with this case history, the therapist is then able to tailor the most effective treatment regime to suit the client. Factors that need to be considered when formulating a treatment approach include endangerment sites, absolute contra-indications, pre-existing disease states or syndromes and medications being administered. By developing a general working knowledge of such factors, the massage therapist will be able to make an informed assessment about the best treatment for each individual client. This will ensure that as a therapist they minimise any harm, thereby providing the best possible care for all clients at all times.

Questions and activities

1. When performing a full body massage, what endangerment sites would a therapist need to be aware of and why?
2. Using examples to illustrate your answer, discuss why massage therapy should be avoided when absolute contraindications exist.
3. Describe what conditions massage may be cautioned in and why.
4. Compare and contrast osteoarthritis and rheumatoid arthritis.
5. Compare and contrast fibromyalgia and chronic fatigue syndrome.

Recommended reading

Rattray, F. S. and Ludwig, L. M. (2000) *Clinical Massage Therapy: Understanding, Assessing and Treating Over 70 Conditions*. Talus Inc., Toronto.

Rhind, J. and Greig, J. (2002) *Anatomy and Physiology Applied to Health Professions* (7th edn). Churchill Livingstone, London.

Thibodeau, G. A. and Patton, T. (2003) *Anatomy and Physiology* (5th edn). Mosby, St Louis.

REFERENCES

Curties, D. (1999) *Breast Massage*. Curties-Overzet Publications, Toronto.

Salvo, S. G. (1999) *Massage Therapy: Principles and Practice*. W. B. Saunders, Philadelphia.

BIBLIOGRAPHY

Arthritis Foundation of NSW (1996) *The Arthritis Handbook* (2nd edn). MacLennan & Petty Pty Ltd, Sydney.

Clancy, J. and McVicar, A. J. (1995) *Physiology & Anatomy — A Homeostatic Approach*. Edward Arnold, London.

Glanze, W. D. (ed.) (1990) *Mosby's Medical, Nursing & Allied Health Dictionary* (3rd edn). Mosby, St Louis.

Hertling, D. and Kessler, R. M. (1996) *Management of Common Musculoskeletal Disorders: Physical Therapy Principles and Methods* (3rd edn). Lippincott-Raven Publishers, Philadelphia.

Katzung, B. G. (ed.) (1992) *Basic & Clinical Pharmacology*. Appleton & Lange, Stamford, Connecticut.

Kisner, C. and Colby, L. A. (1996) *Therapeutic Exercise: Foundations and Techniques* (3rd edn). F. A. Davis & Company, Philadelphia.

McCance, K. L. and Huether, S. E. (2002) *Pathophysiology — The Biological Basis for Disease in Adults and Children* (4th edn). Mosby, St Louis.

Moll, J. M. H. (1997) *Rheumatology — Colour Guide* (2nd edn). Churchill Livingstone, London.

Murtagh, J. (1998) *General Practice* (2nd edn). McGraw-Hill, Sydney.

Premkumar, K. (1996) *Pathology A to Z: A Handbook for Massage Therapists*. VanPub Books, Calgary.

Starlanyl, D. and Copeland, M. E. (1996) *Fibromyalgia & Chronic Myofascial Pain Syndrome*. New Harbinger Publications Inc., Oakland.

Tortora, G. J. and Grabowski, S. R. (1996) *Principles of Anatomy and Physiology* (8th edn). HarperCollins, New York.

chapter 13

Pharmacological considerations for massage

Michael Nott

Learning outcomes

- Describe potential interactions between massage and therapeutic drugs
- Be aware of specific interactions for commonly used drugs
- Discuss management procedures for adverse effects of drugs in massage therapy

INTRODUCTION

A massage therapist will see clients from different walks of life, representing a broad cross section of the community. Consequently many of them will be taking prescribed medications as directed by their primary care physician. Others may be taking proprietary medicines that they have purchased 'over the counter' at pharmacies and supermarkets. Others still may be taking herbal or other preparations provided by their complementary medicine practitioner or purchased from a health food store. This chapter deals with the issues that arise when clients who are taking medicines present for massage treatment. In addition to understanding any underlying medical conditions that clients may present with for massage (see Chapter 12), the therapist should also have knowledge of any medications that clients may be taking and the resultant considerations for the application of massage therapy. By taking a preliminary medication record of the client as part of the ASTER process (see Chapter 11) and considering the consequences for massage, the therapist will be equipped to prepare a treatment approach that is optimal for the client.

INTERACTIONS BETWEEN MASSAGE THERAPY AND DRUG THERAPY

It is widely proposed that massage therapy affects the release of endorphins in the brain and that these naturally occurring opiates, when in circulation, contribute to such beneficial effects as relaxation and pain reduction. There is conflicting evidence to support the contention that massage releases endorphins. In one study no increase in blood levels of endorphins were found after massage (Day et al., 1987) whereas, in another, small increases (which might of course indicate larger increases at neuronal sites of action) were recorded (Kaada and Torsteinbo, 1989). Tuchtan reviews more evidence for the implication of endorphins in modulating pain and consequences for massage (see Chapter 4).

If it is supposed that massage does release endorphins, or other neurotransmitters or hormones, then it is possible that any drugs the patient is taking might enhance or reduce the beneficial effects of massage by interacting with these natural chemicals. It could also be possible that the application of massage may affect the way in which the drug acts in the body.

At this stage it is wise to consider the known effects of drugs and massage and to be careful of an interaction, even if not at a pharmacological level. For example, if the client is taking a sedative drug the practitioner would warn the client that the massage may make them too relaxed and inattentive to drive home safely after the consultation.

THE IMPORTANCE OF A CLIENT'S MEDICATION HISTORY

A client's medication record should constitute part of the formal pre-massage history taking (see Chapter 11). Such a record will give clues to conditions the client may be experiencing. The client may be taking prescribed drugs, or those purchased over the counter in a pharmacy or supermarket. Herbal remedies and nutritional supplements should also be considered. In some cases adverse effects of drugs may impact on the quality and safety of the massage. It is therefore incumbent on the practitioner to be aware of any such reactions, and to be ready to advise and take action when needed.

In this chapter commonly used drugs (see Table 13.1) are described according to the diseases for which they are used. These diseases are generally chosen on the basis of frequency in the population, but with a bias towards those that would be likely to bring a client to massage. Emphasis is given to drugs used in diseases that, though not frequent in the population, present particular challenges for the massage therapist. For each drug, adverse effects that have a bearing on the comfort and safety of the massage treatment are emphasised, even though they may not be the most serious adverse effects overall. Advice is also provided on how to manage any potential problems if they arise (see Table 13.2).

Angina

Typically prescribed drugs for angina are nitrates, β-adrenoceptor antagonists, and calcium channel blockers.

Drug treatment of angina pectoris aims to address the imbalance between blood supply to the heart muscle (the coronary vessels being constricted or blocked) and the amount of work the heart has to do. Such drugs act to reduce force and rate of contractions of the heart or dilate peripheral blood vessels so that the heart has less work to do (for a review see Kerins et al., 2001).

The nitrates are the mainstay of treatment (glyceryl trinitrate being the most common, but isosorbide nitrates are also used). Nitrates act by dilating peripheral arterial and venous blood vessels (Harrison and Bates, 1993). β-adrenoceptor antagonists (β-blockers; e.g., metoprolol, atenolol and many others ending with 'olol') reduce sympathetic drive to the heart, thus lowering rate and force of contraction (Kerins, et al., 2001). They also dilate the peripheral blood vessels (Oates and

Table 13.1 Drug types and some common generic and trade names

DRUG TYPE	GENERIC NAME	TRADE NAMES
angiotensin converting enzyme (ACE) inhibitor	captropil	Captopen
angiotensin II receptor antagonist	losartan	Cozaar
anticontractile drug	dantrolene	Dantrium
	carbamazepine	Tegretol, Teril
antiseizure drugs	phenobarbitone	Phenobarbitone, Prominal, Mysolone
	phenytoin	Dilantin
	sodium valproate	Epilim, Valpro
antihistamines	diphenhydramine	Benadryl, Benacine, Dramamine etc.
	fexofenadine	Telfast
	loratidine	Claratyne
	promethazine	Promethazine, Pothazine, Phenergan, Aromine etc.
	terfenadine	Teldane
anti-inflammatory analgesics	aspirin	Aspro, Bex, Disprin etc.
	aspirin plus codeine, celecoxib	Codral, Aspalgin, Codiphen, Celebrex etc.
	ibuprofen	Brufen, Raphen
	indomethacin	Indocid, Arthrexin
	paracetamol	Panadol, Tylenol
	paracetamol plus codeine	Codral, Panadeine, Codalgin etc.
	prednisolone	Solone, Predsol etc.
antimanic drug	lithium	Lithicarb
β-adrenoceptor antagonists	atenolol	Tenormin, Noten, Anselol
	fenoterol	Berotec
	metoprolol	Betaloc, Lopresor, Minax
	orciprenaline	Alupent
	salbutamol	Ventolin
	terbutaline	Bricanyl
benzodiazepines	alprazolam	Xanax, Kalma, Ralozam
	bromazepam	Lexotan
	clonazepam	Rivotril
	diazepam	Valium, Ducene, Diazapam etc.
	lorazepam	Ativan
	oxazepam	Serepax, Murelax, Alepam
calcium channel blockers	amlodipine	Norvasc
	diltiazem	Cardizem, Coras, Dilzem
	felodipine	Plendil, Agon
	nifedipine	Adalat, Oros, Nifecard
	verapamil	Isoptin, Cordilox, Veracaps, Anpec
GABA	agonist baclofen	Lioresal, Clofen

Table 13.1 Drug types and some common generic and trade names (continued)

DRUG TYPE	GENERIC NAME	TRADE NAMES
insulin	various formulations	various names
nitrates	glyceryl trinitrate	Anginine, Deponit, Nitradisc etc.
	isosorbide	Isordil, Isogen, Sorbidin,
oral hypoglycaemic drug	chlorpropamide	Diabenese
phenothiazine	chlorpromazine	Pericyazine
selective serotonin reuptake inhibitor (SSRI)	fluoxetine	Prozac
serotonin antagonist	sumatriptan	Imigran
stimulant anorectic	diethylproprion	Tenuate
thiazide diuretic	acetazolamide	Diamox
tricyclic antidepressants	amitriptyline	Tryptanol, Endepo, Tryptine
	imipramine	Tofranil, Imiprin, Melipramine
	trimipramine	Surmontil

Brown, 2001). The calcium channel blockers (like verapamil, diltiazem, amlodipine, felodipine and nifedipine) similarly affect peripheral blood vessels yet also dilate the coronary vessels and directly reduce heart contractility (Serruys et al., 1981).

All drugs used to treat angina are prone to cause postural hypotension (Kerins et al., 2001). Thus clients are likely to feel dizzy or faint upon changing from the recumbent to standing position. Practitioners should caution clients to return to a standing posture at a slow rate and with care after the massage. It is also advised that the therapist remain close by during this period and provide assistance as required.

Anorexia nervosa and bulimia nervosa

Typically prescribed drugs for anorexia nervosa and bulimia nervosa are selective serotonin reuptake inhibitors (SSRI), and benzodiazepines.

Psychoneurotic eating disorders such as anorexia nervosa and bulimia nervosa are commonly associated with anxiety and depression (see Chapter 12). Such conditions are treated by antidepressants such as fluoxetine (a selective serotonin reuptake inhibitor; see section on depression below) or an anti-anxiety drug like benzo-diazepines (e.g. diazepam). Fluoxetine does not dry the skin as do other antidepressant drugs such as the tricyclic antidepressants (see section on depression below) and its use should not affect massage. A common outcome of treatment with benzodiazepines is tiredness so the massage therapist should caution the client about driving home after the massage.

Anxiety

Typically prescribed drugs for anxiety are benzodiazepines, and β-adrenoceptor antagonists.

Clients suffering from anxiety may be receiving drug therapy in addition to other support such as counselling, particularly if the anxiety is acute or prolonged. Anxiety may also accompany depression. Drug therapy may be aimed at the anxiety itself, in which case specific anti-anxiety drugs such as a benzodiazepine may be prescribed, or at symptoms, such as heart palpitations, in which case a β-adrenoceptor antagonist may be prescribed. The benzodiazepines are the most commonly used anti-anxiety drugs, and of these alprazolam, bromazepam, diazepam, lorazepam, and oxazepam are commonly chosen because of their relatively long duration of action (Baldessarini, 2001). As the benzodiazepines cause sedation the massage therapist should caution the client about driving home after the massage if they are feeling sleepy post-treatment.

Asthma

Typically prescribed drugs for asthma are mast cell stabilisers, anti-inflammatory steroids, and β-adrenoceptor agonists.

Asthma is treated with drugs such as mast cell stabilisers (cromoglycate and nedocromil) to prevent the initial response to allergens. The inflammatory response of asthma is treated with anti-inflammatory steroids such as beclomethasone. The mainstay of treatment is β-adrenoceptor agonists such as salbutamol, terbutaline, fenoterol and orciprenaline that relax the smooth muscle of the bronchioles.

To minimise systemic side effects, anti-asthma drugs are preferably administered by inhalation, rather than orally. Even so, the β-adrenoceptor agonists still commonly cause skeletal muscle tremor (Securs, 2002). Clients should be reassured that this would not cause a problem in massage.

Attention deficit hyperactivity disorder (ADHD)

Typically prescribed drugs for ADHD are psycho-stimulants.

About one per cent of children are diagnosed as suffering from ADHD with the incidence in boys being ten times greater than in girls. Attention deficit hyperactivity disorder usually becomes apparent between the ages of three to seven years (Findling and Dogin, 1998). The condition may persist into adulthood. Drug treatment relies on paradoxical effects of the psychostimulants dexamphetamine and methyl-phenidate, which are given for extended periods. It is unlikely that clients will have adverse effects that impact on massage.

High doses of psychostimulants, such as those taken illicitly, may cause excitement, palpitations and tremor and, over time, psychosis and chorea (jerky and explosive fidgety movements around the body).

Chronic fatigue syndrome (CFS)

Typically prescribed drugs are selective serotonin reuptake inhibitor (SSRI) antidepressants.

Clients suffering from CFS may be prescribed a selective serotonin reuptake inhibitor (SSRI) antidepressant like fluoxetine (see section on depression below).

Depression (minor) and affective disorders (major depression)

Typically prescribed drugs for affective disorders are selective serotonin reuptake inhibitors (SSRI), reversible inhibitors of monoamine oxidase (RIMA), tricyclic antidepressants, and lithium.

A herbal remedy for affective disorders is St John's wort.

At any time it is estimated that around 20 per cent of the population is suffering from depression (McLennan, 1997). For some clients, depression may be associated with chronic pain or a neurotic or personality disorder. If a client reports that they are receiving treatment for depression then they may be experiencing a short-term personal response to a set back in life and relationships. They may be having counselling with or without a short period of drug therapy.

At the extreme the client may be experiencing major depression (monopolar affective disorder) or, much less commonly, manic depression (bipolar affective disorder). The affective disorders are so-named because of characteristic marked mood (affect) changes. Psychosis is another characteristic. There are also atypical affective disorders, and severe depression associated with neurotic and personality disorders. In all cases, clients may be undergoing prolonged and intense medication with antidepressants, along with other treatments.

The drugs of first choice for affective disorders are the selective serotonin reuptake inhibitors (SSRI) such as fluoxetine, sertraline, fluvoxamine, paroxetine and citalopram, along with moclobemide which is a reversible inhibitor of monoamine oxidase (RIMA), and the newer compounds nefazodone, and venlafaxine. Due to their more marked side effects, the tricyclic antidepressants such as imipramine, amitryptiline, trimipramine and clomipramine are generally reserved for more refractory cases, as is mianserin. The irreversible monoamine oxidase inhibitors (MAOI), such as phenylzine and tranylcypromine, because of their serious side effects and life-threatening food interactions, are drugs of last resort. Extracts of St John's wort also have been shown to be effective in treating depression though less so than the tricyclic antidepressants. Lithium is used for treating the mania of bipolar affective disorder. For a review of the use of antidepressants in Australia and New Zealand see Chapter 19 of Bryant et al. (2003).

None of these drug treatments alone would preclude massage therapy. The tricyclic antidepressants are noted for their atropine-like activity (Leonard and Richelson, 2000) which tends to dry the skin and raise its temperature. In this regard the therapist may choose to use, as a lubricant for massage, oil that is hydrating and nourishing to the skin, such as sweet almond oil and, in consultation with the client, reduce the intensity of the massage. Among other effects of the tricyclics is sedation and the practitioner should caution the client about driving home afterwards if they are feeling sleepy.

Diabetes

Type I diabetes mellitus (juvenile onset; insulin dependent diabetes mellitus; IDDM)

Typically prescribed drugs are insulins (human and bovine).

Clients experiencing type I diabetes mellitus warrant particular attention due to the condition itself (see Chapter 12). They will have injected insulin sometime that day before presenting for the massage. Hypoglycaemia, due to inadequate food intake before the massage, or to the increase in muscle activity during the massage (Davis and Granner, 2001), is the most likely complication and must be dealt with immediately. Symptoms will be recognised by the client and therapist as feelings of faintness, clammy skin and tremor. The therapist should make sure the client is seen on time so as not to interfere with the balance of their insulin/food schedule, and should make sure they have a glucose source (such as marshmallows or jelly beans) at hand before the massage begins (and have one handy in the clinic just in case).

Type II diabetes mellitus (known also as maturity or adult onset; non-insulin dependent diabetes mellitus; NIDDM)

Typically prescribed drugs are oral hypoglycaemic drugs, and insulins.

Depending on the severity of the disease, type II diabetes mellitus may be controlled by diet and exercise; by oral hypoglycaemic drugs; by injections of insulin or a combination of these strategies (Davis and Granner, 2001). Refer to Chapter 12 for symptoms of the disease itself and how the massage should proceed.

Clients generally warrant the same attention as those with type I diabetes mellitus although clients receiving insulin should be considered most prone to hypoglycaemic episodes. Clients receiving oral hypoglycaemic drugs (alone) would be less likely to experience a hypoglycaemic attack (or 'hypo'), and the least likely would be those whose diabetes is controlled by diet and exercise.

The therapist should be alert to symptoms of hypoglycaemia in the client: feelings of faintness, clammy skin and tremor. It is advisable for the massage therapist to schedule the client in advance and see them promptly to avoid interfering with the balance of their drug/food regimen. As in cases of type I diabetes, a glucose source should be kept at hand.

Drug dependence and abuse

Drugs typically abused in society are alcohol, opiates, stimulants, cannabis and hallucinogens.

Clients may present for massage while they are taking drugs (but not being treated for drug dependence), or as part of a drug rehabilitation program. Much will depend on whether the client has volunteered the information about drug taking in the pre-massage history taking. The experienced practitioner should be aware of cues and take precautions accordingly.

Alcohol and opiates such as heroin (and methadone which is used in rehabilitation) are central nervous system depressants, which cause sedation. The client should be cautioned about the possibility of sedative effects of massage adding to the effects of the drug, particularly if they are intending to drive a car afterwards.

Stimulants such as amphetamine and cocaine can cause psychotic episodes. It is possible that massage could induce such an episode, thus endangering the client and practitioner and it would be reasonable to refuse a consultation in such cases.

Cannabis (particularly after chronic use) and hallucinogens may induce psychoses and the practitioner should be prepared to refuse a consultation in such cases where required. Drug counselling may be proposed if the occasion arises.

For further information on adverse effects of drugs of dependence and abuse see O'Brien (2001).

Dysmenorrhea

Typically prescribed drugs for dysmenorrhea are anti-inflammatory analgesics.

Women suffering from dysmenorrhea may be taking anti-inflammatory analgesics such as aspirin or paracetamol to relieve pain. Thus their perception of musculoskeletal pain may be reduced.

Endometriosis

Typically prescribed drugs for endometriosis are anti-inflammatory analgesics.

Precautions and likely drug and massage implications are as for dysmenorrhea (see above).

Epilepsy

Typically prescribed drugs for epilepsy are phenobarbitone (one of the long acting barbiturates), carbamazepine, clonazepam (a long acting benzodiazepine), phenytoin and sodium valproate.

Epilepsy presents a range of potential problems to the massage therapist, the main one being a seizure episode during treatment. This issue, and the therapist's appropriate response, are described in Chapter 12.

Anti-seizure drugs generally cause sedation, in addition to other specific side effects. The practitioner should caution the client about driving home after the massage if they are feeling sleepy.

For specific adverse effects of particular anti-seizure drugs see *MIMS Annual* (2003).

Fibromyalgia

Typically prescribed drugs for fibromyalgia are anti-inflammatory analgesics, anti-anxiety drugs, and tricyclic antidepressants or selective serotonin reuptake inhibitors.

Clients experiencing fibromyalgia characteristically complain of tenderness and pain in skeletal muscles. This chronic condition may induce anxiety and depression. Typical medications include anti-inflammatory analgesics such as aspirin, paracetamol and indomethacin. Long acting benzodiazepines, such as diazepam and lorazepan, are favoured as anti-anxiety drugs. Occasionally an antidepressant such as fluoxetine, or amitryptiline (which has a sedative and atropine-like effect), is required (see section on depression above). See Chapter 12 for more details of fibromyalgia.

Hay fever

Typically prescribed drugs for hay fever are antihistamines, nasal vasoconstrictors and nasal anticholinergics.

Hay fever (allergic rhinitis) is particularly common in Australasia and approximately 20 per cent of the population experiences it (Australian Institute of Health and Welfare, 2001). Hay fever follows an immune response to allergens whereupon autacoids, such as histamine, serotonin and prostaglandin, are released from mast cells to cause inflammation, nasal congestion and hypersecretion.

Clients with hay fever may have been prescribed an orally administered antihistamine or obtained an over-the-counter preparation. Antihistamines block the action of a number of the autacoids released by the immune response (not just histamine) and are thus very effective. The older drugs, such as diphenhydramine and promethazine, are sedative and may be useful at night, but they pose a risk for drivers and users of machinery. Newer antihistamines such as loratidine, terfenadine and fexofenadine are less sedating.

Some antihistamines have marked atropine-like activity and cause the skin to become dry and feel hot. The therapist may choose to use a lubricant that is hydrating and nourishing to the skin such as sweet almond oil and reduce the intensity of the massage.

Hay fever may also be treated by spraying drugs into the nose. Drugs administered this way are vasoconstrictors such as xylometazoline, corticosteroids, mast cell stabilisers, and nasal anticholinergics such as ipratropium, which dry up secretions. Generally, drugs administered by nasal spray act locally and will not produce sufficient systemic concentrations to cause concern with massage.

For more information on allergic rhinitis and its treatment see Chapter 32 of Bryant et al. (2003).

Headache

Typically prescribed drugs for *occasional headaches* are anti-inflammatory analgesics.

Typically prescribed drugs for *persistent headaches* are tricyclic antidepressant, and benzodiazepines.

Typically prescribed drugs for *migraines* are β-adrenoceptor antagonists (β-blockers), antihistamines, and serotonin antagonists.

Normal headache is usually self-treated with a common over-the-counter anti-inflammatory analgesic such as aspirin or paracetamol.

Persistent headaches, depending on the history of the client, may require prescriptions for a tricyclic antidepressant such as amitryptiline, or a long acting benzodiazepine anti-anxiety drug such as diazepam or lorazepam. Such clients often gain relief from massage (see Chapter 12).

Clients experiencing a migraine headache with nausea and vomiting are unlikely to present for massage. The migraine condition and its associated drug treatment are as complex as it is common. Prophylaxis may involve treatment with a β-adrenoceptor antagonist (β-blocker), or an antihistamine, or a serotonin antagonist such as the new drug sumatriptan.

For a review of current treatment strategies for migraine and other headaches see Chapter 21 of Bryant et al. (2003).

Heart failure

Typically prescribed drugs for heart failure are digoxin, angiotensin converting enzyme (ACE) inhibitors, anti-arrthymic drugs, cardiac stimulants, diuretics and anti-hypertensive drugs.

Heart failure is the condition where the heart becomes incapable of pumping sufficient blood to satisfy body tissue demands. Heart failure may be due to hypertension causing the heart to enlarge and become less efficient. In some cases it may be due to poor perfusion or death of heart muscle itself, both due to coronary ischaemia, or alternatively there may be an arrhythmia which underlies the problem.

Until recently digoxin was the drug of first choice in treating heart failure. Digoxin directly increases cardiac contractility and slows heart rate if there is excessive activity coming from the pacemaker region of the atria. Digoxin is still used if heart failure is associated with atrial tachycardia, however current treatment focuses on reducing the oedema associated with the disease. The main drugs used for this are the angiotensin converting enzyme

(ACE) inhibitors such as captropril and enalapril (Ooi and Colucci, 2001).

In this complex and life-threatening condition anti-arrhythmic drugs, cardiac stimulants, diuretics and anti-hypertensive drugs are also used depending on the underlying pathology.

Clients suffering from heart failure and presenting for massage will commonly experience dizziness and feelings of faintness due to the underlying poor cardiac output. As such the massage therapist should advise the client to get up from the table slowly after the massage. The drugs used to treat heart failure may themselves cause central effects leading to sedation, confusion and tremors, but these are not as significant as the underlying circulatory problems (Ooi and Colucci, 2001). The massage therapist can reassure the client if these effects occur and advise the client not to drive home after the massage if they are feeling sleepy or confused.

Hypertension

Typically prescribed drugs for hypertension are thiazide diuretics, β-adrenoceptor antagonists, calcium channel blockers, angiotensin converting enzyme (ACE) inhibitors and angiotensin II receptor antagonists.

Many different drug types are used to treat hypertension or high blood pressure. If the condition is mild a single drug may be prescribed. For more severe hypertension a combination of drugs, each at a relatively low dose, is chosen. The intention is to act at a number of points of blood pressure control and thus minimise the side effects profile of any one drug.

Clients presenting with hypertension are likely to be taking one or more of the following: a thiazide diuretic (e.g. acetazolamide), a β-adrenoceptor antagonist (e.g. alprenolol, metoprolol and many others all ending in 'olol'), a calcium channel blocker (e.g. amlodipine, felodipine or nifedipine), an angiotensin converting enzyme (ACE) inhibitor (captropril and many others, all ending in 'pril') or an angiotensin II receptor antagonist (e.g. losartan and others, all ending in 'artan'). For a review of current treatment practice see Chapter 25 of Bryant et al. (2003).

To a greater or lesser extent all anti-hypertensive drugs may cause postural hypotension, so that clients feel dizzy or faint upon changing from the recumbent to standing position. Practitioners should caution clients, and remain aware and prepared to act during the vulnerable period after the massage when the client, whose blood pressure control is adjusted to the recumbent position, is about to stand up.

Immunosuppressant therapy

Typically prescribed drugs for immunosuppressant therapy are corticosteroids and specific immunosuppressants.

High doses of corticosteroids such as cortisone or prednisolone are used (along with other medications) to suppress the immune response in autoimmune disorders, and in clients who have undergone an organ transplant. Such therapy is usually long term and inevitably leads to adverse effects, some of which may impact on massage.

Corticosteroids cause protein breakdown so that muscles become thinner and weaker, and skin develops striae and a tendency to bruise. Corticosteroids cause negative calcium balance in bone, resulting in fragile bones and osteoporosis. Fungal infection of the skin and nails also may occur. For a review of immunosuppressant therapy see Schimmer and Parker (2001).

The client should first seek advice from their primary care practitioner. Massage may then proceed gently and with constant feedback from the client. If the skin is infected then the practitioner should wear gloves, and infected areas should be avoided (see Chapter 10).

Menopause

Typically prescribed drugs for menopause are oestrogen and progestogen hormone replacement therapy (HRT).

The predominant treatment for the unpleasant symptoms of menopause, and the longer-term issue of osteoporosis, is HRT involving serial courses of an oestrogen and a progestogen (Belchetz, 1994). As osteoporosis, and associated weakening of bone, is an issue for safety in massage (see Chapter 12), it is reasonable (but not demonstrated) that older post-menopausal women on HRT would be less prone to inadvertent fracture during massage. However, with recent warnings on adverse effects, particularly regarding HRT being a risk factor for dementia (Tattersal, 2003), long-term HRT therapy is likely to diminish.

HRT is unlikely to cause adverse effects of consequence for massage. Rather, HRT will reduce hot flush and skin sensitivity associated with menopause, which might otherwise make massage intolerable.

Multiple sclerosis

Typically prescribed drugs for multiple sclerosis are benzodiazepines, GABA agonist and dantrolene.

Drugs used to reduce the symptoms of multiple sclerosis are centrally acting antispastic drugs such as the benzodiazepine diazepam, and the GABA agonist baclofen (GABA being a central nervous system transmitter which acts to reduce neuronal activity to skeletal muscle), and drugs such as dantrolene, which act directly on the muscles to reduce contractility. The centrally acting drugs are likely to cause sedation and practitioners should warn patients about the danger of tiredness if driving home after massage. The anti-contractile drug dantrolene lowers muscle tone, without causing sedation, (Kita and Goodkin, 2000) and should not affect massage.

Obesity

Typically prescribed drugs for obesity are stimulant-anorectics, sibutramine, and antidepressants.

Drugs used as adjuncts to the treatment of obesity typically are the stimulant anorectics such as diethylpropion and phenyldimetrazine (Hoffman, 2001). The centrally acting neurotransmitter uptake inhibitor sibutramine is now being used (Sanders-Bush and Mayer, 2001). Adverse effects of both groups of drugs include anxiety and agitation but, apart from the need to reassure the client, no problems with massage are likely.

Antidepressants such as fluoxitine (Prozac) are also prescribed occasionally. Reported effects of dizziness, nervousness and tremor may be noted by the client but again present no major concern for the massage therapist.

Osteoarthritis

Typically prescribed drugs for osteoarthritis are anti-inflammatory steroids, and non-steroidal anti-inflammatory analgesics.

Drugs used in treating osteoarthritis typically are anti-inflammatory steroids such as prednisolone, and non-steroidal anti-inflammatory analgesics such as aspirin, indomethacin and ibuprofen (see Chapter 55 in Bryant et al., 2003, for treatment regimens). As with analgesics, generally the threshold for pain in the client may be elevated and the practitioner must restrain the limits of the massage to avoid tissue damage.

Paget's disease (osteitis deformans)

Typically prescribed drugs for Paget's disease are non-steroidal anti-inflammatory analgesics, calcitonin, and phosphonates.

Drugs used for treatment of Paget's disease are the non-steroidal anti-inflammatory analgesic, such as aspirin, indomethacin and ibuprofen, and drugs to help re-mineralise bone, such as calcitonin and phosphonates (Marcus, 2001). As with analgesics, generally the threshold for pain in the client may be elevated and the practitioner should restrain the intensity of the massage to avoid tissue damage.

A gentle massage would be required anyway, as the bones of sufferers of Paget's disease are very prone to fracture (see Chapter 12).

Premenstrual syndrome

Typically prescribed drugs for premenstrual syndrome are non-steroidal anti-inflammatory analgesics, calcitonin, and phosphonates.

The pain of premenstrual syndrome may be treated with prescription or over-the-counter anti-inflammatory analgesics (such as those containing aspirin or paracetamol). The massage therapist should restrain the intensity of the massage as pain perception in the client may be reduced with these medications.

Rheumatoid arthritis

Typically prescribed drugs for rheumatoid arthritis are anti-inflammatory steroids, non-steroidal anti-inflammatory analgesics, gold salts, penicillamine, and sulfasalazine.

Drugs used in rheumatoid arthritis are the anti-inflammatory steroids such as prednisolone, and non-steroidal anti-inflammatory analgesics such as aspirin, indomethacin and ibuprofen. As with analgesics generally, the threshold for pain in the client may be elevated and the practitioner should restrain the intensity of the massage to avoid tissue damage.

These days rheumatoid arthritis is often treated at source by drugs that apparently interfere with the underlying autoimmune response. These include gold salts, penicillamine and sulfasalazine. It is unlikely that their effects would interfere with massage treatment.

For details of drugs used to treat rheumatoid arthritis see Chapter 25 of Bryant et al. (2003).

Schizophrenia

Typically prescribed drugs for schizophrenia are phenothiazines and other antipsychotic drug groups.

Antipsychotic drugs are used to treat schizophrenia, and the mainstays are the phenothiazines such as chlorpromazine (Baldessarini and Tarazi, 2001). A variety of other drugs is used in order to gain control with the minimum of side effects, however given that the disease is so serious, major side effects are tolerated in the quest for control.

Schizophrenia is increasingly treated on outpatient principles and clients who are controlled by drugs no doubt will present for massage. They are likely to exhibit a range of side effects with implications for massage, including sedation, hypotension, drying and heating of the skin, and when drug dosage is high, extrapyramidal effects which cause limb stiffness, twitching, muscle tremor and spasms (Baldessarini and Tarazi, 2001).

The massage therapist should counsel the client about tiredness after the massage, adjust the massage to account for the hot and dry skin, account for tense muscles which are under excessive neuronal drive, and be prepared for postural hypotension when the client gets up from the table.

Topical steroid therapy

Typically prescribed drugs for topical steroid therapy are corticosteroids.

Topical corticosteroids are used to treat persistent inflammatory skin conditions such as eczema and psoriasis. These underlying conditions may present issues to be dealt with in massage and the drugs themselves cause important adverse effects (Schimmer and Parker, 2001). Topical corticosteroids tend to thin and weaken the skin so that it becomes easy to bruise. For this reason the intensity of massage in susceptible areas should be restrained. Topical corticosteroids also encourage fungal infections. If the skin is infected then gloves should be worn and the infected areas should be avoided.

Table 13.2 Drug types, possible adverse effects and appropriate actions

DRUG TYPE	POSSIBLE CONSEQUENCE FOR MASSAGE	APPROPRIATE ACTIONS
angiotensin converting enzyme (ACE) inhibitor	mild postural hypotension; giddiness; potential to faint	advise to stand up slowly; be prepared for fainting
angiotensin II receptor antagonist	mild postural hypotension; giddiness; potential to faint	advise to stand up slowly; be prepared for fainting
anti-anxiety drugs	sedation	warn of danger in driving after massage
anticontractile drugs	reduced muscle spasm	no action
antiepileptic drugs	sedation	warn of danger in driving after massage
antihistamines	dry hot skin	hydrating oils; gentle massage
	sedation	warn of danger in driving after massage
anti-inflammatory analgesics	reduced pain response	control intensity of massage
antipsychotic drugs	involuntary movements	reassure patient
antispastic drugs (acting on muscle)	reduced muscle spasm	no action
antispastic drugs (CNS acting)	reduced muscle spasm	no action
	sedation	warn of danger in driving after massage
β-adrenoceptor agonists	muscle tremor	reassure patient; no other action
β-adrenoceptor antagonists	mild postural hypotension; giddiness; potential to faint	advise to stand up slowly; be prepared for fainting
benzodiazepines	sedation	warn of danger in driving after massage
calcium channel blockers	mild postural hypotension; giddiness; potential to faint	advise to stand up slowly; be prepared for fainting
corticosteroids (inhaled)	nil	no action

Table 13.2 Drug types, possible adverse effects and appropriate actions (continued)

DRUG TYPE	POSSIBLE CONSEQUENCE FOR MASSAGE	APPROPRIATE ACTIONS
corticosteroids (oral)	wasting of muscle protein; reduced bone strength; skin wasting and possible fungal infection	take particular care to control intensity of massage; use hydrating oils; take precautions for infected skin
corticosteroids (topical)	thinning of skin, possible fungal infection of skin	control intensity of massage; use hydrating oils; take precautions for infected skin
insulin	hypoglycaemic episode: faintness, clammy skin, tremor	oral glucose or sucrose (jelly beans, one or two candy bars or two bananas); in emergency call ambulance
lithium (antimanic)	acne	skin infection control
	tremor	reassure patient
nitrates	severe postural hypotension with potential to faint	advise to stand up slowly; be prepared for fainting
oral hypoglcaemic drugs	hypoglycaemic episode: faintness, clammy skin, tremor	oral glucose or sucrose (one or two candy bars or two bananas); in emergency call ambulance
phenothiaxines	muscle stiffness	be aware that muscle stiffness and movement is neuronal in origin and not ameliorated by massage
phenothiazines	tremor	reassure patient
	dry hot skin	hydrating oils; gentle massage
phenothiazines	extrapyramidal syndrome: tremor, akinesia, twitching, stiffness, spasms	reassure patient; syndrome is CNS in origin and massage will palliate only
phenothiazines	postural hypotension; giddiness; potential to faint	advise to stand up slowly; be prepared for fainting
	sedation	warn of danger in driving after massage
psychostimulants	low therapeutic doses no problem; high illicit doses cause excitement, palpitations, tremor, chorea, psychotic episode	reassure patient; emergency procedures if required
reversible inhibitors of monoamine oxidase (RIMA)	no common marked adverse effects	no action
selective serotonin reuptake inhibitors (SSRI)	dizziness, nervousness, tremor	reassure patient
St John's wort	occasional serotonin syndrome (confusion, tremor, diarrhoea)	seek medical help
thiazide diuretic	postural hypotension; giddiness; potential to faint	advise to stand up slowly; be prepared for fainting
tricyclic anti-depressants	dry hot skin	hydrating oils; gentle massage
	sedation	warn of danger in driving after massage

CONCLUSION

Many massage clients will be taking prescribed or other medications. Such medications may have an impact on the safety and therapeutic outcome of massage therapy. The therapist should take a preliminary medication record of the client, be equipped to advise clients, be ready to modify the massage accordingly and to take action to prevent adverse outcomes. Knowledge of typical effects of currently used drugs, and the ability to source information on newer drugs, is the necessary precondition for appropriate actions.

Questions and activities

During pre-massage history taking your clients may report they are taking various medications. For each of the following clients record:

(a) further information (if any) you would seek from the client;
(b) advice or warnings (if any) you would give to the client; and
(c) actions you should be prepared to take during the consultation.

Client 1 — Reports he is taking pain killers for arthritis.

Client 2 — Says she is being treated with blood thinners for clotting problems.

Client 3 — Says he is being treated by the doctor for high blood pressure.

Client 4 — Reports she is being treated with Tofranil for depression.

Client 5 — Seems agitated and wants the massage to calm herself down but does not recall taking any prescribed medications.

Further reading

Bryant, B., Knights, K. and Salerno, E. (2003) *Pharmacology for Health Professionals*. Mosby, Sydney.

Hardman, J. G. et al. (2001) *Goodman and Gilman's The Pharmacological Basis of Therapeutics* (10th edn). McGraw Hill, New York.

Katzung, B. et al. (2001) *Basic and Clinical Pharmacoogy* (8th edn). Mosby, London.

MIMS Annual (2003) MediMedia, St Leonards.

MIMS New Zealand on CD (2003) MediMedia, NZ.

Upfal, J. (2002) *The Australian Drug Guide* (6th edn). Black Inc, Melbourne.

REFERENCES

Australian Institute of Health and Welfare (2001) *Chronic Diseases and Associated Risk Factors*. Australian Institute of Health and Welfare, Canberra.

Baldessarini, B. J. (2001) 'Drugs and the treatment of psychiatric disorders: depression and anxiety disorders', in *Goodman and Gilman's The Pharmacological Basis of Therapeutics* (10th edn), J. G. Hardman et al. (eds), McGraw Hill, New York, Chapter 19.

Baldessarini, B. J. and Tarazi, F. I. (2001) 'Drugs and the treatment of psychiatric disorders: psychosis and mania', in *Goodman and Gilman's The Pharmacological Basis of Therapeutics* (10th edn), J. G. Hardman et al. (eds), McGraw Hill, New York, Chapter 20.

Belshetz, P. E. (1994) 'Hormone treatment of postmenopausal women', *New England Journal of Medicine*, 330, 1062–71.

Bryant, B., Knights, K. and Salerno, E. (2003) *Pharmacology for Health Professionals*. Mosby, Sydney.

Davis, S. N. and Granner, D. K. (2001) 'Insulin, oral hypoglycemic agents, and the pharmacology of the endocrine pancreas', in *Goodman and Gilman's The Pharmacological Basis of Therapeutics* (10th edn), J. G. Hardman et al. (eds), McGraw Hill, New York, Chapter 61.

Day, J. A., Mason, R. R. and Chesrown, S. E. (1987) 'Effect of massage on serum level of beta-endorphin and beta-lipotropin in healthy adults', *Physical Therapy*, 67, pp. 926–30.

Findling, R. L. and Dogin, J. W. (1998) 'Psychopharmacology of ADHD: children and adolescents', *Journal of Clinical Psychiatry*, 59, Supplement 7, 42–9.

Harrison, D. G. and Bates, J. N. (1993) 'The vasodilators. New ideas about old drugs', *Circulation*, 87, pp. 1461–7.

Hoffman, B. B. (2001) 'Catecholamines, sympathomimetic drugs, and adrenergic receptor antagonists', in *Goodman and Gilman's The Pharmacological Basis of Therapeutics* (10th edn), J. G. Hardman et al. (eds), McGraw Hill, New York, Chapter 10.

Kaada, B. and Torsteinbo, O. (1989) 'Increase of plasma β-endorphins in connective tissue massage', *General Pharmacology*, 20, pp. 487–9.

Kerins, D. M., Robertson, R. M. and Robertson, D. (2001) 'Drugs used for the treatment of myocardial ischemia', in *Goodman and Gilman's The*

Pharmacological Basis of Therapeutics (10th edn), J. G. Hardman et al. (eds), McGraw Hill, New York, Chapter 32.

Kita, M. and Goodkin, D. E. (2000) 'Drugs used to treat spasticity', *Drugs*, 59, 487–95.

Leonard, B. E. and Richelson, E. (2000) 'Synaptic effects of antidepressants', in *Schizophrenia and Mood Disorder: The New Drug Therapies in Clinical Practice*, P. F. Buckley and J. L. Waddington (eds), Butterworth–Heinemann, Boston.

Marcus, R. (2001) 'Agents affecting calcification and bone turnover', in *Goodman and Gilman's The Pharmacological Basis of Therapeutics* (10th edn), J. G. Hardman et al. (eds), McGraw Hill, New York, Chapter 62.

McLennan, W. (1997) *Mental Health and Wellbeing; Profile of Adults*. Australian Bureau of Statistics, Canberra.

MIMS Annual (2003) MediMedia, St Leonards.

O'Brien, C. P. (2001) 'Drug addiction and drug abuse', in *Goodman and Gilman's The Pharmacological Basis of Therapeutics* (10th edn), J. G. Hardman et al. (eds), McGraw Hill, New York, Chapter 24.

Oates, J. A. and Brown, N. J. (2001) 'Antidiuretic agents and the drug therapy of hypertension', in *Goodman and Gilman's The Pharmacological Basis of Therapeutics* (10th edn), J. G. Hardman et al. (eds), McGraw Hill, New York, Chapter 33.

Ooi, H. and Colucci, W. S. (2001) 'Pharmacological treatment of heart failure', in *Goodman and Gilman's The Pharmacological Basis of Therapeutics* (10th edn), J. G. Hardman et al. (eds), McGraw Hill, New York, Chapter 34.

Sanders-Bush, E. and Mayer, S. E. (2001) '5-Hydroxytryptamine (serotonin): receptor agonists and antagonists', in *Goodman and Gilman's The Pharmacological Basis of Therapeutics*, (10th edn), J. G. Hardman et al. (eds), McGraw Hill, New York, Chapter 11.

Schimmer, B. P. and Parker, K. L. (2001) 'Adrenocorticotropic hormone; adrenocortical steroids and their synthetic analogs; inhibitors of the synthesis and actions of adrenocortical hormones', in *Goodman and Gilman's The Pharmacological Basis of Therapeutics* (10th edn), J. G. Hardman et al. (eds), McGraw Hill, New York, Chapter 60.

Securs, M. B. (2002) 'Adverse effects of β-agonists', *Journal of Allergy and Clinical Immunology*, 110, S322–8.

Serruys, P. W., Brower, R. W, ten Katen, H. J. Bom, A. H. and Hugenholtz, P. G. (1981) 'Regional wall motion from radiopaque markers after intravenous and intracoronary injections of nifedipine', *Circulation*, 63, 584–91.

Tattersal, M. (2003) Report of the Expert Committee convened by the Therapeutic Goods Administration to assess the findings of a report on the safety of the US Women's Health Initiative (combined Hormone Replacement Therapy) trial and presented to the Commonwealth of Australia Minister for Health and Ageing. Online: *http://www.health.gov.au/tga/docs/pdf/hrtyreport.pdf*

chapter 14

Special needs

Margaret Hutchison

Learning outcomes

- Identify clients with particular needs or physical disabilities
- Sensitively communicate with a client with a physical disability
- Describe ways of modifying and adapting massage techniques to suit the client's condition and methods of adapting the massage environment to suit the situation

INTRODUCTION

Technology and medical science are enabling people to live longer and to overcome many of the health challenges that previously limited the extent of people's useful abilities and lifespan. As access to complementary health care options is broadening there is an increasing demand for massage therapists to widen their client base to include clients who have special health-related needs due to a normal life stage, such as pregnancy or ageing, or a temporary or long-term disability. This chapter will identify some of these special needs, and suggest approaches for dealing with those situations most likely to be encountered in practice. It will provide the massage therapist with useful recommendations on how to modify their techniques and approaches to best cater for clients with special needs. Massage therapists who can modify and adapt their techniques and sensitively and safely accommodate a variety of special needs will be in increasing demand over coming years.

SPECIAL NEEDS AND MASSAGE

As discussed in Chapter 5, the importance of touch cannot be overstated. Touch in the form of massage therapy has been shown to be beneficial to human wellbeing as it connects people with their bodies in a way that nothing else does. As such, massage therapy is in the unique position of having the ability to use the transformative power of touch to respond individually to client needs.

This privilege brings with it great responsibilities for the therapist. Firstly, a massage therapist must be able to identify those clients with special requirements and be aware of the importance of communicating sensitively with those who may have particular disabilities or challenges. It also requires the therapist to be flexible in their approach to the situation, and to have the skill to be able to adapt the massage environment and modify the massage techniques to be used in each situation.

From a massage perspective, clients with special needs are those who require an adaptation of either the massage techniques or other special considerations, due to their unique health-related challenges or circumstances. This may involve positioning the person to suit their needs, as in the case of pregnancy or when the client needs extra support for stiff, paralysed or disabled limbs, or performing the massage on a client in a wheelchair. It may require the therapist to employ the same massage techniques as they would for a regular massage but the adaptation would be the amount of pressure used, or the duration of the massage.

Special needs may relate to varying stages of life and development (see Box 14.1).

> **Box 14.1** The seven stages and ages of life
>
> Stage 1 — prenatal
> Stage 2 — infants
> Stage 3 — children
> Stage 4 — teens
> Stage 5 — adults
> Stage 6 — elderly
> Stage 7 — frail, aged

Other types of special needs may be due to physical disabilities or challenges related to differences in size, loss of sensory abilities or loss of physical abilities through birth, accident or illness. Some psychological disorders such as clinical depression may place the person in a special needs category. Still other special needs may result from a client having a diagnosed medical condition or a surgical intervention of some kind (see Box 14.2).

> **Box 14.2** Physical, psychological, medical and surgical reasons for special needs
>
> - Size, body shape, physical imbalances
> - Sensory impairment — vision, hearing, speech
> - Conditions present from birth
> - Paraplegia, quadriplegia, hemiplegia
> - Disfigurement, trauma — accidents, burns
> - Chronic illness/terminal illness
> - Confinement to a wheelchair
> - Major surgery
> - Amputation — prostheses
> - Implants — breast augmentation, pacemakers
> - Reconstruction surgery
> - Renal dialysis
> - Cerebral palsy, multiple sclerosis, Parkinson's disease, dementia and Alzheimer's disease
> - Developmental and learning disabilities — autism and dyslexia
> - Addictions/withdrawal
> - Psychiatric disorders — clinical depression, bipolar disorder, schizophrenia
> - Post traumatic stress disorders
> - Psycho/sexual trauma — abuse, rape, abortion

THE IMPORTANCE OF COMMUNICATION

As a professional the massage therapist is responsible for communicating effectively with all clients and developing a manner that is friendly; one that makes the client feel comfortable and secure at all times. Communication that is over compensatory or patronising will make for difficult relations. At times a client with special needs may require a carer who would attend the massage treatment with the client to assist with their functioning and perhaps even facilitate communication. If this occurs the therapist must take care not to ignore the special needs client altogether by speaking directly with the carer. Such communication is degrading and demeaning to the client and is not recommended. A therapist should interact with a special needs client as they would any client and provide them the respect and dignity they deserve when attending for massage therapy (see Box 14.3).

> **Box 14.3** Guidelines for communication
>
> - Remember that if you are uncomfortable the client will sense your discomfort and may misinterpret your reactions as disgust.
> - Recognise the source of your discomfort and deal with it.
> - Honest communication is best. Find a way to express your feelings openly. Discussion will lead to understanding.
> - Do not ignore the disability or disfigurement; you might say 'I notice that you have ... tell me how you deal with it'.
> - Speak directly to the client, unless you know that they are unable to comprehend or communicate appropriately.
> - If you are unable to deal with your issues, refer the client to another therapist.

Many people who need full-time care for a medical or physical problem such as multiple sclerosis or motor neurone disease may have speech that is slow and difficult to understand but their intellectual abilities are unimpaired. It is important for the massage therapist to remember that all clients should be treated with equal dignity and respect and even if the client appears to have an intellectual disability and seems unable to understand what is said, it is still essential to speak directly to the client. The carer will usually answer for the client if they feel it is necessary.

When treating any client it is imperative that the massage therapist discuss all issues relating to the massage with the client — what, why, how, when and where. This approach is no different for a client presenting with special needs. Some clients will be seated or in wheelchairs. To enhance communication between client and therapist the therapist should be seated during the initial consultation and speak to the client at eye level — having to look up at the therapist may place strain on a client's neck and may create feelings of inferiority in the client.

As with any client the therapist must gain informed consent before commencing any massage treatment. If the treatment plan changes during the consultation, it is imperative that the therapist relays this to the client and, again, gains consent. During the treatment the therapist should ask the client about their limitations; nothing should be assumed.

Feedback should be requested from the client in relation to pressure, heat and pain and such factors should be continually monitored throughout the massage. In the case of clients who are partially paralysed, sensation may be dulled or heightened in certain areas. Paralysis does not mean the area is devoid of feeling.

ADAPTING TECHNIQUES FOR ACCOMMODATING SIZE AND SHAPE

Unlike clients, who come in all shapes and sizes, massage tables are fairly standard in size. The massage therapist should assess whether the client will be comfortable and safe on the massage table. Where the table is not long enough for a tall client nor strong enough for a large client it is advised that the massage should be performed seated in a chair. The therapist could also massage the client on the floor, with good padding (such as a shiatsu futon), if it is comfortable for both the therapist and client (see Figure 14.1). However, this option would not be a preferred option as it poses its own problems for both client and therapist.

Clients who are pregnant, have had breast augmentation or may be larger than most are likely to be uncomfortable lying prone because of pressure on the front of the body. This may cause them to feel suffocated and experience breathing difficulties. Placing rolled towels under the armpits or a small pillow or bolster in front of the chest may make it more comfortable for such clients. Another option is to perform the massage in a seated position. Specific considerations for massaging pregnant clients are discussed in Chapter 19.

A common misconception among beginning massage therapists is that larger clients require deeper pressure on the part of the therapist. This is not necessarily the case, as their sensitivity to pain is often very high. The therapist should use firm,

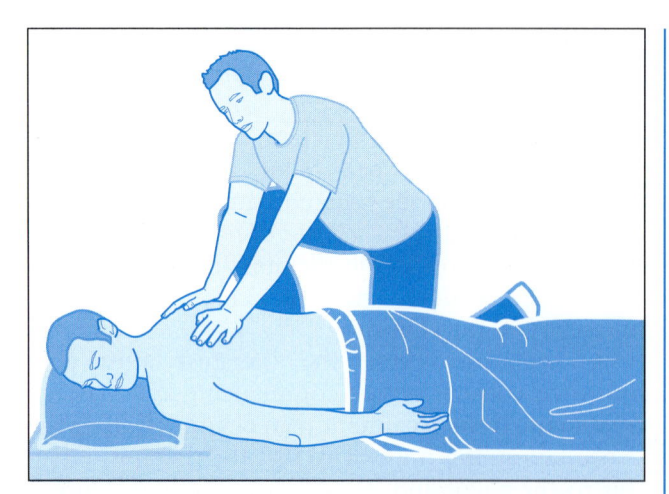

Figure 14.1 Client face down on a futon and therapist performing massage in kneeling position

rhythmic strokes and apply pressure slowly and sensitively, while monitoring the client's reaction to treatment.

When accommodating for differences in size and shape the therapist should focus particularly on posture and positioning, comfort and support. It is important to remember the client must be able to breath and feel comfortable, with no pressure on vulnerable areas. The massage therapist should ensure that affected limbs are supported and the head, neck and spine maintain good alignment. At all times the dignity and privacy of the client are paramount and the therapist should go out of their way to ensure these are maintained.

ADAPTING MASSAGE POSITIONS

As previously mentioned, there are occasions when a massage therapist may choose to treat the client in a seated position. Examples are when:
- the table is too small or narrow for patient comfort — size or shape of client;
- the therapist is unable to get the client onto the table — too high or too difficult;
- space is too small to use a table;
- no other position is comfortable;
- the client is unable to lie down — frailty or respiratory, heart or digestive problem, or pregnancy;
- the client does not want to move from their wheelchair;
- there is lack of mobility — paralysis, frailty, obesity;
- the client is unable to transfer from chair to table;
- there is unacceptable pain on movement;
- the situation is unsuitable — e.g. no privacy; and
- there is not the time required to move the client.

When it comes to the choice of whether to use a table or a chair for a massage it will depend firstly on where the massage is to take place — and this may not always be in a clinical setting. Clients with special needs may often be treated in their homes or in hostels, nursing homes, hospitals, respite facilities or palliative care units. Secondly, it will depend on the client's condition and specific requirements for comfort and the amount of assistance available.

If the client is elderly or has a disability, the location may be a private home, a special unit, hospital, or a nursing home. The therapist may often find an elderly or physically disabled client in a wheelchair or in a bed. In these instances it may be more convenient to treat the client in their chair or bed, as opposed to moving them. Client comfort is of utmost importance. Provided the client is comfortable, it is recommended that the easiest option for all parties is often the best option; the client should not be made to feel that organising them to receive a massage poses a problem for anyone.

When choosing to provide seated massage the therapist should be mindful of the three Cs (see Box 14.4).

Box 14.4 The three Cs of choosing a seated massage

- Condition
- Comfort
- Convenience

The convenience and ease of using a chair for massage has resulted in a range of specifically designed portable massage chairs. Although very useful for seated massage, they are often costly to purchase and would not be appropriate for some clients.

A massage therapist can quite easily adapt a situation to cater for a client requiring a seated massage using any of the following options:
- a solid chair without arms (such as a kitchen chair), a stool, or a wheelchair — with the client leaning over a table;
- client seated and facing the back of a kitchen chair;
- reclining armchair;
- bed — with upper body raised or propped up with pillows;
- massage table against the wall — client seated with pillows behind for support;

- wheelchair — client leans forward using armrests for support; and
- desktop massager (see Chapter 8).

It is quite easy to adapt a situation to cater for a client requiring a seated massage. With creative thinking, it is quite simple and inexpensive to use any available chair and to adapt it with supports for the comfort of the client. The massage table can also be modified for clients who are unable to lie down but do not necessarily need to sit in a chair; this also makes it easier for the therapist to work on the lower limbs. With a kitchen or dining chair the client can either lean forward onto a table with a towel or pillow for comfort (see Figure 14.2) or straddle the chair with their arms resting over a towel or soft pillow placed across the chair back for comfort (see Figure 14.3). This is often the best option for the latter stages of pregnancy.

In order for the therapist to be able to massage the lower limbs of a client who is seated straddling a dining chair, the client should be repositioned seated normally on the chair facing the therapist. The therapist would be seated in a chair opposite the client if comfortable, or on a small stool or cushion placed on the floor at the feet of the client. The therapist would support the client's legs on a towel on the therapist's lap (see Figure 14.4).

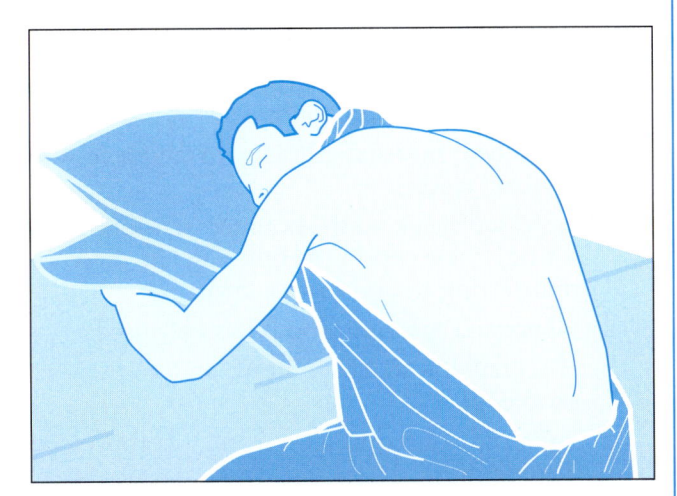

Figure 14.2 Adapted seated massage — client leaning on table with pillow for comfort

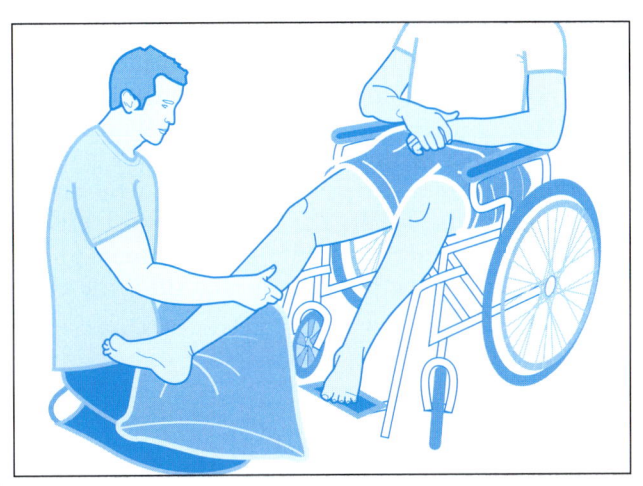

Figure 14.4 Massaging a client's lower limbs when the client is in a seated position

At times a client may be able to receive massage treatment on a massage table but is unable to lie down due to heart disease, digestive ailments or problems associated with breathing. In such cases the client's upper body should be elevated. To do this the head of the massage table should be positioned against a solid wall. Pillows behind their back can then support the client's upper body (see Figure 14.5). A similar position may also be used if the client is to be massaged on a bed, especially if the bed can be adjusted for height and the head of

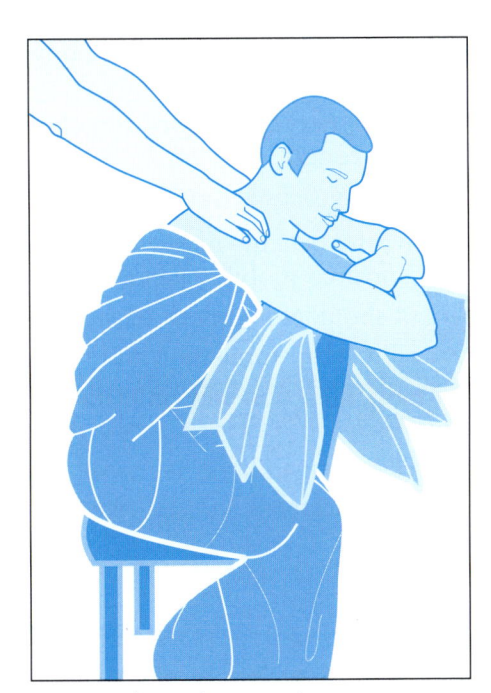

Figure 14.3 Adapted seated massage — client straddling dining chair with added support

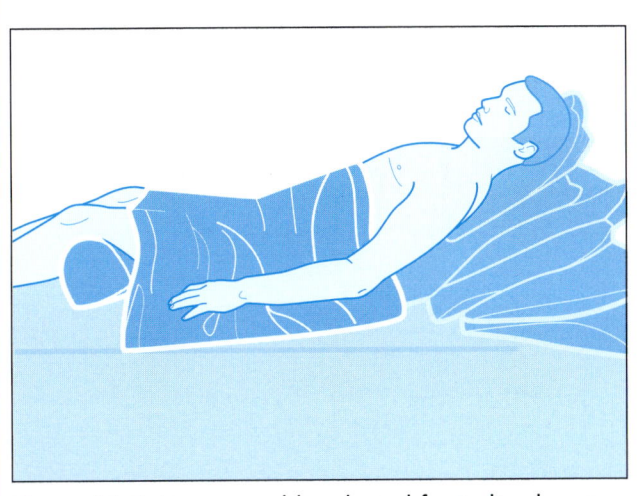

Figure 14.5 Massage table adapted for inclined posture with upper body elevated

the bed can be inclined. In this situation, the therapist must consider their own posture and comfort as well as that of the client. It is more difficult to massage a client on a bed that cannot be adjusted. Beds that can be raised allow the therapist to maintain correct postural alignment.

When massaging a client in a wheelchair and when, for reasons of comfort and convenience for the client, it is easier not to move them, the therapist will only be able to massage those parts of the body that are able to be reached easily. If the client can lean forward, and there is enough space, most of the buttock area can usually be reached (see Figure 14.6). They may even be able to allow a little more access by leaning sideways. In most cases the only part of the body beyond reach will be the posterior, superior thigh area.

When choosing to massage a client whilst they are in their wheelchair, the therapist must ensure that the brakes are on if the client is seated in a manual chair, or the power is turned off if the chair is motorised. The wheels of the chair should be aligned and facing forward. The therapist may wish to remove armrests, neck supports or footplates to ensure client comfort and enhance access for massage. If attachments are removed from the wheelchair the therapist must ensure these are properly replaced immediately after the massage is completed. The therapist should respect the client's right to independence and autonomy, by not attempting to transfer a client from a wheelchair or push a client in their wheelchair without first seeking their consent (see Box 14.5).

MASSAGE AND DISABILITIES

Clients with impaired mobility

Regular massage therapy may prove useful for people who spend a great deal of time sitting in a wheelchair, as they are likely to experience some of the following physical problems:

- weakened postural muscles in thoracic and lumbar regions;
- increased neck and shoulder tension from lifting their body weight up in bed or transferring to and from a chair;
- 'depressed' posture, shoulders collapsed;
- potential for scoliosis, heart and respiratory problems;
- impaired breathing from compressed diaphragm;
- susceptibility to chest infections;
- indigestion, constipation and incontinence from compressed abdomen;
- diminished circulation to lower body leading to skin breakdown;
- diminished nerve function, muscle atrophy, contracture; and
- chronic pain, depression, low self-esteem.

Specifically, the benefits massage may bestow to clients with impaired mobility include:

- relief of shoulder and neck tension;
- postural muscle stimulation and toning;
- breathing, digestion and circulation improvement;
- pain reduction; and
- mood enhancement and self-esteem improvement.

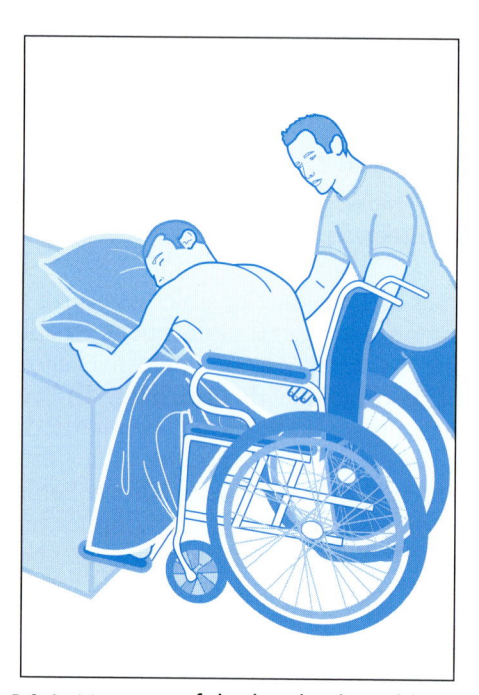

Figure 14.6 Massage of the low back and buttock on a client seated in a wheelchair

---

Box 14.5 Reminders for clients in wheelchairs

- Manual chair — brakes on.
- Motorised chair — power off.
- Wheels aligned and facing forward.
- Replace armrests, neck supports and footplates.
- Never push a wheelchair without permission.
- Informed consent must be obtained to transfer a client.
- Respect the client's right to be independent.

The intellectually challenged client

Intellectual dysfunction may result from a stroke, an accident or birth trauma and can manifest in many ways. It is often accompanied by behaviour that is beyond the person's control and outside the boundaries of what is considered 'normal' or socially acceptable.

People with an intellectual dysfunction are often very energetic and find it difficult to keep still for long periods of time. They may have difficulty in concentrating and following the spoken word. They may even have speech problems and the massage therapist may find it challenging to understand what they are saying. Physically, they may be very stiff and require a great deal of assistance. It requires great sensitivity on the part of the therapist who chooses to work with clients who have an intellectual dysfunction. However, for those who do the rewards are many as these clients are special people with many wonderful attributes.

When treating clients who have an intellectual impairment the therapist should:

- speak slowly and clearly rather than loudly;
- use short, clear sentences;
- remember that lack of speech (aphasia) or difficulty with speech (dysphasia) does not mean the person cannot understand or comprehend what another person is saying;
- use gestures, writing or pictures to help communicate; and
- repeat words or instructions where necessary.

Sensory impairment

Visual impairment

A person may be classified as 'legally blind' for pension purposes and yet have some vision; very few people have no vision at all. A visually impaired person needs to know exactly where everything is, so the therapist should never move any objects the client has placed in a particular spot. The visually impaired person also requires very precise verbal directions when being assisted, such as, 'the massage table is two steps forward and to the right'.

When communicating with clients who have a visual impairment the therapist should:

- speak in a normal tone, they can hear normally — unless they have a hearing problem;
- introduce themselves and address them by name;
- not move anything from where the client has put it;
- describe accurately what is being done and outline clearly their requirements of the client;
- stand on the left-hand side of the client and allow the client to touch their right elbow if they are guiding the movement of the client — the therapist should never push or pull them; and
- never feed or fuss over a guide dog — it is a working dog, not a pet.

Speech impairment

For the person with a severe speech impairment, it can be very frustrating trying to communicate, especially when the people they are speaking to can't understand what they are saying and keep asking them to repeat it or try to help by completing their sentences. When treating clients who have speech impairments, the massage therapist should:

- repeat what is heard to make sure it is what was said;
- ask them to repeat anything that they don't understand;
- ask them to write it down if they still don't understand; and
- not finish their sentences for them.

Hearing impairment

A client with hearing loss has difficulty differentiating sounds and may misunderstand what is being said. As hearing aids amplify sound the therapist should speak in a normal tone and remember to keep background noises to a minimum. When massaging around the neck, shoulders and head of the client the therapist should keep in mind that their hands may interfere with a hearing aid and cause it to 'squeal' in the client's ear. Pressure on a hearing aid will cause similar interference and the client may choose to remove it and rely solely on lip-reading as a means of communication. In this situation, the therapist must remember to allow the client to see their lips move. Of course, if the client is lying prone they will be unable to lip-read, yet if the therapist has fully informed them about the procedure, and a signalling system (such as tapping on the shoulder) is arranged prior to the massage, it should present no problems. Instructions could also be written down for the client.

When consulting with a hearing impaired client the therapist should:

- speak in a normal tone and rhythm;
- tap the client on the shoulder to gain their attention;
- ask if they wish to remove their hearing aid;
- avoid touching the area close to the hearing aid;
- remember that hearing aids amplify sound: they do not make it clearer;

- find the right distance between themselves and the client: getting too close will make the hearing aid 'scream';
- reduce background noise — especially music;
- face the client and keep their mouth visible when speaking to the client; and
- write things down if required.

When treating clients with disabilities it is important that the therapist not fall into the trap of misconception and assumption with regard to disabilities. For instance, it is inaccurate to assume that a person with a disability is helpless, ill or weak, or that simply because someone speaks slowly they are mentally retarded or deaf. Many people considered to have a disability are in excellent health, with perfect sight and hearing and as such consider themselves extremely able and do not wish to be thought of as 'disabled'.

AGED CARE

Ageing is a natural, lifelong process that begins at birth and is the sum of all the changes that occur with the passage of time. Diseases associated with ageing are not a part of normal ageing; they are a secondary process or symptomatic of the ageing process.

The main challenge associated with ageing is remaining physically and mentally fit and healthy, and able to function independently, especially past the age of 70 when everything starts to slow down or break down.

Mentally, physically, financially and socially there is a gradual sense of loss, and the opportunity for loving touch is often a major one. For a growing number of the elderly without a partner and no one to care for them it may mean giving up their home and moving into a hostel or nursing home. As an increasing number of the population approach their mature years many will no doubt be seeking the benefits of regular massage treatment to keep their muscles and joints mobile and pain free.

Physical aspects of ageing

There are many physical changes that accompany the ageing process. A major visual sign of ageing is that the skin becomes thinner and more wrinkled. As one ages the kidneys take longer to clear certain drugs from the body, and the blood circulation is less efficient than in earlier years. Bones become less flexible and joints start to wear; muscle tissue is lost and replaced by fat and connective tissue. The immune system of the older person is less efficient and therefore the body becomes more susceptible to infections.

Conditions associated with ageing include heart and circulatory dysfunctions, urinary and bowel disorders, and problems associated with mobility and balance. Diseases such as arthritis, stroke and osteoporosis become more prevalent. Due to muscle and bone declines, and changes in mobility and balance, falls in the older adult are not uncommon and may become more frequent with age. Walking sticks or walking frames are often used to minimise the risk of falls. Hearing and sight also deteriorate and devices such as magnifying glasses and hearing aids are often used to assist function. Changes in mental capacity may also be observed and some may experience depression.

> **Box 14.6** General signs of ageing
>
> - Generalised deterioration in all systems.
> - Body tends to collapse in stages.
> - Skin becomes thin, dry, wrinkled and prone to bruising and tearing.
> - Muscle tissue replaced by fat and connective tissue.
> - Bones less flexible, prone to breaking — osteoporosis.
> - Joints become worn and inelastic — osteoarthritis.
> - Muscle weakness develops; falls; fractures; loss of independence; increased dependency on others.
> - Reproductive organs cease to function, oestrogen depletion, and menopause.
> - Circulation less efficient.
> - Heart, blood vessels, lungs and kidneys undergo changes.
> - Vision and hearing problems develop.
> - Reactions are slower.

Benefits of massage for the elderly and frail

Massage can be of immense benefit in maintaining health, reducing pain and stiffness, alleviating stress and anxiety and promoting relaxation and restful sleep. It is also valuable because it provides nurturing touch plus physical and emotional stimulation, which may be lacking in an ageing person's life. For someone living alone massage is a pleasurable experience to look forward to, providing an opportunity for positive, social interaction and an attentive, caring presence.

Frail bones may be osteoporotic, so the massage therapist should take care with the amount of pressure used on ribs and the upper back. Osteoarthritis is common among the elderly and massage has been shown to improve joint flexibility and mobility. A study conducted in the UK in 1996 found that elderly people in residential homes, who had a weekly massage, reported a reduction in arthritic pain and muscular tension and experienced an improvement in mobility. Massage may also prove useful for people with dementia. A 1999 study found that slow-stroke massage reduced the agitated behaviour of Alzheimer's patients (Rowe and Alfred, 1999).

Other benefits of massage therapy for the elderly and frail clients include:

- improved overall wellbeing;
- increased circulation;
- reduced pain and stiffness;
- relief for tight muscles;
- reduced risk of injuries from falls;
- reduced stress and anxiety;
- improved skin and relief from dry skin conditions;
- enhanced relaxation and restful sleep;
- social interaction and physical and emotional stimulation; and
- touch as a form of caring communication and a pleasurable experience to look forward to.

Considerations for massaging the elderly and frail

The elderly or frail client may have problems with mobility, and as such the recommendations previously outlined would also apply for these clients. When treating frail or elderly clients, the massage therapist must keep in mind that more sensitivity is needed when it comes to their comfort. For example, comfort is paramount if the client has had a stroke. A client who has experienced a stroke may be partially paralysed and their limbs may be stiff and contracted, or limp and flaccid. The therapist must ensure they use adequate pillows, cushions, or rolled towels as bolsters to give full support to the client's affected limbs.

When consulting with the elderly client the massage therapist needs to explain what the massage entails and ensure that the client fully understands and gives their consent to all procedures. When providing massage therapy to the elderly client the therapist should observe the following general considerations:

- monitor comfort and warmth;
- support weak, contracted, painful areas;
- administer short massage sessions — they tire easily;
- be flexible and adaptable;
- adjust rate, rhythm, pressure, and touch;
- modify massage techniques as needed;
- do not rush them;
- take time to build trust and rapport;
- listen empathetically and show interest, allow them to talk;
- be sensitive to their emotional needs;
- adapt the massage to the client and situation;
- avoid deep work and be careful around the neck and chest;
- obtain permission to massage sensitive areas;
- ask what sort of help they need and support them;
- remember massage therapy is not trying to fix things or cure them; and
- ensure safety on and off the table and, to prevent falling, clean all oil off the client's feet to ensure they are not slippery.

CHRONIC ILLNESS AND TERMINAL ILLNESS

A client may present for massage experiencing a chronic illness or disease or may even be suffering from a terminal illness. A chronic disease or disorder is one that persists for a long period and for which there is treatment to manage the symptoms of the disease yet there exists no known cure. Chronic disease states are commonly termed incurable.

Chronic disease states are often progressively debilitating, developing insidiously and becoming evident after a number of years. Two such conditions are Parkinson's disease and multiple sclerosis. Others, such as chronic back pain, may have been caused by an injury, which despite treatment has left the person to bear or manage the pain for the rest of their life.

A terminal illness is one where nothing further can be done to prolong life. The progression of the illness is largely dependent on the type of condition; it may be slow resulting in a gradual breakdown of body systems, as in the case of AIDS, or it may develop rapidly as with a brain tumour. For clients with a terminal illness, massage may assist in improving their quality of life. For example, a client diagnosed with a terminal illness such as cancer may receive massage therapy to assist with pain relief or cope with depression. The terminally ill person may ultimately require palliative care to make the dying process peaceful and supportive for all concerned.

Considerations for massaging chronically and terminally ill clients

For the massage therapist, massaging clients who are chronically or terminally ill can be very rewarding, as is the case when working with any special needs clients. The chronically or terminally ill client may have problems with mobility, and as such the recommendations previously outlined would apply for these clients also.

If the disease state is one that compromises the immune system then the therapist must ensure they are scrupulous with hygiene. If the massage therapist is unwell and contagious, they are advised not to consult with such clients, as they may be susceptible to the slightest infection. Massage therapy is best postponed until another time when the risk of cross infection is not present.

It is important for the massage therapist working with the terminally ill to recognise that the dying person in our culture confronts us with our own mortality. When people are facing death they often have issues surrounding grief and abandonment to work through and they also may feel very vulnerable. The therapist who intends to work in a palliative care environment will need to be able to deal with their own feelings in relation to grief and death and be prepared to make a commitment to support the client to the end of their life. If a commitment cannot be made then for the sake of the client it would be best for them to be referred to another therapist.

When first dealing with a client with a terminal illness the massage therapist may find it difficult to communicate with the client. How does one talk to a person who is dying? The therapist needs to be honest and open in all communications. Should the client choose to broach the subject of their death the therapist needs to allow them to do so and, where comfortable, reflect what they have heard back to the client in a sensitive manner. There may be times when the client may not wish to receive a massage treatment, perhaps due to unbearable pain or depressive emotional states. If the therapist has a broad scope of practice and has had the relevant training, they may be able to use other approaches with the client, such as aromatherapy, reflexology or energy techniques like therapeutic touch, healing touch or reiki. If the client experiences a sudden release of emotion during the treatment, it may be appropriate to simply hold their hand; words may not be necessary.

When consulting with a client who has a chronic or terminal illness the therapist should:

- be scrupulous with hygiene, especially if the disease compromises immune function;
- reschedule a consultation if they are unwell, as clients may be susceptible to the slightest infection;
- ensure their knowledge of the client's condition is up to date;
- work within their scope of practice;
- provide shorter, more frequent massages;
- remember that such clients' energy levels fluctuate and they fatigue easily;
- use slow, gentle, relaxing techniques — a nurturing touch provides valuable temporary pain relief;
- communicate in an honest and open manner to make the client feel comfortable; and
- remember that death is not the enemy — not recognising our common humanity is.

CONCLUSION

People who are not physically or psychologically challenged may feel uncomfortable around those who are, and some may find it difficult to accept others who are different.

Differences can make people fearful, or insecure. As a caring health professional, it is essential that the massage therapist puts aside personal prejudices, dislikes, and judgments and treats all clients equally, with compassion and respect. This involves the therapist keeping an open mind, being sensitive, tolerant and compassionate, and maintaining consistent personal and professional boundaries. In addition, the massage therapist must exhibit good listening skills, possessing the ability to listen with respect and make clients feel comfortable and at ease.

The massage therapist who demonstrates the above traits and is equipped to easily and professionally adapt their skills and equipment to meet the unique and varying needs of clients provides a very important service to their community. Massage therapy has enormous potential to be of benefit for clients with special needs, whether these needs centre on mobility, physical impairment, dementia, chronic illness or terminal disease. When working with clients with special needs the massage therapist must remember:

- that each client is unique; the impairment is part of how the person functions;
- not to assume that the client is helpless and needs assistance;
- the client will give the best directions, if asked (the therapist needs to ask the client if they need any kind of assistance and should not presume to know what the client needs);

- to recognise and deal with their own feelings if they intend consulting with clients who are terminally ill;
- that fear of a disability is not an excuse — the therapist should learn more about the disability and the best source of knowledge is the client themselves;
- to think of the client first, not the disability; and
- that all clients should be respected and treated equally.

Irrespective of training, any qualified massage therapist has the skills to work with clients who have special needs. The techniques of massage therapy are universal, and as such should be enjoyed by all members of the community, regardless of ability or functional capacity. With minimal imagination and ingenuity, the caring, compassionate and accepting massage therapist can adapt their skills, massage equipment and clinical environment to accommodate the needs of any client. When adapting their practice to accommodate for clients presenting with special needs, the massage therapist will open a new world of experiences, and gain benefit in the process of providing service to this important sector of the community. When consulting with clients who present with special needs, the therapist will enjoy the many rewards of working with this unique group of people.

Questions and activities

1. An elderly client with bilateral hearing attends for a massage treatment. He says he would like to take out his hearing aids to be more comfortable. As the massage therapist, explain how you would communicate with him.
2. You have been asked to give massage to a terminally ill client who has been diagnosed with inoperable bowel cancer. Would you accept? If you accept, what sort of massage techniques might you choose to use? What would you need to consider?
3. Max is a 24-year-old paraplegic client who you decide to massage in his wheelchair. As you are talking to Max you notice that he has quite a few bruises on his legs and Max tells you that he has no feeling in them. When you are interviewing Max, how would you communicate with him? What must you remember to do before you commence the massage? Explain why Max may have bruises on his legs and state what that should alert you to in relation to your massage.

REFERENCE

Rowe, M. and Alfred, D. (1999) 'The effectiveness of slow-stroke massage in diffusing agitated behaviours in individuals with Alzheimer's disease', *Journal of Gerontology and Nursing*, 25, pp. 22–34.

BIBLIOGRAPHY

Campbell, L. Pollard, A. and Roeton, C. (2001) 'The development of clinical practice guidelines for the use of aromatherapy in a cancer setting', *The Australian Journal of Holistic Nursing*, April, 8(1).

De Domenico, G. and Wood, E. C. (1997) *Beard's Massage* (4th edn). W. B. Saunders, Philadelphia.

Holmes, N. H.(1999) *Handbook of Geriatric Care*. Springhouse Corporation, Pennsylvania.

Kent, H. (1985) *Yoga for the Disabled: A Practical Self-Help Guide to a Happier Healthier Life*. Thorsons Publishing Group, London.

Petersen, S. (1999) 'Self-massage empowers seniors', *Massage Magazine*, March/April.

Premkumar, K. (1996) *Pathology A to Z*. VanPub Books, Calgary.

Rattray, F. and Ludwig, L. (2000) *Clinical Massage Therapy: Understanding, Assessing and Treating Over 70 Conditions*. Talus Inc., Toronto.

Tortora, G. J. and Grabowski, S. R. (2002) *Principles of Anatomy and Physiology* (10th edn). John Wiley & Sons, New York.

Ufema, J. (1987) 'How to talk to dying patients', *Nursing*, 87, August pp. 43–6.

section 6

The Massage Treatment – Hands On

chapter 15

Positioning and draping the client

Lisa Casanelia

Learning outcomes

- Demonstrate accepted practice and procedure for draping, pillowing and positioning of clients
- Adapt draping and positioning of clients for massage according to individual needs

INTRODUCTION

There is much for a student to learn in their pursuit to become a professional massage therapist. Although the application of the massage techniques is of utmost importance, a skilled therapist has abilities that extend well beyond their technical skills of performing the massage strokes. For example, a professional therapist would have knowledge of the modern health care system and the roles that many other health professionals play in today's multi-disciplinary approach to wellness and health. They would be aware of the many legal and ethical issues that surround their massage practice, and would be sensitive to the multitude of needs of the client. The professional massage therapist would acknowledge their scope of practice and have an awareness of the evidence surrounding their practice. Such a therapist would work from a suitable practice environment, have the ability to communicate effectively with clients from a broad range of backgrounds, whilst administering their massage treatments in a manner which appears effortless and well organised and orchestrated.

When a client is receiving a massage for the first time they may feel awkward lying on the massage table, exposed in their state of semi-nakedness. So as to ensure the client feels safe, secure and adequately covered, the professional therapist must have the ability to drape (or cover) the client, and move the client from one position to another during the course of the massage treatment, in a manner which appears easy and natural to the client, and does not disrupt the flow of the massage. The purpose of this chapter is to describe simple methods of draping and manoeuvring the client so as to promote the effects of the massage and maximise treatment benefits for the client, in an environment that is safe and secure.

THE IMPORTANCE OF DRAPING

A full body relaxation massage requires the therapist to skillfully manage movement from one body area to another and the draping and undraping of each part of the body without disrupting the flow of the massage. When used effectively, draping will appear effortless to the client and create a natural flow in the massage sequence. The procedure of draping is important for the maintenance of privacy and warmth of the client during the massage treatment.

Before putting draping into practice the therapist should give careful consideration to the draping guidelines described in Box 15.1.

DRAPING MATERIALS

The therapist can choose to use a variety of draping materials, such as towels, sheets and blankets, disposable linens, fitted linens that fit snugly onto the massage table, or any combination of all of these things. Whatever the therapist chooses, they must ensure that draping materials are freshly laundered, stored in a clean and dry environment and only used for single use. To launder massage linens some therapists choose to use a linen service that supplies and launders their linens. In a busy practice this may be a practical idea as laundering linens every day can be time consuming. The draping materials required by the massage therapist in practice are outlined in Box 15.2.

Box 15.1 Draping guidelines

- Only the area being massaged should be undraped.
- Only the areas the client has consented to massage should be undraped.
- Ensure feet are adequately draped, as the extremities are likely to feel the cold.
- Instil trust in the client with efficient, confident and secure draping practices.
- Create a firm and secure boundary — a 'draping line'.
- Do not place your hands beyond the draping line.
- Use freshly laundered draping materials.
- If choosing to work with towels ensure they are large enough to make the client feel adequately covered, or use more than one towel.
- Keep a blanket at hand to ensure the client can be warmed at any time.

Box 15.2 Draping materials

- Fitted sheet, a towel or other suitable covering to completely cover the massage table.
- Fitted cover, a handtowel or disposable cover to protect the face cradle.
- Towels or sheets to cover the client.
- Blankets to drape over linens to keep the client warm.
- Pillowcases to protect pillows.
- Handtowels to cover bolsters, create towel rolls, or drape the chest.
- Handtowels for the therapists' hands, to remove excess oil and to use as a barrier between client and therapist.

Despite regular laundering, draping materials will have a tendency to accumulate massage oil. They may become heavy with the oil as it builds up over time and develop a greasy feel. As a result of this build-up, linens develop an unpleasant odour, and therefore will need to be replaced regularly. To increase the longevity of linens, the therapist should adhere to the guidelines outlined in Box 15.3.

> **Box 15.3** Laundering massage linens
>
> - Cold-pressed vegetable oils are superior to the heat-extracted oils and will wash out more readily.
> - Water soluble massage oils are designed to wash out well from linens.
> - The use of Epsom salts, lectric soda, eucalyptus oil or specialised detergents in the washing process can aid the removal of oils from the linen.
> - All linens should be laundered promptly after use. Do not let them sit in a linen basket for days before washing.

MASSAGE TABLE PREPARATION

Before the client arrives the therapist should take the time to prepare the massage table with fresh linens. The massage table should be completely covered with a towel, sheet or fitted sheet so that the client's skin does not come into contact with the surface of the massage table. Where the therapist is using a face cradle attachment, fitted covers or disposable covers can be used. Handtowels or pillowcases can cover the bolsters or pillows required during the massage. Towels can be placed at the end of the massage table for the client to drape himself or herself with or if a sheet is being used, it should be placed over the massage table with the edge folded back so the client may climb in between.

After the consultation, the therapist must give clear instructions to the client about how to position themselves on the massage table, as it can be confusing for those who are new to massage. When covering the client the therapist should adopt draping techniques that cover areas of the body that are not being massaged. Such draping techniques will define the physical boundaries or parameters of the massage, and ensure the client feels secure, well covered and warm during the massage treatment. To maximise client warmth throughout the massage it may be necessary to add extra draping such as blankets.

DRAPING TECHNIQUES

Draping that is performed with ease, and a minimum of tucking and adjusting, instils in the client a sense of confidence about the therapist's level of skill and professionalism.

The following draping techniques aim to provide the massage therapist with easy-to-use methods of draping the client, whilst maintaining the security and comfort of the client. Although there are many different ways to drape, the following methods of draping have been chosen because of their simplicity for both the client and the therapist.

Client fully draped in prone position

Adjust the draping on the client when first entering the massage room, as it is often difficult for the client to drape fully when arranging themselves on the massage table. Cover the body completely from neck to toes and if necessary cover this draping again with a blanket for extra warmth. Ensure the client is comfortable with bolsters and pillowing and is adequately warm before commencing the massage (Figure 15.1).

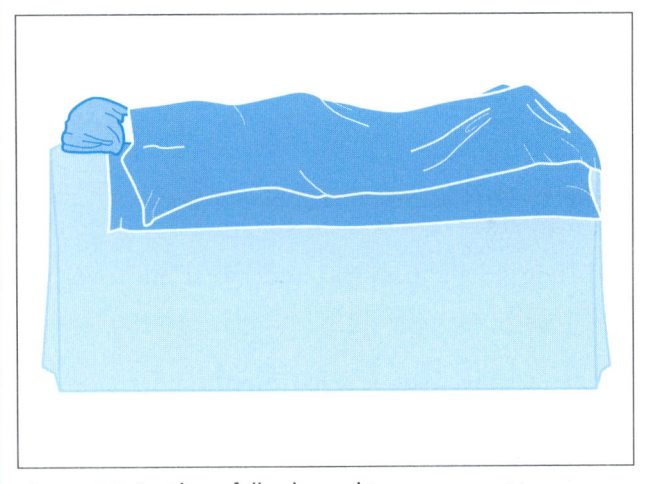

Figure 15.1 Client fully draped in prone position

Undraping the back

When a blanket covers the draping, fold this back over the legs. With the draping that is directly covering the client, pick it up at the low back and tuck this section into the waist of the client's underwear (Figure 15.2.a). Slide the underwear and draping down to the base of the sacrum and fold the top part of the draping down to this drape line to create a flap (Figure 15.2b). This flap can be used to cover the lower part of the back whilst working the upper part of the back. It can be easily flipped back and forth over the back without needing to interrupt the flow of the massage or the need to tuck and untuck the draping. To redrape the back, fold the flap back over the client's back

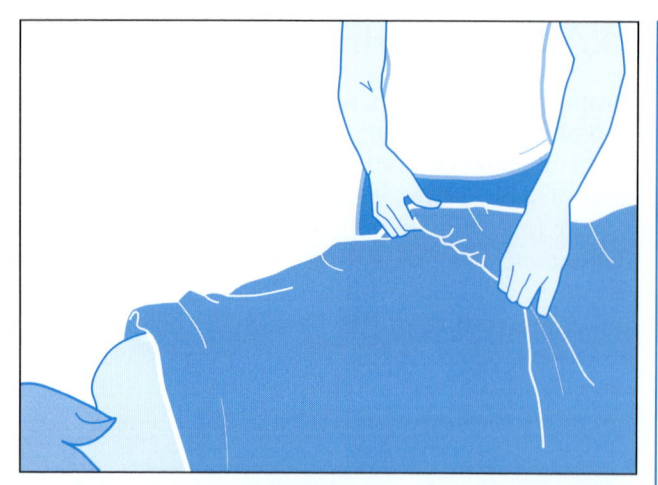

Figure 15.2a Tucking the draping into the underwear

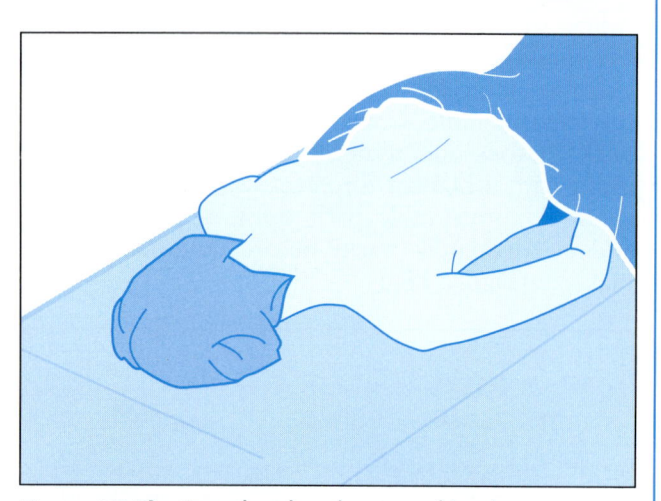

Figure 15.2b Completed undraping of back

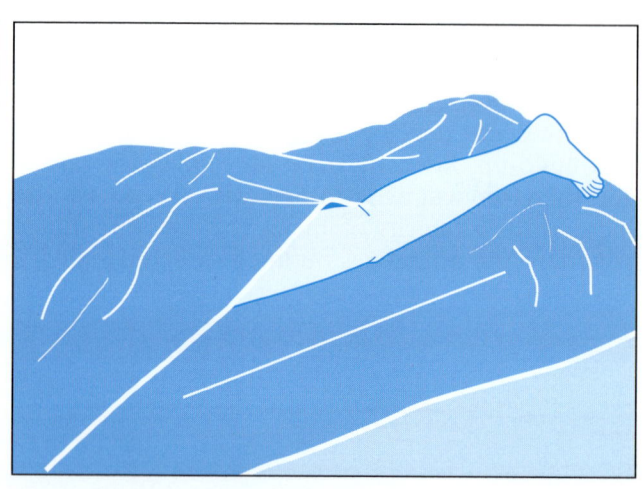

Figure 15.3a Draping folded back over the lower limbs towards midline

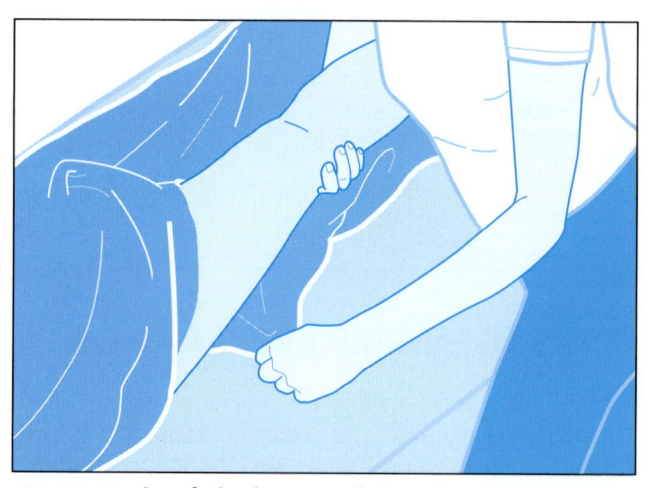

Figure 15.3b Lift the leg to pull the edge of the draping under the thigh

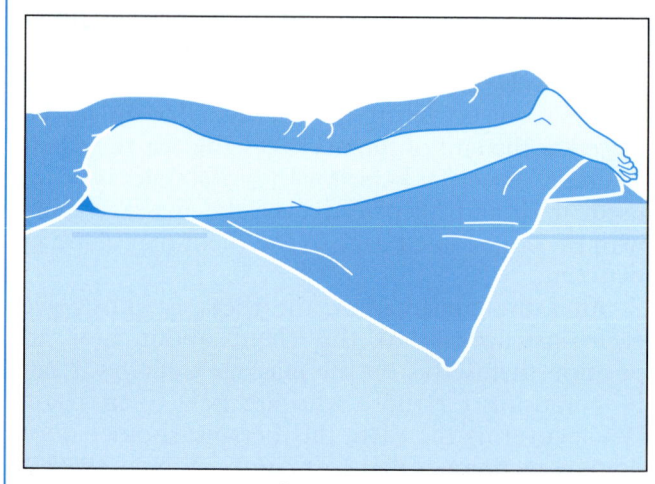

Figure 15.3c Posterior lower limb undraped

and slide it out from the underwear and over the back.

Undraping the lower limb

The same draping procedures are used for undraping the lower limb for both the anterior and posterior aspects. When a blanket covers the draping, fold this back over the leg not being massaged. With the draping that is directly covering the client, fold it back over the leg so that the edges fall to the midline between the legs (Figure 15.3a). Lift the leg that is undraped by supporting it around the inside of the lower leg with the inside arm (facing the head of the table). The other hand reaches under the leg being lifted to pull the drape from the midline of the thigh to the side of the table towards the hip (Figures 15.3b and d). The draping should sit high on the inner thigh and be firm for the client to feel its presence. The top part of the draping at the hip can be tucked into the leg of the client's underwear or anchored under their hip (Figures 15.3c and e). This method of draping for the lower limb is also ideal for the client who prefers not to wear underwear when receiving a massage as it creates a firm and secure draping line around the inner thigh.

Access to the inner thigh will require the therapist to maneuver the lower limb into flexion, external rotation and abduction. The therapist must also adjust the client's draping in this new position

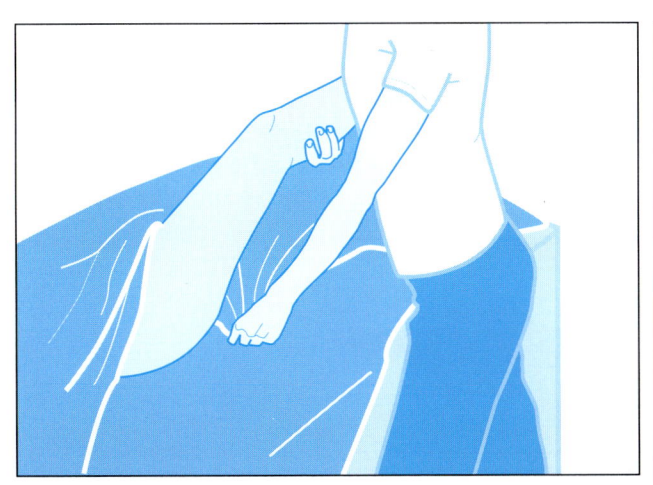

Figure 15.3d Lift the lower limb to pull the edge of the draping under the thigh

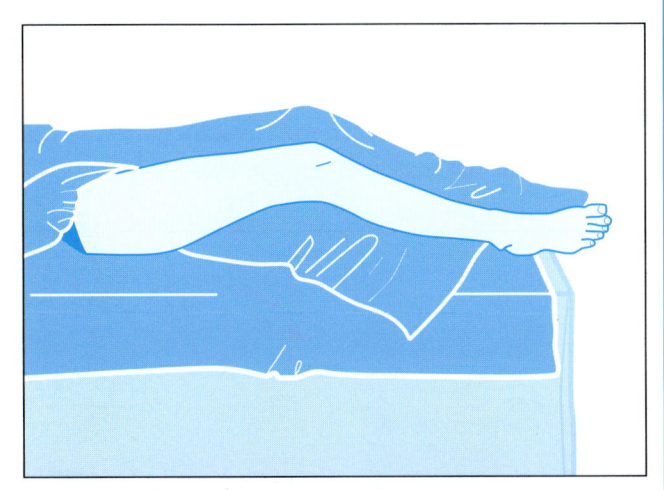

Figure 15.3e Anterior lower limb undraped

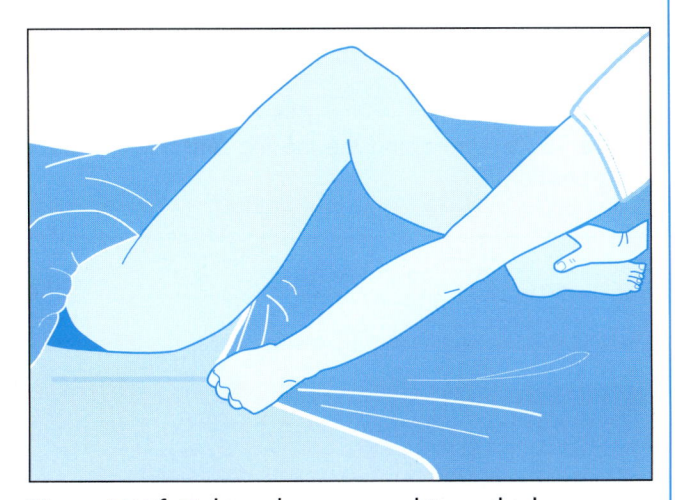

Figure 15.3f Tighten drape around inner thigh

by pulling tight on the edge of the drape at the hip to ensure the drape is tight around the client's inner thigh (Figure 15.3f).

To redrape the lower extremity, lift the leg as done before to drape, and slide the draping out from below the leg.

Undraping the arm

With the client in supine position and completely draped, fold the draping back at the shoulder on the diagonal to reveal the arm. Slide the client's arm out from beneath the draping, lift their arm and replace the drapes. The arm now rests on top of the draping (Figure 15.4). To redrape the arm, reverse the undraping process.

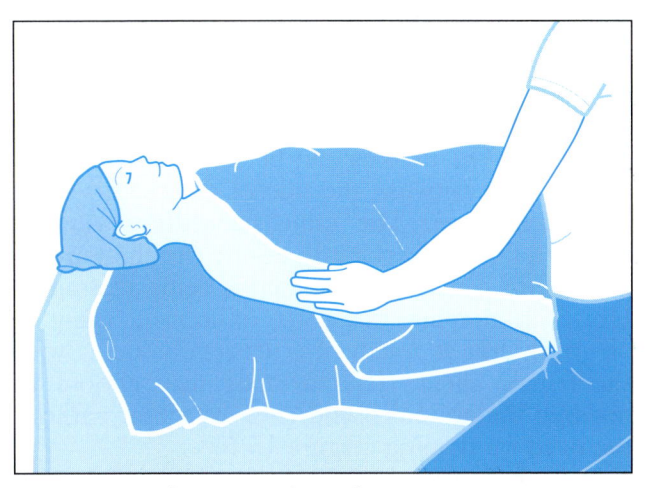

Figure 15.4 The arm undraped

Undraping the abdomen and chest

Standards in professional practice recommend appropriate draping of breasts during a massage. To access the abdomen and maintain the draping of the chest and breasts a handtowel is used. The handtowel is placed over the chest and secured by the therapist at the top edge with one hand. The therapist's free hand slides the main drape from

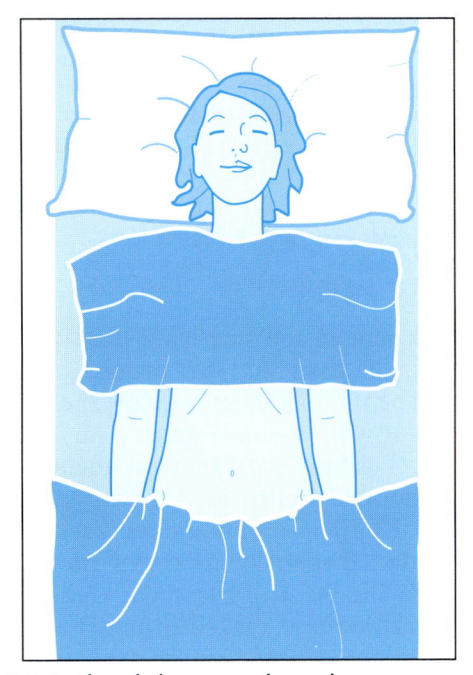

Figure 15.5 The abdomen undraped

under the handtowel and this is then folded back to expose the abdomen. The handtowel can be secured in under the client's arms and folded accordingly to reveal as much of the abdomen and ribs as possible whilst maintaining secure, adequate draping of the breast area. The main drape can be secured by tucking it into the client's underwear at the hips. Whilst massaging the abdomen the handtowel can be extended to cover the top of the shoulders and chest to keep these areas warm (Figure 15.5).

When massaging the top of the chest the abdomen can be redraped and the top of the towel at the chest folded back to the level of the underarm. The draping can be secured by tucking the towel in between the side of the client's body and their arms. The same procedures can be followed for a male client to ensure the chest area is kept warm whilst the abdomen is being massaged. However, draping the chest of a male client is obviously not as much of a sensitive issue as with the female client. The therapist may choose to massage the abdomen and chest as a unit without the need for draping (Figure 15.6).

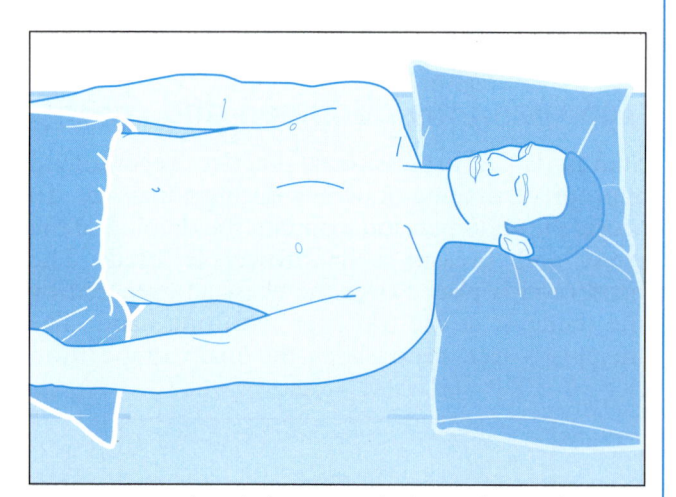

Figure 15.6 The abdomen and chest of a male client undraped

Draping of a client in side-lying position

Draping a client in the side-lying position is often more difficult than in the prone and supine positions. The use of a sheet to drape the client may be easier as it will provide a greater surface area to work with. Position the client on their side with pillows positioned to provide support and comfort (see Figure 15.20). To undrape the back the drape can be folded diagonally to reveal the back and secured into the waist of the client's underwear at the low back and also tucked in under the client's upper arm to prevent exposure of the anterior torso. To add greater security for a female client provide a pillow to hold against their chest which they can also use for added comfort and support (Figure 15.7a).

To undrape the top leg, bring the draping material over the leg from anterior to posterior, support and lift the leg as the draping is tucked in

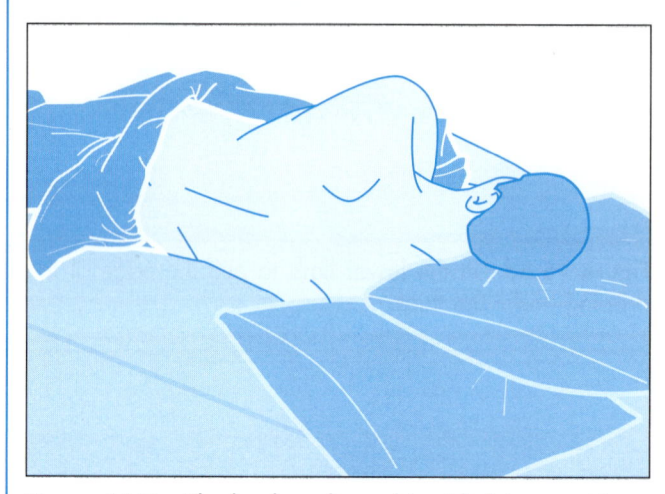

Figure 15.7a The back undraped in side-lying position

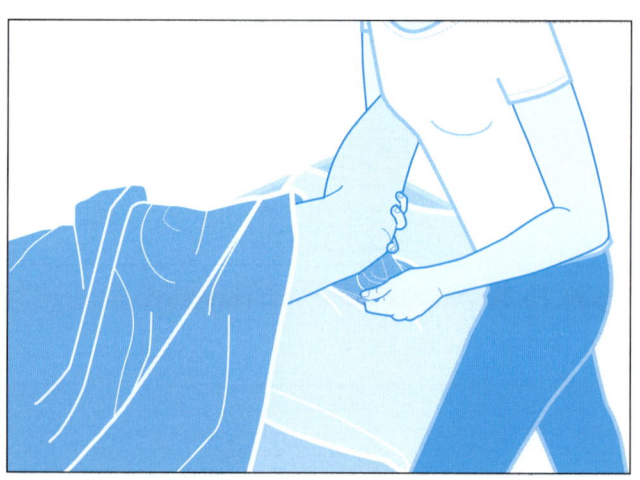

Figure 15.7b Undraping the top leg and thigh in side-lying position

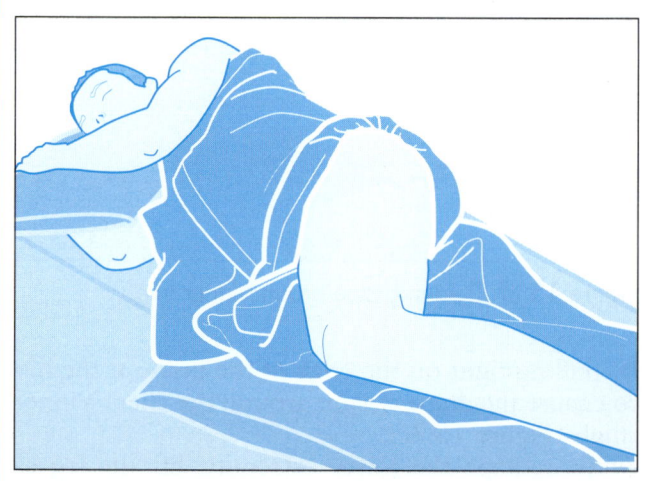

Figure 15.7c The top leg and thigh undraped in side-lying position

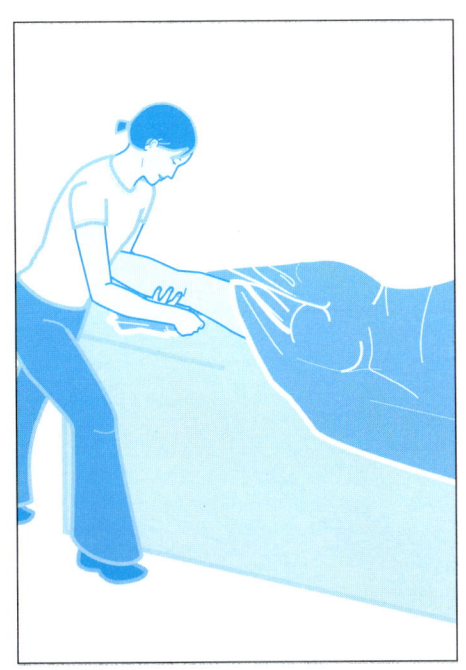

Figure 15.7d Undraping the bottom leg and thigh in side-lying position

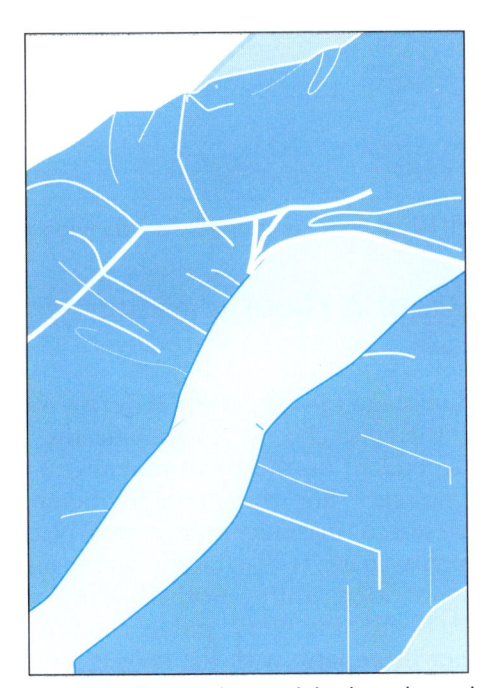

Figure 15.7e The bottom leg and thigh undraped in side-lying position

under the thigh and brought toward the hip to meet the other corner of the draping (Figure 15.7b).

Holding both edges of the draping slide the draping up the leg and thigh to reveal the area to be massaged (Figure 15.7c).

To undrape the bottom leg and thigh, the top leg must first be flexed at a 90 degree angle at the knee and hip, moved anterior and supported with a pillow. The draping is folded back over the leg toward the midline (Figure 15.7d).

The therapist lifts the limb to tuck the draping in under the thigh and brings the edge back to meet the corner of the draping at the hip (Figure 15.7e).

Undraping the buttocks

Standard draping procedures in this text undrape the back to include the superior aspect of the gluteal muscles. More detailed massage to the gluteal muscles may be required when a client presents with a specific problem and massage to these muscles would be indicated as part of the treatment plan. With the client's consent, the draping to the buttocks can be done in several ways.

Option 1: Access to buttocks via back

With the client in prone position, commence the procedure for undraping the back. With the draping that is directly covering the client, pick it up at the low back and tuck this section into the waist of the client's underwear. Slide the underwear and draping down to the gluteal fold (Figure 15.8a). The top flap of the draping is still covering the low

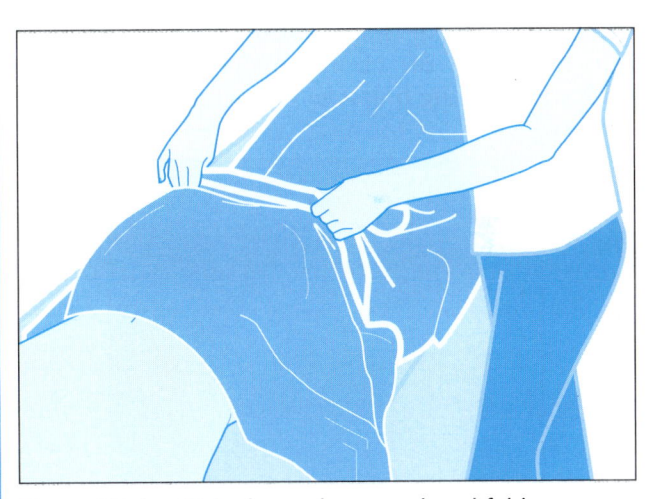

Figure 15.8a Slide drape down to gluteal fold

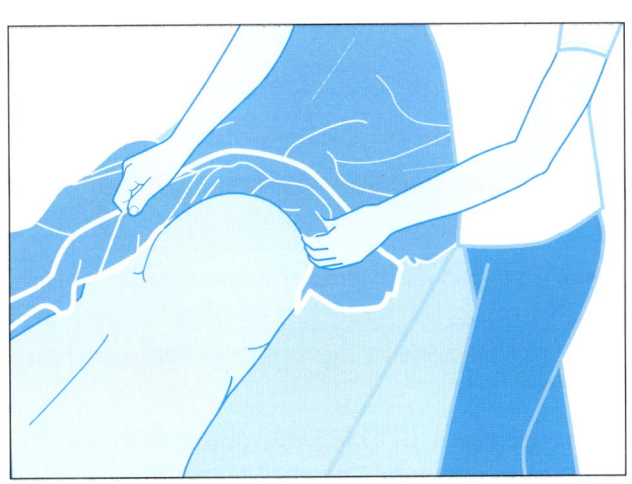

Figure 15.8b Fold drape back to reveal one side of buttocks

back and buttocks and can be folded back on the diagonal to reveal one side of the buttocks (Figure 15.8b). The gluteal cleft remains draped and only one side is undraped at a time. Repeat the undraping procedure on the opposite side once the massage has been completed and the buttocks have been redraped. The client's back can be covered with a drape whilst the therapist is focused with the massage on the buttocks.

Option 2: Access to buttocks via the posterior lower limb

With the client in the prone position follow the procedures for undraping the posterior lower limb. Fold the drape back over the leg so that the edges fall to the midline between the legs (see Figure 15.3a). Lift the leg that is undraped by supporting it around the inside of the lower leg close to the knee with the inside arm (facing the head of the table). The other hand reaches under the leg being lifted to pull the drape from the midline of the thigh to the side of the table towards the hip (see Figure 15.3b). The draping should sit high on the inner thigh and be firm for the client to feel its presence. The top part of the draping at the hip can be tucked into the leg of the client's underwear and drawn back to reveal the buttocks (Figure 15.9).

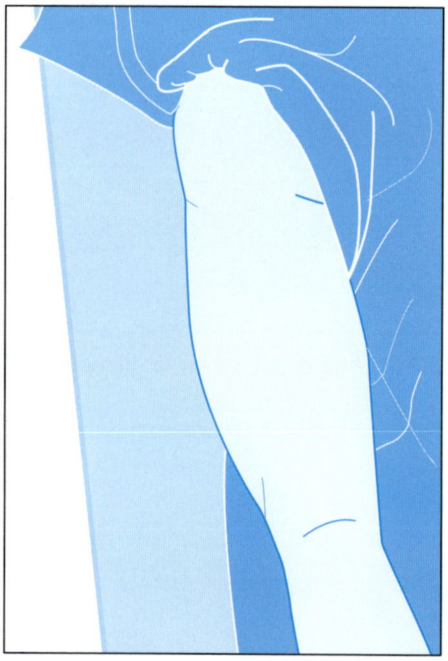

Figure 15.9 Buttocks undraped via posterior lower limb

Option 3: Access to the buttocks via side-lying position

With the client in side-lying position follow the procedures for undraping the lower limb.

To undrape the upper leg, bring the draping material over the leg from anterior to posterior, support and lift the leg as the draping is tucked in under the thigh and brought toward the hip to meet the other corner of the draping (Figure 15.7b and c). Slide the draping up the leg and thigh and toward the iliac crest to reveal the buttocks (Figure 15.10). To access the other side the therapist must turn the client over and repeat the draping procedure on the opposite side.

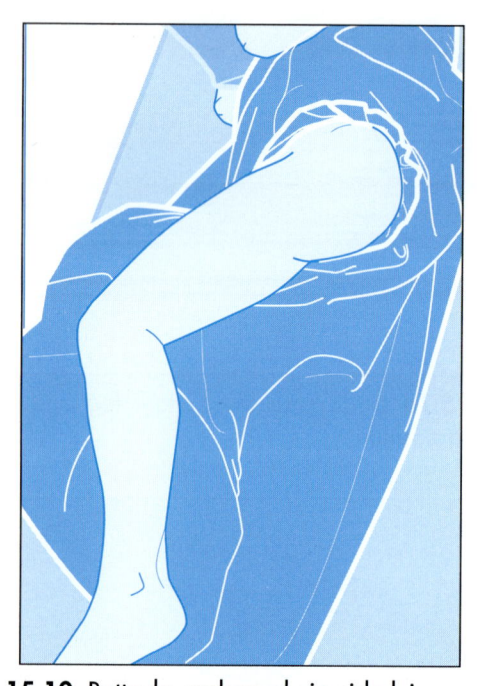

Figure 15.10 Buttocks undraped via side-lying position

Draping of a client in a seated position

A seated massage can take many different forms and how the therapist chooses to provide the massage will be dependent on the environment and purpose of the massage. For the massage therapist who performs seated massage in the workplace or at events such as markets or exhibitions, the massage is usually provided fully clothed due to time constraints and the very public nature of the massage environment; with the massage techniques performed through the client's clothing. By contrast, when operating from a private clinic or the like, and time permits, the massage therapist may require the client to disrobe to a certain degree in order to perform the massage. In such instances a large sheet would be the preferred choice of draping material as it can be easily tucked and tied into place. To access the client's back the sheet can be tied loosely at the back of the client's neck with the opening at the back of the body. The sheet can be secured at the waist of the client's underwear to hold it in place and provide access to the whole back (Figure 15.11a). To access the back of the client's neck and shoulders the therapist can untie the sheet

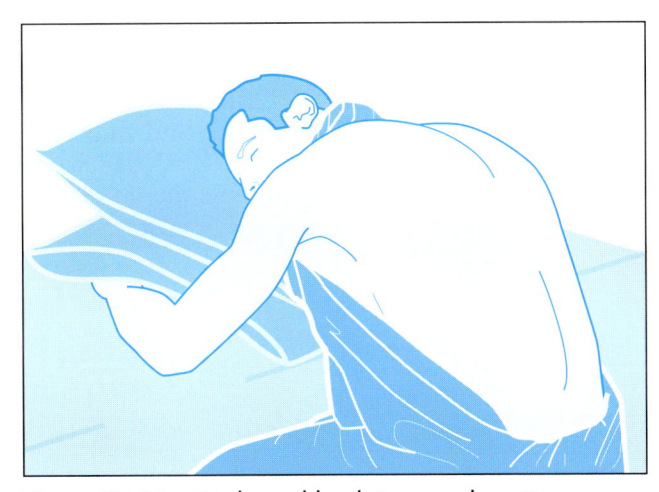

Figure 15.11a Undraped back in seated position

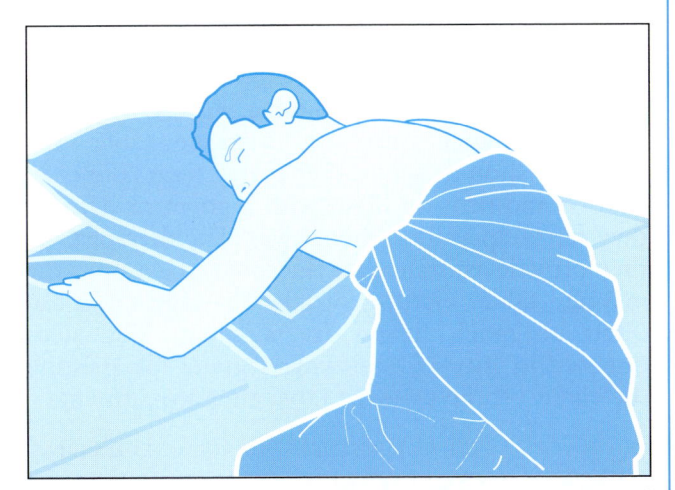

Figure 15.11b Undraped shoulders and neck in a seated position

and wrap it around the client's chest and torso, 'toga' style (Figure 15.11b).

TURNING THE CLIENT FROM PRONE TO SUPINE

The client has two direction options for turning over on the massage table. The therapist should be practiced at both options and be prepared for the client to turn either way. Often clients are too relaxed to take in instructions clearly and may misunderstand which way the therapist has asked them to turn.

When turning the client, excess draping or blankets are removed from the client and put aside for the turning process, and then repositioned when the turning is complete. This means that if two towels are being used to drape a client remove one when the client is turning. The towel covering the torso of the client should be positioned lengthways along the client to cover as much of the body as possible and be used as the draping towel for turning. The draping should not be lifted completely off the client, as they will feel exposed and perhaps startled from their relaxed state.

Here is one method. The therapist stands at the side of the massage table and holds the draping at the top edges near the client's neck. The client is asked to turn onto their back slowly. As they begin to change their position from prone to supine the therapist adjusts their hands on the draping in one of the following ways to suit the direction the client has chosen to turn. These scenarios also work equally as well for the client that is turning from supine to prone or from a side-lying position to prone or supine.

Option 1 — the client turns toward the therapist. The therapist holds the side of the draping nearest to them and allows for the draping to slide over the client as they turn (Figure 15.12).

Option 2 — the client turns away from the therapist. The therapist holds the edges of the draping furthest from them and allows for the draping to slide over the client as they turn. The edge of the draping can be slightly raised to allow room for the client to turn (Figure 15.13).

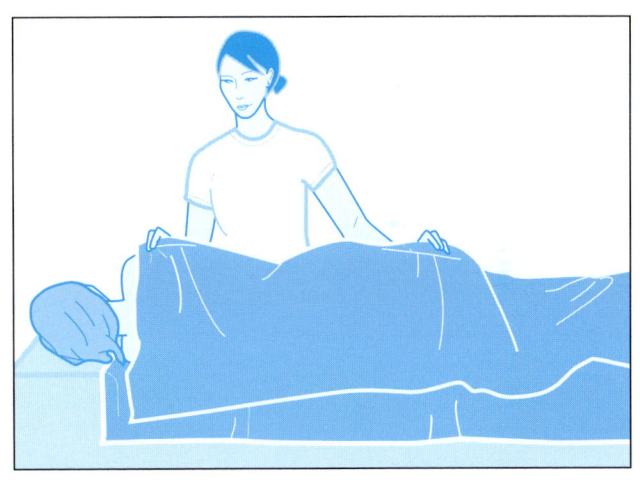

Figure 15.12 Holding the draping for client turning toward the therapist

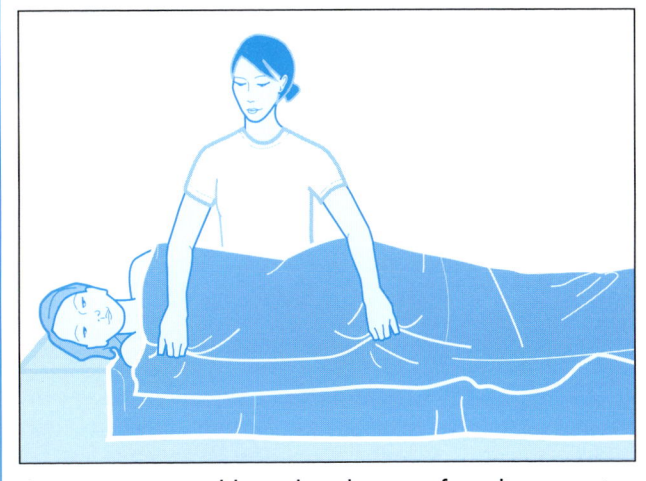

Figure 15.13 Holding the draping for client turning away from the therapist

SECTION 6 THE MASSAGE TREATMENT

The therapist anchoring the draping between the massage table and the therapist's body can further secure the draping in this second turning option.

HELPING THE CLIENT ON AND OFF THE MASSAGE TABLE

The therapist should not be expected to lift a client onto the massage table for the safety of the therapist as well as the client. When a client is unable to move themselves onto a massage table, a seated massage may be more appropriate.

At times, situations will arise when the therapist needs to assist the client on and off the massage table. A client may be elderly and not very agile, have an injury such as a fractured leg, or may have dizzy spells. These and many other reasons may require the therapist to provide minor assistance to the client. A therapist who has an electric or hydraulic table will have an advantage as they can lower the table closer to the floor, making it easier for the client to get on or off the table. A step or footstool can also be of assistance to help the client up onto and off a massage table. Where the client needs assistance onto the massage table, the therapist should allow the client time alone to disrobe and provide them with a gown or draping they can wrap around themselves. The therapist can then provide assistance for the client to get onto the massage table. Getting off the massage table can often be much harder for a client. The steps outlined in Box 15.4 provide a guide for assisting the client off the massage table after a treatment.

> **Box 15.4** Assisting the client off the massage table
>
> - Ask the client to roll onto their side, and bend their knees and hips to 90 degrees of flexion.
> - Stand close to the table, facing the table.
> - Allow the client to reach up to hold onto your shoulders.
> - Place one hand behind the client's neck on the upper back and the other hand behind their thighs (Figure 15.14a).
> - Assist the client to a seated position by swinging the client's legs off the massage table whilst simultaneously lifting their upper body. The momentum of the legs will aid the movement into a seated position (Figure 15.14b).
> - Assist the client down off the massage table.

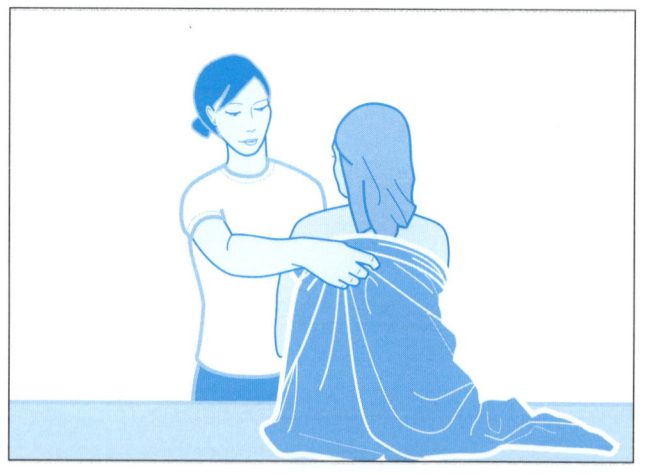

Figure 15.14b Assisting the client into a seated postion

CLIENT POSITIONING

Part of the whole effect of achieving relaxation during a massage is ensuring that the client is comfortable and able to relax their body whilst on the massage table. With the addition of bolsters, pillows and towels the therapist can support the natural contours of the client's body. Additional supports or alternative positions may be required for some clients. The following illustrations provide a guide for the therapist setting up their massage

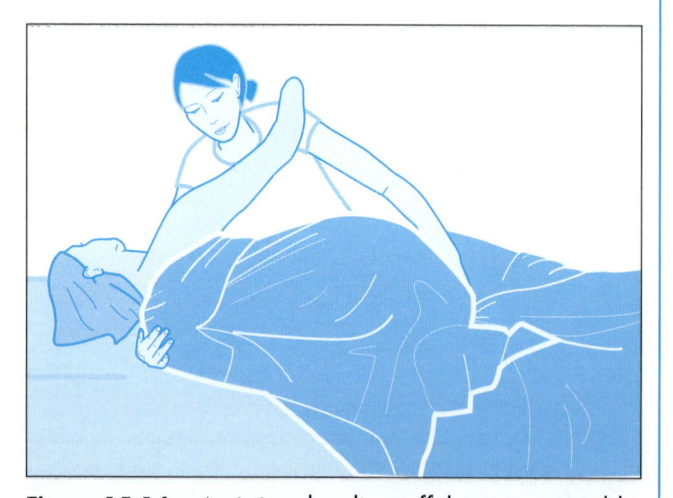

Figure 15.14a Assisting the client off the massage table

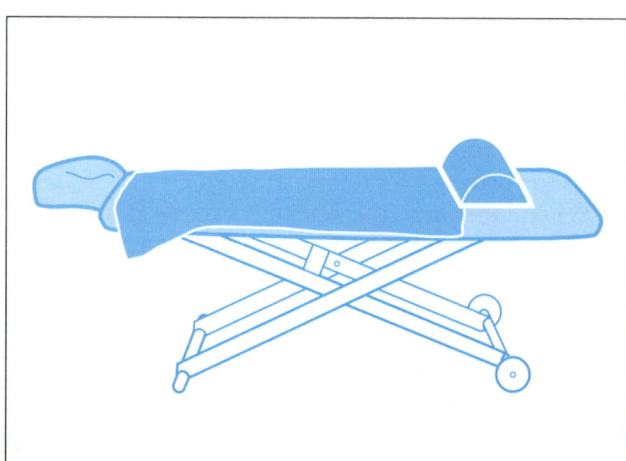

Figure 15.15 Basic prone positioning

table and adapting their pillowing or positioning to suit individual needs (see Figures 15.15 – 15.21).

Figure 15.15 shows an illustration of a massage table with bolster for placement under the front of the ankles.

Figure 15.16 shows prone position with extra support for the lower back. Place a pillow under the client's abdomen between the hips and the chest. A flat pillow may be preferred to the bolster under the ankles.

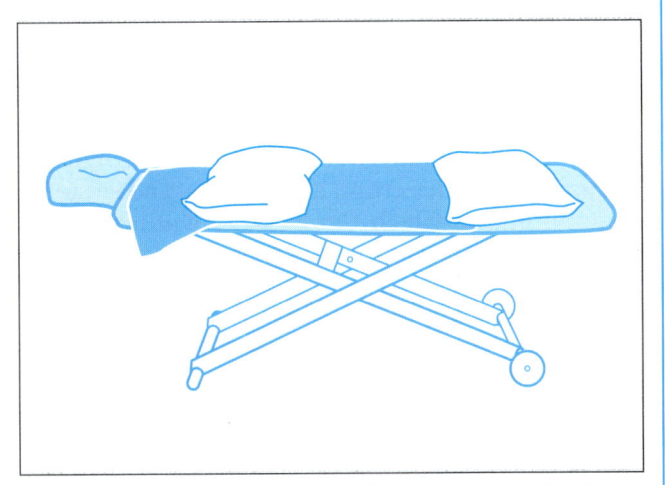

Figure 15.16 Prone position with extra support for lower back

Figure 15.17 shows prone position for reducing breast discomfort. Place a handtowel rolled into a sausage shape below the client's clavicles at the top of the pectorals.

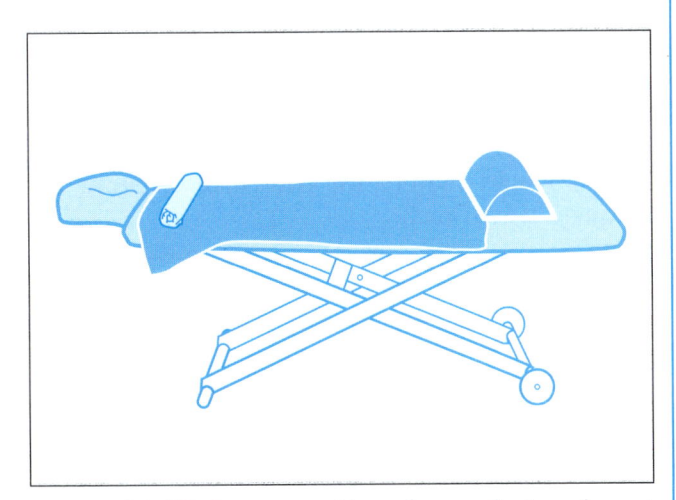

Figure 15.17 Prone position for reducing breast discomfort

In a supine position a pillow can be placed under the client's head for extra support and comfort (Figure 15.18). Some clients may prefer to have no pillow and others may prefer to have several. Observe your client's level of comfort and adjust to suit. The bolster is placed beneath the client's knees. For clients with lower back complaints an

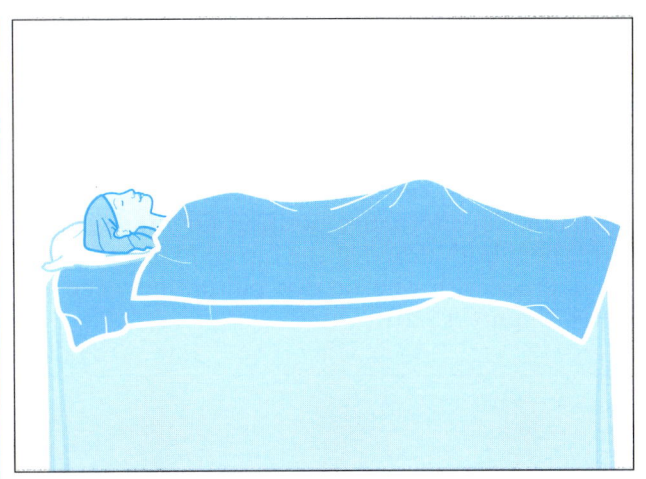

Figure 15.18 Supine position

added pillow under the knees may make them more comfortable.

The therapist will need to position the bolster under the client's knees when they turn from prone to supine. To lift the client's legs in a supported manner, wrap the feet and legs in the draping they are lying on (Figure 15.19a), grasp this draping and lift the client's legs as you slide the bolster under the client's knees (Figure 15.19b).

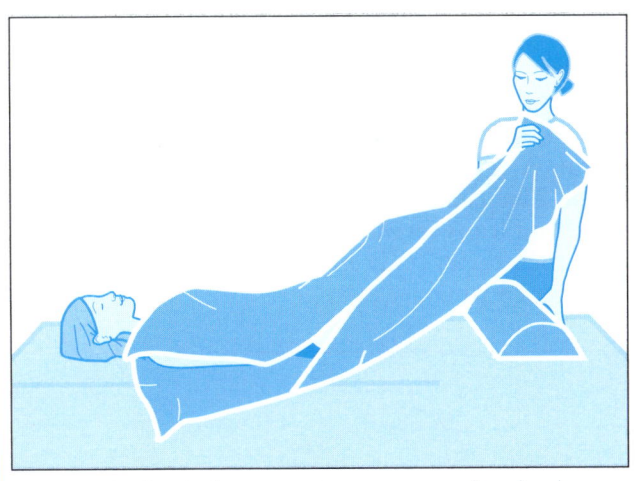

Figure 15.19a Bolster position to support low back

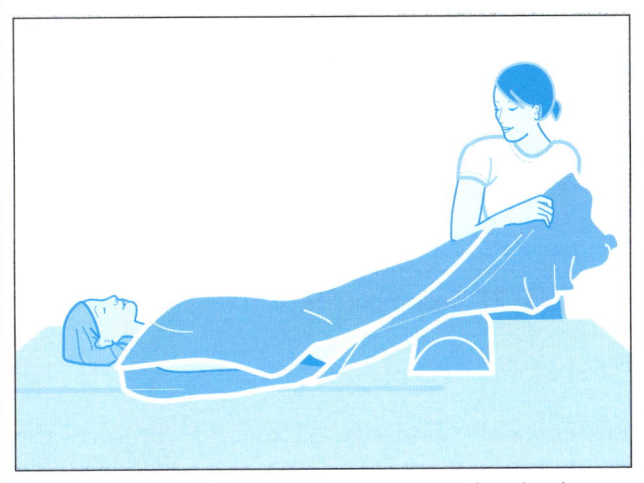

Figure 15.19b Bolster position to support low back

The side-lying position is useful for the pregnant client, the elderly and any client that may have difficulty lying prone. Use a pillow or two for the client's head and a pillow or two under the knee of the client's upper leg whilst the leg the client is lying on is outstretched and slightly posterior. An alternative position for the legs is to have them both flexed at the hip and knee to about 90 degrees with one or two pillows between the knees (Figure 15.20).

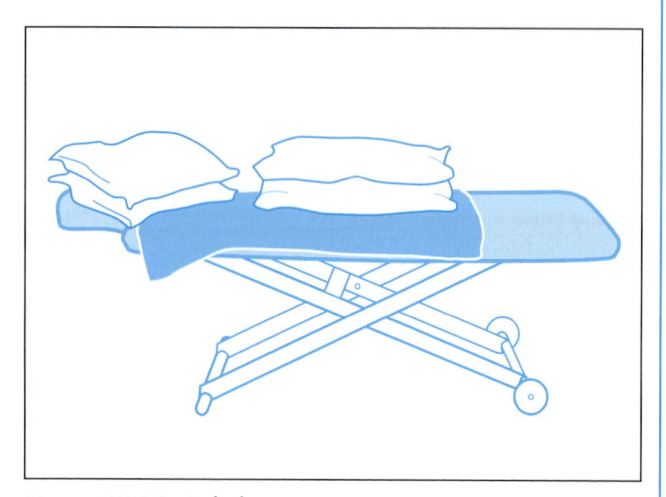

Figure 15.20 Side-lying position

The seated position may be appropriate for clients that have mobility issues, are wheelchair bound, or have difficulty being comfortable lying down. A regular chair, stool or wheelchair can be used. The client sits down close to the massage table and leans forward over the massage table and rests their upper body and head onto several pillows (Figure 15.21).

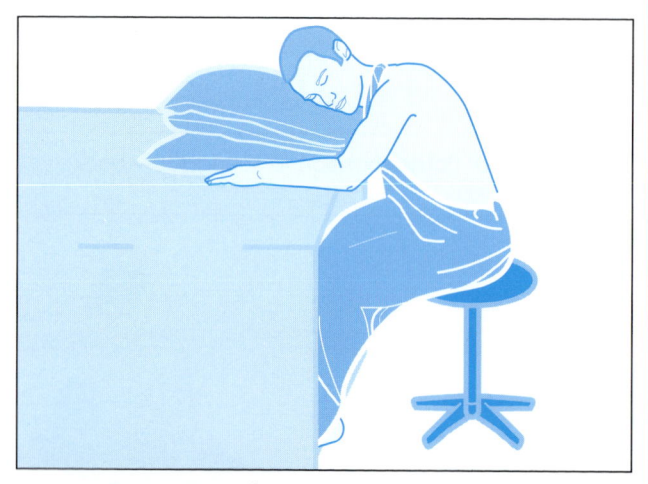

Figure 15.21 Seated position

CONCLUSION

Professional standards of practice require the massage professional to provide adequate draping for a client, whereby the areas of the body that are not being massaged or have not been consented to for massage will remain covered throughout the treatment. Like massage techniques, draping also requires a degree of skill and sensitivity. Gaining access to parts of a client's body throughout the course of a massage means that the therapist may need to lift limbs and tuck the draping to anchor it in place. The draping should be secure without the need for the therapist to readjust it throughout the massage and the area to be massaged should be sufficiently undraped to gain proper access without the need for the hands to go beyond the draping line.

Draping may be considered a form of non-verbal communication with a client about the area that is about to be massaged. When used correctly, draping techniques create a definite boundary and a defining line in which the massage will take place. In addition, draping provides warmth for the client, and in maintaining privacy helps create a sense of security, allowing the client to feel relaxed and comfortable throughout the massage treatment. By draping confidently and efficiently the massage professional will allow a greater sense of trust and security to be felt by the client. Draping that is performed swiftly and with ease will go a long way to ensuring the massage treatment is one that is effective, efficient and professional, and provides a high level of warmth, security and comfort to the massage client.

Questions and activities

1. You are commencing a clinic, and anticipate consulting with up to five patients per day for four days a week. You plan to do all your own laundering daily, and need to purchase draping materials. Detail exactly what draping materials you would require for your clinic, stating the quantities of each.
2. To ensure clients return to receive massage from you, write a statement relating to draping and privacy that can be given to first-time clients that explains the process of, and considerations given to, draping in your professional massage practice.

Further reading

Andrade, C. and Clifford, P. (2001) *Outcome-Based Massage*. Lippincott Williams & Wilkins, Baltimore.

De Domenico, G. and Wood, E. C. (1997) *Beard's Massage* (4th edn). W. B. Saunders, Philadelphia.

Fritz, S. (2000) *Mosby's Fundamentals of Therapeutic Massage* (2nd edn). Mosby, St Louis.

Salvo, S. G. (2003) *Massage Therapy: Principles & Practice* (2nd edn). W. B. Saunders, Philadelphia.

chapter 16

Body mechanics and massage

Chris Bennett

Learning outcomes

- Describe the importance of good body mechanics
- Describe the five principles of good body mechanics
- Discuss the importance of leverage when performing a massage
- Discuss the significance of foot positioning and wrist angle when performing a massage

INTRODUCTION

The application of massage is strenuous. Any massage therapist will attest to the fact that the repetitive nature of performing massage after massage can be exhausting. For the professional massage therapist who makes a living from performing massage on a daily basis, such a career choice can often leave them feeling fatigued and may result in injury. To avoid fatigue and injury, it is vitally important that the massage therapist employ good body mechanics whilst performing massage.

For a massage therapist, the conservation of their energy throughout the day is necessary to ensure they are able to perform massage consistently and to a high standard. By ensuring they use correct body mechanics, they are more efficient in their movements and thus fatigue less. Conserving energy while performing massage enables the therapist to be more attentive to the client's needs. When the therapist is feeling fresh, they are better able to make judgments regarding the type of strokes to use as well as the depth and speed of application and the duration of treatment. A therapist who is 'fatigue-free' also has the mental clarity and energy required to perform an appropriate assessment of the condition of the client's tissues and evaluate the effectiveness of massage techniques used.

For the busy massage therapist who may consult with a great number of clients and sometimes massage for as many as eight to ten hours a day, good body mechanics are essential to conserve energy and minimise the risk of injury to themself. Common sites of injury for a massage therapist include the soft tissues and joints of the hands, arms, shoulders, knees, hips and spine. Such injuries often result from the use of poor body mechanics. For example, a therapist may rotate and flex their lumbar spine whilst performing deep manipulations to a client's back. Such a posture, when repeated and sustained, may lead to injury of the therapist's low back, and thus should be avoided.

When performing the repetitive movements associated with the application of massage, the therapist must adopt correct technique and avoid fatiguing their body — by ensuring they always perform massage using correct body mechanics. This chapter outlines the principles associated with good body mechanics, and describes the use of good body posture when applying massage. By adopting such good postures, the massage therapist will minimise fatigue and reduce the risk of injury, thereby improving their career longevity as a professional massage therapist.

GENERAL PRINCIPLES OF GOOD BODY MECHANICS

The structural system of the human body is made up of bones and muscles, which are supported by ligaments. The way in which this mechanical system moves depends on the joints and muscles that are recruited, and such movement may be highly efficient or very inefficient. When the body moves in an efficient way, it moves with ease and requires little energy to perform the movement. In contrast, an inefficient movement is one that is awkward, unnatural and requires considerable energy. Although one may assume the body would naturally move in an efficient manner, this is not always the case, as the person driving the body may succumb to poor habits of posture or place themselves in positions that do not promote efficient movement.

> **Box 16.1** Remember
>
> A body that moves freely, efficiently and with ease is moving with good body mechanics.

When the body moves with efficient movement it is employing good body mechanics. As described previously, such efficient movements conserve energy and minimise the risk of injury. When performing massage, the therapist should adopt efficient movements, and the following five principles of good body mechanics will assist with their practice.

Principle 1 — use body weight, not muscular strength, to apply pressure

Most massage strokes can be applied with sufficient pressure simply by the massage therapist leaning their weight onto their hands with little or no effort. The stroke can then be moved along the body part being worked by the therapist appropriately shifting their weight, usually from one leg to the other in a manner determined by the stroke itself.

Principle 2 — keep the back comfortably upright and straight wherever possible

The back, especially the lower back, is vulnerable to injury while massaging. Keeping the back straight helps ensure its safety. Avoid reaching or moving forward by bending the back — always use the legs to move around the patient.

Principle 3 — use correct alignment of torso and limbs while performing strokes

For strokes that require pushing or pressing of the therapist's hands, fingers or thumbs onto the body, the elbows should be straight but not locked. For strokes where the direction of force changes continuously, such as circular finger kneading or C-scoop, the elbows should be bent to avoid shearing forces to the elbow joint. For most strokes the wrists should be kept straight.

Principle 4 — the hands, fingers or thumbs should always be appropriately supported while applying pressure

The therapist should fix and support smaller joints and muscles (for example in the fingers and hands), while using the muscles of larger body parts, like the legs, to do the work. If the fingertips or thumbs are being used to manipulate the tissues the therapist should not rely on the strength of the small hand muscles to do this. It is safer and more effective to fix or lock the position of the fingers, hands and wrist and move the body weight into the stroke by using the legs. The therapist should use two hands instead of one wherever possible.

Principle 5 — wherever possible perform strokes with a rhythmical, fluid, whole-body movement

The therapist should keep the stroke moving and flowing smoothly and continuously, and avoid stopping and starting or jerking movements. Flowing movements require less effort because of the continuous momentum (and feel more relaxing to the client), whereas to restart a movement after it has stopped requires effort to overcome inertia.

> **Box 16.2** The five principles of good body mechanics
>
> 1. Use body weight, not muscular strength to apply pressure.
> 2. Keep the back comfortably upright and straight wherever possible.
> 3. Use correct alignment of torso and limbs while performing strokes.
> 4. The hands, fingers or thumbs should always be appropriately supported while applying pressure.
> 5. Wherever possible, perform strokes with a rhythmical, fluid, whole-body movement.

THE IMPORTANCE OF LEVERAGE FOR EFFORTLESS PRESSURE

Leverage involves utilising maximum force with minimum effort. For example, it would be very difficult to remove a large boulder from the ground by simply using the arms, but when a crowbar is used it has the effect of increasing the leverage of the arms and increases the force, thus allowing the boulder to be shifted from its resting place with minimal effort.

When performing massage, it is difficult to generate pressure by simply using the fingers. By contrast, a therapist who uses the leverage of their body weight and leans into the movement of their fingers with the weight of the body behind them is able to generate greater force and pressure.

If correct leverage is used for the application of massage, performing the massage stroke should feel effortless. If it doesn't, the stroke is not being performed correctly and the massage therapist should check their body mechanics, find the fault and make the necessary adjustments. When good leverage and body mechanics are being used the therapist does not have to 'work harder' by pushing harder; all that is required to increase pressure is a shift in the body weight achieved by leaning into the stroke.

Using leverage during massage

When adopting a stride or wide stance, leverage is gained by shifting the body weight between the feet. Figures 16.1 and 16.2 show the leverage and

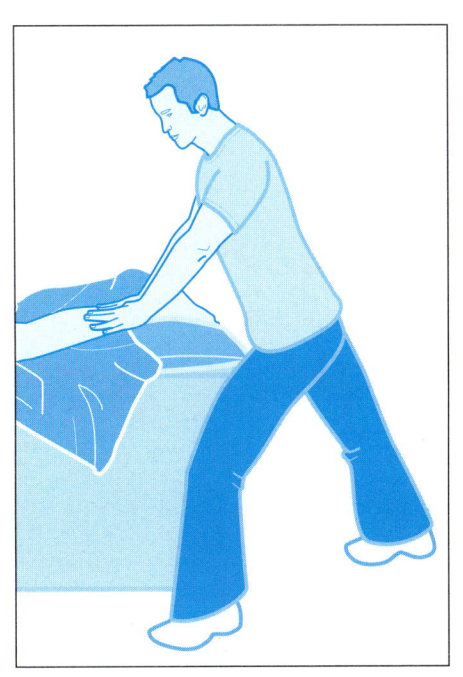

Figure 16.1 Rowing stroke, forward moving part of stroke

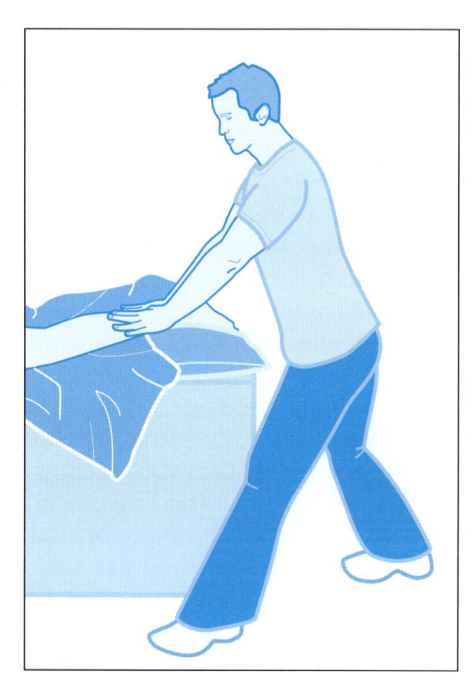

Figure 16.2 Rowing stroke, backward moving part of stroke

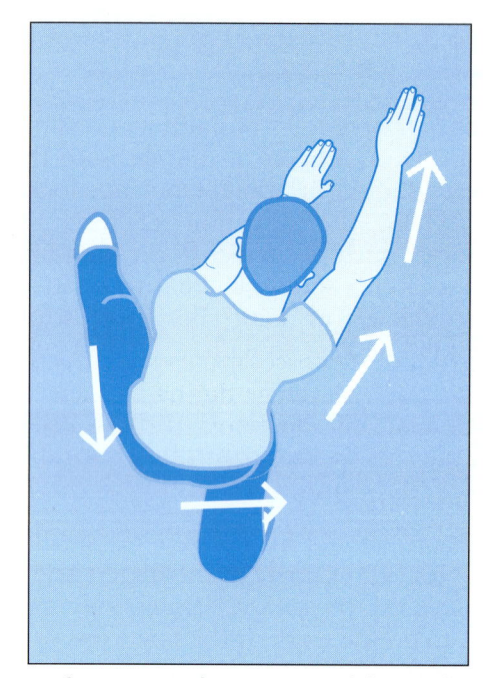

Figure 16.3b Rotational movement of the trunk

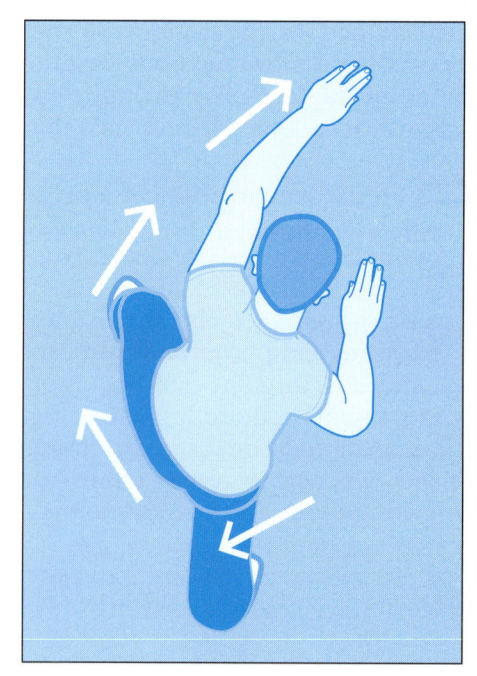

Figure 16.3c Opposite rotational movement of the trunk

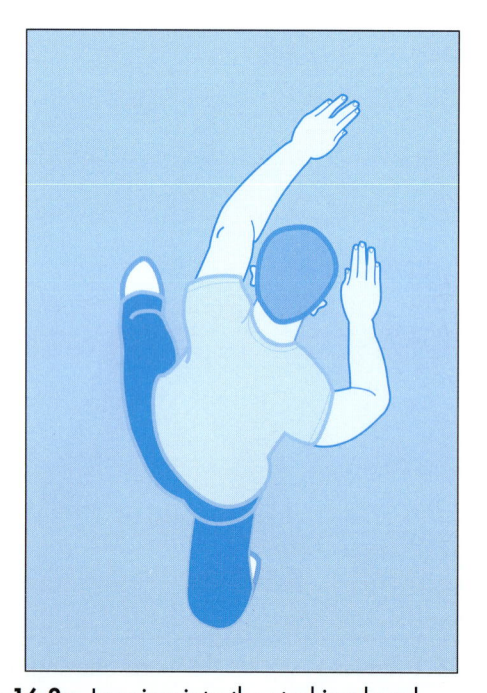

Figure 16.3a Leaning into the stroking hand

lines of force applied when correctly performing 'rowing strokes'. The same principles apply to all strokes that use the stride or wide stance.

For strokes that alternate hand movements, such as 'hand-after-hand' or 'side pulls', a rotational movement must occur through the central axis of the body for the stroke to be effective and easy to perform. In Figure 16.3, pressure is applied when performing the 'hand-after-hand' stroke by leaning into the stroking hand. A rotational movement of the trunk allows the shoulder and then the hand to move forward. At the same time as the trunk rotates, the pelvis rotates in a counter clockwise direction, causing the forward knee to extend and the back knee and hip to flex (see Figures 16.3 a and b). Such movement at the knees and hips is important for the force and reach of this stroke. If the knees were held tight and did not move with the stroke, the effectiveness of the stroke would be lost and the lower back would be subjected to undue torsion and strain. As the hand finishes its stroke the other hand begins to move forward, again facilitated by the rotation of the trunk, this time in the opposite direction (see Figure 16.3c). When learning this movement it often seems difficult to coordinate, yet simply paying attention to the bending and straightening of the front knee makes it easier to do.

The position of the feet

When a person performs a throwing action, the direction that the foot of the leading leg is pointing is the direction the ball is thrown in. Likewise when performing massage, the direction the feet face is the direction of the force of the stroke. As the body weight is used for leverage during massage, the feet should point in the direction of the stroke, as the body weight will be shifted forwards and backwards over the feet. If the feet are not aligned to the direction of the stroke, then the movement of the body will result in the knees shearing laterally. Such a movement creates shearing forces that detract from the efficiency of the stroke and may result in injury of the knee or hip.

> **Box 16.3** Remember
>
> As a general rule for most strokes the feet should be facing forward in the same direction the pelvis is facing and in the same direction the stroke is moving, unless it is a 'pulling' stroke.

The angle of the wrist

The flat of the hand is commonly used to perform effleurage stroking. When doing so, the angle of the wrist is important to ensure undue pressure is not placed on the joint and the many structures that cross the wrist joint. Holding the wrist in 90 degrees of extension and placing downward pressure on the joint to perform massage is not advisable (see Figure 16.4 a). The optimal joint angle is midway between neutral and 45 degrees of extension (see Figure 16.4 b).

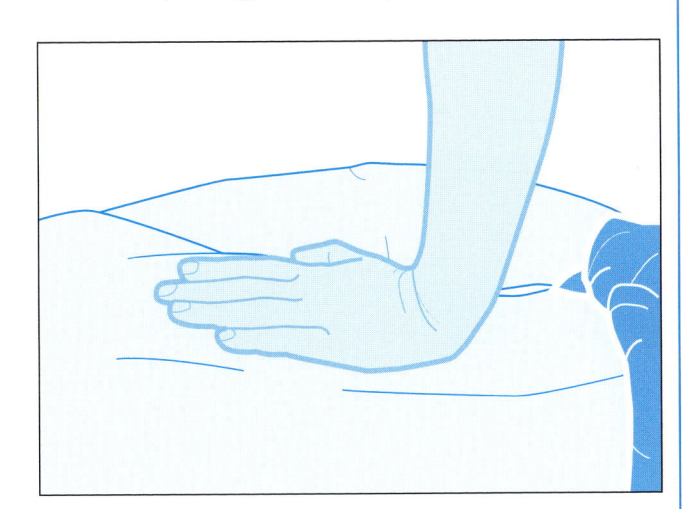

Figure 16.4a A poor wrist angle

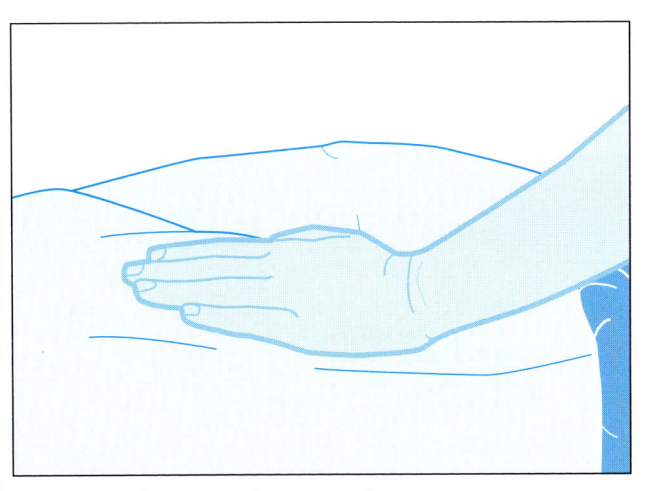

Figure 16.4b Optimal wrist angle

> **Box 16.4** Remember
>
> The optimal angle of the wrist for flat-hand stroking is midway between neutral and 45 degrees of extension.

Using the forearm

When performing deep effleurage, the forearm is often used as opposed to the flat of the hand. When using the forearm to stroke, it is important to remember that the weight of the upper body should be directly over the elbow joint. Ideally the elbow joint should be flexed to 90 degrees, and the shoulder or glenohumeral joint abducted 45 degrees from the body (so as to avoid undue strain on the deltoid muscles and shoulder joint).

The body stance used with forearm stroking is a modified stride position, where the therapist bends slightly forward from the waist. In this position it is important to maintain a flat or straight back, and bending both knees slightly may assist this (see Figure 16.5). To provide additional stability the free

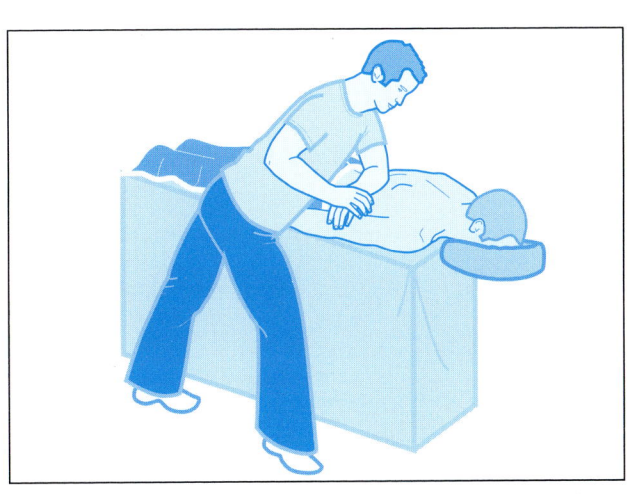

Figure 16.5 Leverage for ulna edge or forearm strokes

hand may grasp the wrist to reinforce the position, or rest on the table to provide additional support to the back.

> **Box 16.5** Remember
>
> When performing forearm stroking the elbow joint should be flexed to 90 degrees, and the glenohumeral joint abducted 45 degrees from the body.

CONCLUSION

When pushing a heavy weight a person instinctually adopts good body mechanics. For example, if a broken down car needs to be pushed to the side of the road, a person would tend to adopt a stance that would include the body leaning into the car with straight arms, erect spine and legs pushing against the ground; the whole body aligned for maximum leverage. Such a position would allow for maximal strength with minimal effort.

The massage therapist should adopt a similar approach when performing a massage stroke. Using correct body alignment, the therapist should lean into the posture and use their body weight for leverage in the direction of the stroke they are performing. The force should come from the body behind the stroke, and not be generated simply by the smaller muscles of the hands and forearms.

By adopting the principles of good body mechanics and being aware of their posture, the professional massage therapist will be better able to perform repeated massages with minimal effort and fatigue. With good body mechanics they will be able to minimise their risk of injury and prolong their career as a professional massage therapist. As with any physical endeavour, correct technique is paramount to performance. When performed with ease and efficiency the application of massage is a most enjoyable and rewarding occupation that serves to challenge and exercise both body and mind.

Questions and activities

1. When you performed your last massage, were there any movements you performed that felt awkward, difficult or ineffectual? Did these relate in any way to how you were using your body? If so, how can you adapt your movement to better perform the massage next time?
2. Do you have any injuries or limitations of movement that affect the way you perform massage? If so, how do you adjust to ensure the movement is easier? Are these adjustments the best you can make?
3. Imagine yourself providing up to eight massages a day for six days a week. What strategies could you put in place to ensure you maintain optimal energy levels and minimise the risk of injury to yourself?

Further reading

Cassar, M. (1999) *Handbook of Massage Therapy: A Complete Guide for the Student and Professional Massage Therapist*. Butterworth–Heinemann, Oxford.

Fritz, S. (2000) *Mosby's Fundamentals of Therapeutic Massage*. Mosby, St Louis.

Greene, L. (1995) *Save Your Hands! Injury Prevention for Massage Therapists*. Gilded Age Press, Colorado.

chapter 17

Massage manipulations

Charles Tuchtan

Learning outcomes

- Describe the major Swedish massage strokes
- Discuss the techniques of application of each of the Swedish massage strokes
- Discuss the contraindications and precautions of application of each of the Swedish massage strokes
- Describe the effects of each of the Swedish massage strokes

INTRODUCTION

The massage manipulations of Per Ling, often referred to as the father of Swedish massage, have now been taught and performed for over two centuries. These techniques have been and are still being used by massage therapists, other manipulative therapists and health care workers throughout the world. According to *Dorland's Illustrated Medical Dictionary* (2000) a manipulation is applied skilfully as a form of treatment via the hands or with the use of mechanical means. Thus a therapist who uses massage manipulations as a form of treatment could be described as having the ability to treat with their hands in a skilful manner. Such manipulations would include the various 'strokes' or manipulations introduced throughout this chapter.

Johann Mezger (1838–1909) has been credited for the classification of Swedish massage manipulations and the introduction of their French terms: *effleurage, pétrissage, tapôtement* and *massage à friction* (Calvert, 2002; Kamenetz, 1980; Palmer, 1912; Ellison, 1904). In the late nineteenth century vibration was added to this inventory (Kellogg, 1895). Many authors have used additional or differing terms to classify the various strokes. James Menell (1917) classified massage manipulations as stroking, compression and percussion. He subcategorised stroking into two distinct manipulations, superficial stroking and deep stroking or effleurage. Kellogg (1895) described the massage strokes in English and defined them into seven categories: touch, stroking, friction, kneading, vibration, percussion and joint movements.

This text classifies the massage strokes into five distinct categories as described in Box 17.1. The purpose of this chapter is to define each of the strokes, discuss their usage and critically analyse the reported effects of the strokes. It should be noted that in addition to the five stroke classifications outlined in Box 17.1, Ling described two additional techniques referred to as passive and active movements. These two techniques are outside the scope of this text, thus will not be discussed in this chapter.

EFFLEURAGE

Definition

Effleurage is a gliding manipulation of the superficial tissues.

Effleurage is derived from the French verb *effleurer*, meaning 'to brush against, to skim over or to touch lightly'. Some authors equally refer to this manipulation as stroking or gliding (Cassar, 1999; Loving, 1999; Tappan and Benjamin, 1998), whilst others describe stroking and effleurage as two different manipulations (Rattray and Ludwig, 2000; Hollis, 1998; DeDomenico and Wood, 1997; Holey and Cook, 1997).

The major difference between stroking and effleurage relates to the depth of pressure applied. Stroking is usually performed slowly with gentle pressure that is firm enough for the client to feel yet light enough so that there is minimal deformation of the subcutaneous tissue (Andrade and Clifford, 2001; DeDomenico and Wood, 1997). It is believed that stroking offers little direct mechanical effect, as the depth of technique is too superficial. However, significant reflexive effects have been observed with the application of stroking. Effleurage is applied with greater pressure than stroking, and its effect on the subcutaneous tissue could be described as deforming. Effleurage by contrast has a greater mechanical effect and may also produce the same reflexive effects as stroking. Effleurage is said to have a major effect on venous and lymphatic return.

The therapist generally applies effleurage with the flat palms placed on the client's body. The therapist then uses their body weight to 'lean into' the superficial tissues, pushing the stroke forwards. Traditionally, this technique is performed in the direction of venous and lymphatic flow in the direction of the heart (Kellogg, 1895; Palmer, 1912; Beard and Wood, 1964; Andrade and Clifford, 2001). There is a belief amongst some authors that structural damage may occur to the valves within the veins if effleurage is applied in a centrifugal direction (Tappan, 1998). However, no evidence exists to substantiate this claim, yet if the treatment goals are to increase venous and lymphatic flow, then the direction of the technique should be aligned to the direction of fluid flow.

Box 17.1 Classification of massage manipulations

Effleurage	Superficial stroking
	Superficial effleurage
Pétrissage	Pétrissage
	Skin rolling
	Compression
Vibration	Vibrations
	Shaking
	Rocking
Tapôtement	
Friction	

Description

The application of stroking and effleurage can be likened to the affectionate caress of a loved one or the petting of a favourite animal. The stroke is applied purposefully with gliding movements that follow the contours of the body. It is applied over large areas, and usually moves distal to proximal in the direction of venous (blood returning to the heart) and lymphatic flow to enhance their effects. In order to maintain flow and continuity, the return stroke travels in the opposite direction with light stroking pressure to the starting position, however, if the goal of the treatment is to augment circulation then the return stroke may be omitted.

Throughout the stroke, the contoured palms, hands, fingers or fingertips mould to the shape of the body region being treated (De Domenico and Wood, 1997). The hands are relaxed and the stroke is performed in a smooth and rhythmic fashion. The pressure employed is derived from the therapist leaning their body weight into the stroke.

Effleurage manipulations may be used for a variety of reasons. As previously described, effleurage is an ideal stroke to use as an introduction of the therapist's touch, and is used to aid the spread of lubricant. As it enhances circulation, effleurage warms the underlying tissues in preparation for deeper manipulations. Effleurage may be used to soothe an area after the application of deep work, and is used as a transitional or connecting stroke for other manipulations (Salvo, 1999).

Techniques

The therapist can vary the way in which effleurage manipulations are applied by using differing hand techniques. Depending on the region being treated and the desired effect, the therapist may apply effleurage with the forearms, palms, contoured hands, fingers or fingertips, and even the side or the back of the hand.

To decrease the risk of therapist injury, it is important to ensure that there is minimal pressure placed on the wrist. Excessive wrist movement (in extension or deviation) may lead to a repetitive strain injury. It is recommended that the fingers face the direction of the movement, thus reducing the amount of deviation at the wrist. The angle of the wrist should remain between neutral and 45 degrees of extension (see Chapter 16).

Rowing stroke

Rowing stroke is performed by placing open palms on the tissues. The palms then glide toward the top of the trunk or limb, where the hands then separate and perform a return gliding stroke down the sides of the trunk or limb (see Figure 17.1).

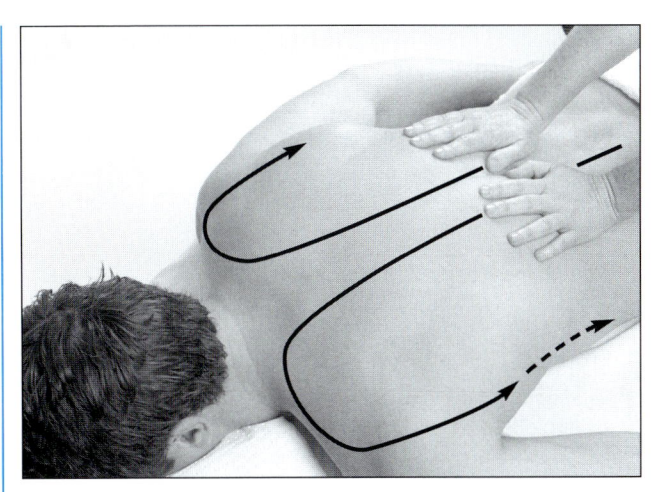

Figure 17.1 Rowing stroke

Half rowing stroke (reinforced effleurage)

Reinforced techniques allow the therapist to penetrate the deeper tissues of the body. The half rowing stroke is performed by placing a reinforced hand (one hand placed over the other) on the tissues. The hand glides toward the top of the trunk or limb and then moves towards the side of the trunk or limb and performs a return gliding stroke to the starting position (see Figure 17.2).

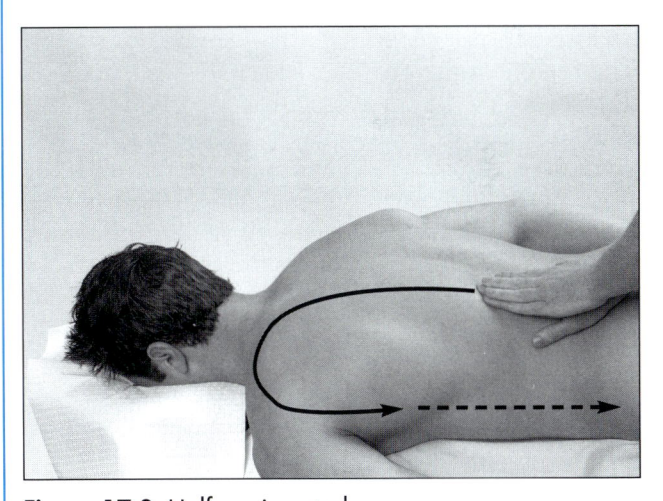

Figure 17.2 Half rowing stroke

Forearm effleurage

Forearm effleurage is normally used when deep pressure is required. This technique engages both the deep and superficial fascia. If the stroke is performed slowly it may soften and lengthen the fascial tissue. As the name suggests, forearm effleurage is a gliding stroke performed with the forearm of the therapist. Using the arm that is closest to the client, the therapist rests their forearm on the tissue to be massaged, making sure to avoid body areas such as the scapula and spine. With the shoulder placed directly over the forearm, the therapist uses their body weight to glide the

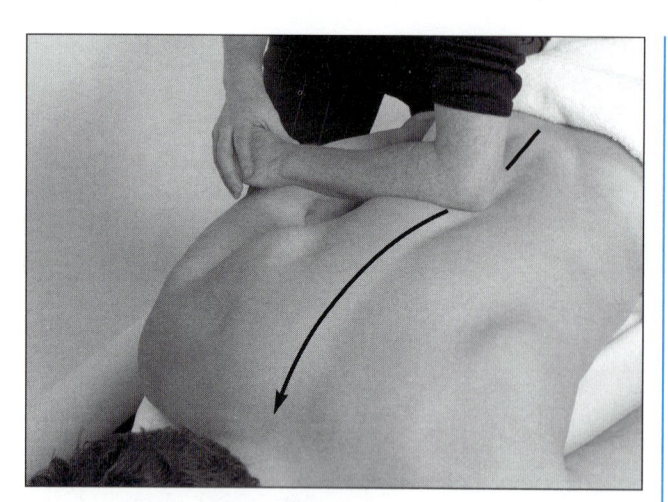

Figure 17.3 Forearm effleurage

forearm along the tissue, easing off the pressure towards the end of the stroke (see Figure 17.3).

Fist effleurage

Loose fist effleurage is a deep effleurage technique primarily used on well-developed or very tight muscles. This technique engages both the deep and superficial fascia. If the stroke is performed slowly it may soften and lengthen the fascial tissue. The therapist makes a fist with the hand of the arm that is closest to the client. The 'flat' surface of the fist (the region of the proximal phalanges) is placed on the tissue to be massaged (as opposed to the knuckles). The technique is reinforced by the therapist's other hand, which wraps around the wrist of the massaging hand. The therapist uses their body weight to glide the fist along the tissue, easing off the pressure towards the end of the stroke (see Figure 17.4).

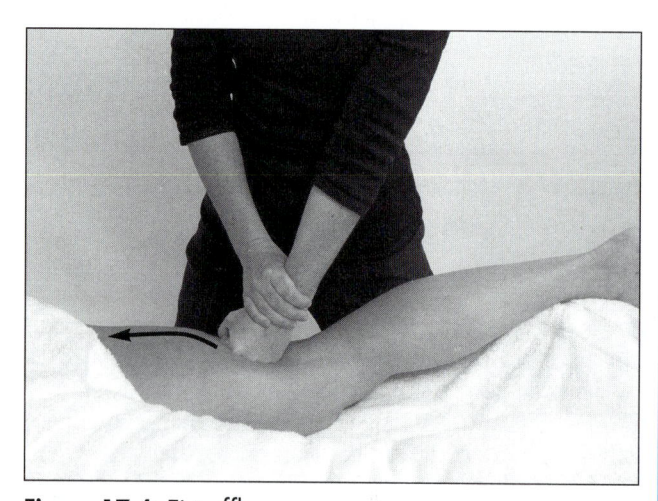

Figure 17.4 Fist effleurage

Hand after hand

One hand glides up the trunk or limb for a short distance followed by the other hand. The leading hand is lifted off as the other hand follows through and the massage therapist continues to alternate hands as they move up the trunk or limb. At the top of the trunk or limb the hands come together in a reinforced position. The technique restarts when the therapist performs a return stroke to the beginning position (see Figure 17.5).

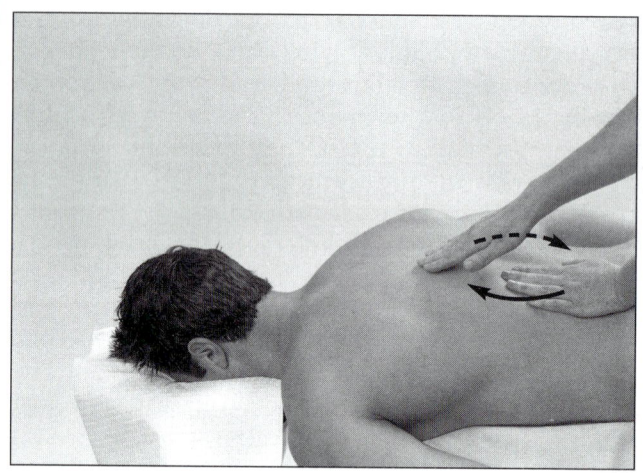

Figure 17.5 Hand after hand

Side pulls

Side pulls are performed by reaching both hands across to the far side of the client's trunk or limb. One hand glides toward the midline of the trunk or limb. The other hand begins the same action when the first hand is halfway through its stroke (see Figure 17.6).

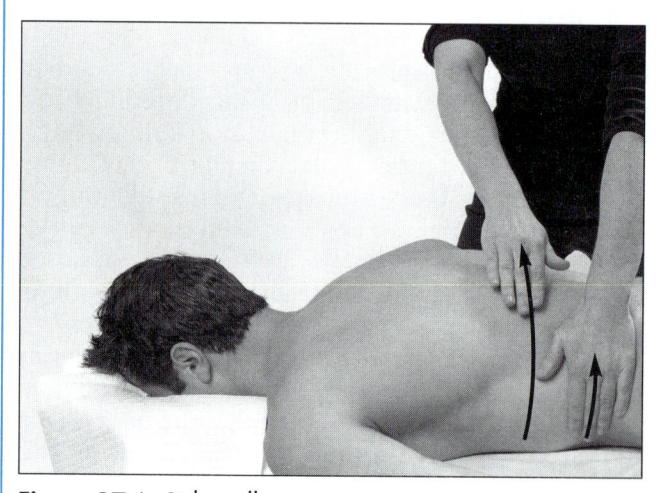

Figure 17.6 Side pulls

Nerve strokes (light stroking)

Nerve strokes (also known as cat or feather strokes) are a light stroking technique and are performed slowly with very light pressure, using the fingertips or even fingernails. With the fingertips stroke down the spine in a continuous alternating pattern (see Figure 17.7).

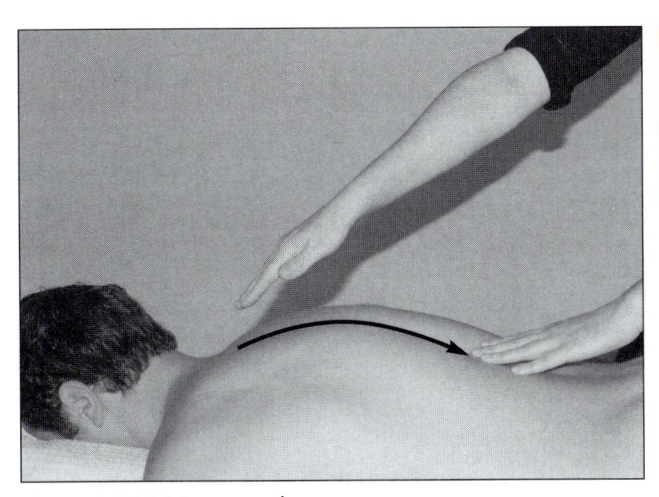

Figure 17.7 Nerve stroke

Contraindications and precautions

The use of stroking and effleurage requires a suitable amount of clinical training and supervised practice to ensure its correct application. More advanced training is necessary for those wishing to use these manipulations for more specific pathologies. All absolute contraindications as noted in Chapter 12 should be adhered to when using effleurage. Deep effleurage over marked varicosities may result in damage to the vein wall and should be avoided. Stroking is locally contraindicated on areas of acute inflammation as it may exacerbate the pain and inflammation (Andrade and Clifford, 2001). It is also contraindicated on areas of acutely damaged tissue, such as burns or wounds or areas of gross oedema, where splitting of the skin is a risk (DeDomenico and Wood, 1997). Effleurage is also best avoided over infected areas, newly formed scars, cellulitis and thrombus (Andrade and Clifford, 2001).

PÉTRISSAGE

Definition

Pétrissage is a group of techniques that repetitively lift, roll, stretch compress or squeeze the underlying tissue.

Pétrissage is derived from the French verb *pétrir* meaning 'to knead'. The intention when performing pétrissage manipulations is to lift and squeeze (or 'milk') or compress the tissue. When performing pétrissage, the therapist lifts, rolls, stretches, compresses, kneads or squeezes the underlying tissue or structures between their hands (Salvo, 2003). Some authors equally refer to this manipulation as kneading (Fritz, 2000; Rechian, et. al, 1998), while others use the term kneading as one of the techniques of kneading (Hollis, 1998; Holey and Cook, 1997). Pétrissage consists of several techniques; namely, kneading, squeezing, compression and skin rolling (DeDomenico and Wood, 1997; Cassar, 1999; Loving, 1999), some texts add shaking (Holey and Cook, 1997; Hollis, 1998) whilst others exclude compression (Rattray and Ludwig, 2000; Salvo, 2003). Over time and with practice, the therapist is able to develop the skill to perform pétrissage in a smooth and rhythmical manner.

Description

There are many pétrissage manipulations and, as previously mentioned, they involve lifting, rolling, stretching, compressing, squeezing or kneading underlying tissues. Each technique has its own unique action and its own effect.

The most common pétrissage attribute is known as kneading. This attribute is much like the kneading of bread dough. One or both hands compress, lift and twist the muscles and subcutaneous tissues, often in an alternating fashion. Pétrissage manipulations involve the use of the whole hand, as the entire palmar surface, the fingers and the thumb, as well as the tips of every digit, are recruited. With practice, the therapist will find it is easier to grasp the tissue when kneading is performed slowly (allowing approximately 2–3 seconds for every pétrissage stroke). As proficiency increases, the therapist can begin to use a more rapid kneading action to produce a stimulating effect on the nervous system. Chaitow and DeLany (2000) recommend the kneading technique rhythm be delivered at around 10–15 cycles per minute for relaxation or around 35 cycles per minute for stimulation.

Pétrissage is said to encourage peripheral blood flow, and may assist with the resolution of oedema. It may be useful in situations of abnormal muscle contracture or soft tissue adhesions (Liston, 1995). Through muscular lengthening and relaxation, pétrissage manipulations may assist painful conditions and relieve muscular fatigue (Chaitow and DeLany, 2000; Salvo, 2003).

Techniques

There are many variations of pétrissage — each having its unique movement and employing the hands in differing ways. Despite the altered dynamics, the unique kneading motion of pétrissage manipulations remains a constant.

C-scoop kneading

The hands are placed on the surface of the skin with thumbs and fingers separated, creating a 'C' shape. The hands alternately glide back and forth grasping and picking up and squeezing the muscle between the fingers and thumbs. This two-handed technique can be performed on all large surface areas such as calves, thighs, back and abdomen. For smaller surface areas, such as the arms, a single-hand technique can be performed (see Figure 17.8).

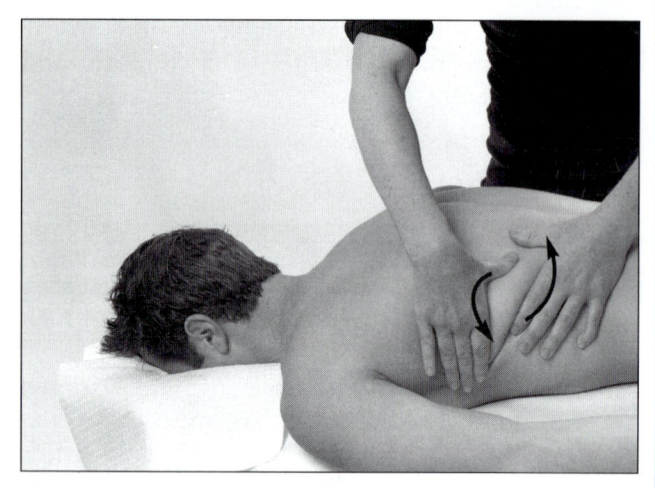

Figure 17.8 C-scoop kneading

Circular kneading

Circular kneading is comprised of circular motions synchronised with compression. Performed with one or both hands, circular kneading consists of short rhythmic circular movements of the finger pads, thumbs, palms or forearms. If both hands are used the technique may be performed either simultaneously or with alternating movements. During the technique the pressure increases to peak mid-way, then with pressure reducing to complete the stroke. This technique can be performed stationary on a large surface area (such as using the forearms to knead the calf muscles) or can travel during the movement to cover the entire tissue with small circles (see Figures 17.9 and 17.10).

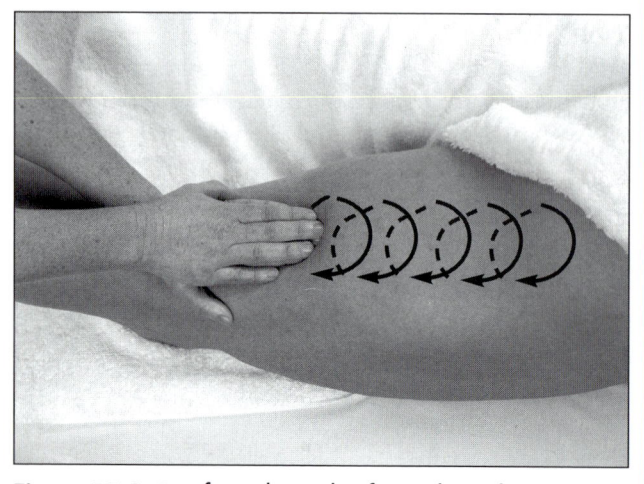

Figure 17.9 Reinforced circular finger kneading

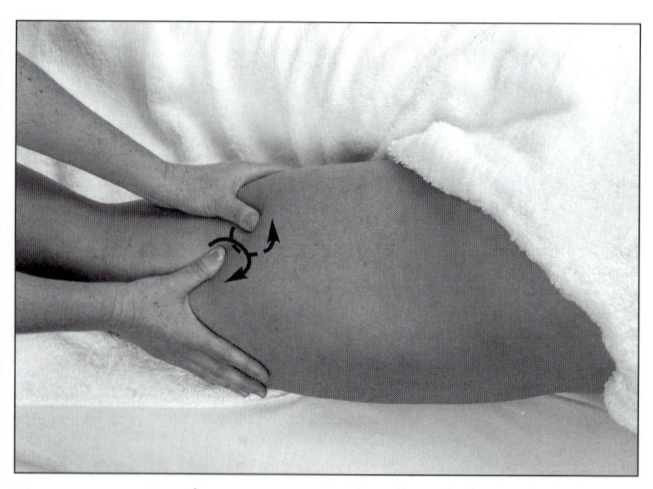

Figure 17.10 Alternating circular thumb kneading

Squeezing

This is a non-gliding technique; therefore the use of oil is unnecessary. One or both hands grasps, lifts and squeezes the muscle or muscle group. The hands then relax and, whilst maintaining skin contact, glide slightly along the limb, where the technique is repeated (see Figure 17.11). For smaller or individual muscles, squeezing may be performed

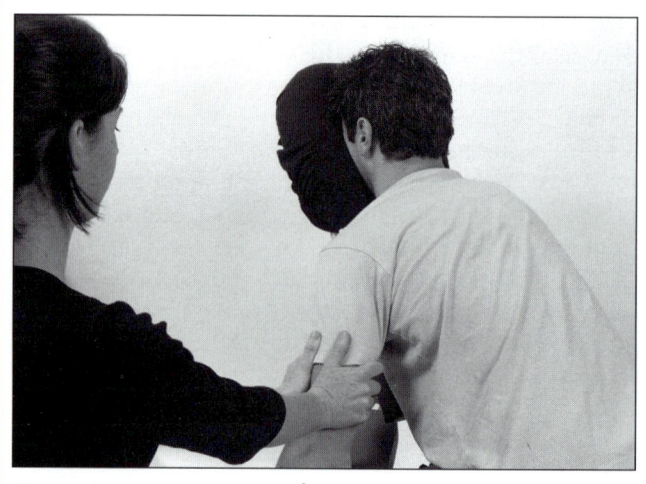

Figure 17.11 Squeezing the arms

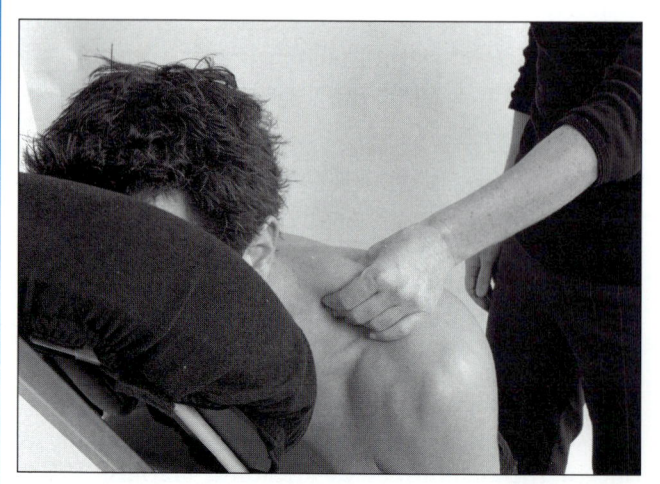

Figure 17.12 Squeezing the trapezius muscle

using the thumb and fingers. This technique is also known as pincer compressions (see Figure 17.12).

Wringing

Wringing is performed with the therapist facing the client. Each hand is placed on either side of the trunk or limb to be manipulated. The hands simultaneously glide, lift and shear between the muscles as they pass each other moving from one side of the body to the other in opposite directions (see Figures 17.13 and 17.14).

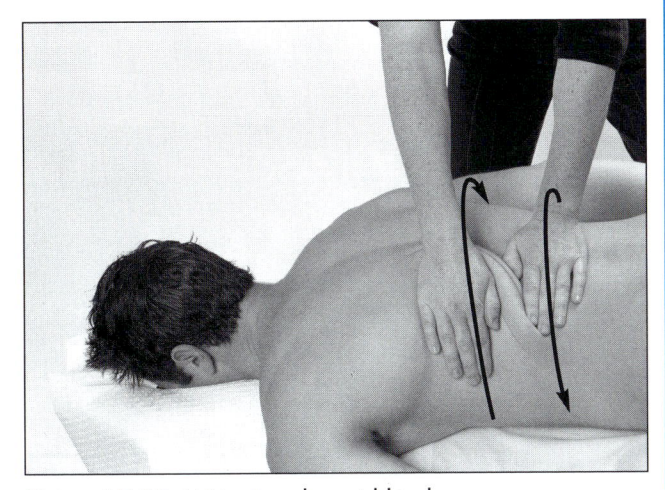

Figure 17.13 Wringing the mid back

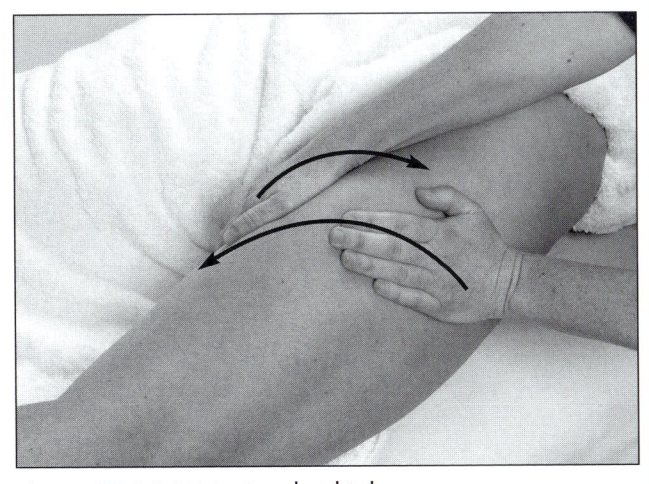

Figure 17.14 Wringing the thigh

Skin rolling

Skin rolling is a pétrissage technique that is used for assessment and treatment. It can be used to assess the mobility of the superficial fascia. Restricted superficial fascia is noted where the skin is difficult to lift off the underlying tissue. It may be an indication of underlying problems such as underlying connective tissue or joint dysfunction (Fritz, 2000). As a treatment technique skin rolling improves the mobility of the superficial fascia and, indirectly through its attachments to the deeper structures, may influence motion at a deeper level (Andrade and Clifford, 2001). This involves a pincer-like grip that places the thumb and forefinger (in the shape of a 'C') on the skin, then using a rolling action the finger and thumb lift the skin to loosen it from the subcutaneous tissue (see Figure 17.15).

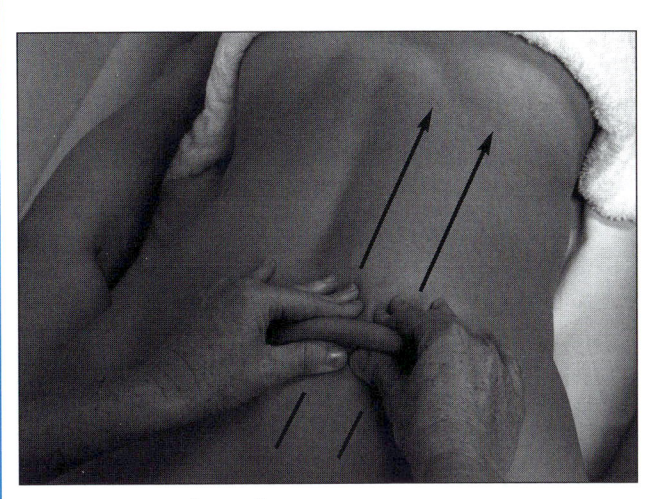

Figure 17.15 Skin rolling

Compression

According to some authors, compression has been developed into a distinct manipulation (Fritz, 2000; Salvo, 1999). Fritz (2000) classifies compression as a Swedish massage technique whereas Salvo (1999) and Rattray and Ludwig (2000) classify compression as ancillary or non-Swedish massage technique. Dr James Menell (1917; refer Chapter 2) classifies both pétrissage and friction manipulations as compression techniques. Because most massage manipulations involve an element of compressive force and therefore constitute a compression technique, a separate compression category may be deemed superfluous.

There are two types of compression used in massage — broad compression and specific compression. *Broad compression* is a non-gliding technique, using a broad surface such as the palm or fist, applied perpendicular to the muscle belly (Fritz, 2000; Salvo, 1999). It is often used as an introductory stroke that can assess the level of tension present within the tissues and occasionally the depth of the tension. It is also believed that broad compression has effects on circulation, muscle resting tension, and rib cage mobility. Gentle broad compressions are used over the lymphatic nodes in manual lymph drainage to encourage lymphatic flow (Casley-Smith, 1997). An osteopathic model of lymphatic drainage also uses gentle compression over the ribs and over the soles of the feet to encourage lymphatic return (Greenman, 1996). Broad compressions are used in pre-event sports massage, as no oil is required, and can be performed through clothing. Broad compressions may increase or stimulate muscle tone and stimulate arousal and therefore will benefit the athlete preparing for sport (Loving, 1999; Fritz, 2000). Broad compressions are often used in conjunction with rocking manipulations and therefore have a combined effect (see rocking).

The hands, the flat of the fists or forearm are applied over a broad contact region. Perpendicular pressure is slowly applied to the tissue and sustained and then gradually released. For a more stimulating effect the therapist completes the technique more vigorously (see Figures 17.16 to 17.18).

Specific compressions are a non-gliding technique using a specific surface such as the thumbs, knuckles or elbow and applied perpendicular to a particular surface, such as muscle, tendon or connective tissue (Andrade and Clifford, 2001). Specific compressions are used in many massage modalities such as Shiatsu, oriental massage, trigger-point therapy and myofascial release techniques. Specific compression, also known as trigger-point pressure release, is an effective treatment of central myofascial trigger points (see Box 17.2) (Simons, Travell and Simons, 1999). Trigger-point pressure release is normally applied to lengthened muscle and then

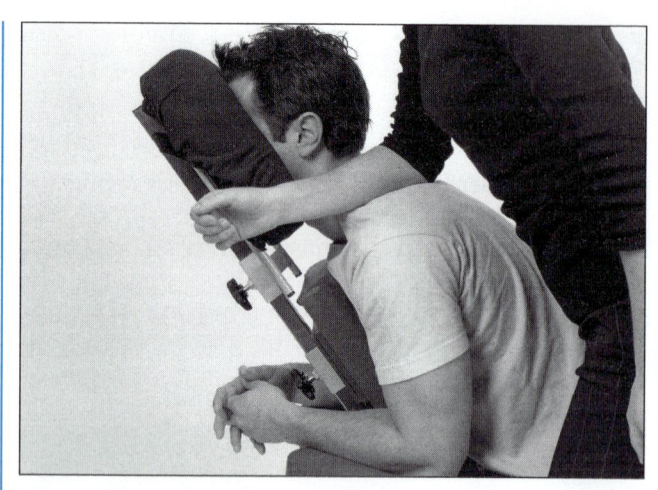

Figure 17.18 Broad compression using the forearm on the trapezius muscle

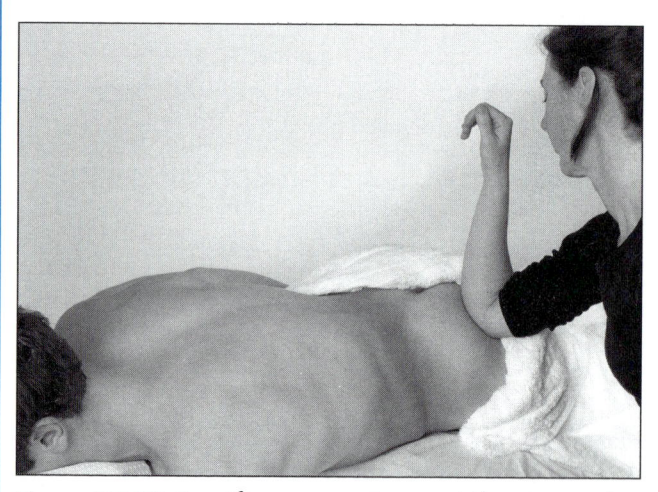

Figure 17.19 Specific compression to piriformis muscle

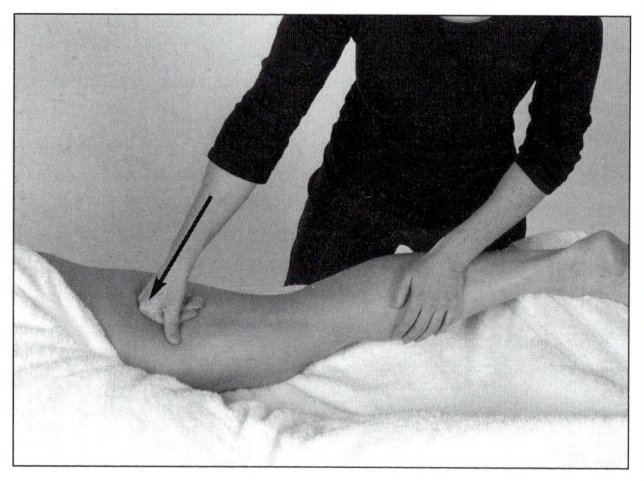

Figure 17.16 Broad compression using the flat of the fist over the hamstring

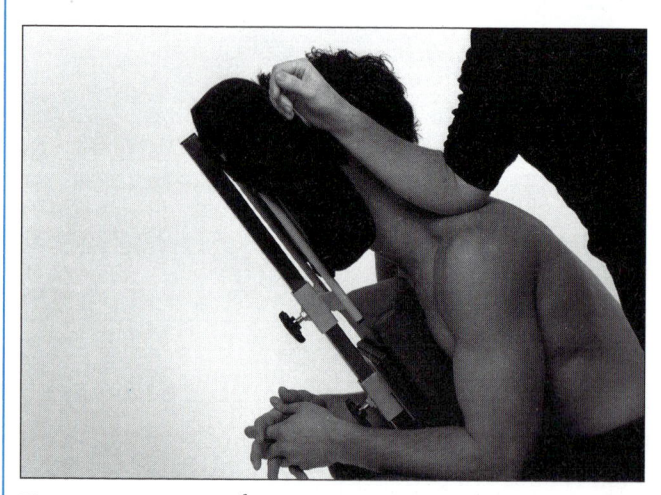

Figure 17.20 Specific compression to trapezius muscle

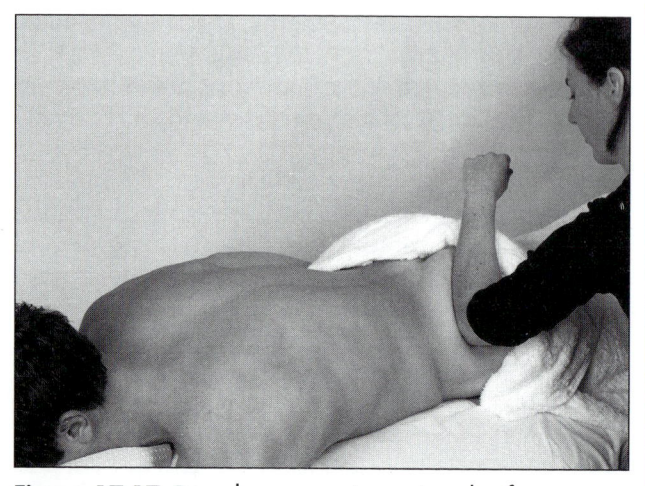

Figure 17.17 Broad compression using the forearm on the buttocks

gentle, gradual pressure is applied to the trigger point until tissue resistance is met. The client may feel some discomfort but not pain. A pain scale such as the visual analogue scale (see Chapter 18) may be used to ensure the pressure of the technique is not excessive. Once the barrier slacks off, additional pressure may be added until a new barrier is reached (see Figures 17.19 and 17.20). As this technique

> **Box 17.2** Myofascial trigger points
>
> Definition: A hyperirritable spot in skeletal muscle that is associated with a hypersensitive, palpable nodule in a taut band. The spot is painful on compression and can give rise to referred pain, referred tenderness, motor dysfunction and autonomic phenoma (Simons, Travell and Simons, 1999).
>
> Types of myofascial trigger points:
>
> | | |
> |---|---|
> | Active | A clinical pain complaint where the pain refers in a characteristic pattern. |
> | Latent | A clinically silent trigger point that only responds in a characteristic pattern on palpation. |
> | Central | Located near the centre of the muscle at the motor end plates. |
> | Attachment | Located at the musculotendinous junction or at the enthesis as a result of unrelenting tension of the taut band produced by the central trigger point. |
> | Primary | The muscle develops a trigger point due to its overuse. |
> | Key | Responsible for activating satellite trigger points. |
> | Satellite | Activated neurogenically or mechanically by the key trigger point. |

may cause some discomfort, it is often interchanged temporarily with pétrissage or effleurage.

Contraindications and precautions

The use of pétrissage manipulations requires a suitable amount of clinical training and supervised practice to ensure its correct application. More advanced or specialist training is needed for those wishing to use friction manipulations for the treatment of specific pathologies. When applying pétrissage all absolute contraindications, as noted in Chapter 12, should be adhered to, as well as the following:

- Pétrissage should be avoided in the acute state of healing, however caution should still be used when using pétrissage in the subacute stage of healing — vigorous pétrissage or deep compression may re-damage the tissue causing pain and inflammation (DeDomenico and Wood, 1997; Kissner and Colby, 2002).
- Pétrissage should be avoided with confirmed or suspected thrombophlebitis, thrombosis or moderate to severe varicosities. Pétrissage over these areas may dislodge a blood clot from the wall of the blood vessel (DeDomenico and Wood, 1997; Rattray and Ludwig, 2000).
- Caution should be used when applying pétrissage over hypertonic muscles (spasm) and hypotonic (atrophic) muscles or over osteoporotic bone, to avoid damaging underlying structures (Andrade and Clifford, 2001; Rattray and Ludwig, 2000).

TAPÔTEMENT

Definition

Tapôtement is a repeated, rhythmical, firm-striking manipulation of the superficial and/or deep tissues that is followed by a quick rebound.

Tapôtement is derived from the French verb *tapôter* meaning 'to tap'. Many texts also equally refer to this manipulation as percussion (Andrade and Clifford, 2001; Fritz, 2000; Cassar, 1999; Menell, 1920).

Description

Just like playing a percussion instrument such as a leather-skin drum, the hands apply a rhythm or beat to the body. Such percussive rhythms may be applied using the palms, ulnar surface of the hands, the fists or even 'cupped' and curved fingers. The hands usually strike the body alternately, and the elbow performs small bending and straightening movements whilst the wrists are kept relaxed throughout the movement. When performing these techniques, ensure excessive movement does not occur at the wrists, as this may lead to wrist strain. The repeated striking of the tissue with percussive strokes serves to stimulate the underlying tissue, yet also induces a reflexive response on the whole body.

Tapôtement manipulations are effective for nervous stimulation, and may enliven or increase the alertness of the recipient. Such techniques are often employed during short-duration massage treatments, like those performed in a seated position in the workplace of the recipient. They may also prove effective in stimulating an athlete prior to competition. Due to this stimulating effect, tapôtement manipulations are often omitted during a relaxation massage sequence. The beginning massage student will enjoy practising this highly effective and entertaining manipulation, considered the showpiece of Swedish massage.

Techniques

There are five main types of percussive strokes that may be applied with varying depth of pressure.

These are hacking, pummelling, cupping, plucking and tapping.

Hacking

Hacking is performed with loosely spread hands and fingers that strike with the ulnar side of the hand, and the little finger. After striking the skin the fingers cascade together but only the side of the hand, little finger and the tips of the third and forth fingers make actual contact with the tissue. The fingers quickly rebound off the tissue rather than landing heavily — as in a chopping action. This technique is usually performed in a quick and rhythmic alternating fashion (see Figure 17.21).

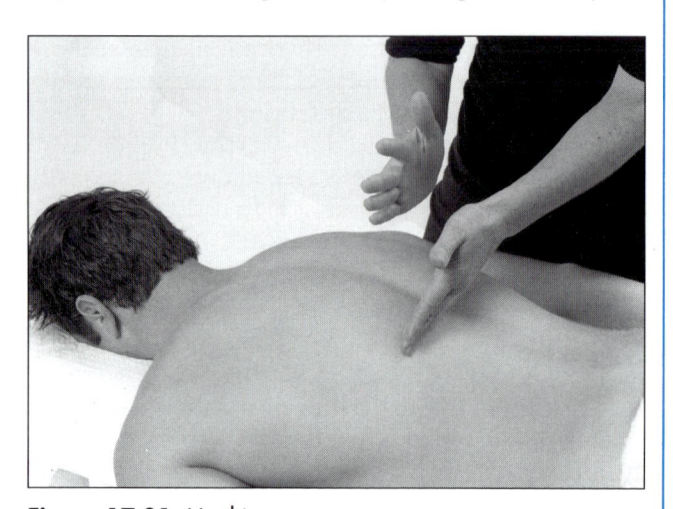

Figure 17.21 Hacking

Pummelling

Pummelling, also known as pounding, has a similar movement to hacking — again the ulnar surface of the fingers and hands are used. The technique is performed with loose alternating fists that strike and rebound off the tissues (see Figure 17.22).

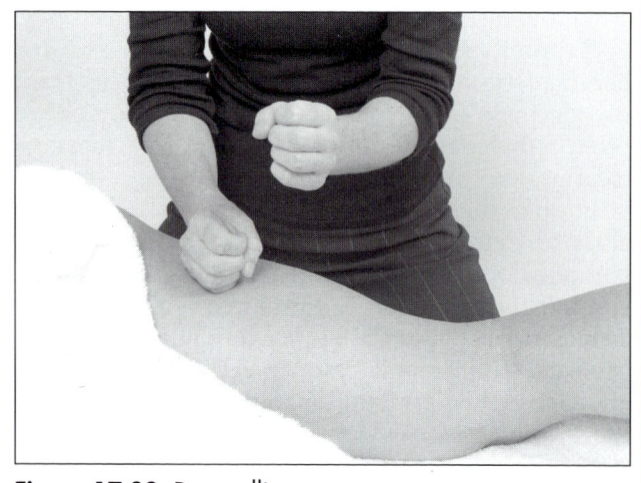

Figure 17.22 Pummelling

A variation of pummelling is called beating. It has an identical action to pummelling. Alternating between the left and right hands, this technique is performed with lightly closed fists and palms facing down. The therapist strikes and rebounds off the tissues.

Cupping

Cupping is performed with cupped hands, formed by holding the fingers and thumb close together with the fingers and palm curving to allow the hand to form a hollow. When the hand strikes the tissue, only the edges of the 'cup' come into contact. Upon lifting the hand from the skin, a vacuum is created. This technique is usually performed on broad surfaces such as the back or thigh. It is also the stroke of choice for loosening mucous and phlegm from the respiratory system. This stroke is performed with rhythmic alternating hands (see Figure. 17.23).

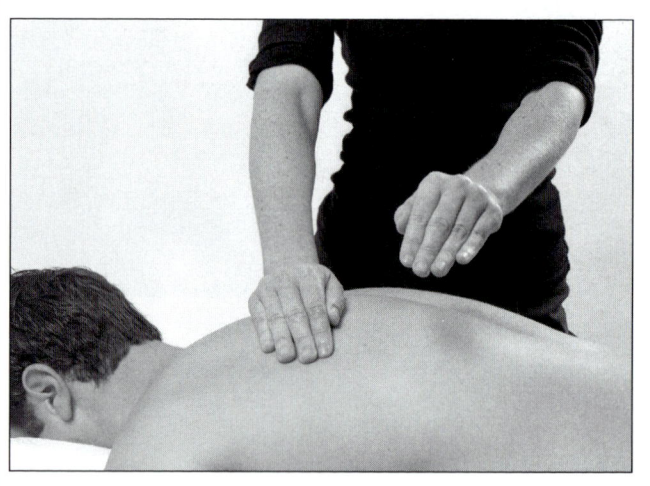

Figure 17.23 Cupping

A variation to cupping is known as slapping. Slapping is performed with an open palm and fingers, creating a loud smacking sound when it strikes the skin. This technique is performed on broad surfaces such as the back and thigh or tough surfaces such as the soles of the feet. Again this technique uses quick rhythmic alternating strokes.

Plucking

Plucking, also known as pecking or pincement, is a light and springy technique where the superficial tissues are picked up between the thumb and first two fingers. The fingers and thumb glide over the tissues until they come together. This technique is performed as a rapid, gentle and rhythmic stroke alternating the left and right hands (see Figure 17.24).

Tapping

Tapping is applied with slightly bent fingers allowing the fingertips to 'tap' the tissue. Again a

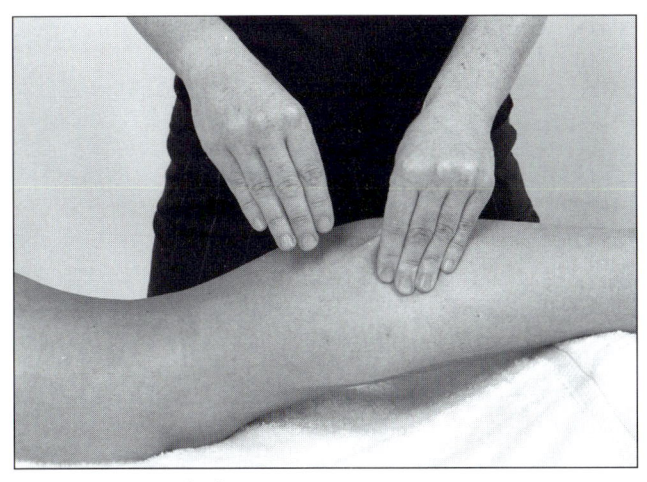

Figure 17.24 Plucking

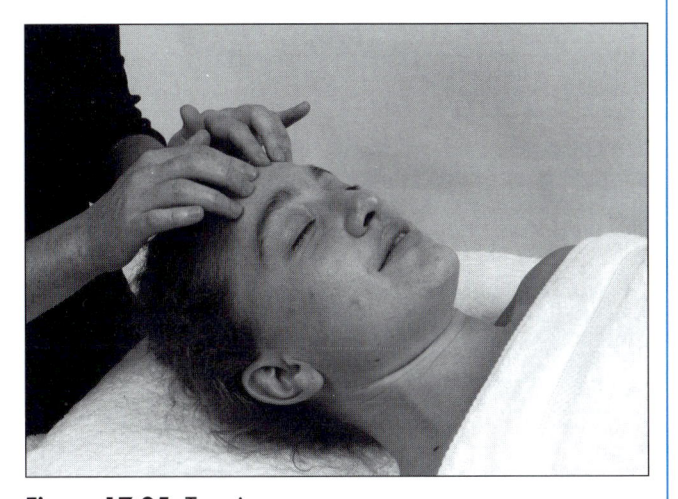

Figure 17.25 Tapping

rhythmic alternating stroke is used. Tapping is the lightest and most superficial tapôtement technique. It can be used on delicate and sensitive areas such as the face, chest and arms (see Figure 17.25).

Contraindications and precautions

The use of tapôtement requires a suitable amount of clinical training and supervised practice to ensure its correct application. More advanced or specialist training is needed for those wishing to use tapôtement manipulation for mucus clearance, and for use with specific pathologies. When applying tapôtement, all absolute contraindications as noted in Chapter 12 should be adhered to, as well as the following:

- Tapôtement should not cause the client pain or discomfort; post-treatment erythema (reddening of the skin) and client discomfort is considered poor application of technique (Andrade and Clifford, 2001). To prevent discomfort or irritation of the skin, use a barrier such as a towel, sheet or even clothing between the therapist's hands and the client's skin (Kisner and Colby, 2002; Salvo, 1999; DeDomenico and Wood, 1997; Holey and Cook, 1997).
- Tapôtement is locally contraindicated during the early stages of injury repair as it may further damage the tissues involved or affect the formation of scar tissue (DeDomenico and Wood, 1997). Tapôtement should not be used over bony areas such as the head, neck, back of the knee, or on the spine (Cassar, 1999).
- Tapôtement should be used with caution or avoided altogether over areas where muscle bulk is lacking, such as the kidney area, and over the lower and floating ribs. Caution should also be used on areas of hypersensitivity (Cassar, 1999; DeDomenico and Wood, 1997).

There are specific contraindications and precautions to percussion used in conventional chest physiotherapy. These include the avoidance of cupping over fractures, spinal fusion or osteoporotic bone. Cupping is also contraindicated if a client has a pulmonary embolus (blood clot in the chest region), any unstable cardiac conditions such as angina, and following recent chest or spinal surgery (Kisner and Colby, 2002; DeDomenico and Wood, 1997).

FRICTION

Definition

Friction is a specific, repetitive, non-gliding technique where superficial tissues are moved over the underlying structures and it produces improved mobility, increased local blood flow and decreased pain.

According to Turchaninov (2000), Hippocrates was the first author to describe friction manipulations and the guidelines for application. Claudius Galen (AD 130–199) used a system of friction manipulations as a doctor at a gladiator school (see Chapter 2) to prepare and/or rehabilitate injured gladiators. The term friction is derived from the Latin *fricto*, meaning 'to rub'.

The aim of friction manipulations is to mobilise the superficial tissues over the underlying structures for the purpose of improving mobility (Simons, Travell and Simons, 1999), increasing local blood flow (Cyriax, 1984) and decreasing pain (de Bruijn, 1984). Friction manipulations commence superficially and progress more deeply, affecting muscular and fascial tissues (Salvo, 1999). The way in which such rubbing strokes are applied will greatly alter their effectiveness.

Description

Friction manipulations are most commonly performed in a linear or circular fashion. Such strokes may be applied with the fingers, fingertips, palms, knuckles, the forearm or even the elbow. Friction manipulations are usually administered over defined, local areas of tissue, and are often used to relieve a contraction in a muscle and reduce pain. Such relaxation of musculature will encourage the lengthening of the tissue, and lead to enhanced movement. Some therapists employ friction strokes during the rehabilitation of injuries to facilitate the proper parallel alignment of collagen during the repair process.

Techniques

It is imperative that when performing friction manipulations with the intent of penetrating deeper tissue, one must progress slowly. When practising friction strokes, it is important to reduce the depth and pressure if the recipient counteracts the technique with a 'muscular guard response'. By progressing slowly, the sensory receptors of the recipient will have time to adjust to the pressure and depth, and will be less prone to responding via muscular contraction for protection. The type of friction manipulations the therapist chooses will depend on the situation at hand and the therapist's preference for style.

Linear friction

Linear or longitudinal friction is usually done in a straight line along with the direction of muscle fibres. If done on the surface, linear frictions can be done to generate heat, as in heat rubbing. If done to penetrate more deeply into tissue, it moves along as the resistance of tissue is met and yields. Linear friction is usually applied with reinforced fingers and tips, or the palms of the hands. If done more deeply, the therapist will use their elbow (see Figure 17.26).

Circular friction

Circular friction is performed with the tips of the middle three fingers or the thumb. It is important for therapists to always reinforce their hands when applying this technique. Apply obliquely into tissue with slow movement at the beginning and, moving in circles, increasing depth with each successive movement. When the desired depth is reached, the therapist gradually decreases pressure and uses an effleurage stroke to move to the next area to be treated (see Figure 17.27).

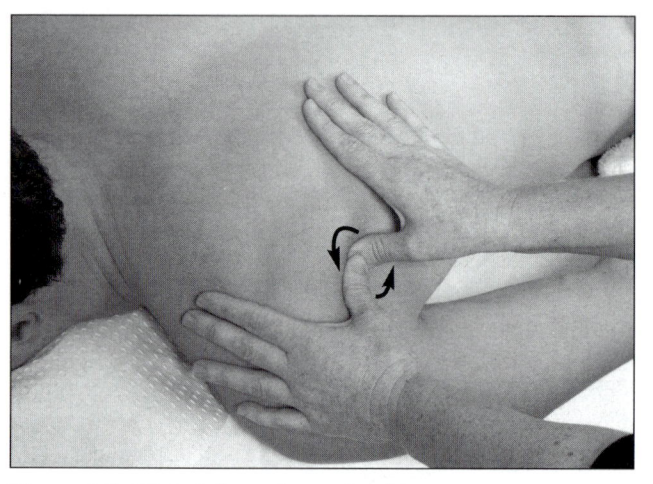

Figure 17.27 Reinforced circular frictions

Transverse or cross-fibre friction

James Cyriax (1904–85) commonly regarded as the father of orthopaedic medicine, popularised transverse or cross-fibre friction. He advocated the use of this manipulation in the treatment of musculoskeletal conditions such as sprains, strains and tendonitis. Cross-fibre friction can be administered slowly or vigorously in a one-directional sawing 'back and forth' motion to eventually break down, separate and numb the affected tissue or structure. Such a technique can be very painful to the person receiving it, and therefore caution must be used when delivering this technique (see Figures 17.28 to 17.30).

Cyriax insisted that this technique be applied using the following principles:

- The exact location of tissue dysfunction must be found.
- Friction manipulations are performed at a right-angle to the length of the muscle or structure involved.
- The therapist's fingers and client's skin move as one.

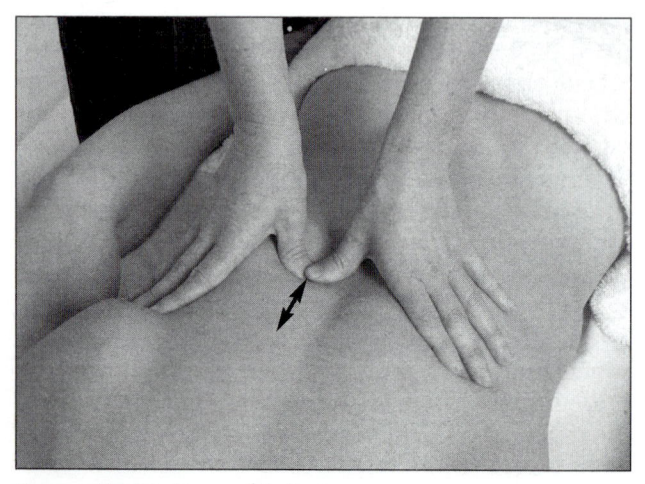

Figure 17.26 Linear frictions

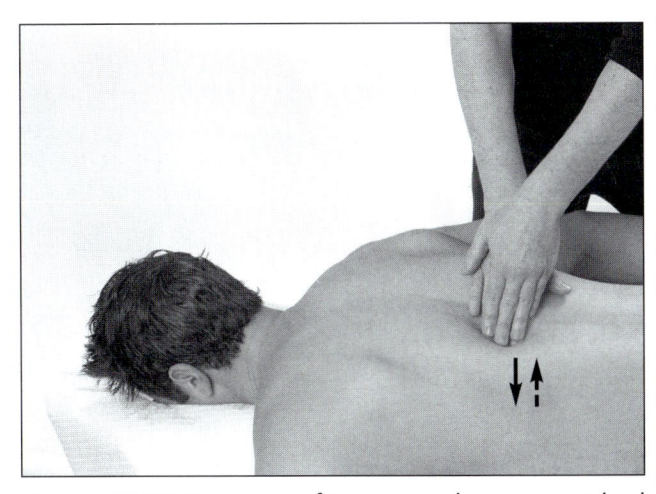

Figure 17.28 Transverse frictions to the paravertebral muscles

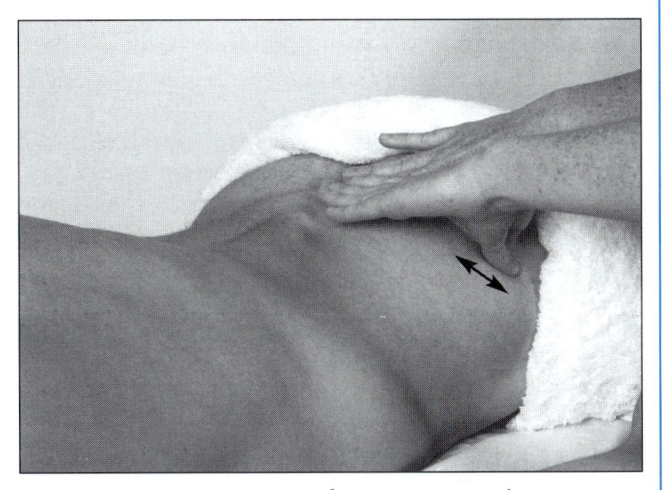

Figure 17.29 Transverse frictions over the superior gluteal insertions

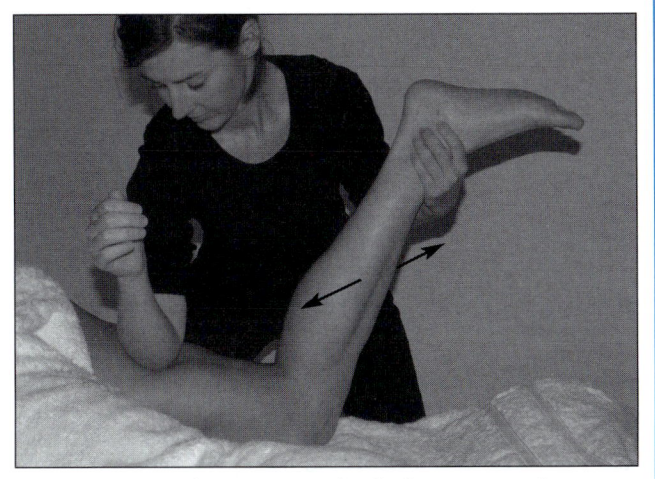

Figure 17.30 Alternative method of transverse friction to the hamstring muscles

- The technique must be deep enough and have enough movement to directly affect the specified tissue.
- The client must be in a comfortable position (Chamberlain, 1982; Cyriax, 1984).

In Figure 17.30 the therapist begins with deep local compression on the hamstring muscle. The therapist then medially and laterally rotates the femur, creating transverse friction between elbow and the tissue. The therapist's elbow compresses the tissue and then rotates the joint so that the transverse movement occurs through passive client movement rather than therapist movement.

Contraindications and precautions

The use of friction manipulations requires a suitable amount of clinical training and supervised practice to ensure its correct application. More advanced or specialist training is needed for those wishing to use friction manipulations for the treatment of tendonitis, sprains and other specific pathologies. When applying friction all absolute contraindications as noted in Chapter 12 should be adhered to, as well as the following:

- Friction manipulations should not be used on acutely inflamed tissue, where acute signs and symptoms such as heat, redness, pain, spasm and oedema should be resolved before its application (Hammer, 1999; Hertling and Kessler, 1996).
- Friction manipulations should be avoided over acute muscle tears, haematomas, calcifications and peripheral nerves (Hammer, 1999). Frictions over skin diseases such as acute dermatitis and psoriasis may aggravate these conditions and therefore should be avoided (DeDomenico and Wood, 1997).
- Caution should be used when applying friction manipulations to the tissues of unstable joints as this may exacerbate the condition (Andrade and Clifford, 2001). Caution should also be used when treating clients with osteoporosis; deep techniques may damage the potentially weak bone.

VIBRATIONS

Definition

Vibrations are a group of techniques that consist of rhythmic manipulations of the soft tissues.

Vibration manipulations encompass a collection of strokes that include vibration, rocking, shaking and jostling. Such movements are rhythmic and trembling or oscillating in nature, and may be applied by using the whole hand, the fingertips or even a mechanical device. Vibration manipulations differ from tapôtement strokes in that the hands do not usually break contact with the skin, with the exception of the 'rocking' technique. As simple as they may sound, vibration manipulations are one of the most physically challenging strokes a massage therapist can perform. When performed skilfully, through much practice, vibration strokes are useful for inducing a sense of relaxation.

Description

All vibration manipulations commence with some degree of compression. After a desired depth of compression is achieved, the hands tremble or oscillate, thus transmitting a 'vibration' into the underlying tissues. Such manipulations are often employed as distraction techniques for the suppression of pain. Turchaninov (2000) believes vibratory techniques are useful for nervous system dysfunctions, such as cerebrovascular accidents (or strokes). It is said that the application of gentle vibration manipulations may aid recovery from conditions such as stroke, as it may improve motor function (Turchaninov, 2000).

Techniques

There are three groups of vibrations, namely static and dynamic, rocking, and shaking. Each of these groups may have many variants. A few will be described here.

Static and dynamic vibration

Vibration techniques can be performed statically or with movement, either using a single hand or reinforced hands. The muscles of the forearm alternately contract and relax, creating a rhythmic movement transmitted through the hand onto the tissue treated (see Figure 17.31).

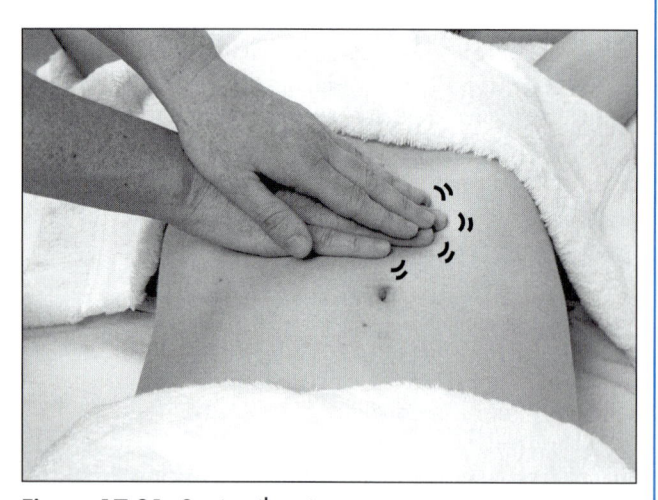

Figure 17.31 Static vibrations

Shaking vibration

Shaking is very effective with clients who have the propensity to muscle guard. With limb shaking there is a lift and pull component to the technique. A muscle group or limb is grasped, lifted and shaken. The shake can be up and down or side to

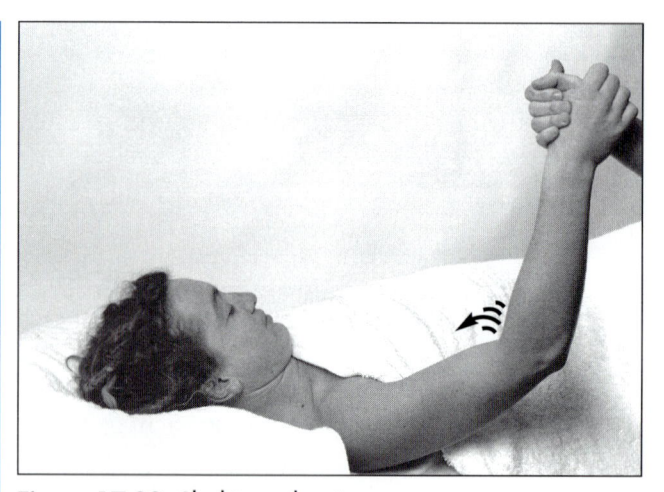

Figure 17.32 Shaking vibrations

side. Attempt to shake with a sense of rhythm, and attempt to feel how much resistance there is in the limb. Feel the weight of the limb, apply a slight traction with coarse shaking and after the application feel the difference in the limb (see Figure 17.32).

Rocking vibration

Rocking is a popular form of vibration. It is gentle and once the therapist achieves a desired rhythm, it lulls the client into deep relaxation. Rocking is rhythmic and should be applied with a deliberate full-body motion. Rocking involves the up-and-down and side-to-side motion of shaking, but no flick or throw-off occurs at the end of the movement. The action moves the body as far as it will go, allowing it to return to its original position (see Figure 17.33).

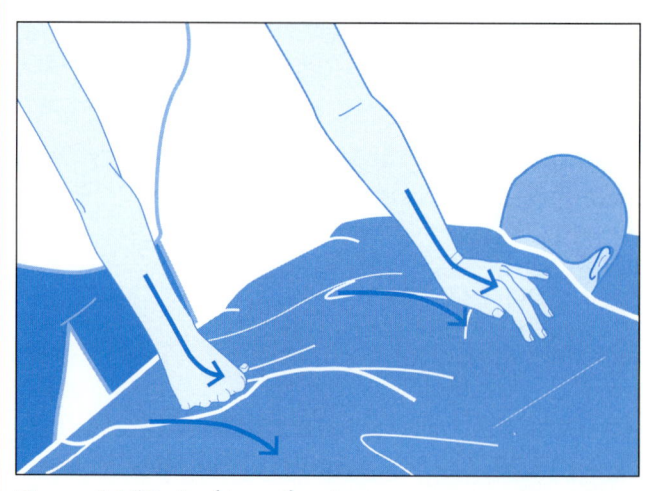

Figure 17.33 Rocking vibrations

With a tense or anxious client who may initially resist the rocking movement, begin with more deliberate shaking vibration and then move in to rocking vibration. Attempt to find a movement that is flowing, and avoid anything abrupt.

Contraindications and precautions

The use of vibration techniques requires a suitable amount of clinical training and supervised practice to ensure its correct application. More advanced or specialist training is needed for those wishing to use these manipulations for mucus clearance, and for use with specific pathologies. When applying vibrations, shaking and rocking, all absolute contraindications as noted in Chapter 12 should be adhered to, as well as the following:

- Vibration and shaking should be avoided on any muscle that contains an acute injury. However, light vibration may be used for pain relief provided caution is taken during its application to ensure that the weight of the hand does not aggravate the pain (Andrade and Clifford, 2001).
- Shaking and vibrations may exacerbate spasm, spasticity or hyperreflexia when applied to a client exhibiting these signs (DeDomenico and Wood, 1997; Rattray and Ludwig, 2000).
- Rocking should be used with caution on clients with reduced motion or where pain aggravates movement. Fast or abrupt rocking may cause nausea, and should not be used on clients suffering from vertigo or motion sickness (Andrade and Clifford, 2001).

EFFECTS OF THE MANIPULATIONS

There is much written on the claimed effects of the major Swedish massage strokes. A beginning massage therapist might be lead to believe that all strokes potentially share the same therapeutic capabilities, as the reputed benefits of the major massage manipulations are great, and in many instances such usage and effects overlap for each stroke.

The purpose of this section is to critically analyse some of the claimed effects of the major massage manipulations, and contrast such beliefs with theories supported by research investigating the effects of massage manipulations. Although the application of massage has been observed in clinical practice and benefits of massage such as pain reduction and enhanced circulation have been noted, the underlying mechanical or physiological mechanisms for such benefits are not understood. As such, the effects of massage are poorly described and at best unclear. The so-called purported effects are presented here for the purposes of stimulating review and academic debate.

Effleurage

According to many of the popular massage books, effleurage strokes are capable of enhancing blood and lymph circulation, inducing relaxation, improving the quality of sleep, reducing the pain experience, uplifting mood and reducing abnormal muscle contraction (Salvo, 2003; Fritz, 2000; DeDomenico and Wood, 1997; Tappan and Benjamin, 1998). Despite these claims there exists little research to validate such claimed effects of effleurage. Much of the research investigating the effects of effleurage centres on what are referred to as 'superficial stroking' and 'effleurage'.

Superficial stroking has been used to stimulate and relax mood, relieve anxiety, reduce resting muscle tension and facilitate regression of sensory analgesia (Hollis, 1998; DeDomenico and Wood, 1997; Holey and Cook, 1997). As previously described, stroking is often used as an introductory or closing technique during a massage routine (Rattray and Ludwig, 2000). Its effect on arousal is dependent upon the speed of the stroke: a slow stroke may have a more relaxing effect whereas a fast stroke tends to stimulate (DeDomenico and Wood, 1997).

One particular use of superficial stroking is known as the slow-stroke back massage (SSBM). The slow-stroke back massage is a specific nursing protocol which consists of slow, gentle, rhythmical strokes using two hands simultaneously over the client's/patient's back two inches out from the spine, from the crown of the head to the sacral area, and has been used in nursing since the mid 1960s (Holland and Pokorny, 2001). Several studies have used SSBM and have found it to be a successful nursing intervention for promoting relaxation and thus promoting sleep (Holland and Pokorny, 2001; Labyak and Metzger, 1997; Meek, 1993; Fakouri and Jones, 1987).

Fakouri and Jones (1987) examined the effectiveness of SSBM in promoting relaxation. The researchers measured blood pressure, heart rate and skin temperature prior to and immediately after a three minute SSBM. Heart rate and skin temperature were again measured ten minutes post-treatment. According to the data collected, blood pressure and heart rate decreased with the application of SSBM, whilst skin temperature increased. According to the authors, the findings from this study suggest that SSBM promotes relaxation.

Similar results were recorded by Meek (1993) who investigated the effects of SSBM on systolic and diastolic blood pressure, heart rate and skin temperature in a population of 30 adult hospice patients. Results showed that blood pressure and heart rate decreased and skin temperature increased for five minutes after the treatment, suggesting that SSBM promotes relaxation.

Holland and Pokorny (2001) examined the effects of three consecutive days of SSBM on adult patients in a rehabilitation setting. The Huchstadt

Touch Instrument (HTI) was used to assess the patient's physiological and psychological responses to touch and was administered each day prior to SSBM. Blood pressure, pulse and respiratory rate were assessed immediately prior to and post-treatment. The HDI scores were reduced over the three days of treatment, indicating a positive response to SSBM. The authors noted a significant decrease in blood pressure and heart rate, and concluded that SSBM induced relaxation.

Rowe and Alfred (1999) investigated the effects of slow-stroke massage on the agitation behaviours of individuals with Alzheimer's disease. The Agitated Behaviour Rating Scale Scoring Guide (ABRSSG) was used by caregivers to record all agitated events such as pacing, walking, tapping, banging, searching and wandering. The findings from this study showed that physical expressions of agitation were decreased when patients received slow-stroke massage, suggesting that slow-stroke massage is a useful relaxation intervention to reduce agitation in adult hospice patients.

It has long been postulated that light touch has the effect of modulating pain (see Chapter 4). As theorised by Melzack and Wall (1965), the application of light stroking irritates pressure and touch receptors and in some way affects nerve conduction and reduces messages of pain going to the central nervous system. Although theorised, the exact mechanism underlying the gate-control theory is not well understood (Rechtien et al., 1998; Hertling and Kessler, 1996).

Ueda, Katatoka and Sagara (1993) examined the effect of gentle epigastric massage on the regression of the sensory analgesia of epidural block. Superficial stroking was performed on 16 patients who had undergone minor obstetric or gynaecologic surgery under epidural anaesthetic. The patients were divided into two groups, a control group that received no stimulation and an experimental group that received 30 minutes of gentle stroking to the epigastric region. The authors noted that stimulation as weak as superficial stroking caused significant regression of sensory analgesia approximately 30 minutes after the massage. The authors concluded that gentle massage of the epigastric region might reduce the effect of analgesia by accelerating the removal of analgesic medication from the system, and proposed that this could occur due to an increase in blood flow.

Like superficial stroking, superficial effleurage is an adaptable massage manipulation that is known for its circulatory effects. In the massage literature, superficial effleurage has been reported to assist in venous and lymphatic return (Hollis,1998; Loving, 1999; Tappan, 1998). Despite these claims, some studies suggest that effleurage has little or no effect on increasing venous return (Shoemaker, Tiidus and Mader, 1997; Tiidus and Shoemaker, 1995; Hansen and Kristensen, 1973) whilst others do support the ability of massage to enhance circulation of the blood and lymph.

In an early study, Hansen and Kristensen (1973) evaluated the effects of massage on Xenon (Xe) disappearance rate from muscles and subcutaneous tissue. Twelve healthy subjects were injected with Xe (a washout marker) into the right calf and in the subcutaneous tissue of the left calf. Effleurage, short-wave diathermy and ultrasound were applied in random order for five minutes each. The authors found that during the massage period Xe clearance in muscle increased, suggesting that massage enhanced circulation.

Specific massage of the lymphatic system is referred to as manual lymph drainage (MLD). Manual lymph drainage is designed to stimulate the lymphatic system by clearing oedema in the tissue spaces, increase uptake of the initial lymphatics and increase lymphatic flow throughout the system (Mason, 1993). Superficial effleurage is often part of MLD and is used to remove oedema and assist with the drainage of lymphs through its system (Mason, 1993). External compression on the lymphatic vessels, such as massage, has been shown to increase peripheral lymphatic pressure and drain the lymphatic vessels of the limbs (Schmid-Schönbein, 1990).

Secretory immunity is part of the first-line defence against invading micro-organisms. It has been suggested that stress may cause immunosuppression, thus increasing the risk of infection (Jemmott and McClelland, 1989). Groër et al. (1994) assessed the effects of a 10 minute nursing back rub (effleurage) on salivary secretory immunoglobulin A (s-IgA) and state anxiety in well older adult subjects. The Spielberger State/trait Anxiety Inventory (STAI) was used pre- and post-test to measure the level of anxiety. A saliva sample was also collected pre- and post-test to examine the levels of the s-IgA. Two groups were formed — a control group (n=14) who rested on a bed for 10 minutes and an experimental group (n=18) who received a 10 minute effleurage-based massage. Salivary secretory immunoglobulin A was found to significantly increase in the experimental group, suggesting that effleurage elevates immune function and assists in reducing stress.

Several authors claim that effleurage may have the ability to reduce muscle tone (Holey and Cook, 1997; Cassar, 1999). Sullivan et al. (1993) examined the effects of effleurage on H-reflex amplitude to the triceps surae in 16 neurologically healthy subjects. The H-reflex or Hoffman reflex is an indirect measure of motorneuron excitability (Hollis, 1998) (see Chapter 4). Effleurage was applied to the belly of the triceps surae in a centripetal direction over a distance of 20–25 cm

Table 17.1 Summary of the effects of effleurage manipulations

	SUPERFICIAL STROKING				SUPERFICIAL EFFLEURAGE			
	Supported by research	Likely	Questionable	Unlikely	Supported by research	Likely	Questionable	Unlikely
Induces relaxation	•							
Improves the quality of sleep	•							
Uplifts mood		•				•		
Increases arousal		•				•		
Relieves anxiety		•				•		
Enhances blood flow		•					•	
Enhances lymphatic flow		•				•		
Reduces oedema		•				•		
Induces muscle relaxation				•	•			
Relieves pain		•				•		
Elevates immune function					•			
Reduces stress					•			

for three minutes. H-reflex recordings were obtained from the left triceps surae muscle using two disposable surface electrodes and were recorded pre-, during and post-treatment. The authors found a mean reduction in H-reflex amplitude of 25 per cent during the massage, suggesting that effleurage may induce muscle relaxation when applied to a healthy muscle (see Table 17.1).

Pétrissage

The claimed effects of pétrissage are wide and varied. Such purported effects include enhanced blood flow, increased lymphatic return, removal of chemical irritants, increased connective tissue extensibility, reduced local swelling, recovery from general fatigue, muscle relaxation, reduced muscle soreness and reduced pain (Salvo, 2003; Fritz, 2000; Tappan and Benjamin, 1998; Holey and Cook, 1997; DeDomenico and Wood, 1997). An exhaustive search of the research in this area uncovered very little evidence to substantiate such claims.

For example, it is often considered that pétrissage improves both lymph and blood flow. In clinical practice pétrissage techniques such as gentle kneading and compressions are often included in manual lymph drainage due to supposed effects on enhancing circulation. As such, authors suggest that pétrissage may enhance lymphatic return (Mason, 1993; Wallace et al., 2003). Despite the existence of data to support the effects of mechanical pétrissage (Yamazaki et al., 1988), no studies exist to support the use of pétrissage manipulations to improve lymph flow.

In relation to the effects of pétrissage on blood flow, studies exist that are contrary to the beliefs of popular massage texts. Hovind and Nielsen (1974) investigated the effects of pétrissage on blood flow in skeletal muscle of the forearm and thigh, using a xenon washout method for determining blood flow. The findings from this study showed that pétrissage had little effect when it came to increasing tissue perfusion of Xenon. As such the authors concluded that pétrissage had no effect on increasing blood flow in skeletal muscle of the forearm and thigh. A study conducted by Shoemaker, Tiidus and Mader (1997), using a Doppler ultrasound to measure blood flow, also concluded that pétrissage had no effect on increasing blood flow.

In light of such findings, it appears unlikely that pétrissage enhances lymph or blood circulation. To validate the use of such techniques in clinical practice, further investigation is required to confirm the effects observed by therapists in the clinical setting.

Research does exist to validate the use of pétrissage techniques for reducing muscle tone via a reduction in motoneuron excitability in both neurologically healthy subjects as well as patients with spinal cord injury (Sullivan et al., 1991; Morelli, Seaborne and Sullivan, 1991; Goldberg et al., 1994). Such investigations have been conducted by physical therapists, with a special interest in identifying the effectiveness of pétrissage for reducing muscle tone in spastic muscles. It is argued that a lack of evidence to validate the effects of pétrissage in other areas and for other conditions does not necessarily correlate to a lack of effect on the part of pétrissage itself, but rather a lack of interest in the academic pursuit of such effects (see Table 17.2).

Tapôtement

Much investigation into the effects of tapôtement has been conducted by physical therapists seeking to validate the use of such techniques for respiratory conditions. The pounding effect of tapôtement manipulations on the ribcage has been used to loosen mucus in clients with respiratory conditions such as asthma and cystic fibrosis (De Domenico and Wood, 1997; Rattray and Ludwig, 2000). Tapôtement also has the effect of quickly increasing local blood flow to the area treated (Liston, 1995).

Much of the research on tapôtement has investigated its effect on loosening mucous secretions and increasing airway clearance in the lungs, primarily in respiratory conditions that are associated with an excessive production of sputum, such as cystic fibrosis.

Mucus clearance is a problem in pulmonary conditions like cystic fibrosis and bronchiectasis (Langenderfer, 1998). In Australia and New Zealand the manual treatment of these conditions is normally performed under the supervision of a specialist physiotherapist. A physiotherapist would employ specialised techniques known as *manual chest percussion*, which have been used for over 40 years, to enhance airway clearance (McIlwaine and Davidson, 1996). Percussion is performed with cupped hands alternately striking the chest wall over the lung segment being drained (see cupping) and is normally used in combination with postural drainage and a pattern of breathing exercises such as the active cycle of breathing techniques (ACBT) (Dallimore, Jenkins and Tucker, 1998; Kisner and Colby, 2002).

A study by Dallimore et al. (1998) investigated the respiratory and cardiovascular effects of manual chest percussion in seven healthy subjects. Whilst lying on their right side, they received three percussion techniques at random with a five minute recovery period between applications. The three different treatments included:

- percussion applied to the lateral chest wall for one minute with the subject breathing at their own rate;
- percussion to the lateral chest wall with the subject performing five thoracic expansion exercises (TEE) (deep breathing); and
- the subject performing five consecutive TEE only (no percussion).

The authors noted all three treatments produced significant increases in inspiration volume and heart rate. Percussion performed with TEE and TEE alone also showed significant increase in the number of breaths per minute, oxygen consumption and arterial oxygen consumption.

Table 17.2 Summary of the effects of pétrissage	Supported by research	Likely	Questionable	Unlikely
Enhances blood flow			●	
Increases lymphatic return		●		
Removes chemical irritants			●	
Increases connective tissue extensibility			●	
Reduces local swelling			●	
Aids recovery from fatigue				●
Induces muscle relaxation	●			
Reduces muscle soreness				●
Relieves pain		●		

These findings suggest that percussion stimulates respiratory and cardiovascular function in healthy subjects.

A study by Gallon (1991) investigated the effects of chest percussion in patients with copious sputum production. Nine stable outpatients with diagnosed bronchiectasis and a minimum of 25 gm of sputum production per day were recruited for participation. Each subject received three different treatment modalities every day over a three-week period. The first treatment modality involved postural drainage (PD), deep breathing exercise (DBE), and forced expiration technique (FET) acted as the control. The second treatment modality comprised of PD, DBE, FET and fast manual chest percussion (FMCP), whilst the third treatment modality consisted of PD, DBE, FET and slow manual chest percussion (SMCP). Both experimental groups, that received manual chest percussion with PD and FET, resulted in significantly higher rates of sputum production in subjects when compared to the control, whilst fast manual chest percussion was more effective for sputum production than slow manual chest percussion.

The findings of Gallon (1991) and Dallimore et al. (1998) are inconsistent with the earlier findings of Van Der Schans et al. (1986). Van Der Schans et al. (1986) investigated the effects of manual chest percussion on airway clearance in patients with chronic airflow obstruction and excessive mucous production. The researchers found that the application of manual chest percussion slightly yet significantly improved tracheobronchial clearance in patients with chronic airflow obstruction and excessive secretion. The authors also reported that postural drainage and coughing with or without manual chest percussion had a greater improvement on airway clearance than manual percussion alone.

Tapôtement not only has an effect on airway clearance, it also has an effect on the neuromuscular system. Bélanger et al. (1989) investigated the effects of muscle tapping on soleus muscle motor neuron excitability. The study involved eight healthy adult subjects between the ages of 19 and 25 years, with no known neurological deficit. Muscle tapping was performed over the soleus muscle, Achilles tendon, hamstring muscles and tibialis anterior muscle for 30 seconds. H-reflex responses were recorded at approximately five-second intervals during the treatment and less frequently post-treatment up to five minutes through electromyography (EMG). It was reported that tapping of these muscles resulted in a reduction of soleus motor neurone excitability. The researchers proposed that muscle tapping activated a range of afferent nerve fibres such as those involved in touch and pressure as well as the muscle receptors — the Golgi tendon organs and muscle spindles. The findings from this study suggest that tapôtement may have an ability to reduce muscle tone in hypertonic muscle in various neurological, orthopaedic and musculoskeletal conditions.

Despite the findings of Belanger et al. (1989) many authors claim that tapôtement can stimulate the stretch reflex, thereby facilitating a contraction or shortening of the muscle when it is applied to the belly or tendon of that muscle (Fritz, 2000; Turchaninov, 2000; Salvo, 1999; Holey and Cook, 1997; DeDomenico and Wood, 1997). Such an effect is opposite to that of pétrissage, in that rather than relaxing the muscle tissue it leads to contraction or improved tone of musculature (Salvo, 2003; Cassar, 1999). It is thought that the percussive manipulations stimulate sensory receptors in the tissues (referred to as mechanoreceptors), thereby inducing a protective contraction of the muscles being manipulated. Such a protective response is known as a reflex contraction (Rattray and Ludwig, 2000). According to Cassar (1999), when incorporated into a massage sequence, such manipulations should be performed for short duration, as excessive stimulation may lead to muscle fatigue and prove counterproductive (Cassar, 1999). Despite such claims, no evidence exists to substantiate the use of tapôtement for improving muscle tone. On the contrary, the body of evidence that currently exists tends to support the use of tapôtement for reducing muscle tone (Bélanger et al., 1989).

Travell and Simons (1992) recommend the use of percussion and stretching to deactivate trigger points, where the muscle is placed in a lengthened position with the onset of passive resistance and a reflex hammer is used to hit the trigger point approximately once every second for ten repetitions. In contrast to the beliefs of Travell and Simons, some authors argue that tapôtement over hypertonic muscle should be avoided (Cassar, 1999; DeDomenico and Wood, 1997).

When one peruses the scholarly texts on the subject of massage, authors claim many additional effects of tapôtement. For example, tapôtement is considered to have a general stimulating effect, therefore the technique is often used at the end of a sedating massage, on client's with generalised fatigue or as part of a pre-event massage to increase the clients level of arousal (Andrade and Clifford, 2001; Rattray and Ludwig, 2000; Fritz, 2000; Tappan, 1998; Holey and Cook, 1997; DeDomenico and Wood, 1997). However, some argue that the opposite may occur when this technique is performed at even rhythm for extended periods (Andrade and Clifford, 2001; Salvo, 1999).

Hovind and Nielsen (1974) examined the effects of tapôtement in their study of 'the effects of massage on blood flow in skeletal muscle'. Skeletal muscle blood flow was measured before, after and

Table 17.3 Summary of the effects of tapôtement

	Supported by research	Likely	Questionable	Unlikely
Enhances blood flow locally	●			
Stimulates respiratory function	●			
Stimulates cardiovascular function	●			
Induces muscle relaxation	●			
Improves muscle tone			●	
Deactivates trigger points		●		
Increases arousal		●		

during two minutes of hacking by a proficient physical therapist using the Xenon washout method for determining blood flow. Nine healthy volunteers were injected in the brachioradialis muscle of the forearm and the lateral vastus muscle of the thigh with isotonic saline containing Xenon (Xe). The findings from this study showed that the application of tapôtement resulted in a significant increase in blood flow during treatment. Superficial hyperaemia was also noted following tapôtement for up to 10 minutes. The authors suggest that the increase in superficial blood flow was due to a local inflammatory response to tissue damage caused through tapôtement (see Table 17.3).

Friction

Friction techniques are often recommended for the management of injuries, when the inflammatory process is controlled (Brukner and Khan, 2001; Lowe, 2003). It is proposed that friction manipulations promote the healing of injuries by encouraging healthy alignment of connective tissue during the healing process. Despite clinical reports into the effectiveness of such techniques during the recovery phase of injuries, no controlled, randomised studies exist to support such claims.

It is believed that friction manipulations have a strong analgesic effect (Hammer, 1999; de Bruijn, 1984). The underlying mechanism of such an effect is still uncertain, however various models have been developed to explain this phenomenon. Hammer (1999) discusses the anaesthetic effect of friction using the gate-control theory of pain (see Chapter 4) stating that 'stimulation of large fibre mechano-receptors will cause presynaptic inhibition at the spinal cord, preventing the small-diameter (slower) fibres from reaching consciousness' (p. 464).

De Bruijn (1984) investigated the analgesic effects of deep transverse friction on 11 patients diagnosed with tenoperiostal lesions using a Cyriax method of assessment. The author noted that the analgesic effect of deep transverse frictions ranged from 0.3 minutes to 48 hours (mean 26 hours). The findings from this study suggest that transverse frictions applied to lesions during the acute and sub-acute phase of treatment relieve pain and thus may improve functional ability (see Table 17.4).

Vibrations

According to Fritz (2000), vibration manipulations are capable of producing reflexive effects if sustained for a sufficient period of time and

Table 17.4 Summary of the effects of friction manipulations

	Supported by research	Likely	Questionable	Unlikely
Promotes connective tissue alignment		●		
Reduces pain	●			
Improves functional ability	●			

performed to a desired intensity. It is believed that when applied for approximately 30 seconds, vibrational strokes will encourage relaxation of muscular tissue. It is proposed that as the sensory input supplied with the application of vibration manipulations is unordered, the central nervous system has difficulty integrating the stimulus, and thus muscular relaxation more often than not results.

Vibrations may stimulate the digestive system by reflexively contracting the smooth muscles of the small and large intestines, encouraging defecation and the elimination of gas (Cassar, 1999; Salvo, 2003; Tappan and Benjamin, 1998). When performed over the ribcage, vibrations loosen mucous from the respiratory system, which is in abundance during respiratory conditions (Cassar, 1999; Kisner and Colby, 2002; Rattray and Ludwig, 2000; Tappan and Benjamin, 1998). Vibrations are also believed to have the effect of relieving pain, possibly via the gate-control theory (Salvo, 1999) (see Chapter 4). According to Cassar (1999), vibration manipulations reduce the viscosity of thick lymph and interstitial fluid, thus allowing increased lymphatic circulation and reduction of oedema.

Shaking is often used during pre-event and post-event sports massage, possibly due to its effects on decreasing muscle tension and increasing arousal (Benjamin and Lamp, 1996). Despite the fact that some authors believe shaking may reduce muscle tone and increase muscle relaxation through a reflex action from the sensory input from proprioceptive nerve afferents in muscles and joints (Hertling and Kessler, 1996; Rattray and Ludwig, 2000), there is no research to substantiate this claim.

Clients who receive a rocking treatment frequently describe their relaxation as very deep and almost trance-like. Mothers have been aware of this phenomenon for decades, as whole-body rocking is a common form of deep proprioceptive stimulation used to calm infants. According to Lederman (1997) studies into the effects of whole-baby rocking have shown it calms and reduces anxiety in infants and small children and is more effective than verbal cues in reducing an infant's crying. In the clinical domain those working with special populations attest to the benefits of rocking for calming disabled or hyperactive children.

It appears the mechanism underlying such effects of rocking are associated with the vestibular apparatus in the semicircular canals of the ear, in addition to proprioceptive receptors of the skin, joints and muscles. Such sensory is processed in the area of the brain called the vestibular nucleus. A continuous flow of impulses from the vestibular nucleus plays a part in the generation of motor tone in postural muscles. Inhibition of this flow usually results in muscle relaxation. It has been suggested that slow rhythmic rocking movements stimulate the vestibular apparatus, thereby resulting in inhibition at the vestibular nucleus. The concurrent stimulation of skin receptors may also add to the overall relaxation response (Lederman, 1997) (see Table 17.5).

It is clear that more investigation is required to determine the way in which the major massage manipulations affect the body. With sound, controlled, randomised clinical trails, the effects of massage may be more delineated and understood. Such academic pursuit will allow for greater application and acceptance of massage across the wider community.

Table 17.5 Summary of the effects of vibration manipulations	Supported by research	Likely	Questionable	Unlikely
Induces muscle relaxation		●		
Stimulates digestion				●
Enhances respiratory function			●	
Relieves pain			●	
Increases lymphatic return			●	
Reduces oedema			●	
Increases arousal			●	
Reduces anxiety	●			

CONCLUSION

This chapter has described in detail the major manipulation techniques used in Swedish massage, and discussed their usage, application, contraindications and precautions, and varied effects. The massage therapist who has practised and skilfully mastered each manipulation and variation will possess a plethora of techniques upon which to draw to create his or her own unique massage sequence.

A sound and well-packaged treatment, such as the one outlined in this text for the beginning therapist, encompasses each and every one of the Swedish manipulations. When performing techniques, the beginning therapist should be sure to practice safely, endeavouring to adhere to the guidelines, scope and ethics of the massage profession. Above all, the beginning therapist should have fun and be playful with the varying strokes, recognising the great art and responsibility they hold at their fingertips.

Questions and activities

1. A regular client of yours attends for a massage. She is seven months pregnant with her second child, and is complaining of fluid retention in her ankles and feet, which her doctor says is perfectly normal at this stage of her pregnancy.
    (a) What massage strokes would be beneficial to apply over her feet and legs during the massage and why?
    (b) What other benefits of this stroke may assist this particular client?
2. A regular elderly client of yours presents for a massage. He is recovering from a bad cough, which has left him with respiratory congestion. He is taking a cough syrup purchased at the chemist, which he says is doing 'little good'.
    (a) What massage strokes may prove useful for this client?
    (b) Describe any contraindications you may need to be aware of with this client.
3. A nurse friend of yours is considering introducing a program of massage into the respite centre she works in, which largely provides short-term accommodation for elderly persons. She states that she is looking for a short protocol that could prove useful to assist with sleep, and requires that it be supported by evidence.
    (a) Suggest a massage stroke suited to this purpose, and describe the evidence to support its use.
    (b) What other benefits of this stroke may be of interest to your friend for the elderly population in respite care?

Further reading

Andrade, C. and Clifford, P. (2001) *Outcome-Based Massage*. Lippincott Williams & Wilkins, Philadelphia.

De Domenico, G. and Wood, E. C. (1997) *Beard's Massage* (4th edn). W. B. Saunders, Philadelphia.

Fritz, S. (2004) *Mosby's Fundamentals of Therapeutic Massage* (3rd edn). Mosby, St Louis.

Holey, E. A. and Cook, E. M. (2003) *Evidence-Based Therapeutic Massage*, (2nd edn): *A Practical Guide for Therapists*. Churchill Livingstone, London.

Salvo, S. G. (2003) *Massage Therapy: Principles and Practice* (2nd edn). W. B. Saunders, St Louis.

REFERENCES

Andrade, C. and Clifford, P. (2001) *Outcome-Based Massage*. Lippincott Williams & Wilkins, Philadelphia.

Beard, G. and Wood, E. C. (1964) *Massage Principles and Techniques*. W. B. Saunders, Philadelphia.

Bélanger, A. Y., Morin, S., Pépin, P., Tremblay, M. and Vachon, J. (1989) 'Manual muscle tapping decreases soleus H-reflex amplitude in control subjects', *Physiotherapy Canada*, 41(4), pp. 192–6.

Benjamin, P. J. and Lamp, S. P. (1996) *Understanding Sports Massage*. Human Kinetics, Champaign.

Brukner, P. and Khan, K. (2001) *Clinical Sports Medicine* (2nd edn). McGraw-Hill, Sydney.

Calvert, R. N. (2002) *The History of Massage: An Illustrated Survey From Around the World*. Healing Art Press, Rochester.

Casley-Smith, J. R. and Casley-Smith, J. R. (1997) *Modern Treatment for Lymphoedema* (5th edn). Lymphoedema Association of Australia, Adelaide.

Cassar, M. (1999) *Handbook of Massage Therapy: A Complete Guide for the Student and Professional Massage Therapist*. Butterworth–Heinemann, Oxford.

Chaitow, L. and DeLany, J. W. (2000) *Clinical Application of Neuromuscular Techniques: Volume 1 – The Upper Body*. Churchill Livingstone, London.

Chamberlain, G. J. (1982) 'Cyriax's friction massage: a review', *Journal of Orthopaedic and Sports Physical Therapy*, 4(1), pp. 16–22.

Cyriax, J. (1984) *Textbook of Orthopaedic Medicine: Volume 2* (11th edn). Baillière Tindall, London.

Dallimore, K., Jenkins, S. and Tucker, B. (1998) 'Respiratory and cardiovascular responses to manual chest percussion in normal subjects', *Australian Journal of Physiotherapy*, 44(4), pp. 267–74.

De Bruijn, R. (1984) 'Deep transverse friction; its analgesic effect', *Int. J. Sports Med*, 5, 35–6.

De Domenico, G. and Wood, E. C. (1997) *Beard's Massage* (4th edn). W. B. Saunders, Philadelphia.

Dorland's Illustrated Medical Dictionary (2000) (29th edn). W. B. Saunders, Philadelphia.

Ellison, M. A. (1904) *Manual for Students of Massage* (2nd edn). Baillière, Tindall & Cox, London.

Fakouri, C. and Jones, P. (1987) 'Slow stroke back rub', *Journal of Gerontological Nursing*, 13(2), pp. 32–5.

Fritz, S. (2000) *Mosby's Fundamentals of Therapeutic Massage* (2nd edn). Mosby, St Louis.

Gallon, A. (1991) 'Evaluation of chest percussion in the treatment of patients with copious sputum production', *Respiratory Medicine*, 85(1), pp. 45–51.

Goldberg, J., Seaborne, D. E., Sullivan, S. J. and Leduc, B. E. (1994) 'The effect of therapeutic massage on H-reflex amplitude in persons with a spinal cord injury', *Physical Therapy*, 74(8), pp. 728–37.

Greenmann, P. E. (1996) *Principles of Manual Medicine* (2nd edn). Lippincott Williams & Wilkins, Philadelphia.

Groer, M., Mozingo, J., Droppleman, P., Davis, M., Jolly, M. L., Boynton, M., Davis, K. and Kay, S. (1994) 'Measures of salivary secretory immunoglobulin A and state anxiety after a nursing back rub', *Applied Nursing Research*, 7(1), pp. 2–6.

Hammer, W. I. (1999) *Functional Soft Tissue Examination and Treatment by Manual Methods: New Perspectives* (2nd edn). Aspen Publications, Gaithersburg.

Hansen, T. I. and Kristensen, J. H. (1973) 'Effect of massage, shortwave diathermy and ultrasound upon Xe disappearance rate from muscle and subcutaneous tissue in the human calf', *Scand J Rehab Med*, 5, pp. 179–82.

Hertling, D. and Kessler, R. M. (1996) *Management of Common Musculoskeletal Disorders: Physical Therapy Principles and Methods* (3rd edn). Lippincott Williams & Wilkins, Baltimore.

Holey, E. and Cook, E. (1997) *Therapeutic Massage*. W. B. Saunders, London.

Holland, B. and Pokorny, M. E. (2001) 'Slow stroke back massage: its effect on patients in a rehabilitation setting', *Rehabilitation Nursing*, 26(5), pp. 182–6.

Hollis, M. (1998) *Massage for Therapists* (2nd end). Blackwell Science, Oxford.

Hovind, H. and Nielsen, S. L. (1974) 'Effect of massage on blood flow in skeletal muscle', *Scand J Rehab Med*, 6, pp. 74–7.

Jemmott, J. and McClelland, D. (1989) 'Secretory IgA as a measure of resistance to infections disease: Comments on Stone, Cox, Valdimimarsdottir, and Neale', *Behavioral Medicine*, 15, pp. 63–70.

Kamenetz, J. M. (1980) 'History of massage', in *Manipulation, Traction and Massage* (2nd edn), J. B. Rogoff (ed.). Williams and Wilkins, Baltimore.

Kellogg, J. H. (1895) *The Art of Massage: Its Physiological Effects and Therapeutic Applications*. Modern Medicine Publishing, Battle Creek, Michigan.

Kisner, C. and Colby, L. A. (2002) *Therapeutic Exercise: Foundations and Techniques* (4th edn). F.A. Davis & Company, Philadelphia.

Labyak, S. E. and Metzger, B. L. (1997) 'The effects of effleurage backrub on the physiological components of relaxation: A meta-analysis', *Nursing Research*, 46(1), 59–62.

Langenderfer, B. (1998) 'Alternatives to percussion and postural drainage: A review of mucus clearance therapies', *Journal of Cardiopulmonary Rehabilitation*, 18, pp. 283–9.

Lederman, E. (1997) *Fundamentals of Manual Therapy: Physiology, Neurology and Psychology*. Churchill Livingstone, London.

Liston, C. (1995) *Sports Physiotherapy: Applied Science and Practice*, M. Zuluaga, et al. (eds). Churchill Livingstone, Melbourne.

Loving, J. (1999) *Massage Therapy: Theory and Practice*. Appleton & Lange, Stamford, Connecticut.

Lowe, W. W. (2003) *Orthopaedic Massage: Theory and Technique*. Mosby, London.

Mason, M. (1993) 'Treatment of lymphoedema by complex physical therapy', *Australian Physiotherapy*, 39, pp. 41–5.

McIlwaine, M. P. and Davidson, A. G. (1996) 'Airway clearance techniques in the treatment of cystic fibrosis', *Curr Opin Pulm Med*, 2(6), pp. 447–51.

Meek, S. S. (1993) 'Effects of slow stroke back massage on relaxation in hospice clients', *Image J Nurs Scholar*, 25(1), pp. 17–21.

Melzack, R. and Wall, P. O. (1965) 'Pain mechanisms: a new theory', *Science*, 150, p. 971.

Menell, J. B. (1917) *Massage: Its Principles and Practice*. J. & A. Churchill, London.

Morelli, M., Seaborne, D. E. and Sullivan, S. J. (1991) 'H-reflex modulation during manual muscle massage of human triceps surae', *Arch Phys Med Rehabil*, 72, pp. 915–19.

Palmer, M. D. (1912) *Lessons on Massage*. Baillière, Tindall & Cox, London.

Rattray, F. S. and Ludwig, L. M. (2000) *Clinical Massage Therapy: Understanding, Assessing and Treating Over 70 Conditions*. Talus Inc., Toronto.

Rechtien, J. J., Andary, M., Holmes, T. G. and Wieting, J. M. (1998) 'Manipulation, massage and traction', in *Rehabilitation Medicine: Principles and Practice* (3rd edn), Delisa, J. A. and Gans, B. M. (eds). Lippincott Williams & Wilkins, Philadelphia.

Rowe, M. and Alfred, D. (1999) The effectiveness of slow-stroke massage in diffusing agitated behaviours in Alzheimer's disease patients', *Journal of Gerontological Nursing*, 25(6), pp. 22–34.

Salvo, S. G. (1999) *Massage Therapy: Principles and Practice*. W. B. Saunders, Philadelphia.

—— (2003) *Massage Therapy: Principles and Practice* (2nd edn). W. B. Saunders, St Louis.

Schmid-Schönbein, G. W. (1990) 'Microlymphatics and lymph flow', *Physiological Review*, 70(4), pp. 478–83.

Shoemaker, J. K., Tiidus, P. M. and Mader, R. (1997) 'Failure of manual massage to alter limb blood flow: measures by Doppler ultrasound', *Medicine and Science in Sports and Exercise*, 29(5), pp. 610–14.

Simons, D. G., Travell, J. G. and Simons, L. S. (1999) *Travell and Simons' Myofascial Pain and Dysfunction: The Trigger Point Manual*, Volume 1, (2nd edn). Williams & Wilkins, Pennsylvania.

Sullivan, S. J., Seguin, S. J., Seaborne, D. E. and Goldberg, J. (1993) 'Reduction of H-reflex amplitude during the application of effleurage to triceps surae in neurologically healthy subjects', *Physiotherapy Theory & Practice*, 9, pp. 25–31.

Sullivan, S. J., Williams, L. R. T., Seaborne, O. E. and Morelli, M. (1991) 'Effects of massage on alpha motorneuron excitability', *Physical Therapy*, 7(8), August, pp. 555–60.

Tappan, F. M. and Benjamin, P. J. (1998) *Tappan's Handbook of Healing Massage Techniques: Classic, Holistic and Emerging Methods* (3rd edn). Appleton & Lange, Stamford, Connecticut.

Tiidus, P. M. and Shoemaker, J. K. (1995) 'Effleurage massage, muscle blood flow and long-term post-exercise strength recovery', *Int. J. Sports Med.*, 16(7), pp. 478–83.

Travell, J. G. and Simons, D. G. (1992) *Myofascial Pain and Dysfunction: The Trigger Point Manual*, Volume 2. Williams and Wilkins, Baltimore.

Turchaninov, R. (2000) *Therapeutic Massage: Scientific Approach*. Aesculapius Books, Phoenix.

Ueda, W., Katatoka, Y. and Sagara, Y. (1993) 'Effect of gentle massage on regression of sensory analgesia during epidural block', *Anesthesia & Analgesia*, 76(4), pp. 783–5.

Van Der Schans, C. P., Piers, D. A. and Postma, D. S. (1986) 'Effect of manual percussion on tracheobronchial clearance in patients with chronic airflow obstruction', *Thorax*, 41(6), pp. 448–52.

Wallace, E., McPartland, J. M., Jones, J. M., Kuchera, W. A. and Buser, B. R. (2003) 'Lymphatic system: lymphatic manipulative techniques', in Ward, R. C. (ed.), *Foundations for Osteopathic Medicine* (2nd edn). Lippincott Williams & Wilkins, Philadelphia.

Yamazaki, Z., Idezuki, Y., Nemoto, T. and Togawa, T. (1988) 'Clinical experience using pneumatic massage therapy for edematous limbs over the last 10 years', *Angiology — the J of Vascular Diseases*, February, pp. 154–63.

chapter 18

Putting massage into practice — the massage sequence

Lisa Casanelia and Charles Tuchtan

Learning outcomes

- Apply the principles of Swedish massage
- Perform a full body massage using the methods and techniques presented
- Demonstrate safe and effective body mechanics when performing massage
- Demonstrate the ability to maintain 'flow' during the massage

INTRODUCTION

A massage sequence is a collection of massage manipulations put together in a particular order to achieve certain predetermined goals. These goals may include relaxation of the body and mind or, more specifically, a reduction of tight or congested soft tissue. Although there are many different approaches one can take to performing a massage sequence, it is often good for the beginning practitioner to learn one approach. As they develop and refine their skills through clinical practice, this can be adapted.

The purpose of this chapter is to present a one-hour full body massage sequence and a 10–15 minute clothed seated massage. These sequences are a starting point for the beginning massage student. Students require the solid grounding provided by a simple sequence that emphasises technique, blending and continuity, and that demonstrates all massage manipulations. Once the student has mastered the basics they can then develop their own style as well as adapt the sequence to suit each client's specific treatment goals.

There are many different variations used in performing a massage; these depend on therapist preference, client needs, therapist palpation skills, client muscle tone, client contraindications and precautions, and time restriction. As long as the general principles of massage are followed, the massage therapist can use their own imagination to create a massage sequence.

This sequence of massage manipulations is presented in a systematic order, which takes into consideration depth, pressure, direction, speed, rhythm, duration and frequency (see Chapter 16).

THE PRINCIPLES OF MASSAGE APPLICATION

The previous chapter explored the major massage manipulations, examined the effects and contraindications of each technique and described how to perform each manipulation. Once each manipulation is mastered the strokes can then be applied in a sequence. Structuring the sequence is as important as mastering each technique. There are some common guidelines that ensure each stroke is placed in an appropriate order, at a suitable depth and in a specific direction to achieve the desired effect.

When performing a massage sequence the strokes need to be ordered so that broad strokes are applied prior to more localised manipulations. For example, when performing effleurage, a broad surface area such as the palm is used. This broad surface has a general effect on superficial muscles, warming and softening the tissues in preparation for more specific massage techniques. A more localised massage technique such as transverse friction is applied with the fingers, thumbs, knuckles or elbows, to a smaller surface area such as a segment of a tight muscle. This technique is often used to relax contracted muscle in localised areas and would only be performed following less specific techniques such as effleurage and pétrissage. As a general rule the progression of stroke from general to specific is as follows — effleurage, pétrissage, vibration, tapôtement, friction, then compression. During a massage sequence the therapist returns to broad techniques like effleurage after the application of specific techniques, and again to conclude the massage sequence. Figure 18.1 demonstrates the *general to specific* rule of massage.

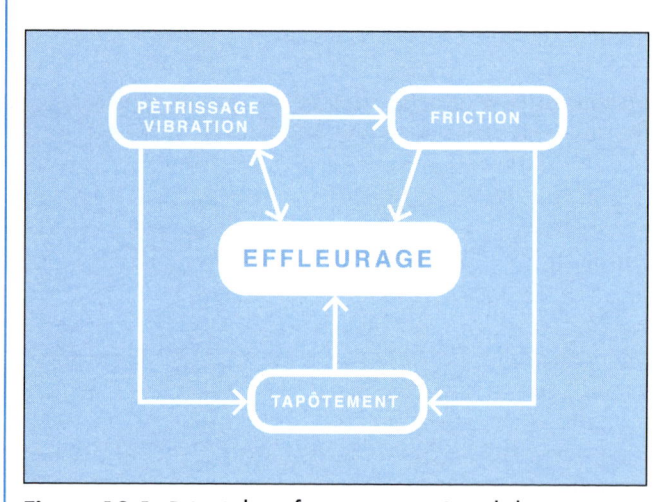

Figure 18.1 Principles of sequencing Swedish massage

Following the same principle of *broad to specific*, superficial strokes are performed prior to deep strokes. Effleurage is performed with a broad surface and also with lighter pressure. In contrast, frictions are performed with a smaller surface area and with firmer pressure.

For many decades, if not centuries, massage strokes were always performed in a direction toward the heart (Mennell, 1917; Tappan and Benjamin, 1998). In fact, some believed that massage away from the heart resulted in harm, as it damaged the valves of the venous system that prevent blood from pooling at the extremities (Tappan and Benjamin, 1998). There has been no evidence to substantiate such claims and, as a result, massage therapists now perform massage in many directions. It should be noted that mechanical stimulus in the direction of blood flow may be beneficial if the intent of the massage is to promote circulation.

Maintaining flow

A proficient and experienced massage therapist is able to blend the massage strokes into a rhythmic flowing style, such that the client receiving the massage is not able to determine the therapist's movement from one side of the table to the other, or the transition from one stroke to another. The client should feel as if the therapist has a multitude of hands performing the massage. When the student is learning the massage sequence each stroke is taught individually. Once the stroke is mastered, and confidence gained, the student can then develop their own style, blending the strokes together.

Many strokes in the following sequence are designed to maximise flow. These include transitional strokes, integrating strokes and return strokes. Transitional strokes such as the reverse rowing stroke enable the therapist to move from one side of the table to the other whilst maintaining continuity throughout the sequence. Integration strokes are designed to reconnect the body after specific areas have been worked. For instance, when massaging the leg the therapist massages the thigh, the leg and then the foot. The integrating strokes are the effleurage strokes that are applied at the beginning, the middle and the end of the sequence to continually reconnect each of these parts to the whole limb. The return strokes are designed to return the technique being performed to the starting position. Rather than removing the hands from the client's body at the end of a massage stroke the therapist's hands continue to massage (usually with effleurage) and return to the stroke's starting position. For example, following the hand-after-hand technique applied to the paraspinal muscles of the back, the hands return to the lower back by coming together at the shoulder and gently gliding down the side of the torso to the starting position.

Maintaining flow also requires maintaining contact throughout the massage. The therapist's hands remain in contact with the client at all times — even during oil application and moving from one body part to another. This principle ensures continuity, instils feelings of security and enhances the overall relaxation effect.

> **Box 18.1** Remember — when in doubt, effleurage
>
> To maintain flow — whether during transitions from one side of the body to the other or from one stroke to another, or if there is hesitation over which stroke to apply next — *use effleurage*.

PAIN THRESHOLD

During the massage there may be times when the massage therapist finds abnormal muscle contraction through palpation and decides, with client consent, to use deep and specific massage manipulations over the area. These techniques may cause the client pain. Pain is an individual and subjective phenomenon, and each person is capable of withstanding a certain amount of pain. The ability we have of being able to 'put up with pain' is referred to as our *pain threshold*. When massaging the soft tissue the therapist will notice that some clients will prefer a light, soft massage, whilst others will happily tolerate, and can withstand, a deeper massage. It is important for the therapist to be

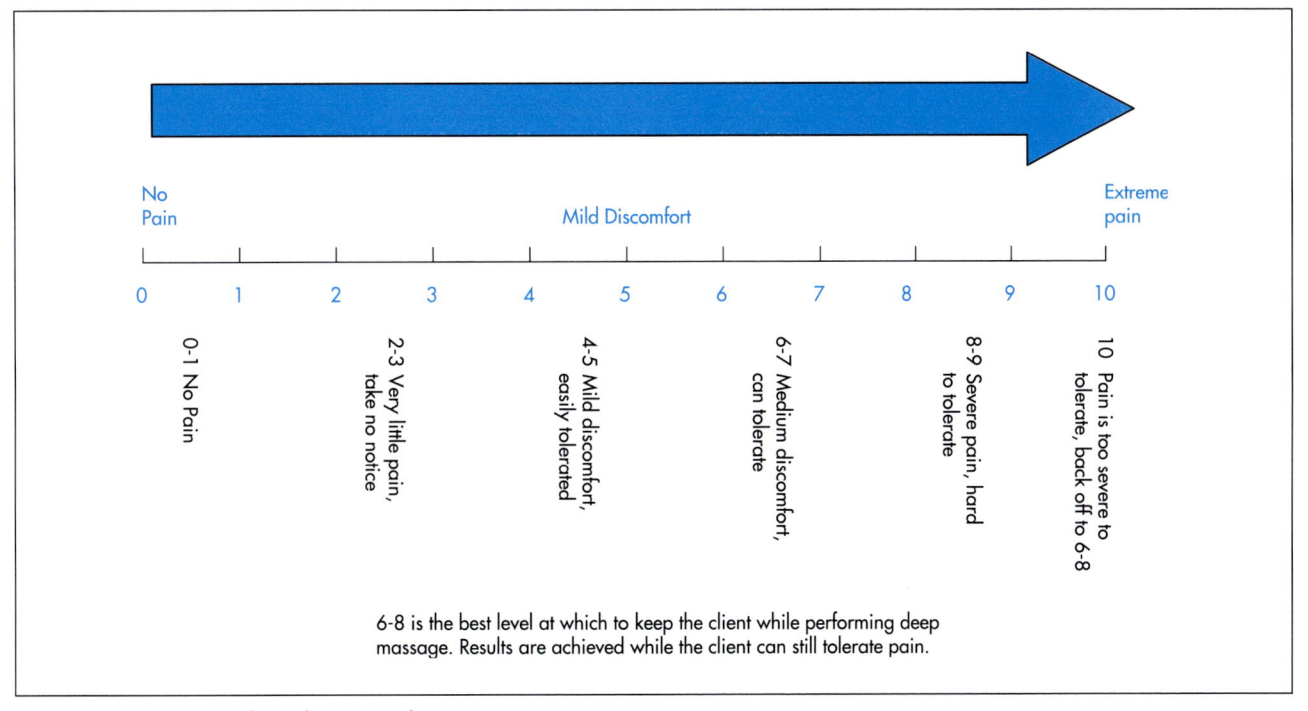

Diagram 18.1 Visual analogue scale

No Pain — Mild Discomfort — Extreme pain

0 — 0-1 No Pain
1
2 — 2-3 Very little pain, take no notice
3
4 — 4-5 Mild discomfort, easily tolerated
5
6 — 6-7 Medium discomfort, can tolerate
7
8 — 8-9 Severe pain, hard to tolerate
9
10 — 10 Pain is too severe to tolerate, back off to 6-8

6-8 is the best level at which to keep the client while performing deep massage. Results are achieved while the client can still tolerate pain.

guided by the client's pain threshold so as to minimise the amount of discomfort experienced during the treatment. Clients who experience pain or severe discomfort during a treatment will protect themselves by contracting musculature, which may negate any treatment benefits. To minimise or prevent severe discomfort or pain, a therapist can employ the use of the visual analogue scale (or pain scale).

The visual analogue scale (VAS) was first developed to measure arthritic pain. It is a simple linear scale that is relatively easy to use as a single measure of pain intensity. The VAS illustrated in Diagram 18.1 has been adapted for use in massage therapy. It should be noted that the VAS:

- is a measure of one's own pain tolerance that cannot be compared to others;
- needs careful explanation, and the numbers on the scale must be clearly defined before use.

THE FULL BODY MASSAGE

It is common for massage therapists to book clients for full body massage appointments that last between 30 minutes and one and a half hours. The sequence presented in this chapter is suited for a one hour session. The following is a guideline of how to allocate time spent on each area of the body:

- back — 15 minutes;
- back of thigh, leg and foot — 5 minutes each side;
- front of thigh and leg — 5 minutes each side;
- abdomen — 5 minutes;
- chest — 3 minutes;
- arm and hand — 3.5 minutes each side;
- shoulders, neck, head and face — 10 minutes.

It is difficult to recommend how may stroke-repetitions should be performed to ensure the sequence is completed within the hour. Many texts recommend three repetitions before moving onto a different approach (Fritz, 2000; DeDomenico and Wood, 1997), however the duration of each stroke is dependent upon the therapist's hand size, the speed at which the technique is performed and the size of the client. A therapist with small hands performing effleurage technique on a large expansive back will take longer to perform each technique, whereas a therapist with large hands performing effleurage on a petite back will complete each stroke significantly quicker if travelling at the same speed. The speed of the technique inevitably has an effect on the duration of the sequence. Students of massage will need to experiment with speed of technique and find a happy medium that suits the outcome of the massage.

Overview of the massage sequence

This section summarises the full body massage sequence. Once each stroke is mastered this overview will allow easy recall during practice. The column on the left indicates positional cues and the therapist's or the client's limb position. For easy reference the numbers in the centre column match the detailed description of each stroke given in the 'massage sequence in detail' section of this chapter.

BACK

Stance	Sequence reference	Description
Stand at side	1	Centering
Stand at side	2	Rocking and compressions to back of body through draping
Stand at side	Ch 15	Undrape back
		Apply oil
Stand at side	3	Rowing stroke
Stand at side	4	Half rowing stroke
Stand at side	5	Hand after hand
Stand at side	6	Long hand after hand
Stand at side	7	Reinforced circular finger kneading along the paraspinal muscles
Stand at side	8	Alternating circular thumb kneading along the paraspinal muscles
Stand facing back	9	Side pulls
Stand at head	10	Reverse rowing stroke (transitional stroke)
Change sides		
Stand facing back	9	Side pulls
Stand at side	4	Half rowing stroke

Stand at side	5	Hand after hand
Stand at side	6	Long hand after hand
Stand at side	7	Reinforced circular finger kneading along the paraspinal muscles
Stand at side	8	Alternating circular thumb kneading along the paraspinal muscles
Stand facing back	11	Figure of 8
Stand facing back	12	C-scoop over the opposite side of the back
Stand facing buttocks	13	Palmar kneading over the top portion of the buttocks, opposite side
Stand facing buttocks	14	Reinforced circular finger kneading over the top portion of the buttocks, opposite side
Stand facing buttocks	15	Alternating circular thumb kneading over the top portion of the buttocks, opposite side
Stand facing back	16	Wringing up to the shoulders and down to the low back (integrating stroke)
Stand facing back	17	Reinforced fingertip frictions to the opposite paraspinal muscles
Stand facing back	16	Wringing up to the shoulders (transitional stroke)
Stand at head	10	Reverse rowing stroke (transitional stroke)
Change sides		
Stand facing back	16	Wringing from the shoulders to the waist (transitional stroke)
Stand facing back	12	C-scoop over the opposite side of the back
Stand facing buttocks	13	Palmar kneading over the top portion of the buttocks, opposite side
Stand facing buttocks	14	Reinforced circular finger kneading over the top portion of the buttocks, opposite side
Stand facing buttocks	15	Alternating circular thumb kneading over the top portion of the buttocks, opposite side
Stand facing back	16	Wringing up and down the back (integrating stroke)
Stand facing back	17	Reinforced fingertip frictions to the opposite paraspinal muscles
Stand at side	3	Rowing stroke (integration stroke)
Stand at side	18	Hand after hand around the scapula
Stand at side	19	One-handed reinforced circular finger kneading around the scapula
Stand at head	18	Hand after hand around the scapula from the head of the table
Stand at head	20	Alternating thumb kneading along the medial border of the scapula
Stand at head	21	Reinforced deep thumb effleurage alternated with hand after hand
Stand at head	22	Reinforced palmer effleurage around the scapula
Stand at head	23	Short reverse rowing stroke to the scapulae
Change sides		
Stand at side	18	Hand after hand around the scapula
Stand at side	19	One-handed reinforced circular finger kneading around the scapula
Stand at head	18	Hand after hand around the scapula from the head of the table
Stand at head	20	Alternating thumb kneading along the medial border of the scapula
Stand at head	21	Reinforced deep thumb effleurage alternated with hand after hand
Stand at head	22	Reinforced palmer effleurage around the scapula
Stand at head	23	Short reverse rowing stroke to the scapula
Stand at head	24	C-scoop to the upper trapezius
Stand at head	25	Knuckle kneading the upper trapezius
Stand at head	26	Finger pad kneading along both sides of the neck
Stand at head	10	Reverse rowing stroke (integration stroke)
Stand facing neck	27	C-scoop the back of the neck
Stand facing back	28, 29	Hacking and cupping over back

Stand facing back	30	Forearm press
Stand at side	3	Rowing stroke
Stand at side	31	Nerve stroke
	32	Redrape the back and press the towel over the back to remove excess oil

POSTERIOR LOWER LIMB

Stand facing thigh and leg	33	Muscle squeezing and compressions to the posterior lower limb through draping
Stand at side	Ch 15	Undrape the posterior lower limb Apply oil
Stand at side level to foot	34	Rowing stroke to the posterior leg and thigh
Stand at side level to foot	35	Half rowing stroke

POSTERIOR THIGH

Stand at side level to leg	36	Hand after hand
Stand facing thigh at angle	37	Side pulls
Stand facing thigh at angle	38	Wringing
Stand facing thigh	39	C-scoop
Stand at side level to leg	40	Two-handed palm-heel kneading
Stand at side level to leg	41	Reinforced circular finger kneading
Stand at side level to leg	42	Alternating circular thumb kneading
Stand at side level to leg	43	Long hand after hand (transitional stroke)
Stand facing thigh	44	Flat of fist along iliotibial band
Stand at side level to leg	45	Rowing stroke to thigh
Stand at side level to foot	34	Rowing stroke to the posterior leg and thigh (integration stroke)

POSTERIOR LEG

Stand at side level to foot	46	Rowing stroke to the posterior leg
Stand at side level to foot	47	Hand after hand with V-stroke
Stand at side level to foot	48	V-stroke
Stand facing leg	49	C-scoop
Stand at side level to foot	50	Alternating circular thumb kneading
Stand at side level to foot	46	Rowing stroke to the posterior leg
Stand at side, bend knee and support foot on therapist's shoulder	51	Two-handed palm-heel kneading
Stand at side, bend knee and support foot on therapist's shoulder	52	Shaking the calf
Stand at side, straighten leg	46	Rowing stroke to the posterior leg
Stand at side level to foot	34	Rowing stroke to the posterior leg and thigh (integration stroke)
Stand facing thigh	28, 53, 54	Hacking, pummelling and plucking to leg and thigh
Stand at side level to foot	34	Rowing stroke to the posterior leg and thigh
Stand at side level to foot	31	Nerve stroke
	32	Redrape the posterior limb and press the towel over the limb to remove excess oil

FOOT

Stand at base of table	55	Superficial stroking over the base of the foot to apply lubricant
Stand at base of table	56	Alternating circular thumb kneading around the heel and base of the foot

Stand at base of table	57	Effleurage each ray of the foot finishing at the toes
Stand at base of table	58	Mobilise rays of the foot
Stand at base of table	59	Fist rolling
Stand at base of table	60	Chafe along the midline of the foot with the side of the hand
Stand at base of table	55	Superficial stroking over the base of the foot
Stand at base of table	32	Redrape the foot and press the towel over the foot to remove excess lotion
		Repeat on the opposite limb
	Ch 15	Turn client from prone to supine

ANTERIOR LOWER LIMB

Stand facing thigh and leg	33	Muscle squeezing and compressions to the anterior thigh and leg through the draping
	Ch 15	Undrape the anterior lower limb
		Apply oil
Stand at side level to foot	61	Rowing stroke to the anterior thigh and leg
Stand at side level to foot	62	Half rowing stroke

FRONT OF THIGH

Stand at side level to shin	63	Hand after hand
Stand facing thigh on angle	64	Side pulls
Stand facing thigh on angle	65	Wringing
Stand facing thigh on angle	66	Reinforced broad circular kneading to the inner thigh
Stand facing thigh	67	C-scoop whole thigh
Stand at side level to shin	68	Two-handed palm-heel kneading
Stand at side level to shin	69	Reinforced circular finger kneading
Stand at side level to shin	70	Alternating circular thumb kneading
Stand at side level to shin	71	Long hand after hand
Stand at side level to foot	61	Rowing stroke to the anterior thigh and leg (integration stroke)

ANTERIOR LEG

Stand at side level to foot	72	Rowing stroke to the anterior leg
Stand at side level to foot	73	Hand after hand with V-stroke
Stand facing shin	74	C-scoop
Stand at side level to foot	75	Alternating circular thumb kneading to the muscles on the outside of the leg
Stand at side level to foot	72	Rowing stroke to the leg
Bend knee	76	Rolling calf
Bend knee	77	Split calf
Bend knee	78	Alternating circular thumb kneading around the knee joint
Straighten leg/stand at side level to foot	72	Rowing stroke to the leg
Stand at side level to foot	61	Rowing stroke to the thigh and leg (integration stroke)
Stand facing thigh	28, 53, 54	Hacking, pummelling and plucking to the thigh
Stand at side level to foot	61	Rowing stroke to the thigh and leg (integration stroke)
Stand at side level to foot	31	Nerve stroke
	32	Redrape anterior lower limb, press towel over limb to remove excess oil

FOOT

Stand at base of table	79	Mobilise the ankle

Stand at base of table	80	Broad compression of the foot
Stand at base of table	81	Thumb stripping between the metatarsals
Stand at base of table	82	Knead the toes
Stand at base of table	83	Rowing stroke over the front of the foot
	32	Redrape foot and press towel over the foot to remove excess oil
		Repeat on the opposite limb

ABDOMEN

Stand facing abdomen	84	Rest one hand on the abdomen and the other on the chest
	Ch 15	Undrape abdomen
Stand facing abdomen	85	Sun and moon stroke
Stand facing abdomen	86	Hand after hand
Stand facing abdomen	87	Side pulls
Stand facing abdomen	88	Rib raking
Stand facing abdomen	89	Broad circles over the ribs
Stand facing abdomen	90	C-scoop opposite and lateral side of the abdomen
Change sides		
Stand facing abdomen	87	Side pulls
Stand facing abdomen	88	Rib raking
Stand facing abdomen	89	Broad circles over the ribs
Stand facing abdomen	90	C-scoop opposite and lateral side of the abdomen
Stand facing abdomen	85	Sun and moon stroke
Stand facing abdomen	91	Reinforced circular finger kneading over the large intestine
Stand facing abdomen	92	Vibrations over transverse colon
Stand facing abdomen	85	Sun and moon stroke
Stand at side at hip level	93	Short rowing stroke lifting the low back
Stand at side at hip level	31	Nerve stroke
	32	Redrape abdomen and press towel over the abdomen to remove excess oil

CHEST

	Ch 15	Undrape chest
Stand facing chest on angle	94	Broad palmer stroke across the chest
Stand facing chest on angle	95	Hand after hand to the opposite side of the chest
Stand facing chest on angle	96	One-handed reinforced effleurage to the opposite side of the chest
Stand facing chest on angle	97	Reinforced circular finger pad kneading to the opposite side of the chest
Stand facing chest on angle	98	Alternating circular thumb kneading to the opposite side of the chest
Stand facing chest on angle	94	Broad palmer stroke across the chest
Change sides		**Repeat on other side**
Stand facing chest	31	Nerve stroke
	32	Redrape the chest and press towel over the chest to remove excess oil

ARM, FOREARM AND HAND

Stand facing arm	33	Muscle squeezing and compressions to the arm through the draping
	Ch 15	Undrape the arm
Stand at side and support at hand	99	Gently shake the arm with the arm bent
		Apply oil
Stand at side support arm at wrist	100	Alternating one-handed rowing stroke

Stand at side support arm at inner elbow	101	One-handed kneading to the front of the upper arm
Stand facing chest support arm at outer elbow	102	One-handed kneading to the back of the upper arm
Stand at side support arm at wrist	103	One-handed C-scoop to the forearm
Stand at side support arm at wrist	104	Alternating circular thumb kneading to the wrist
Stand at side support arm at wrist	105	Alternating circular thumb kneading to the palm
Stand at side support arm at wrist	106	Thumb stripping between the rays of the hand
Stand at side support arm at wrist	107	Kneading to each finger
Stand at side support arm at wrist	100	Alternating one-handed rowing stroke
Stand at side support arm at wrist and hand	108	Gently shake the arm with the arm straight
Stand at side	31	Nerve stroke
	32	Redrape arm and press the towel over the arm to remove excess oil
		Repeat on the other arm, forearm and hand

NECK — SUPINE

Sit at head of table	109	Rowing stroke to the chest, shoulders and neck
Sit at head of table	110	Knuckle kneading to the top of the chest
Sit at head of table	111	Trapezius alternating pinch knead
Sit at head of table	112	Half rowing stroke to the chest, shoulders and neck
Sit at head of table	113	Flat of fist down upper trapezius
Sit at head of table	114	Circular thumb kneading to the posterior triangle
Sit at head of table	115	Finger pad rub to sternocleidomastoid
Sit at head of table	116	Circular fingertip kneading to the base of the skull
		Repeat 112–116 on opposite side
Sit at head of table	111	Trapezius knead
Sit at head of table	109	Rowing stroke
Sit at head of table	117	Sub-occipital release

SCALP AND FACE

Sit at head of table	118	Fingertip kneading to the scalp
Sit at head of table	119	Palmer flat kneading to the sides of the scalp
Sit at head of table	120	Fingertip kneading around the hairline
Sit at head of table	121	Circular thumb kneading along the midline of the head
Sit at head of table	122	Finger pad kneading across the forehead
Sit at head of table	123	Finger pad kneading to the temples and jawline
Sit at head of table	124	Jawline pinch kneading
Sit at head of table	125	Alternate thumb stroking from the nose to the hairline
Sit at head of table	126	Index finger compression under the rim of the upper eye socket
Sit at head of table	127	Downwards thumb compressions on the cheekbone
Sit at head of table	128	Upwards index finger compressions on the cheekbone
Sit at head of table	129	Thumb stroking outward across the cheekbone
Sit at head of table	123	Finger pad kneading to the temples and jawline
Sit at head of table	130	Pinch kneading the ear

Sit at head of table	131	Long prayer stroke
Sit at head of table	132	Heels of the hand stroking across the forehead
Sit at head of table	125	Alternate thumb stroking from the nose to the hairline
Sit at head of table	133	Tapping over the forehead
Sit at head of table	134	Hot hand compressions over the eyes
Sit at head of table	135	Hold the crown
Sit at head of table	136	Stroke fingers through the scalp and hair pulling

THE MASSAGE SEQUENCE IN DEPTH

This section breaks down the massage sequence and outlines each stroke. Each stroke is fully explained in written form and supported with illustration. The therapist's posture is also described with each stroke.

Back routine

Client position: Prone with bolster under ankles.
Draping: Completely covering client from neck to toes (Figure 18.2).
Therapist posture: Standing at the side of the massage table facing the client at mid-torso level.

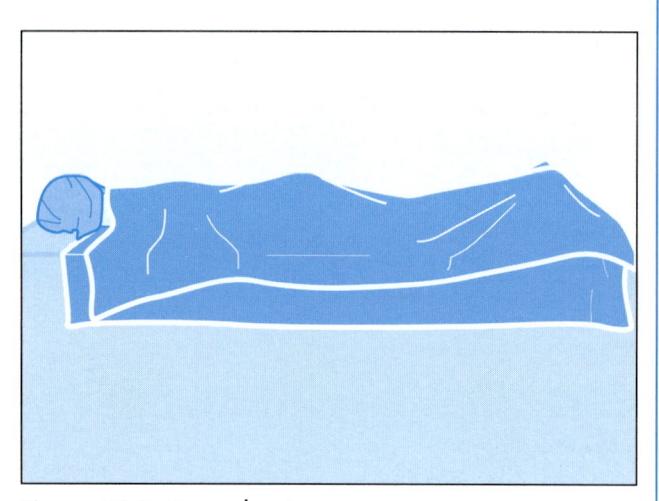

Figure 18.2 Prone draping

1. Centering

Therapist posture: Stand at the side of the massage table facing the client at mid-torso level.
Hands: Place one hand on the sacrum and one at the base of the neck.
Movement: Hold the above position for a moment. Ask the client to take a few deep breaths and use this time to focus in on the client and the massage about to be given.

2. Rocking and compressions

Therapist posture: Stand at the side of the massage table facing the client at mid-torso level.
Hands: Place one hand on the sacrum and one on the opposite paraspinal muscle.
Movement: Gently rock the pelvis from side to side with one hand and use the heel of the other hand to compress and rock the paraspinal muscles from the upper back region to the low back region. The hand rocking the pelvis performs compression and rocking to the buttock on the same side they are standing. Both hands gradually move down the leg and thigh. When one hand is on the back of the thigh the other is on the buttock and when one hand is on the back of the leg the other is on the thigh. Using the heel of the hand, apply compression and rocking. At the feet the therapist moves around the table and moves up the body from the lower limb, reversing the order. The hands finish in the centering position (1) gently rocking the body.

Draping

Tuck the drape into the waist of the client's underwear and fold the drape back to reveal the client's back (refer to Chapter 15, Figures 15.2a and 15.2b, for draping procedures).

Apply oil

Warm the hands by rubbing them together, apply oil to the hands and use gliding effleurage strokes to apply the oil to the back, reapply by turning one hand over so that the back of the hand rests on the client's back, pour the oil into the hand and then reapply using effleurage strokes to the client's back.

3. Rowing stroke to the back

Therapist posture: Stand beside the client's pelvis facing the head of the table, the legs in the stride position — the leg closer to the table is outstretched behind and the other leg forward (Figure 18.3).
Hands: Place the hands on the paraspinal muscles on either side of the spine at the low back, the fingers point towards the head of the table.
Movement: Lunge forward and apply pressure, glide over the paraspinal muscles to the shoulders,

move across the top of the shoulders, around the deltoid muscle and back down the sides of the body to the starting position. This can be repeated several times (Figure 18.4).

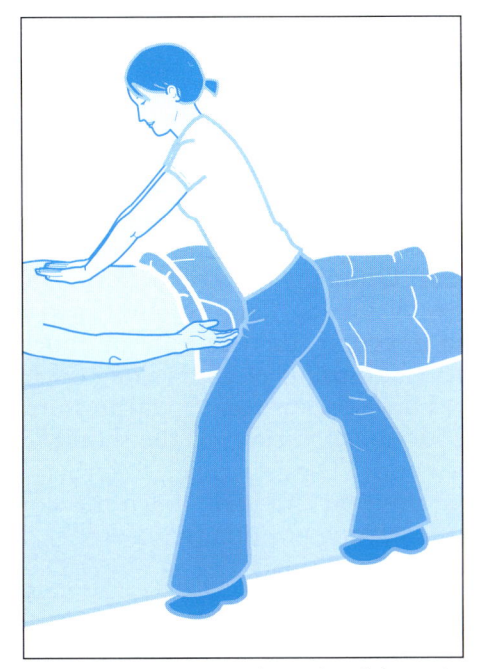

Figure 18.3 Stride stance at the side of the pelvis

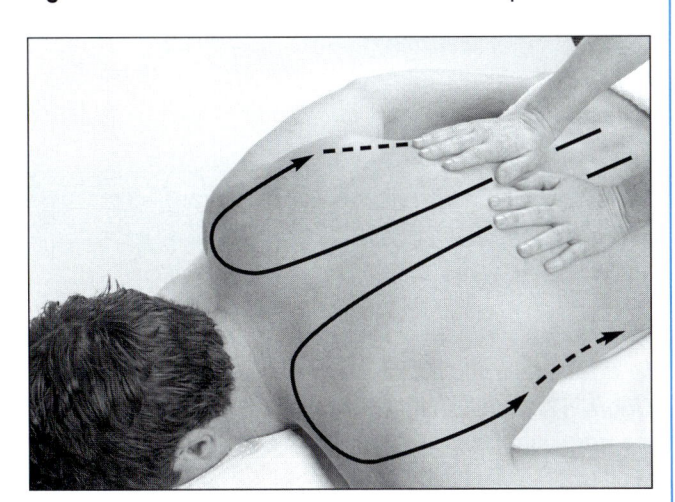

Figure 18.4 Rowing stroke to the back

4. Half rowing stroke to the back

Therapist posture: Stride stance facing the head of the table (Figure 18.3).
Hands: The hand closer to the client's body sits beneath the other hand. This reinforced configuration is placed on the paraspinal muscles of the low back on the same side to which the therapist is standing.
Movement: Lunge forward and apply pressure gliding over the paraspinal muscles to the shoulder, move across the top of the shoulder, around the deltoid and back down the side of the body to the starting position (Figure 18.5). This can be repeated several times.

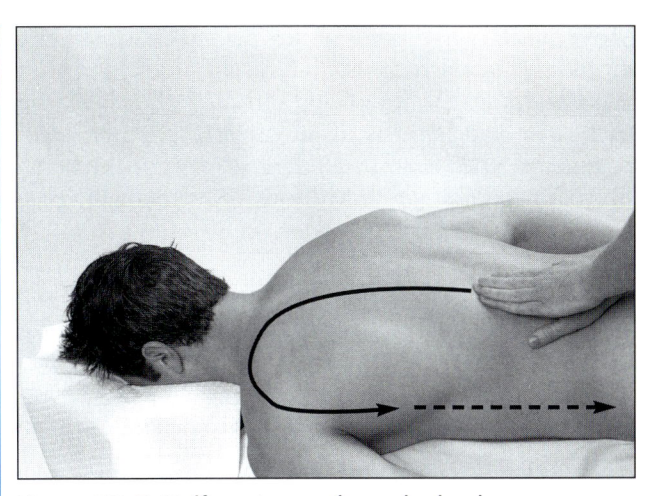

Figure 18.5 Half rowing stroke to the back

5. Hand after hand to the back

Therapist posture: Stride stance facing the head of the table (Figure 18.3).
Hands: Place one hand on the paraspinal muscles of the low back on the same side to which the therapist is standing.
Movement: This hand glides up the back for a short distance followed by the other hand. The top hand is lifted off as the other hand follows through and they continue to alternate as they move up the back. At the shoulder both hands come together in the reinforced position (i.e. the hand closer to the client's body sits below the other hand) and glide down the side of the body to return to the starting position (Figure 18.6). This can be repeated several times.

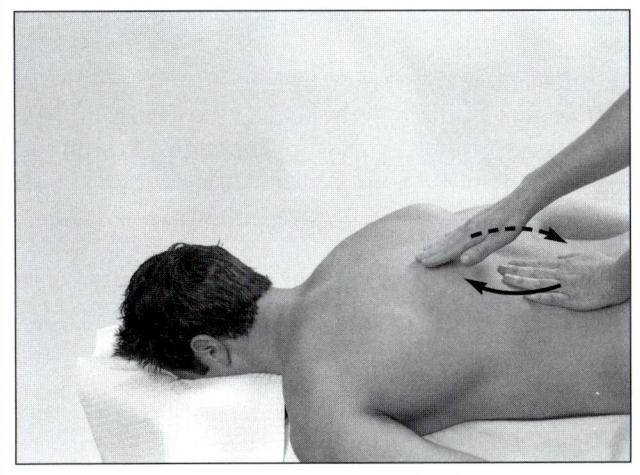

Figure 18.6 Hand after hand to the back

6. Long hand after hand to the back

Therapist posture: Stride stance facing the head of the table (Figure 18.3).
Hands: Place one hand on the paraspinal muscles of the low back on the same side to which the therapist is standing.

Movement: This hand glides up the back to the shoulder; once it has reached the shoulder the other hand starts at the low back and also glides up the back. The top hand is lifted off as the other hand begins at the low back and they continue to alternate to create a continuous movement (Figure 18.7). This can be repeated several times.

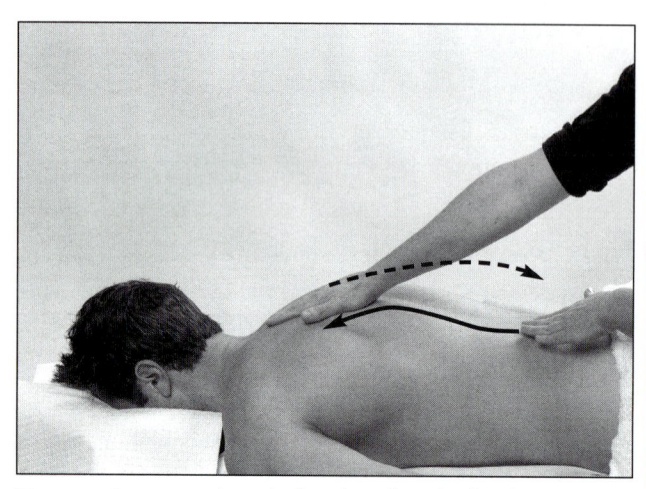

Figure 18.7 Long hand after hand to the back

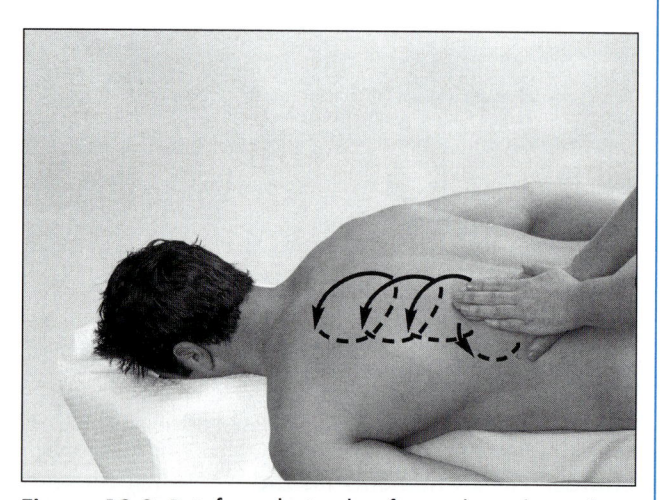

7. Reinforced circular finger kneading along the paraspinal muscles

Therapist posture: Stride stance facing the head of the table (Figure 18.3).
Hands: Place reinforced hands on the paraspinal muscles of the low back on the same side the therapist is standing. The whole hand makes contact with the back but the emphasis of pressure and movement is on the finger pads.
Movement: The finger pads move in a small circle away from the spine. Pressure of the stroke is emphasised at the top of the circle and lightens as the fingers complete the circle to return to the starting position. This movement is continued along the length of the back. At the shoulder both hands in the reinforced position glide down the side of the body to the starting position (Figure 18.8). This can be repeated several times.

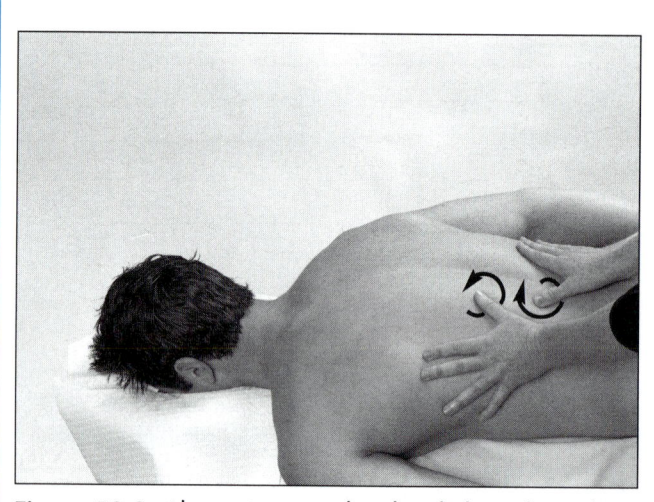

8. Alternating circular thumb kneading along the paraspinal muscles

Therapist posture: Stride stance facing the head of the table (Figure 18.3).
Hands: Both hands are placed on the paraspinal muscles of the low back on the same side to which the therapist is standing. The hands sit side by side with the thumbs meeting in the middle.
Movement: Using the thumbs, perform alternating circular movements, one thumb moving in a clockwise direction, the other in an anticlockwise direction. This movement glides along the length of the back. Lunge forward and apply pressure gliding over the paraspinal muscles to the shoulder. At the shoulder both hands come together in the reinforced position and glide down the side of the body to the starting position (Figure 18.9). This can be repeated several times.

Figure 18.9 Alternating circular thumb kneading along the paraspinal muscles

9. Side pulls to the back

Therapist posture: With a wide stance face the client at mid-torso level (Figure 18.10). During this movement, the therapist bends and straightens the knees to aid the rhythm, movement and pressure of the technique.
Hands: Both hands reach across the client's body to the opposite side of the waist.
Movement: Glide one hand across the client's low back towards the midline. The other hand begins the same action when the first hand is halfway through its stroke. Repeat these strokes as the hands move up the side of the torso and across the top of the shoulder and back down again to the starting position. Repeat once more to end at the shoulder (Figure 18.11).

Figure 18.8 Reinforced circular finger kneading along the paraspinal muscles

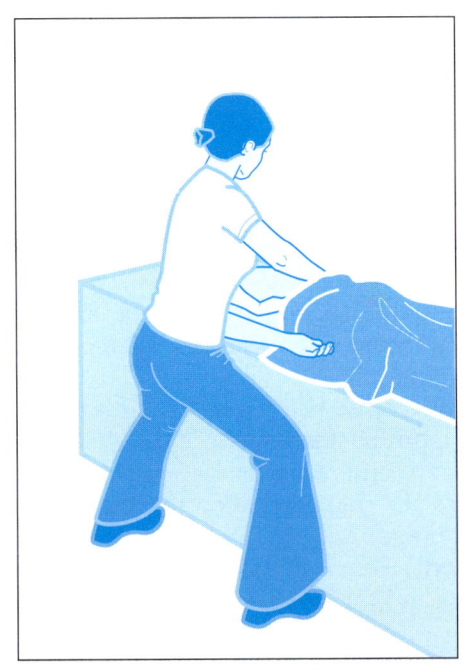

Figure 18.10 Wide stance facing the client at mid-torso level

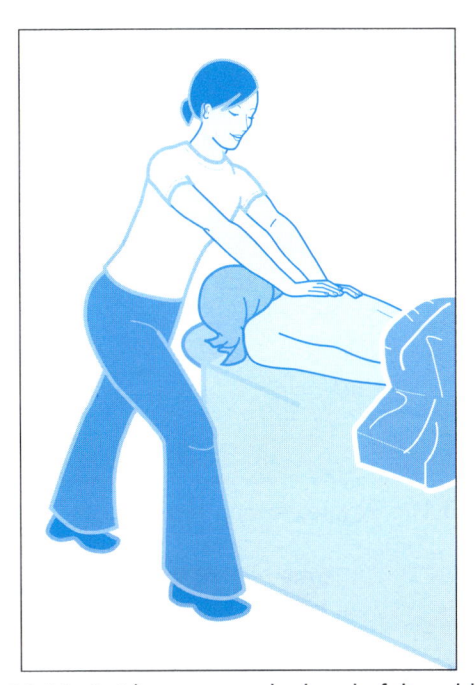

Figure 18.12 Stride stance at the head of the table

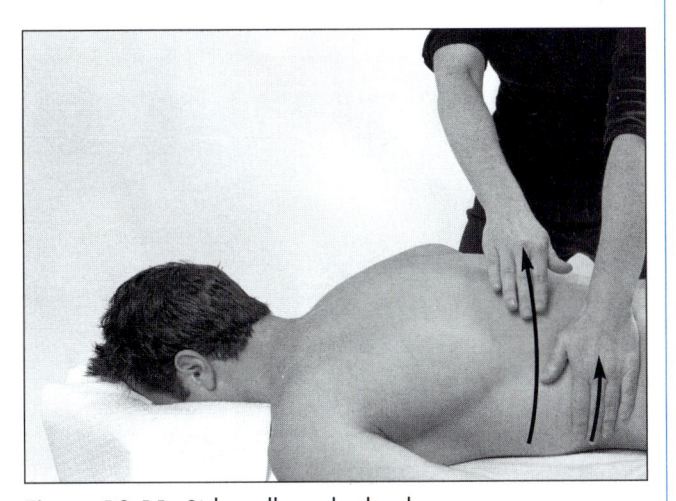

Figure 18.11 Side pulls to the back

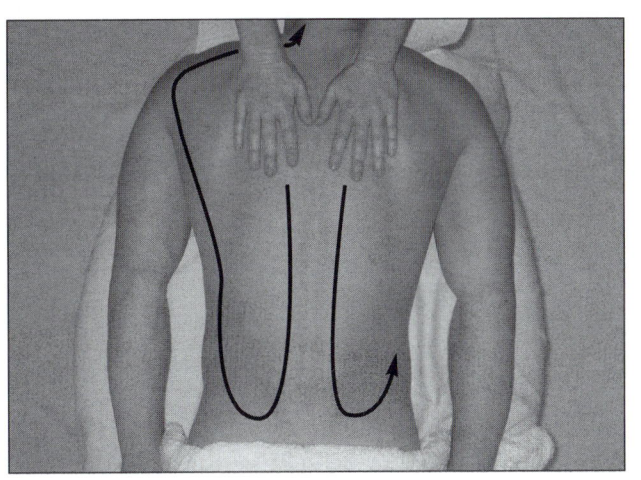

Figure 18.13a Reverse rowing stroke

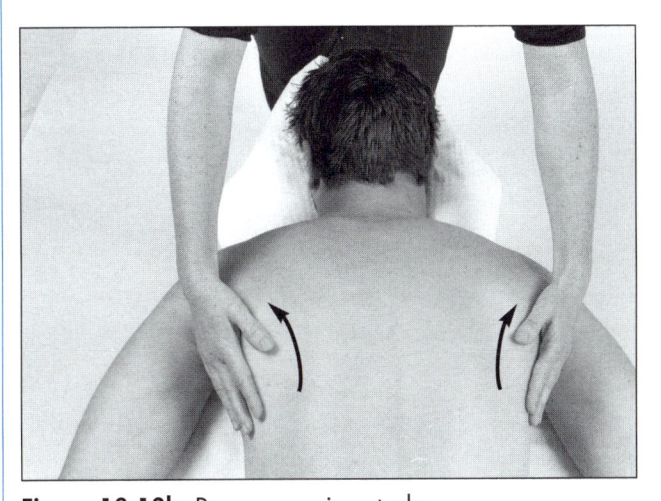

Figure 18.13b Reverse rowing stroke

10. Reverse rowing stroke (transitional stroke)

Therapist posture: Stand at the head of the table with legs in a stride stance. During the technique the body lunges forward as the stroke moves down the back (Figure 18.12).

Hands: Both hands on paraspinal muscles on either side of the spine, at the base of the neck. The fingers face towards the foot of the table.

Movement: Glide the hands down the back towards the buttocks. Glide the hands over the top of the buttocks towards the sides of the body and return along the sides of the torso, around the top of the arms and up the sides of the neck to the base of the skull (Figures 18.13a–d). Repeat this several times. To transit to the next stroke and to the opposite side of the table, glide the hands down the back as the therapist takes a new position on the opposite side.

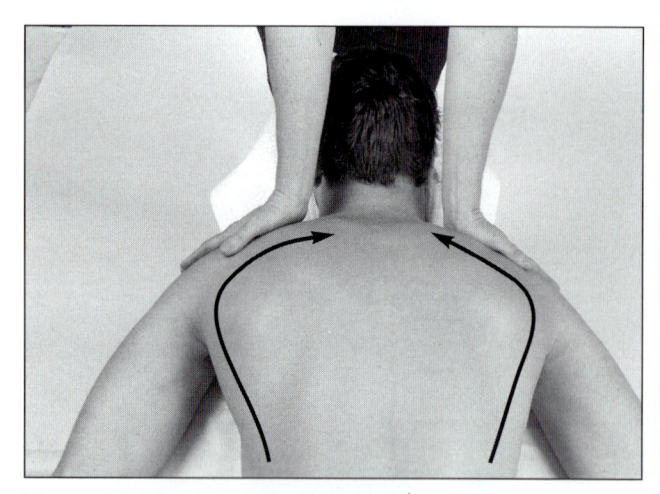

Figure 18.13c Reverse rowing stroke

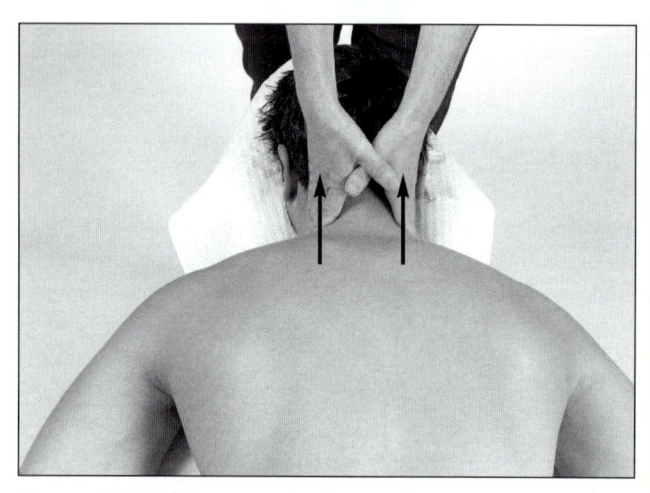

Figure 18.13d Reverse rowing stroke

11. Figure of 8

Therapist posture: With a wide stance face the client at mid-torso level (Figure 18.10).
Hands: Place reinforced hands on the low back.
Movement: Beginning at the client's low back, move the hands across the back in a large sweeping action, transcribe the figure '8' covering the surface of the back (Figure 18.14). Repeat this movement in a fluid motion progressing up and down the length of the back.

12. C-scoop over the opposite side of the back

Therapist posture: With a wide stance face the client at mid-torso level (Figure 18.10). During this movement, the therapist bends the knees and the body sways from side to side to enhance the rhythm of the technique.
Hands: Place the hands on the surface of the back on the opposite side to where the therapist stands. The fingers and thumbs face toward each other creating a 'C' shape between the thumb and index finger.
Movement: Squeeze and lift with one hand using fingertips and thumbs and then with the other, slide these movements back and forth alternating the hands in a rhythmical and gliding fashion to cover the opposite side of the back (Figure 18.15).

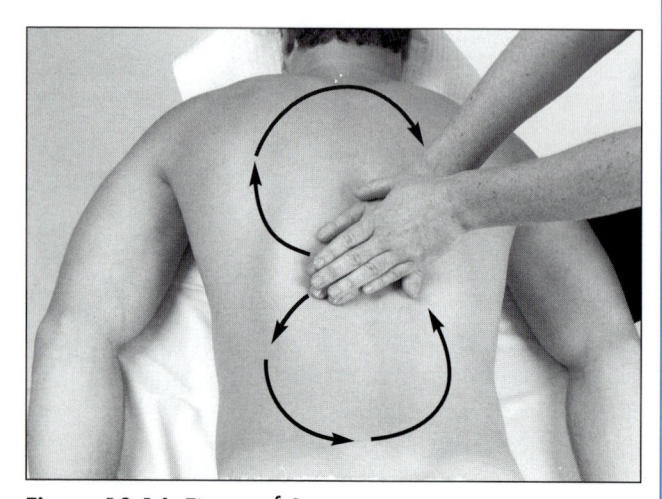

Figure 18.14 Figure of 8

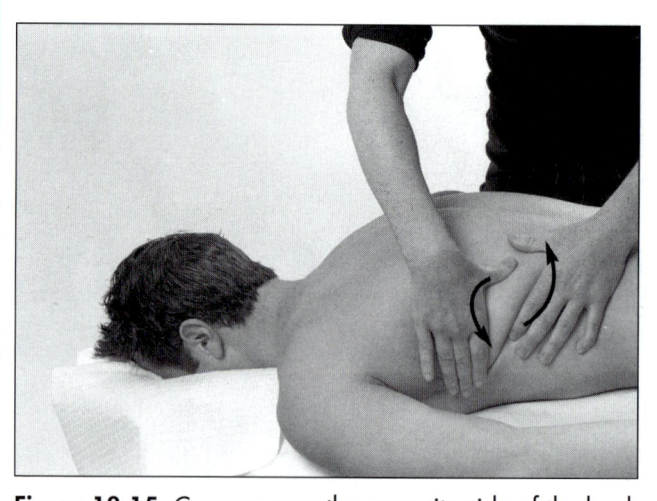

Figure 18.15 C-scoop over the opposite side of the back

13. Palmer kneading over the buttocks

Therapist posture: Standing at the level of the draping line at the low back facing the client, stand with the legs astride, front leg bent and back leg straight. The table may be used as a support for the therapist to lean into and the therapist can lean into the technique to apply added pressure by pushing off on the back foot by lifting the heel and pressing down onto the ball of the foot (Figure 18.16).
Hands: One of the therapist's palms is placed on the top portion of the buttocks on the opposite side to the therapist's standing position.
Movement: The heel of this hand glides over the buttocks followed by the heel of the other hand. The top hand is lifted off as the other hand follows through and they continue to alternate as they move back and forth across the buttocks from medial to lateral (Figure 18.17).

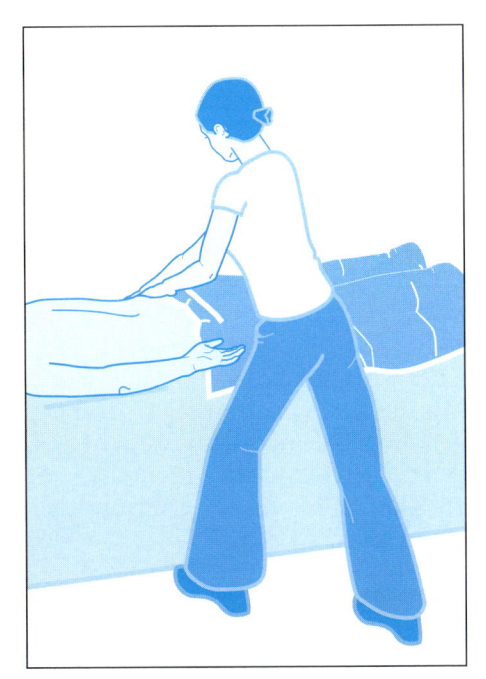

Figure 18.16 Stride stance facing the pelvis

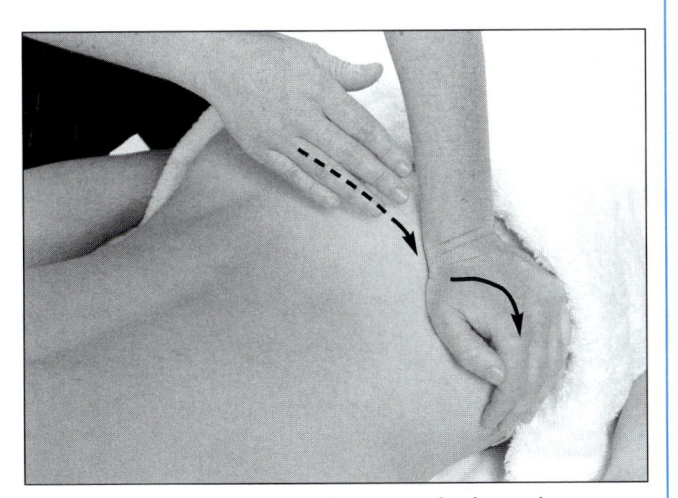

Figure 18.17 Palmer kneading over the buttocks

14. Reinforced circular finger kneading over the buttocks

Therapist posture: Stride stance facing the pelvis (Figure 18.16).
Hands: Place reinforced hands on the top portion of the buttock on the opposite side to where the therapist is standing.
Movement: Perform a variety of broad and small circular movements with the fingertips in a clockwise or anticlockwise direction (Figure 18.18).

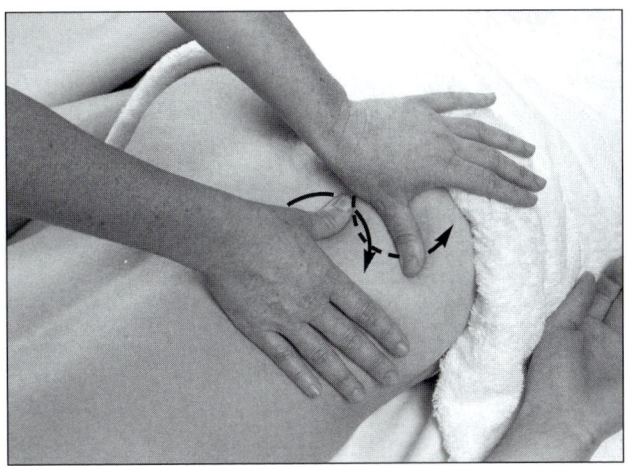

15. Alternating circular thumb kneading over the buttocks

Therapist posture: Stride stance facing the pelvis (Figure 18.16).
Hands: Place the hands on the top portion of the buttock on the opposite side to where the therapist

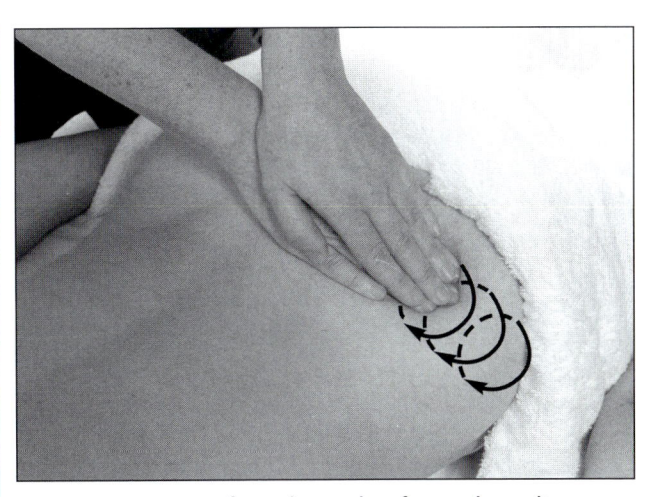

Figure 18.18 Reinforced circular finger kneading over the buttocks

is standing. The hands sit side by side with the thumbs meeting in the middle.
Movement: Using the thumbs, perform alternating circular movements (one thumb moving in a clockwise direction, the other in an anticlockwise direction) covering the buttock (Figure 18.19).

Figure 18.19 Alternating circular thumb kneading over the buttocks

16. Wringing the back

Therapist posture: With a wide stance face the client at mid-torso level (Figure 18.10). During this movement, the therapist bends and straightens the knees (as in a squatting movement) to enhance the rhythm and depth of pressure. The knees are bent when the hands are positioned on the outside of the torso and the knees straighten when the hands are closer to the midline.
Hands: Place one hand on either side of the client's waist with the fingers pointing away from the therapist (i.e. one hand is over the far waist and the other is close to the therapist's body).
Movement: The hands simultaneously glide from one side of the body to the other. At the midline the

hands pass in close proximity to each other. This technique begins at the low back and gradually moves towards the shoulders and then returns to the starting position (Figure 18.20). Repeat this several times.

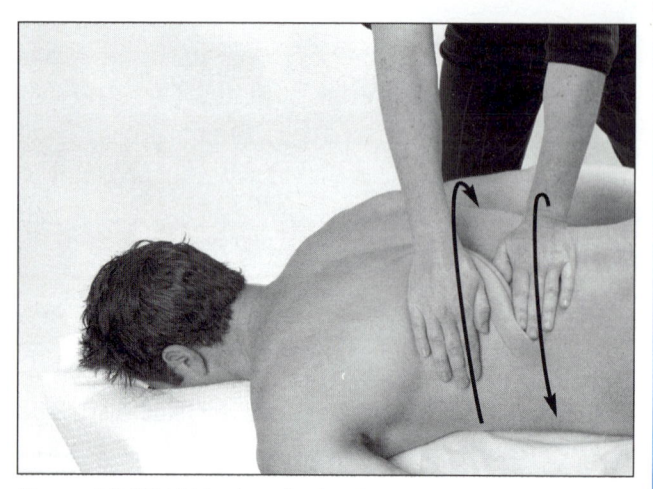

Figure 18.20 Wringing the back

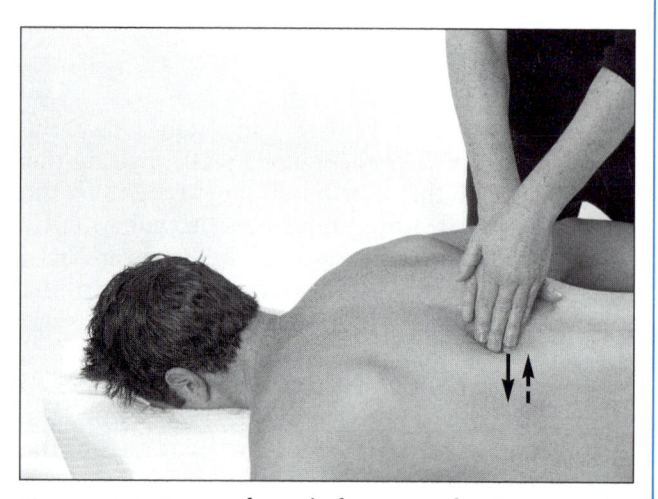

17. Reinforced fingertip frictions to the opposite paraspinal muscles

Therapist posture: With a shortened stride stance face the client at mid-torso level (Figure 18.16). The table may be used as a support for the therapist to lean into and, by pushing down onto the ball of the foot and lifting the heel, can aid in the application of added pressure.
Hands: Place reinforced hands (i.e. one hand sits below the other hand) on the opposite paraspinal muscles at the level of the low back. The fingertips are used to perform the movement.
Movement: The fingertips are pressed down into the paraspinal muscle and move across the muscle fibres to push them away from the spine. Glide the hands back to the spine moving further along the length of the paraspinal muscles. Continuing this same movement, repeat to cover the length of the spine from the low back to the base of neck and return to finish at the low back (Figure 18.21).

18. Hand after hand around the scapula

Therapist posture: Stride stance at the waist facing the head of the table (Figure 18.3).
Hands: Place one hand on the paraspinal muscles of the middle back on the same side the therapist is standing.
Movement: This stroke is the same as the stroke used along the paraspinal muscles. In this variation the hands follow the medial and superior borders of the scapula closer to the therapist, one hand following the other in a continuous flowing movement (Figure 18.22).

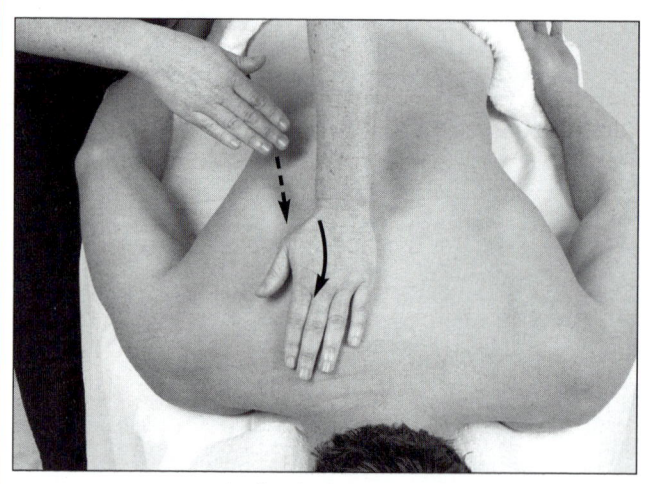

Figure 18.22 Hand after hand around the scapula

19. One-handed reinforced circular finger kneading around the scapula

Therapist posture: Stride stance at the waist facing the head of the table (Figure 18.3).
Hands: Place reinforced hands (i.e. the hand closer to the client's body sits below the other hand) on

Figure 18.21 Reinforced fingertip frictions to the opposite paraspinal muscles

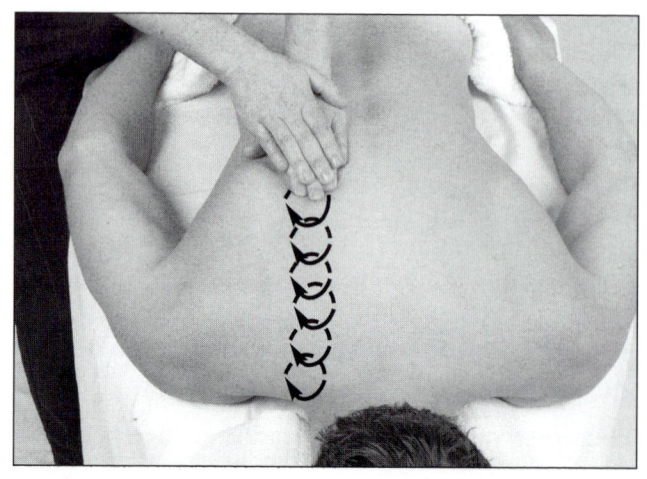

Figure 18.23 One-handed reinforced circular finger kneading around the scapula

the paraspinal muscles of the middle back, the same side to which the therapist is standing.
Movement: This stroke is the same as the stroke used along the paraspinal muscles. In this variation the stroke follows the medial and superior borders of the scapula; the fingers glide along the edges of the scapula in a continuous flowing movement (Figure 18.23).

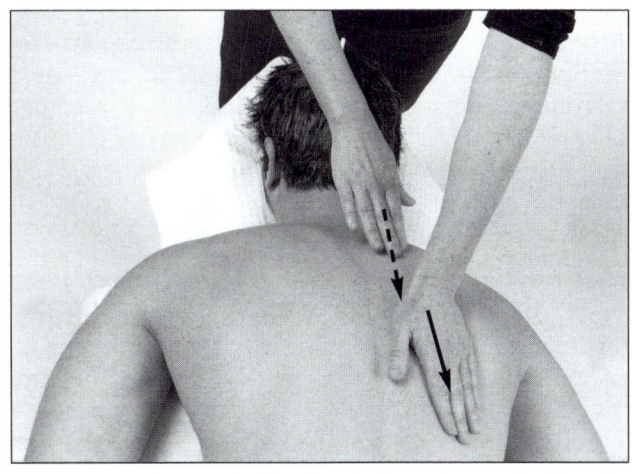

20. Alternating thumb kneading along the medial border of the scapula

Therapist posture: Stride stance at the head of the table facing the foot of the table (Figure 18.12).
Hands: Both hands are placed on one side of the upper back on the muscles between the medial border of the scapula and the spine. The hands sit side by side with the thumbs meeting in the middle.
Movement: Using the thumbs, perform alternating circular movements, one thumb moving in a clockwise direction, the other in an anticlockwise direction. This movement glides back and forth along the muscles between the medial border of the scapula and the spine (Figure 18.24).

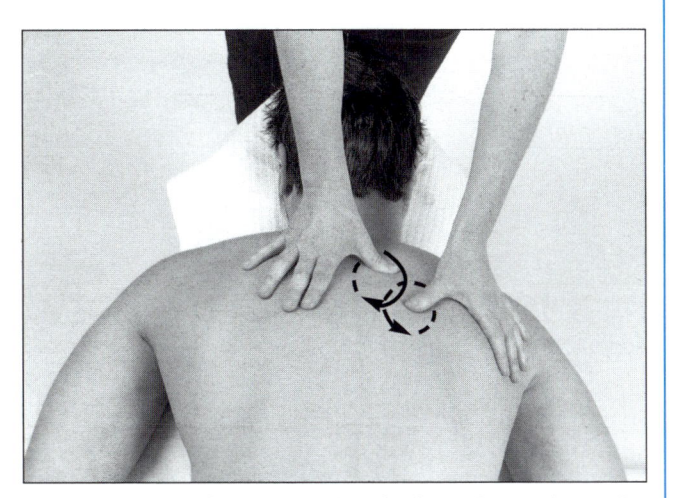

Figure 18.24 Alternating thumb kneading along the medial border of the scapula

21. Reinforced deep thumb effleurage alternated with hand after hand

Therapist posture: Stride stance at the head of the table facing the feet (Figure 18.12).
Hands: Both hands are placed on one side of the upper back on the muscles between the medial border of the scapula and the spine. One thumb is placed on top of the other thumbnail.
Movement: The reinforced thumbs apply deep pressure into the muscle and slowly move caudally in a strip along the medial border of the scapula. After the completion of this strip the hands apply hand-after-hand strokes to the same area (see Figures 18.25a and b). Another strip is applied, this time moving slightly medially from the previous strip and again hand-after-hand strokes follow at its completion. Continue this combination of movements until the thumb strips come close to the spine. The movements should begin at the shoulder and end in line with the inferior angle of the scapula.

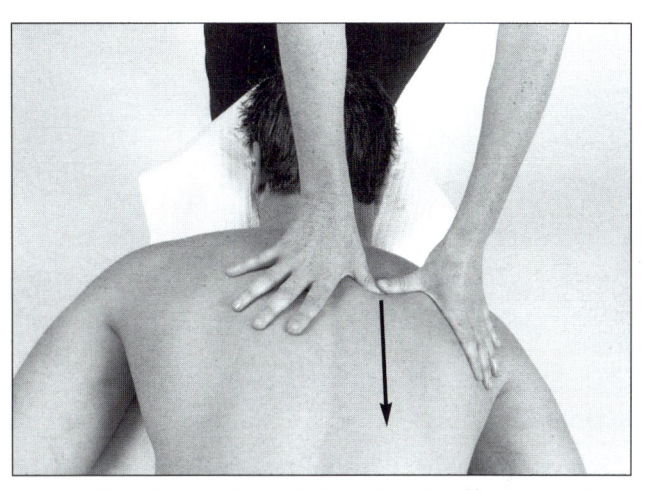

Figure 18.25a Reinforced deep thumb effleurage along the medial border of the scapula

Figure 18.25b Hand after hand along the medial border of the scapula

22. Reinforced palmer effleurage around the scapula

Therapist posture: Stride stance at the head of the table facing the foot of the table (Figure 18.12).
Hands: The reinforced hands are placed on one side of the upper back on the muscles between the medial border of the scapula and the spine.
Movement: The hands trace around the borders of the scapula, beginning at the superior medial aspect, down the medial border around the inferior angle, glide back up the lateral and superior aspects to the starting point. The emphasis of the pressure in this stroke is on the downward movement along the medial border of the scapula. This can be repeated several times (Figure 18.26).

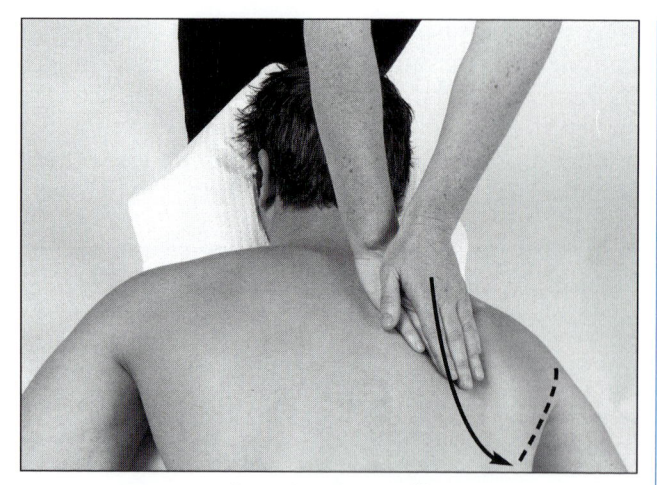

Figure 18.26 Reinforced palmer effleurage around the scapula

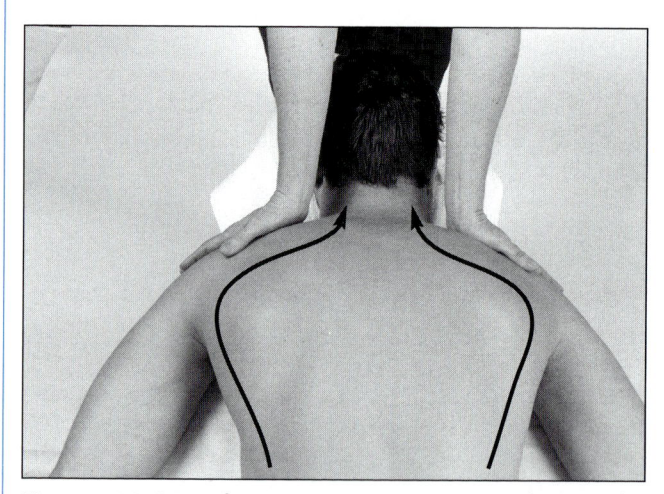

23. Short reverse rowing stroke to the scapulae

Therapist posture: Stride stance at the head of the table (Figure 18.12).
Hands: Place the hands at the base of the neck with the fingers facing down the back and one hand on either side of the spine.
Movement: Perform a reverse rowing stroke, beginning at the base of the neck and only continuing as far as the inferior angle of the scapulae (Figure 18.27a). The stroke continues to glide up the lateral border of the scapulae (Figure 18.27b), over the deltoids, and over the upper trapezius, to finish at the base of the neck (Figure 18.27c).

24. C-scoop to the upper trapezius

Therapist posture: The therapist stands at the head of the table with the legs in a wide stance (Figure 18.28).
Hands: Place one hand on each upper trapezius muscle. The thumbs sit on the anterior aspect of the muscle and the fingertips sit on the posterior aspect.

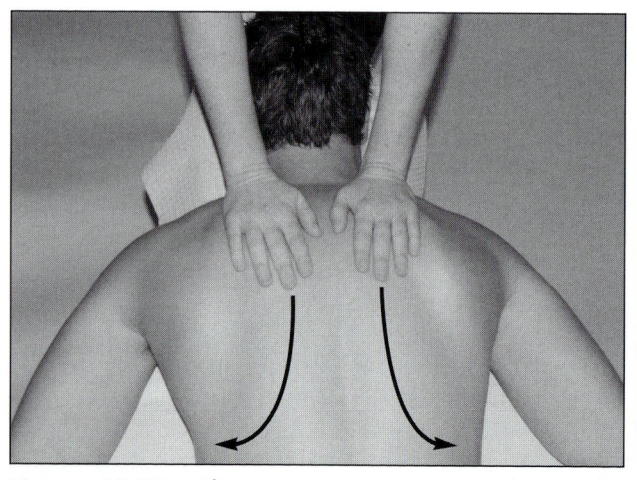

Figure 18.27a Short reverse rowing stroke to the scapulae

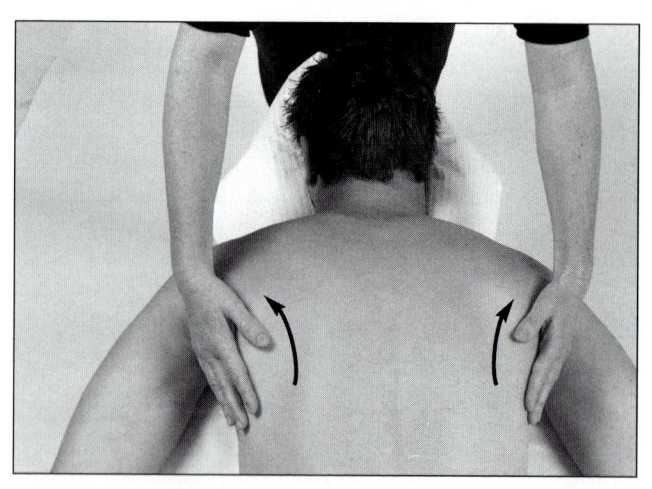

Figure 18.27b Short reverse rowing stroke to the scapulae

Figure 18.27c Short reverse rowing stroke to the scapulae

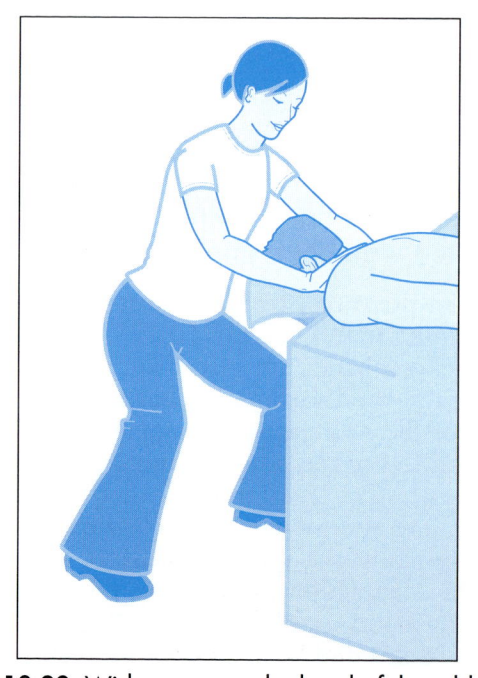

Figure 18.28 Wide stance at the head of the table

Movement: The thumb and fingers of one hand come together to grasp, lift and squeeze the muscle. The stroke is performed in an alternating pattern so that when one trapezius is being squeezed the other is relaxed (Figure 18.29a). The stroke is intensified by using two hands on the one trapezius to knead one side and then the other (Figure 18.29b).

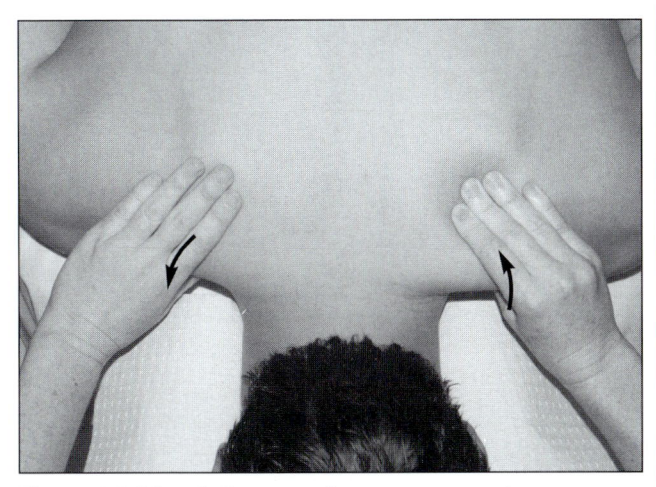

Figure 18.29a C-Scoop to the upper trapezius

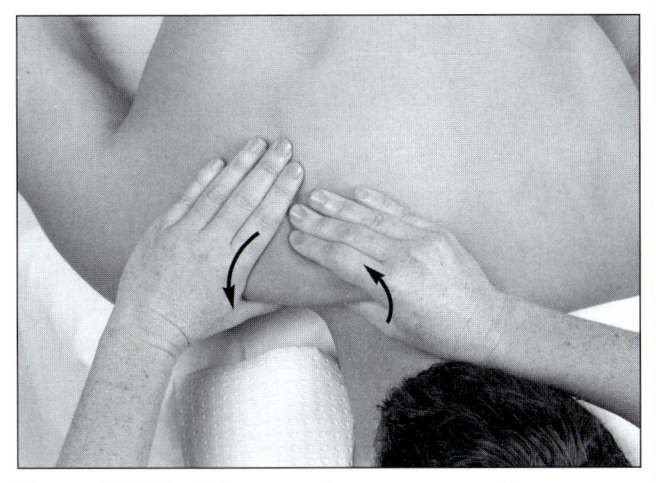

Figure 18.29b C-Scoop to the upper trapezius

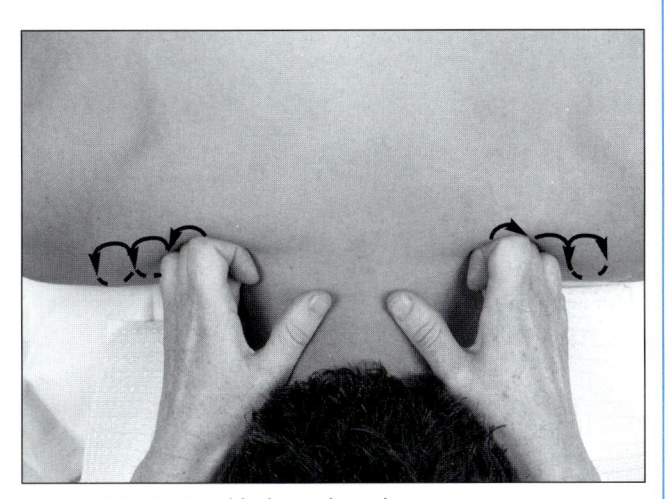

Figure 18.30 Knuckle kneading the upper trapezius

25. Knuckle kneading the upper trapezius

Therapist posture: Wide stance at the head of the table (Figure 18.28).
Hands: Curl the fingers and place the flat part of the middle phalangeal on the upper trapezius muscle. One hand is on either side of the neck and the palms are facing down.
Movement: Gently knead the upper trapezius muscle by rolling the knuckles outward in a circular motion. The thumbs come together behind the back of the neck to provide a pivot point from which the knuckles rotate. Work back and forth along the length of the muscle (Figure 18.30).

26. Finger pad kneading along both sides of the neck

Therapist posture: Wide stance at the head of the table (Figure 18.28).
Hands: The finger pads are placed on either side of the neck with the palms facing in toward each other.
Movement: The finger pads perform circular movements along the side of the neck. The fingers are kept straight and both hands perform the movement in unison (Figure 18.31).

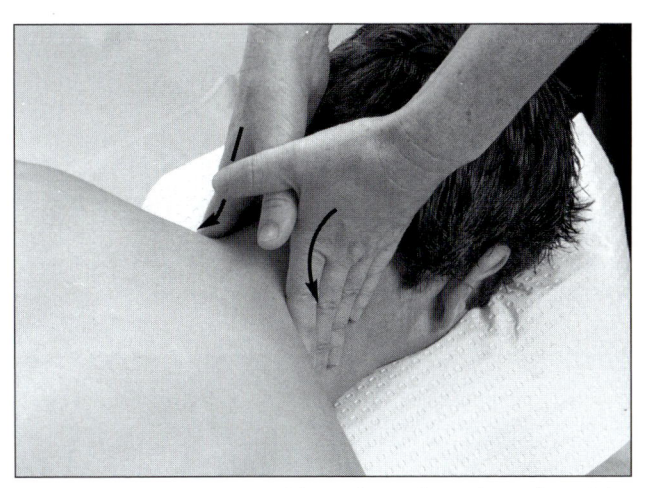

Figure 18.31 Finger pad kneading along the sides of the neck

27. C-scoop the back of the neck

Therapist posture: The therapist stands at the side of the table in a wide stance, facing the client at the level of the neck and shoulders (Figure 18.10).
Hands: The hands are placed around the back of the neck with the fingers on one side and the thumbs on the other side of the neck.
Movement: Grasp the back of the neck with thumbs and finger pads and gently pick up and knead the back and sides of the neck, the hands are working in an alternating pattern (Figure 18.32).

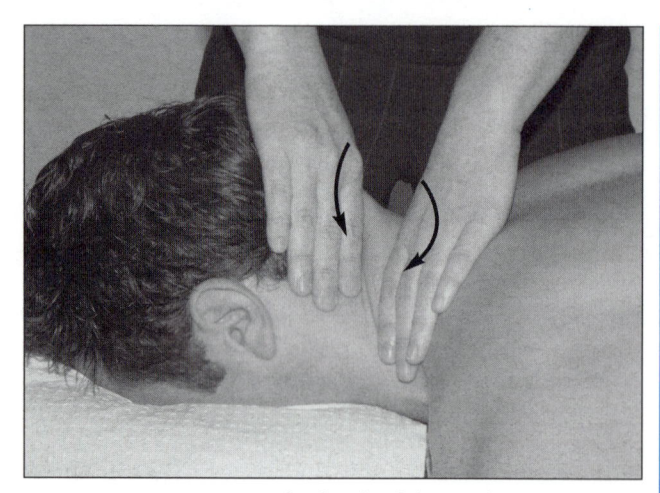

Figure 18.32 C-scoop the back of the neck

28 and 29. Hacking and cupping over the back

Therapist posture: With a wide stance face the client at mid-torso level (Figure 18.10).

Hacking

Hands: Hacking is a form of tapôtement performed with the ulnar side of the hand. Place the hands on the back with the little fingers in contact with the body and the palms parallel about 10 centimetres apart.
Movement: Flick the wrists back and forth alternately so that the tips of the third, fourth and fifth digits come into contact with the back. The fingers are kept relaxed and the wrists are loose so that the fingers spring up off the back rather than landing heavily in a chopping action (Figure 18.33).

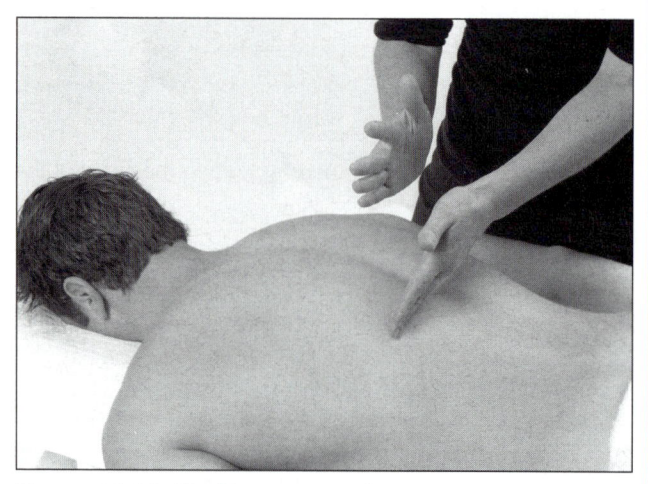

Figure 18.33 Hacking

Cupping

Hands: The therapist makes a cup with each of their hands by squeezing the fingers and thumbs close together with tension in the palms to form a hollow; the cups should be tight enough to scoop water. The hands are placed palm down with the edges of the cup making contact with the client.
Movement: Perform the same alternating action as for hacking, keeping the wrists loose. A deep hollow sound should be heard as each cupped hand strikes the skin (Figure 18.34).

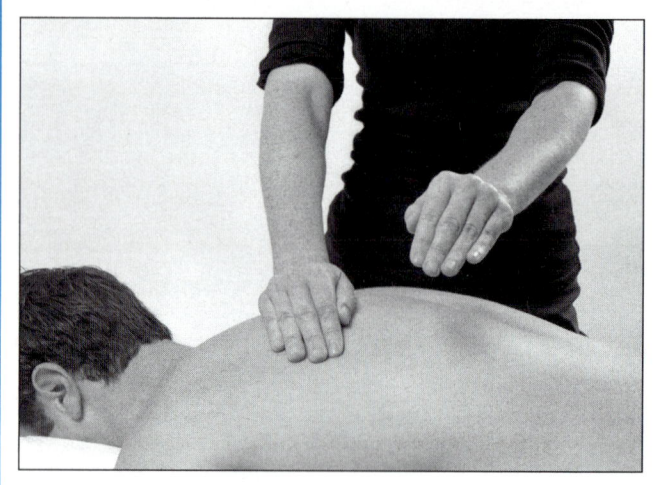

Figure 18.34 Cupping

Note: The biggest challenge with tapôtement strokes is striking evenly with both hands, and coordination. These techniques are performed up and down the paraspinal muscles of the back and across the shoulders, and care is taken to avoid bony prominences and the kidney regions.

30. Forearm press

Therapist posture: With a wide stance face the client at mid-torso level. The therapist bends the knees (as in a squatting movement) and with the trunk leans over the top of the forearms to perform the stroke (Figure 18.10).
Hands: The therapist places the forearms across the middle of the client's back with the palms facing up.
Movement: As the forearms separate and glide to opposite ends of the spine, the palms roll face down

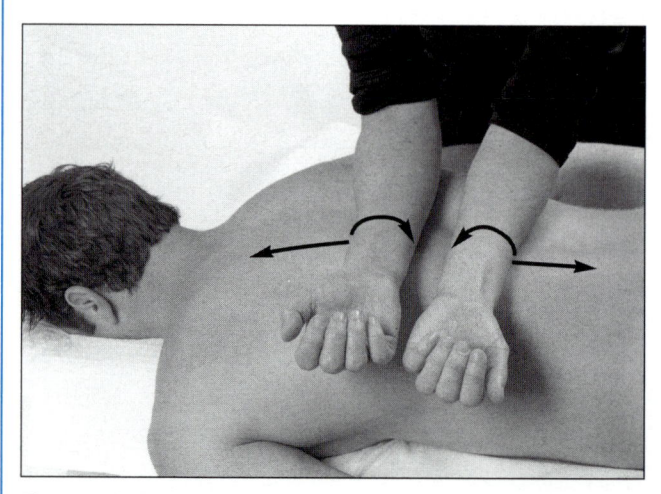

Figure 18.35a Forearm press

CHAPTER 18 THE MASSAGE SEQUENCE   245

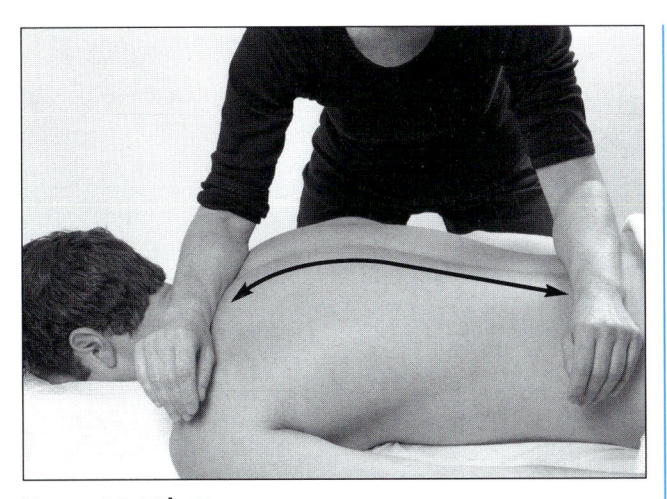

Figure 18.35b Forearm press

and the fleshy part of the forearms make contact with the back (Figure 18.35a and b). The intention of this stroke is to create a sensation of stretching and lengthening of the spine — to make this possible the pressure is exerted outward rather than straight down onto the back.

31. Nerve stroke

Therapist posture: Stride stance facing the head of the table (Figure 18.3).
Hands: The therapist places the fingertips lightly at the base of the neck.
Movement: With the fingertips, stroke down the spine in a continuous alternating pattern. The pressure is light and the speed is slow (Figure 18.36).

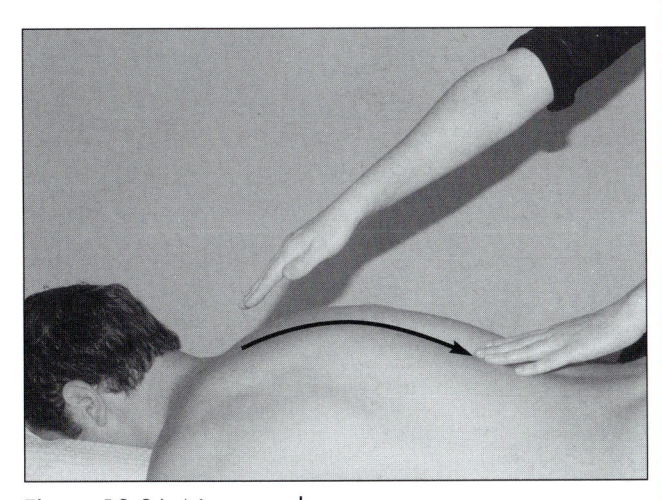

Figure 18.36 Nerve stroke

32. Press towel over the back to remove excess oil

Therapist posture: The therapist faces the client at mid-torso level.
Hands: Untuck the draping at the low back and draw the draping over the back to cover the whole area.

Movement: Squeeze and press the hands over the back through the draping.

Posterior lower limb

Client positioning: The client is lying in the prone position, a pillow or bolster sits under the front of the feet and ankles for support and comfort.

33. Muscle squeezing and compressions

Therapist posture: Standing at the side of the massage table facing the client's thigh.
Hands: Place both hands on the thigh.
Movement: Press the heel of the hands into the muscles of the thigh and hold the pressure momentarily before releasing. Squeeze and release the muscles as the hands move along the thigh and leg to the foot.
Draping: The limb that is to be massaged is undraped and secured under the thigh (refer to Chapter 15, Figures 15.3a, 15.3b and 15.3c, for draping procedures).

34. Rowing stroke to the posterior leg and thigh

Therapist posture: The therapist stands at the side of the massage table at the level of the client's feet, in long stride stance facing the head of the table (Figure 18.37).
Hands: The hands are placed side by side at the ankle, with fingers pointing toward the top of the limb.
Movement: The hands glide up the centre of the limb from the ankle to the buttocks. As the hands

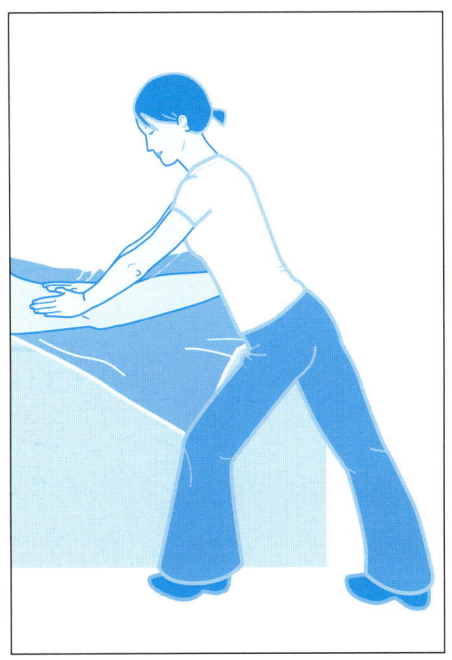

Figure 18.37 Long stride stance for strokes to the length of lower limb

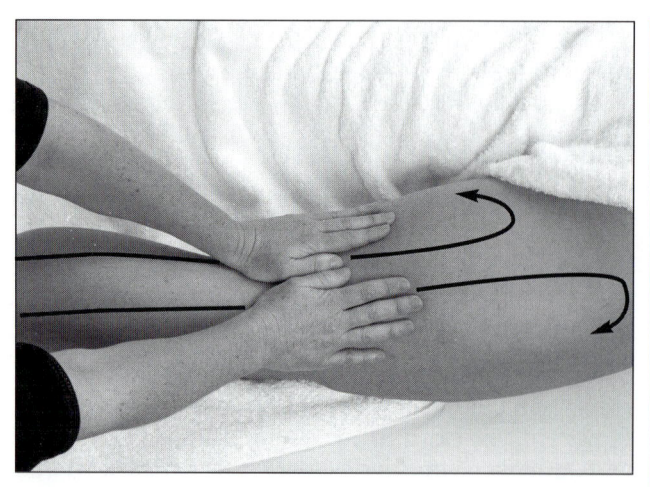

Figure 18.38 Rowing stroke to the posterior leg and thigh

reach the top of the thigh the hands branch off — the inside hand follows the inner thigh and back down the leg, while simultaneously the outside hand glides over the gluteals and back down the lateral side of the thigh and leg, meeting together again at the starting point. Repeat this stroke several times (Figure 18.38).

35. Half rowing stroke to the posterior leg and thigh

Therapist posture: Long stride stance facing the head of the table (Figure 18.37).
Hands: The therapist's leading hand is the one nearer the client's leg. This hand is placed at the client's ankle with the fingers pointing toward the top of the limb. The other hand sits on top of this hand to reinforce the stroke.
Movement: The reinforced hands glide up the back of the leg and thigh, sweep over the gluteals and down the outside of the thigh and leg, returning to the starting point (Figure 18.39). Repeat this stroke several times.

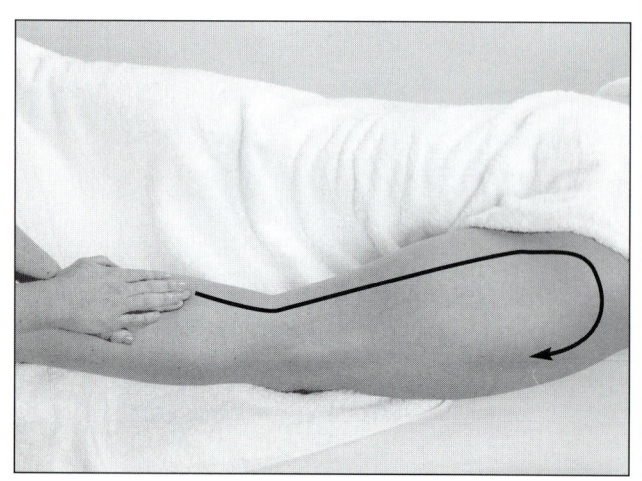

Figure 18.39 Half rowing stroke to the posterior leg and thigh

36. Hand after hand to the posterior thigh

Therapist posture: Stride stance at the level of the client's calf facing the head of the table (Figure 18.40).
Hands: Place one hand behind the knee with fingers pointing to the top of the thigh.
Movement: This hand glides up the thigh for a short distance followed by the other hand, the top hand is lifted off as the other hand follows through and they continue to alternate as they move up the thigh. At the buttock both hands come together in the reinforced position (i.e. the hand closer to the client's body sits below the other hand) and glides down the lateral side of the thigh to return to the starting position (Figure 18.41). This can be repeated several times.

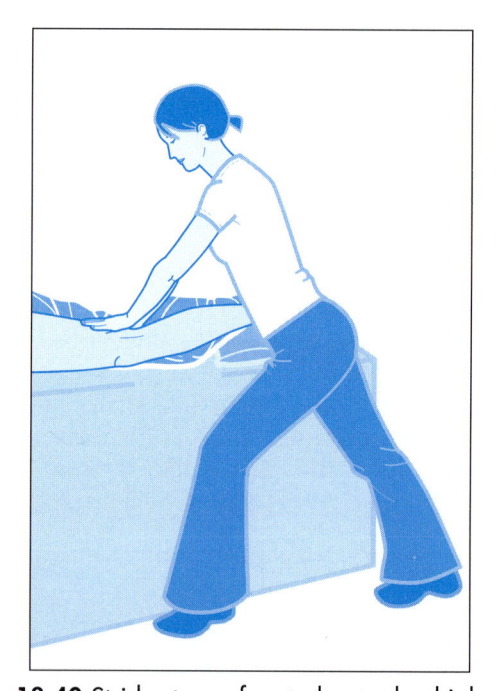

Figure 18.40 Stride stance for strokes to the thigh

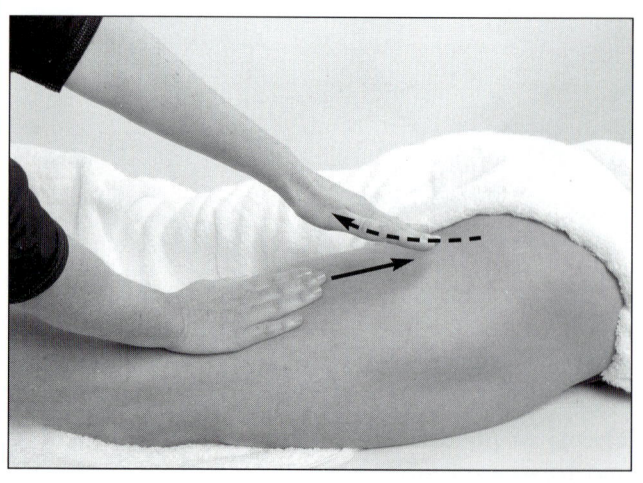

Figure 18.41 Hand after hand to the posterior thigh

37. Side pulls to the posterior inner thigh

Therapist posture: Stride stance at an angle facing client's opposite foot (Figure 18.42).
Hands: Both hands rest on the inner thigh at the knee.
Movement: This stroke is performed to the inner thigh only. Glide one hand across the thigh to the midline on an angle; the angle lines up the inner knee with the outer hip. As this hand reaches the midline of the thigh the other hand follows the same path to create a continuous flowing stroke. This is repeated as both hands move up and down the inner thigh (Figure 18.43).

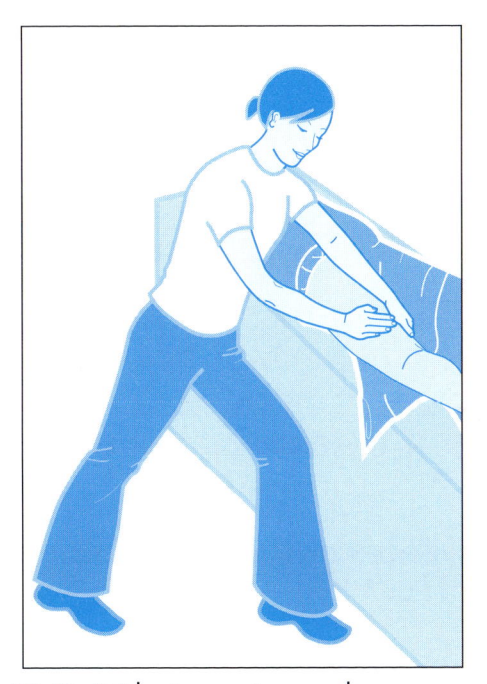

Figure 18.42 Stride stance at an angle

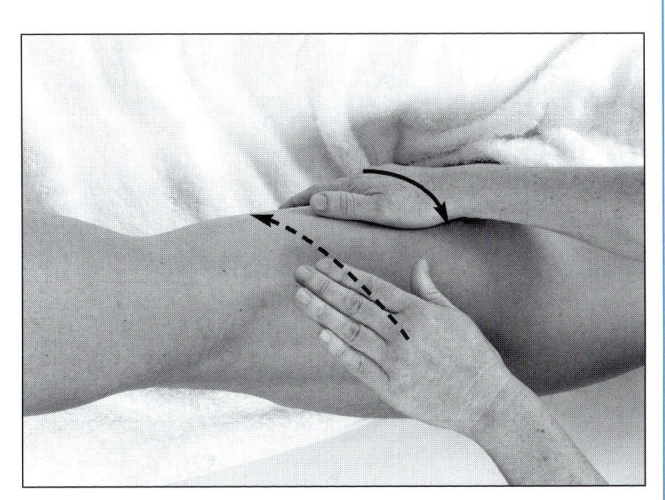

Figure 18.43 Side pulls to the posterior inner thigh

38. Wringing the posterior thigh

Therapist posture: Stride stance at an angle facing client's opposite foot (Figure 18.42).
Hands: Start behind the knee with one hand on the inside of the thigh and the other on the outside.
Movement: Glide the hands across the thigh on a diagonal. The hands cross paths in the middle of the thigh and glide to opposite sides. Progress this pattern up the length of the thigh and back down to the starting position (Figure 18.44).

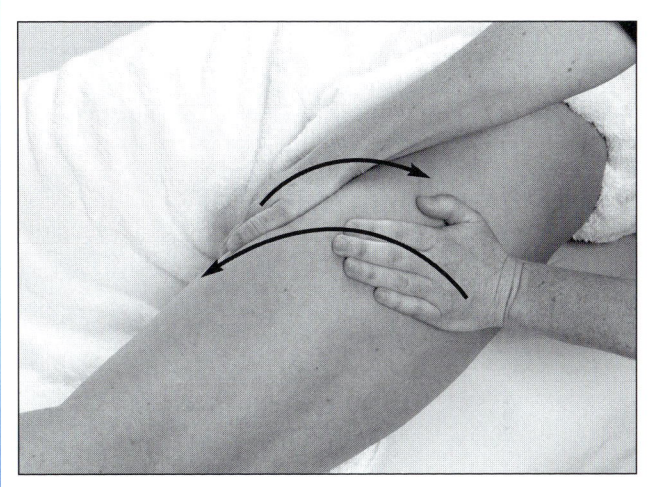

Figure 18.44 Wringing the posterior thigh

Note: the lateral aspect of the thigh has a greater surface area to cover than the inner thigh. Having the therapist's positioning angled allows for greater surface area of the lateral thigh to be covered.

39. C-scoop to the posterior thigh

Therapist posture: The therapist stands in a wide stance facing the side of the massage table at the level of the client's thigh (Figure 18.45).

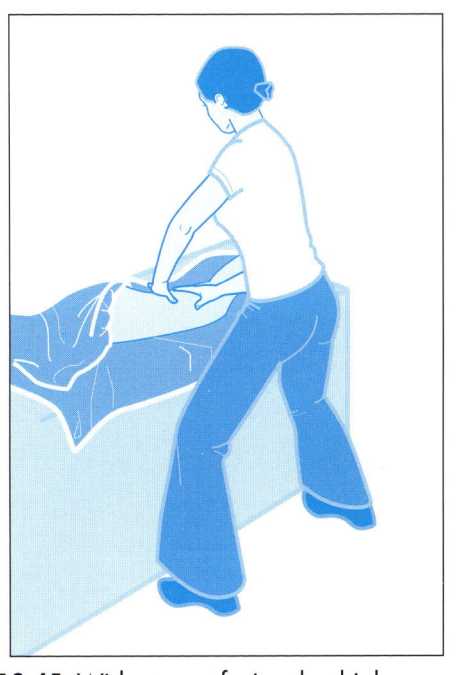

Figure 18.45 Wide stance facing the thigh

Hands: The hands are placed on the thigh facing each other with thumbs and fingers separated creating a 'C' shape.

Movement: The hands alternately glide back and forth grasping and picking up the muscle between the fingers and thumbs. This stroke is performed covering the whole surface area of the thigh (Figure 18.46).

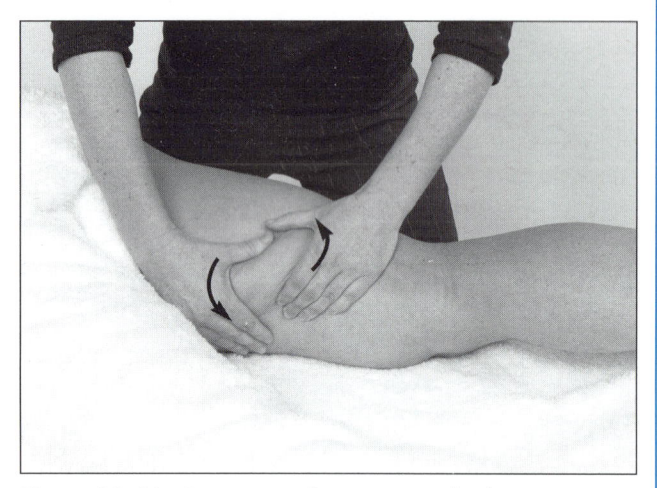

Figure 18.46 C-scoop to the posterior thigh

40. Two-handed palm-heel kneading to the posterior thigh

Therapist posture: Long stride stance at the lower limb facing the head of the table (Figure 18.47).

The leg closest to the massage table is stretched out behind and remains straight, the front leg is stretched out in front and bends to allow the therapist to get close to the thigh without hunching over. The chest should remain open and the back straight.

Hands: The fingers of the therapist's hands are loosely interlocked with the heel of the palms resting on the thigh.

Movement: The pressure of this stroke is exerted from the compressive action of the heel of the hands squeezing the thigh. This action is combined with a circular gliding action up the thigh at the release of each compression. This stroke is performed covering the whole surface area of the back of the thigh (Figure 18.48).

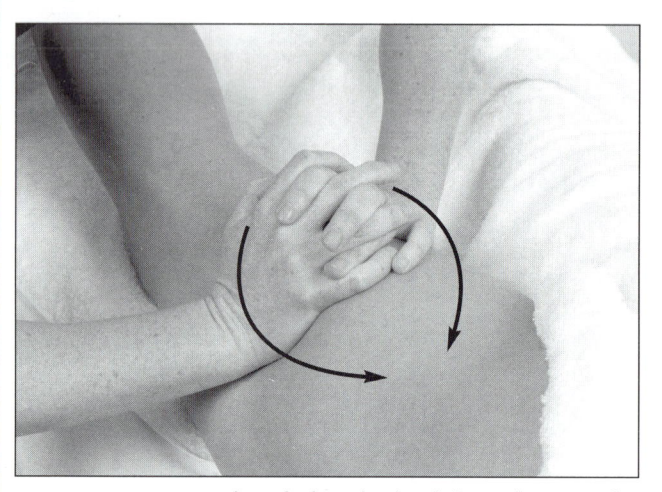

Figure 18.48 Two-handed palm-heel kneading to the posterior thigh

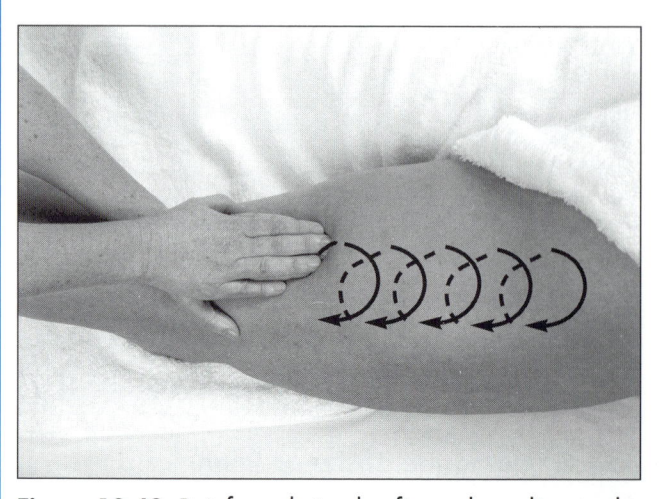

41. Reinforced circular finger kneading to the posterior thigh

Therapist posture: Stride stance at the level of the client's calf facing the head of the table (Figure 18.40).

Hands: The therapist's hand that is closest to the client's body is placed on the thigh with the fingers facing toward the head of the table. The other hand rests on top to provide support and strength to the

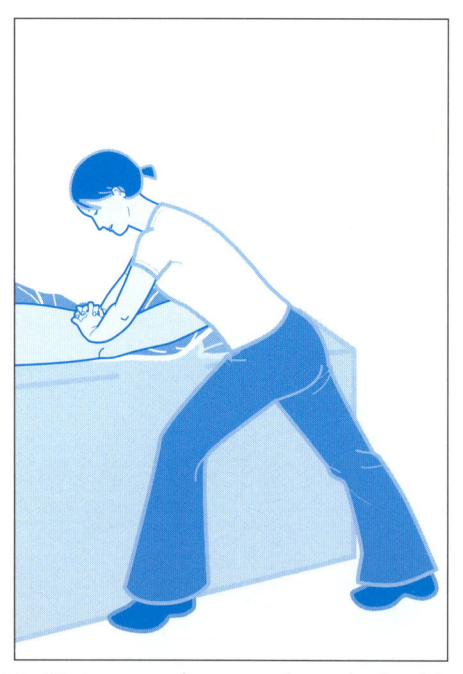

Figure 18.47 Long stride stance for palm-heel kneading

Figure 18.49 Reinforced circular finger kneading to the posterior thigh

stroke. The whole hand remains in contact with the thigh throughout this stroke but the emphasis of the stroke is placed on the finger pads.

Movement: The finger pads move in a small circle away from the inner thigh. Pressure of the stroke is emphasised at the top of the circle and lightens as the fingers complete the circle to return to the starting position. This movement is continued along the length of the thigh. At the top of the thigh both hands come together in the reinforced position and glide down the outside of the thigh to the starting position (Figure 18.49). This can be repeated several times.

42. Alternating circular thumb kneading to the posterior thigh

Therapist posture: Stride stance at the level of the client's calf facing the head of the table (Figure 18.40).

Hands: The therapist's hands are placed on the thigh with the thumbs coming together and the fingers relaxed around the thigh.

Movement: The thumbs perform small alternating circular movements with the thumb pads. One thumb will circle in a clockwise direction and the other anticlockwise. This movement is performed in vertical lines moving up to cover the whole surface of the posterior thigh. For access to the top of the thigh and inner thigh the therapist's fingers may need to be tucked into the palm (Figure 18.50).

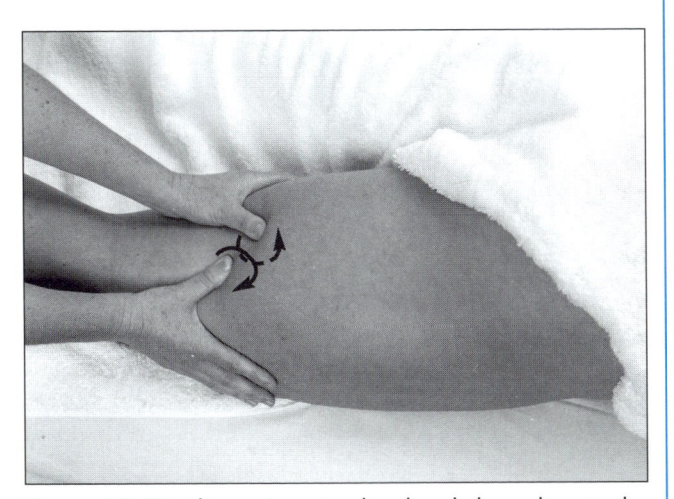

Figure 18.50 Alternating circular thumb kneading to the posterior thigh

43. Long hand after hand to the posterior thigh

Therapist posture: Stride stance at the level of the client's calf facing the head of the table (Figure 18.40).

Hands: Place one hand behind the knee with fingers pointing to the top of the thigh.

Movement: The hand behind the knee glides up the length of the thigh from the back of the knee to the hip. The other hand follows the same path of movement once the first hand has reached the hip. The hands continue to alternate to create a continuous flowing movement (Figure 18.51).

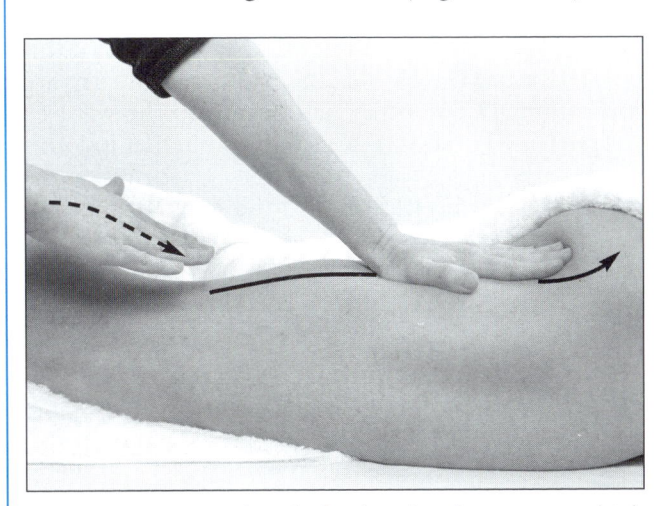

Figure 18.51 Long hand after hand to the posterior thigh

44. Flat of fist along iliotibial band

Therapist posture: The therapist uses a wide stance facing the client's thigh. The foot closest to the head of the table is turned out so that the foot faces the head of the table, allowing the therapist to lunge in the direction of the stroke as it moves up the thigh (Figure 18.52).

Hands: The back of the therapist's hand (hand nearer the head of the table) is placed on the side of the client's leg just above the knee.

Movement: The therapist uses the back surface of the fingers with the knuckles pointing to the top of the thigh and the fingers pointing toward the feet. The back of the fingers glide up the length of the

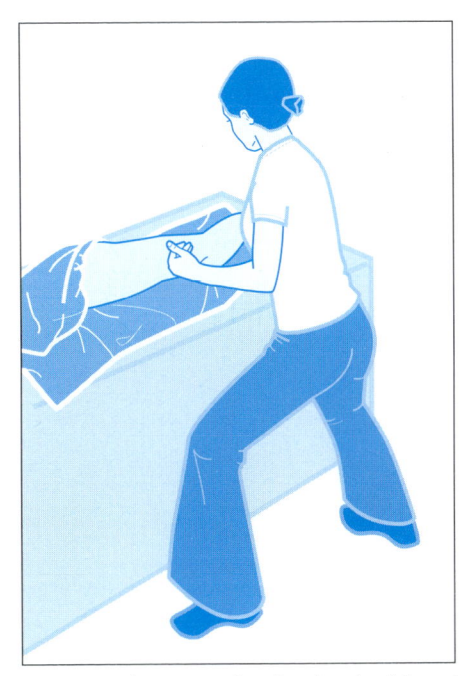

Figure 18.52 Wide stance for the iliotibial band stroke

outside of the thigh to the greater trochanter (a bony prominence of the femur). The hands release at the top and the palm and fingers glide back down the side of the leg to the starting position (Figure 18.53). Repeat several times.

Note: To decrease strain on the wrist with this stroke, ensure the back of the hand and forearm are in alignment. The other hand can grip the wrist to support it. To add your body weight behind this stroke, the elbow of the hand performing the technique can be tucked into the front of the hip. When the body weight is shifted forward this will add pressure to the stroke.

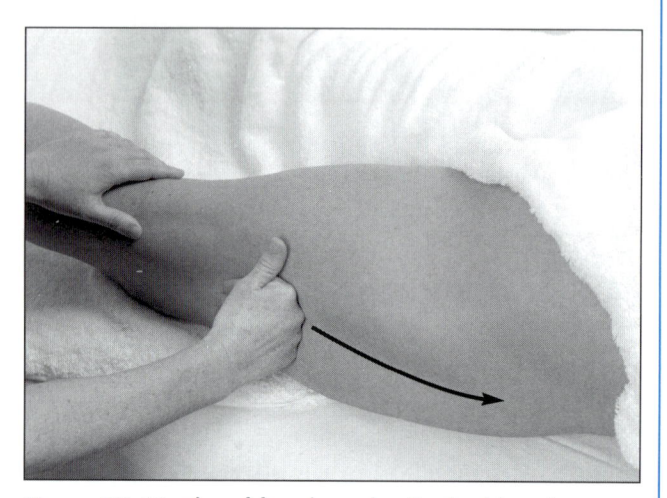

Figure 18.53 Flat of fist along the iliotibial band

45. Rowing stroke to finish the thigh

Therapist posture: Stride stance standing by the client's leg facing the head of the table (Figure 18.40).
Hands: The hands are placed side by side above the knees, with fingers pointing toward the top of the thigh.
Movement: The hands glide up the back of the thigh from the knee to the buttocks. As the hands reach the top of the thigh the hands branch off; the inside hand follows the inner thigh and back down, and simultaneously the outside hand glides over the buttock and back down the outside of the thigh, to meet together again at the starting point. Repeat this stroke several times (Figure 18.54).

46. Rowing stroke to the posterior leg

Therapist posture: Stride stance standing by the client's foot facing the head of the table (Figure 18.55).
Hands: The hands are placed side by side at the ankle, with fingers pointing toward the top of the leg.
Movement: The hands glide up the back of the leg from the ankle to the knee. As the hands reach the knee the hands branch off, the inside hand follows the inside of the leg and the outside hand follows the outside of the leg, returning to the starting point (Figure 18.56). Repeat this stroke several times.

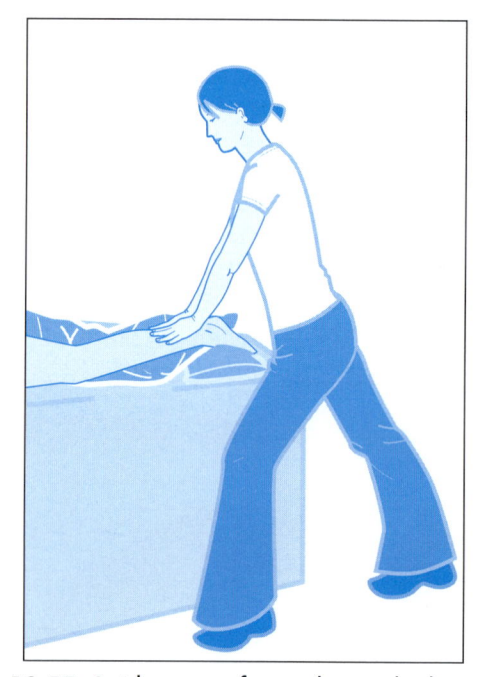

Figure 18.55 Stride stance for strokes to the leg

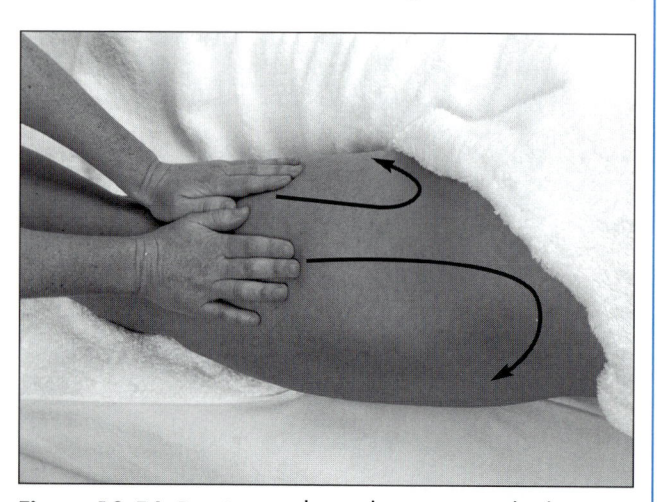

Figure 18.54 Rowing stroke to the posterior thigh

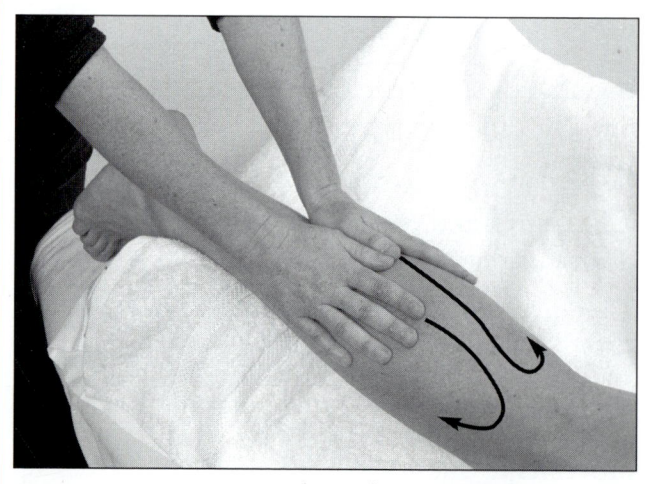

Figure 18.56 Rowing stroke to the posterior leg

47. Hand after hand with V-stroke to the posterior leg

Therapist posture: Stride stance standing by the client's foot facing the head of the table (Figure 18.55).

Hands: At the ankle, place one hand with fingers and thumb spread so that the hand wraps around the ankle, with the space between the thumb and fingers creating a 'V' shape.

Movement: This hand glides up the leg for a short distance followed by the other hand. The top hand is lifted off as the other hand follows through and they continue to alternate as they move up the leg. At the top of the leg the hands branch off — the inside hand follows the inside of the leg and the outside hand follows the outside side of the leg, meeting together at the starting point (Figure 18.57). Repeat this stroke several times.

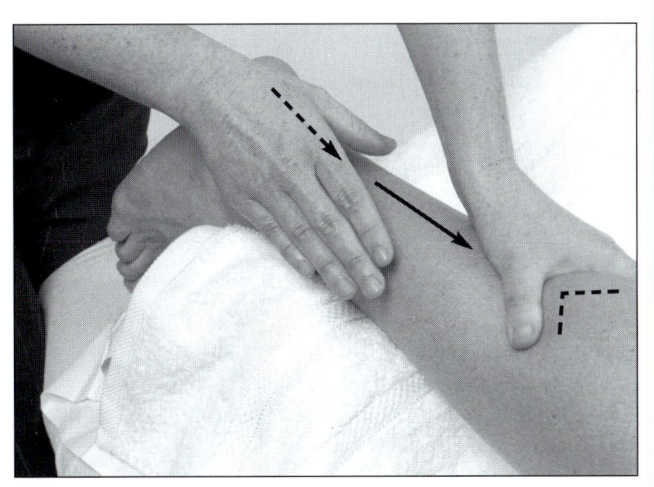

Figure 18.57 Hand after hand with V-stroke to the posterior leg

48. V-stroke to the posterior leg

Therapist posture: Stride stance at the level of the client's foot facing the head of the table (Figure 18.55).

Hands: At the ankle, place one hand with fingers and thumb spread so that the hand wraps around the ankle, with the space between the thumb and fingers creating a 'V' shape. Tuck the other hand in behind it with the same positioning so that the fingers on each hand are wrapped around opposite sides of the leg.

Movement: The hands glide up the leg with a squeezing action. At the top of the leg the hands branch off; the inside hand follows the inside of the leg and the outside hand follows the outside of the leg, meeting together at the starting point (Figure 18.58). Repeat this stroke several times.

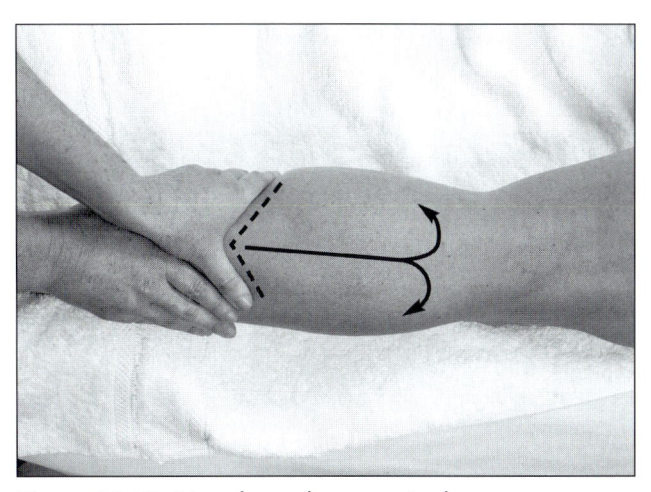

Figure 18.58 V-stroke to the posterior leg

49. C-scoop to the posterior leg

Therapist posture: Wide stance facing the client's leg (Figure 18.59).

Hands: The hands are placed on the leg facing each other with thumbs and fingers separated creating a 'C' shape.

Movement: The hands alternately glide back and forth grasping and picking up the muscle between the fingers and thumbs. This stroke is performed covering the whole surface area of the back of the leg (Figure 18.60).

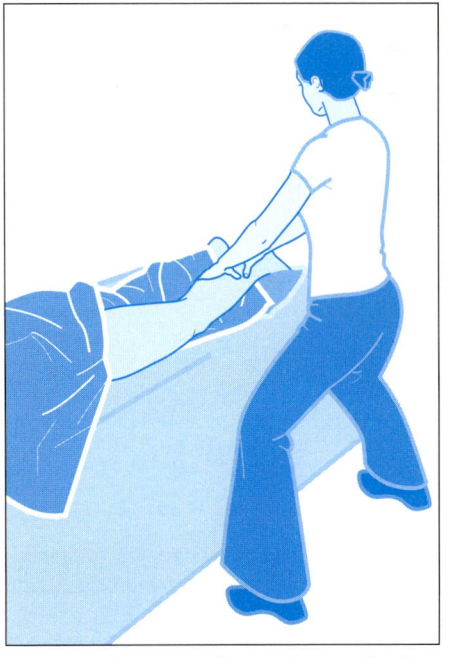

Figure 18.59 Wide stance for strokes to the leg

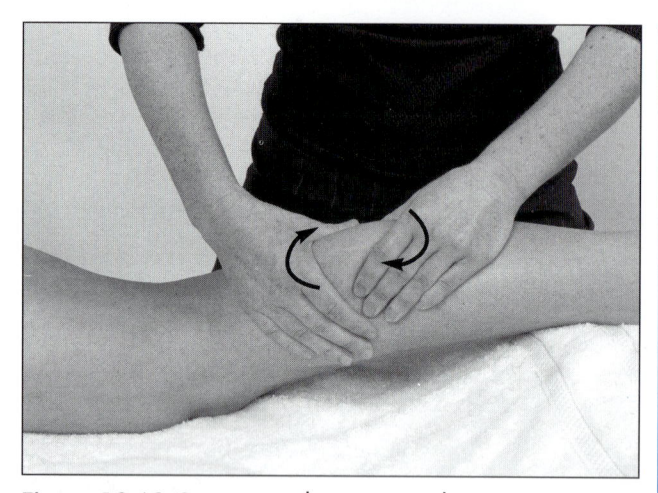

Figure 18.60 C-scoop to the posterior leg

50. Alternating circular thumb kneading to the posterior leg

Therapist posture: Stride stance at the level of the client's foot facing the head of the table (Figure 18.55).
Hands: The therapist's hands are placed on the leg with the thumbs coming together and the fingers relaxed around the leg.
Movement: The thumbs perform small alternating circular movements with the thumb pads. One thumb will circle in a clockwise direction and the other anticlockwise. This movement is performed in vertical lines moving up to cover the whole surface of the back of the leg (Figure 18.61).

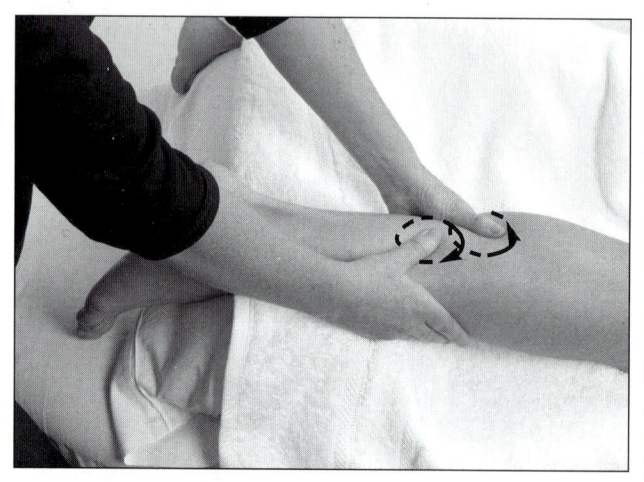

Figure 18.61 Alternating circular thumb kneading to the posterior leg

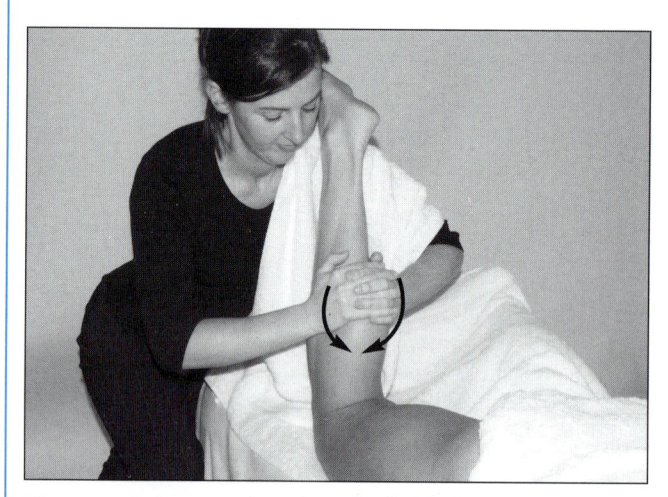

51. Two-handed palm-heel kneading to the posterior leg

Therapist posture: Wide stride stance at the level of the client's foot facing the head of the table. The therapist bends the client's knee and places the client's ankle and foot onto the therapist's shoulder (Figure 18.62).

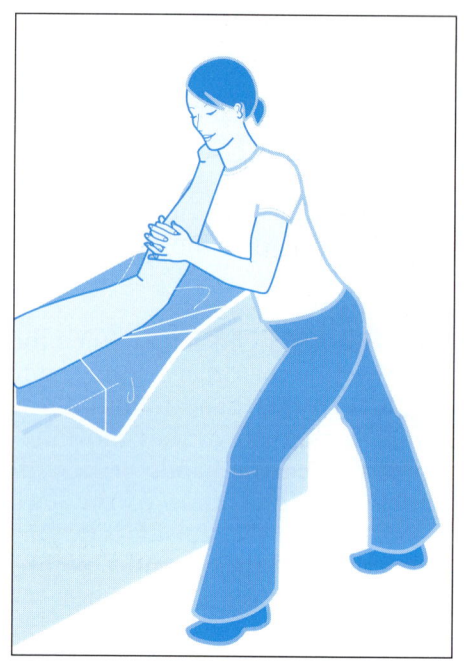

Figure 18.62 Long stride stance for two-handed palm-heel kneading to the posterior leg

Figure 18.63 Two-hand palm-heel kneading to the posterior leg

Hands: A hand towel can be used to protect the therapists clothing. The fingers of the therapist's hands are loosely interlocked with the heel of the palms resting on either side of the leg.
Movement: The pressure of this stroke is exerted from the compressive action of the heel of the hands coming together. This action is combined with a gliding action along the leg at the release of each compression. This stroke is performed covering the whole surface area of the back of the leg (Figure 18.63).

52. Shaking the calf

Therapist posture: Long stride stance at the level of the client's foot facing the head of the table. The therapist bends the client's knee and places the

CHAPTER 18 THE MASSAGE SEQUENCE 253

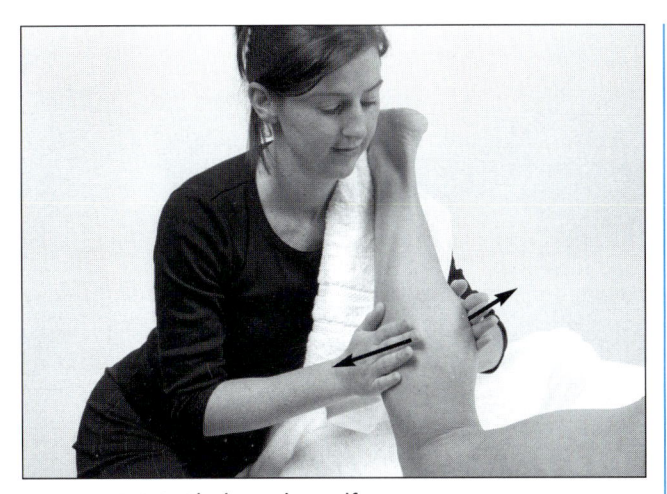

Figure 18.64 Shaking the calf

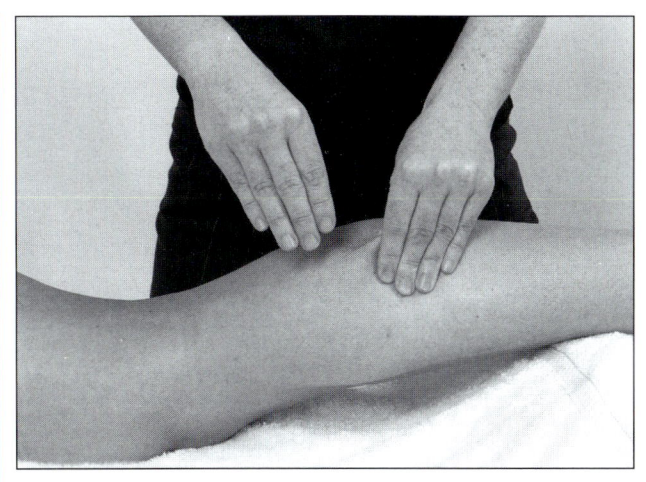

Figure 18.65b Plucking

client's ankle and foot onto the therapist's shoulder (Figure 18.62).
Hands: The therapists' hands are placed on either side of the calf muscle.
Movement: The therapist shakes the calf by rolling the calf back and forth between the hands (Figure 18.64).

28, 53 and 54. Pummelling, hacking and plucking to leg and thigh

Therapist posture: Wide stance facing the client's leg and thigh (Figure 18.45).

Hands

Pummelling: With both hands forming loose fists, place them close together on the thigh (little finger side down) (Figure 18.65a).
Hacking: Both hands are open and fingers relaxed and spread on the thigh, little finger side face down (see hacking on the back, Figure 18.33).
Plucking: The superficial tissues of the thigh are picked up between the thumb and first two fingers (Figure 18.65b).
Movement: Using an even rhythm, alternately raise the hands up and down to contact the thigh and spring back off. The contact with the thigh and leg should be firm and quick.

31. Nerve stroke

Therapist posture: Stride stance standing by the client's foot facing the head of the table (Figure 18.37).
Hands: Place both hands lightly on the top of the thigh.
Movement: Both hands start at the top of the thigh and the finger pads alternately draw down the limb in light feather-like strokes.

Foot

55. Superficial stroking over the base of the foot

Therapist posture: With a wide stance, the therapist stands at the base of the massage table facing the client's foot (Figure 18.66).
Hands: Place one hand on the base of the foot.
Movement: Apply lubricant with gliding strokes to cover the surface of the base of the foot.

56. Alternating circular thumb kneading around the heel and base of the foot

Therapist posture: Wide stance at the foot of the table (Figure 18.66).
Hands: The therapist's hands are placed around the foot with the thumbs coming together at the heel.
Movement: The thumbs perform small alternating circular movements with the thumb pads; one thumb will circle in a clockwise direction and the other anticlockwise. This movement is performed around the base of the heel and then moves over the whole surface of the base of the foot (Figure 18.67).

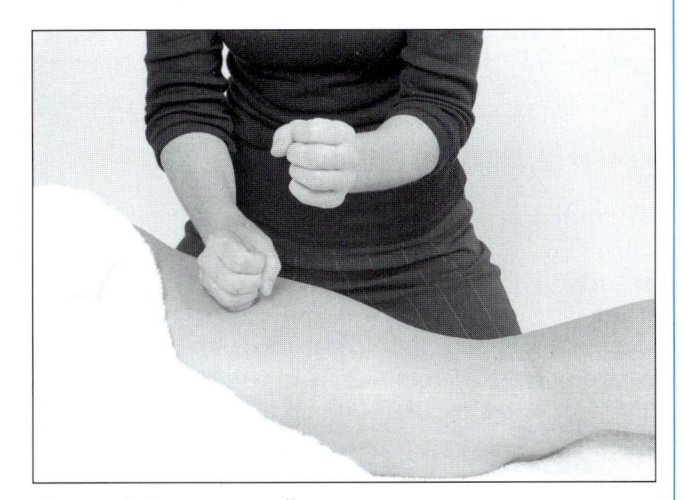

Figure 18.65a Pummelling

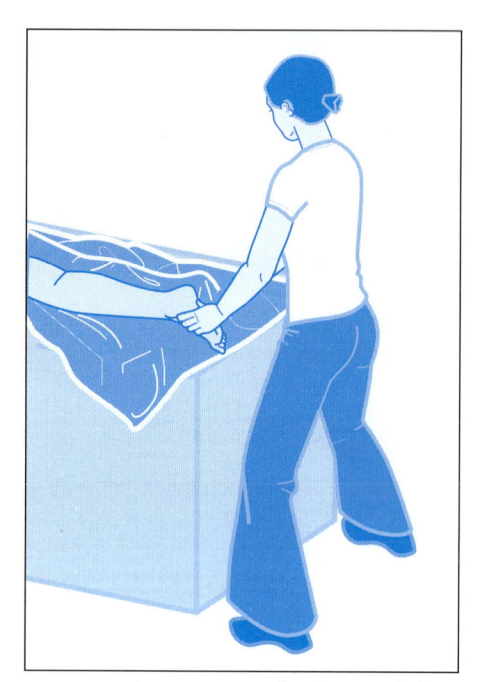

Figure 18.66 Wide stance at the base of the massage table

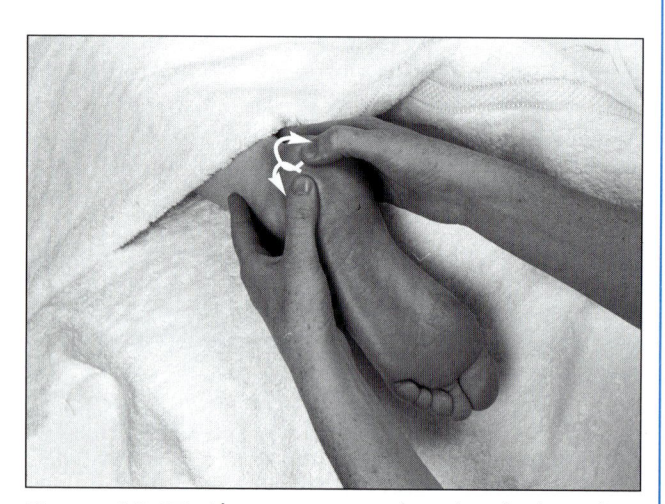

Figure 18.67 Alternating circular thumb kneading around the heel and base of the foot

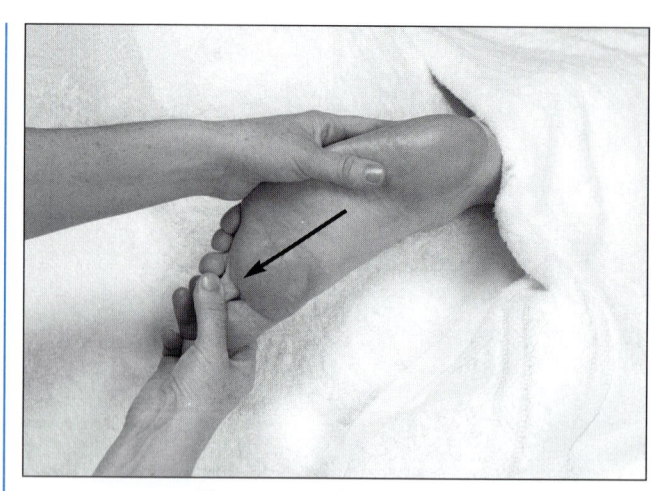

Figure 18.68 Effleurage each ray of the foot finishing at the toes

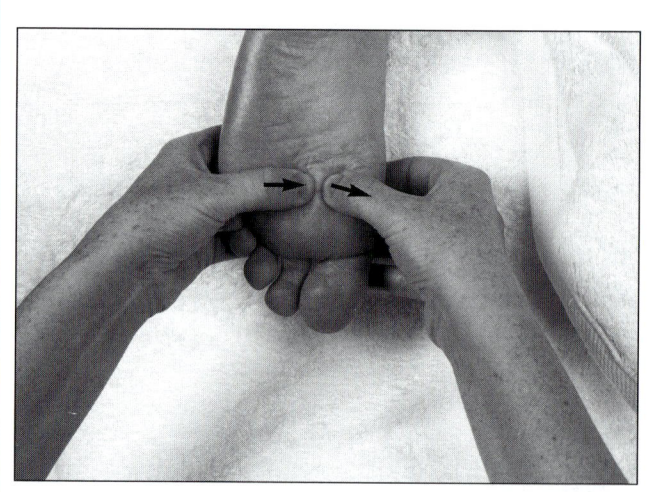

Figure 18.69 Mobilise each ray of the foot

57. Effleurage each ray of the foot finishing at the toes

Therapist posture: Wide stance at the foot of the table (Figure 18.66).
Hands: Fingers reach around the front of the foot and the thumbs rest on the base.
Movement: Slide the fingers along each ray of the foot (the rays are the bones of the foot that lead to the toes, also referred to as metatarsals). When the toe is reached, rotate and squeeze as you move down the toe. Repeat this to each ray of the foot and to each toe (Figure 18.68).

58. Mobilise each ray of the foot

Therapist posture: Wide stance at foot of table (Figure 18.66).

Hands: Fingers reach around to the front of the foot and the thumbs rest on the sole. The fingers and thumb of the mobilising hand grasp each side of the ray to be manipulated. The other hand stabilises the foot to prevent any movement occurring from the other rays.
Movement: The fingers grasp the first ray and mobilise by pushing the ray back and forth. This is repeated several times before moving on to another ray (Figure 18.69). Repeat movement to each ray of foot.

59. Fist rolling to the base of the foot

Therapist posture: Wide stance at the foot of the table (Figure 18.66).
Hands: The therapist's hand supports around the front of the foot while the other hand makes a fist. Push the fist into the arch of the foot.
Movement: Rotate the fist and compress it into the arch as the fist rotates (Figure 18.70).

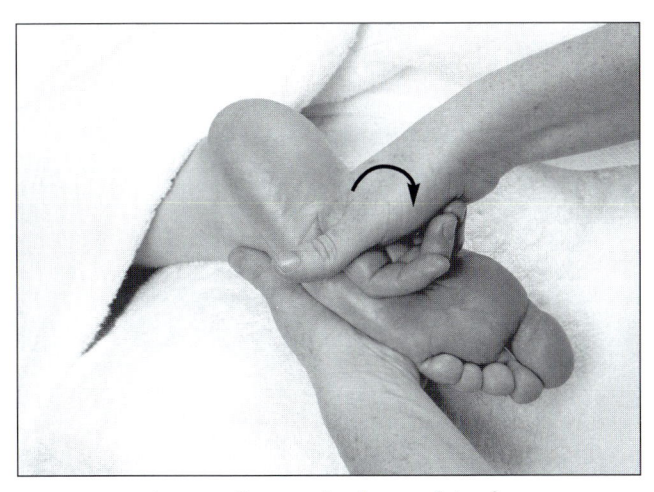

Figure 18.70 Fist rolling to the base of the foot

60. Chafe along the midline of the foot with the side of the hand

Therapist posture: Wide stance at foot of table (Figure 18.66).
Hands: Place a supporting hand underneath the foot to prevent movement. The ulnar side (little finger side) of the other hand is placed on the foot at a diagonal across the arch of the foot.
Movement: Rapidly chafe the foot with the side of the hand, as in a sawing movement (Figure 18.71).

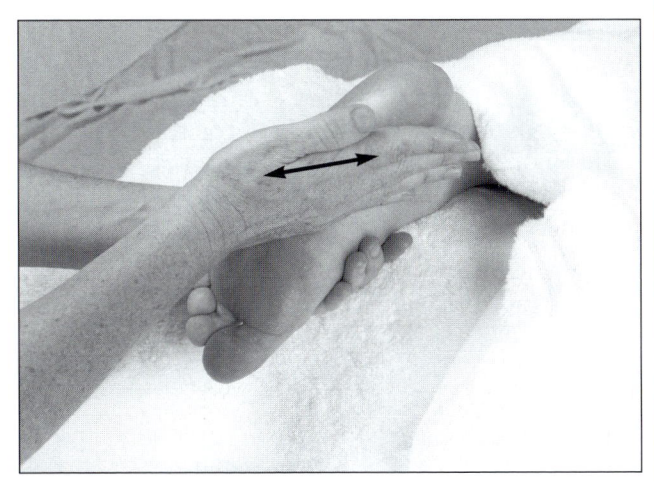

Figure 18.71 Chafe along the midline of the foot with the side of the hand

Anterior lower limb

Client positioning: The client is lying in supine position with a pillow at the head and under the knees for support and comfort.
Draping: The limb that is to be massaged is undraped and secured under the thigh (refer to Chapter 15, Figures 15.3d and 15.3e, for draping procedures).

61. Rowing stroke to the anterior thigh and leg

Therapist posture: The therapist stands at the side of the massage table at the level of the client's feet, in long stride stance facing the head of the table (Figure 18.37).
Hands: Place the hands on the muscles on either side of the tibia (shinbone), near the ankle. The fingers point toward the head of the table.
Movement: Lunge forward and apply pressure gliding over these muscles, glide around the patella (kneecap) onto the quadriceps. As the hands reach the top of the thigh the hands branch off — the inside hand follows the inner thigh and back down the inner leg, while simultaneously the outside hand glides over the hip and back down the lateral side of the thigh and leg, meeting together at the starting point. Repeat this stroke several times (Figure 18.72).

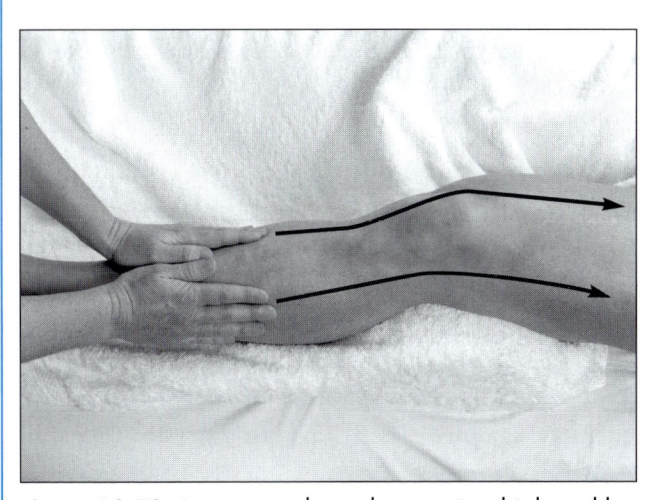

Figure 18.72 Rowing stroke to the anterior thigh and leg

62. Half rowing stroke to the anterior thigh and leg

Therapist posture: The therapist stands at the side of the massage table at the level of the client's feet, in long stride stance facing the head of the table (Figure 18.37).
Hands: The therapist's leading hand is the one closer to the client's leg. This hand is placed at the client's ankle with the fingers pointing toward the top of the leg. The other hand sits on top of this hand to reinforce the stroke.
Movement: The reinforced hands glide up the muscle on the outside of the tibia, around the outside of the patella and onto the quadriceps. As the hands reach the hip they curve and glide down the outside of the thigh and leg, returning to the starting point (Figure 18.73). Repeat this stroke several times.

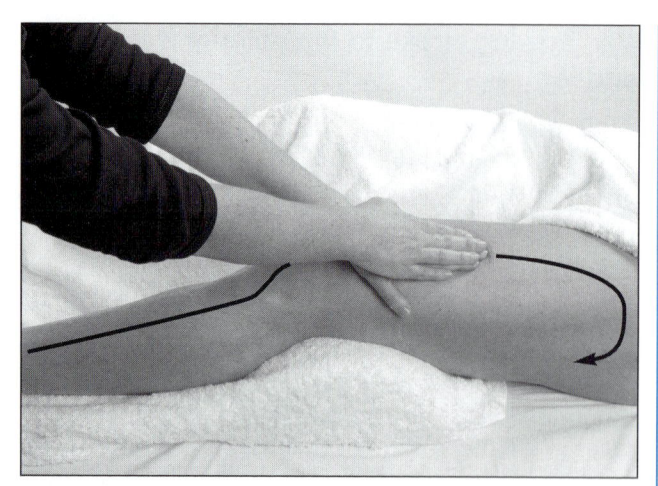

Figure 18.73 Half rowing stroke to the anterior thigh and leg

Front of thigh

63. Hand after hand to the anterior thigh

Therapist posture: Stride stance facing the head of the table standing by the client's leg (Figure 18.40).
Hands: Place one hand with fingers pointing to the top of the thigh just above the knee.
Movement: This hand glides up the thigh for a short distance followed by the other hand; the top hand is lifted off as the other hand follows through and they continue to alternate as they move up the thigh. At the hip both hands come together in the reinforced position (i.e. the hand closer to the client's body sits below the other hand) and glide down the side of the thigh to return to the starting position (Figure 18.74). This can be repeated several times.

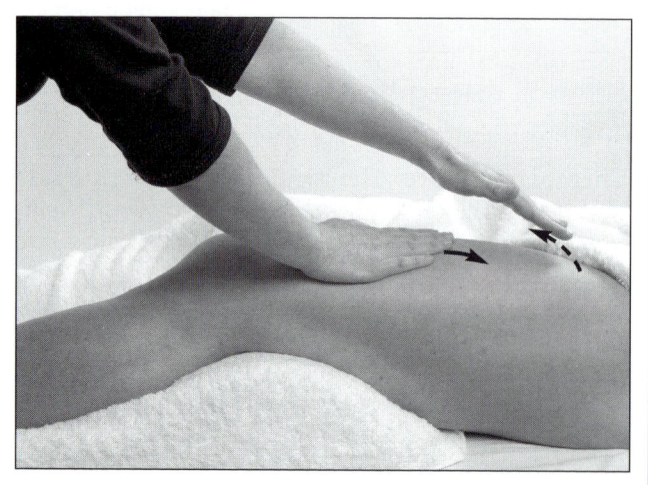

Figure 18.74 Hand after hand to the anterior thigh

64. Side pulls to the anterior inner thigh

Therapist posture: Stride stance at an angle facing the client's opposite foot (Figure 18.42).
Hands: Place one hand on the inner thigh at the knee.
Movement: This stroke is performed to the inner thigh only. Glide one hand across to the midline of the thigh. As this hand reaches the midline the other hand follows the same path to create a continuous flowing stroke that moves up and down the inner thigh (Figure 18.75).

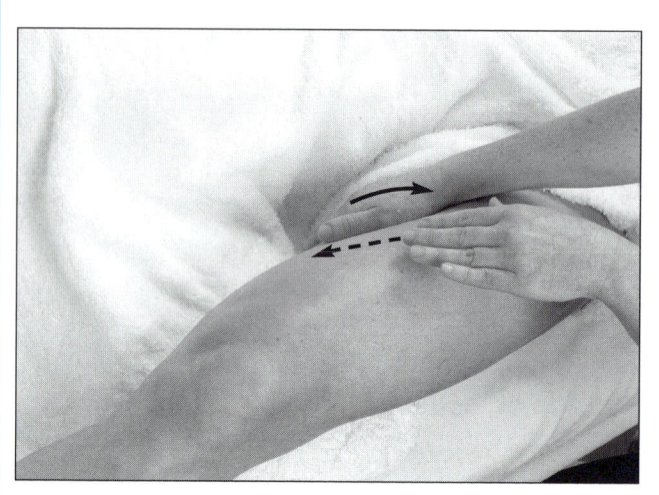

Figure 18.75 Side pulls to the anterior inner thigh

65. Wringing the anterior thigh

Therapist posture: Stride stance at an angle facing client's opposite foot (Figure 18.42).
Hands: Start at the level of the knee with one hand on the inside of the thigh and the other on the outside.
Movement: Glide the hands across the thigh; the hands cross paths in the middle of the thigh and glide to opposite sides. Progress this pattern up the length of the thigh and back down to the starting position (Figure 18.76).

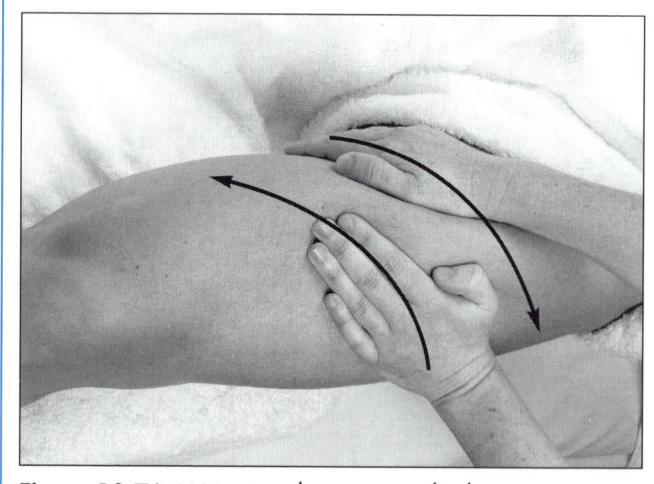

Figure 18.76 Wringing the anterior thigh

66. Reinforced broad circular kneading to the inner thigh

Therapist posture: Stride stance at an angle facing the client's opposite foot (Figure 18.42).

Hands: Starting at the level of the knee, place one hand on the inside of the thigh and the other hand resting on top to provide support and strength to the stroke. The whole hand remains in contact with the thigh throughout this stroke.
Movement: The reinforced hands perform broad sweeping circles over the inner thigh in an anticlockwise direction (Figure 18.77).

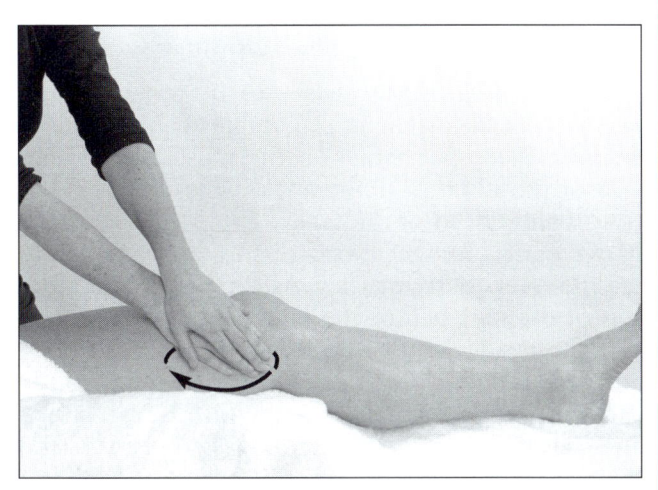

Figure 18.77 Reinforced broad circular kneading to the inner thigh

67. C-scoop to the anterior thigh

Therapist posture: The therapist stands in wide stance facing the side of the massage table at the level of the client's thigh (Figure 18.45).
Hands: The hands are placed on the thigh facing each other with thumbs and fingers separated, creating a 'C' shape.
Movement: The hands alternately glide back and forth grasping and picking up the muscle between the fingers and thumbs. This stroke is performed covering the whole surface area of the front of the thigh (Figure 18.78).

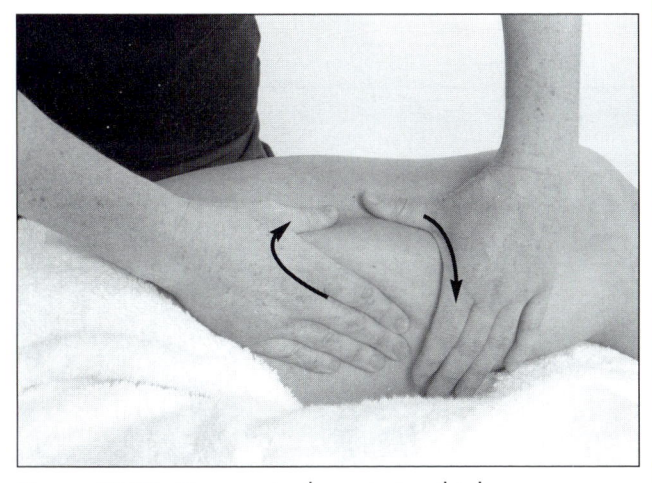

Figure 18.78 C-scoop to the anterior thigh

68. Two-handed palm-heel kneading to the anterior thigh

Therapist posture: Long stride stance at the lower limb facing the head of the table (Figure 18.47).
Hands: The fingers of the therapist's hands are loosely interlocked with the heel of the palms resting on the thigh.
Movement: The pressure of this stroke is exerted from the compressive action of the heel of the hands pressing together. This action is combined with a gliding action up the thigh at the release of each compression. This stroke is performed covering the whole surface area of the front of the thigh (Figure 18.79).

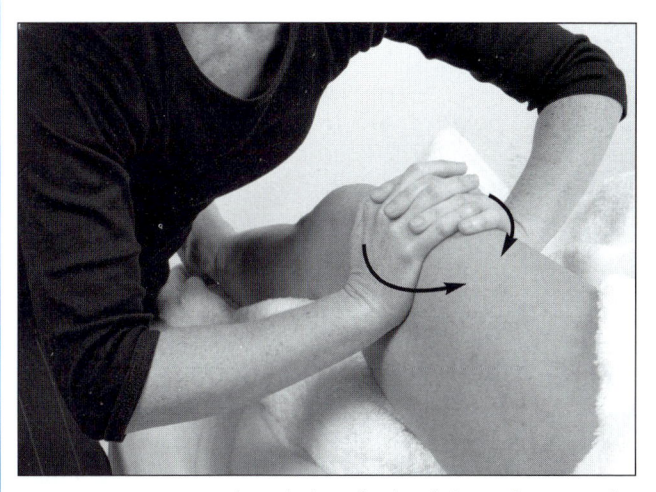

Figure 18.79 Two-handed palm-heel kneading to the anterior thigh

69. Reinforced circular finger kneading to the anterior thigh

Therapist posture: Stride stance at the level of the client's leg facing the head of table (Figure 18.40).
Hands: The therapist's hand that is closer to the client's body is placed on the thigh, with the fingers

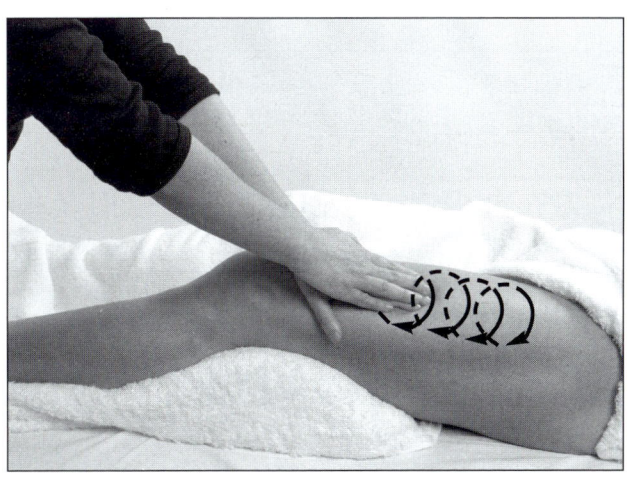

Figure 18.80 Reinforced circular finger kneading to the anterior thigh

facing toward the head of the table. The other hand rests on top to provide support and strength to the stroke. The whole hand remains in contact with the thigh throughout this stroke but the emphasis of the stroke is placed on the finger pads.
Movement: The finger pads move in a small circle away from the inner thigh. Pressure of the stroke is emphasised at the top of the circle and lightens as the fingers complete the circle to return to the starting position. This movement is continued along the length of the thigh. At the top of the thigh both hands come together in the reinforced position and glide down the side of the thigh to the starting position (Figure 18.80). This can be repeated several times.

70. Alternating circular thumb kneading to the anterior thigh

Therapist posture: Stride stance at the level of the client's leg facing the head of table (Figure 18.40).
Hands: The therapist's hands are placed over the thigh with the thumbs together and the fingers relaxed around the thigh.
Movement: Using the thumb pads perform small alternating circles. One thumb circles in a clockwise direction and the other anticlockwise. This movement is performed in vertical lines going up the thigh to cover the whole surface of the front of the thigh (Figure 18.81). For access to the top of the thigh and inner thigh the therapist's fingers may need to be tucked into the palm.

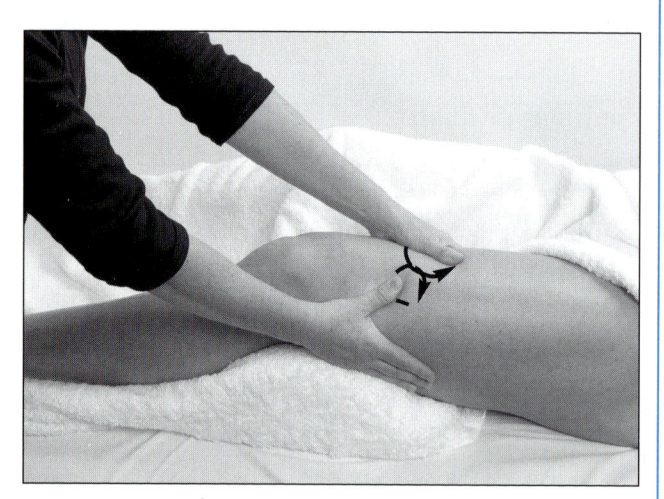

Figure 18.81 Alternating circular thumb kneading to the anterior thigh

71. Long hand after hand to the anterior thigh

Therapist posture: Stride stance at the level of the client's leg facing the head of the table (Figure 18.40).
Hands: Place one hand above the knee with fingers pointing to the top of the thigh.

Movement: This hand glides up the length of the thigh from the top of the knee to the hip. The other hand follows the same path of movement once the first hand has reached the hip. The hands alternate to create a continuous flowing movement (Figure 18.82).

Front of leg

72. Rowing stroke to the anterior leg

Therapist posture: Stride stance at the level of the client's foot facing the head of table (Figure 18.55).
Hands: Place the hands on the muscles on either side of the tibia, near the ankle. The fingers point towards the head of the table.
Movement: Lunge forward and apply pressure gliding over these muscles. As the hands reach the top of the leg (before the knee) the hands branch off, the inside hand follows the inside of the leg and travels back down to the ankle. Simultaneously the outside hand glides over the outside of the leg and travels down to meet the other hand at the ankle. Repeat this stroke several times (Figure 18.83).

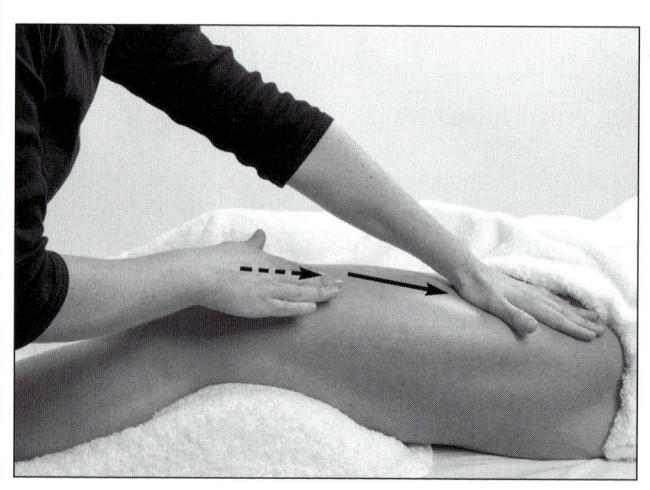

Figure 18.82 Long hand after hand to the anterior thigh

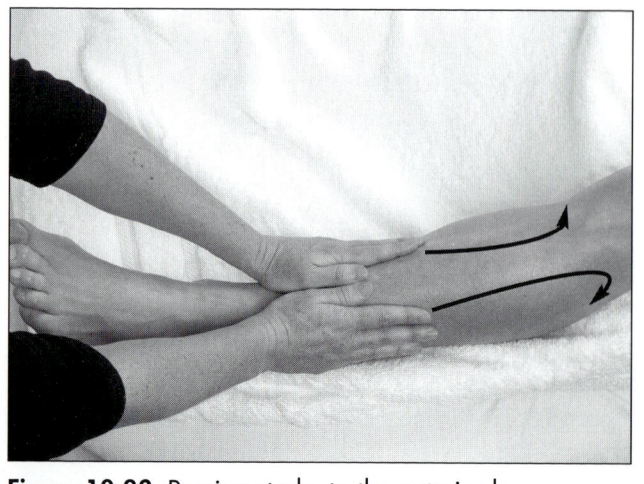

Figure 18.83 Rowing stroke to the anterior leg

73. Hand after hand with V-stroke to the anterior leg

Therapist posture: Stride stance at the level of the client's foot facing the head of the table (see Figure 18.55).
Hands: At the ankle, place one hand with fingers and thumb spread so that the hand wraps around the ankle, with the space between the thumb and fingers creating a V-shape.
Movement: This hand glides up the leg for a short distance followed by the other hand; the top hand is lifted off as the other hand follows through and they continue to alternate as they move up the leg. At the top of the leg the hands branch off — the inside hand follows the inside of the leg and the outside hand follows the outside side of the leg, meeting together at the starting point (Figure 18.84). Repeat this stroke several times.

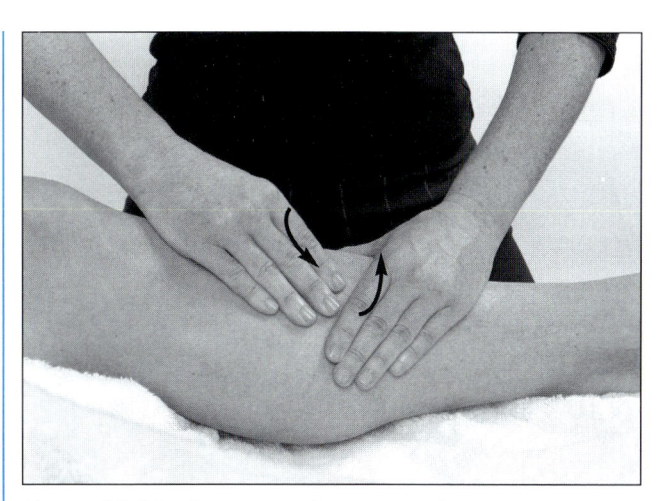

Figure 18.85 C-scoop to the anterior leg

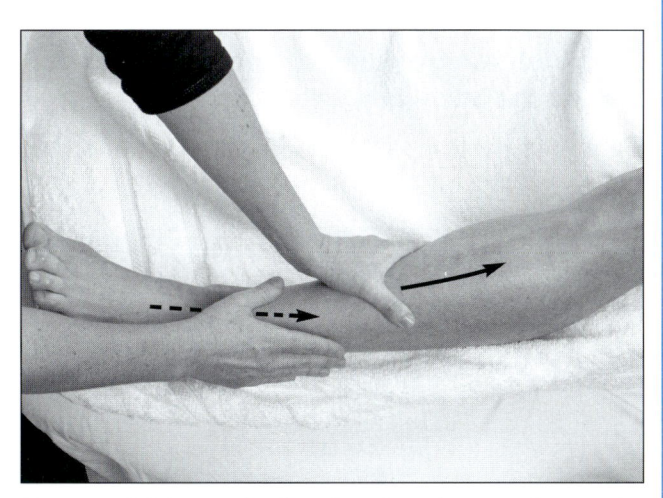

Figure 18.84 Hand after hand with V-stroke to the anterior leg

74. C-scoop to the anterior leg

Therapist posture: Wide stance facing the client's leg (see Figure 18.59).
Hands: The hands are placed on the leg facing each other with thumbs and fingers separated creating a 'C' shape.
Movement: The hands alternately glide back and forth grasping and picking up the muscle between the fingers and thumbs. This stroke is performed covering the whole surface area of the front of the leg (Figure 18.85).

75. Alternating circular thumb kneading to the muscles on the outside of the leg

Therapist posture: Stride stance at the level of the client's foot facing the head of the table (Figure 18.55).
Hands: The therapist's hands are placed on the muscle on the outside of the leg (lateral to the tibia)

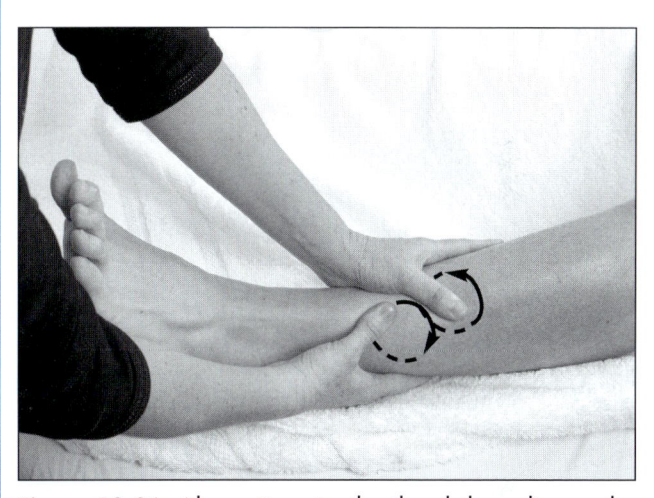

Figure 18.86 Alternating circular thumb kneading to the muscles on the outside of the leg

with the thumbs coming together and the fingers relaxed around the leg.
Movement: The thumbs perform small alternating circular movements with the thumb pads. One thumb will circle in a clockwise direction and the other anticlockwise. This movement is performed in a vertical line moving up to cover the length of the leg (Figure 18.86).

Bend knee and gently sit on foot

The therapist bends the client's knee to rest the foot level with the mid leg of the opposite limb (Figure 18.87a). The therapist then folds the drape over the client's foot and sits on the foot on the edge of the table to prevent movement of the leg (Figure 18.87b)

76. Rolling the calf

Therapist posture: The therapist sits at the edge of the massage table (Figure 18.87c).
Hands: The outside hand supports the knee to prevent the thigh from turning out. The inside forearm sits below the calf muscle. The hand should

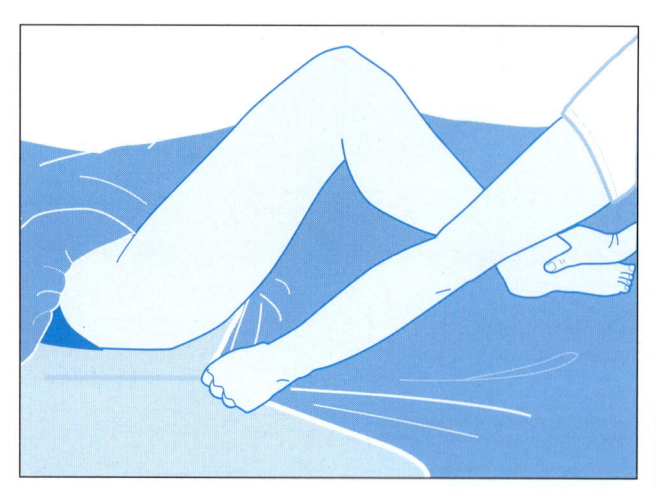

Figure 18.87a Drape and limb positions to manage bent knee

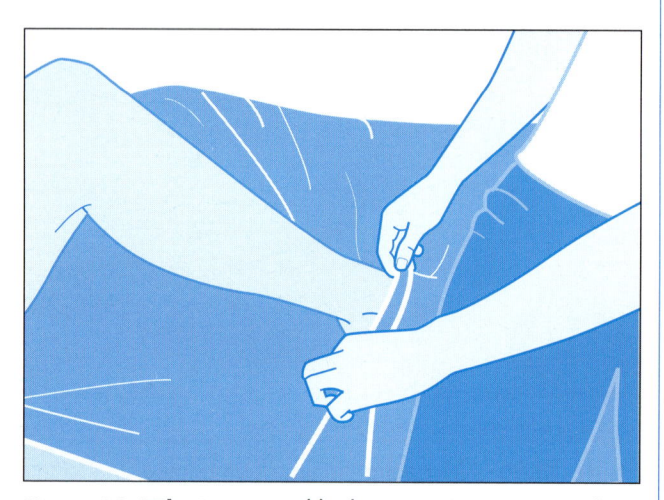

Figure 18.87b Drape and limb positions to manage bent knee

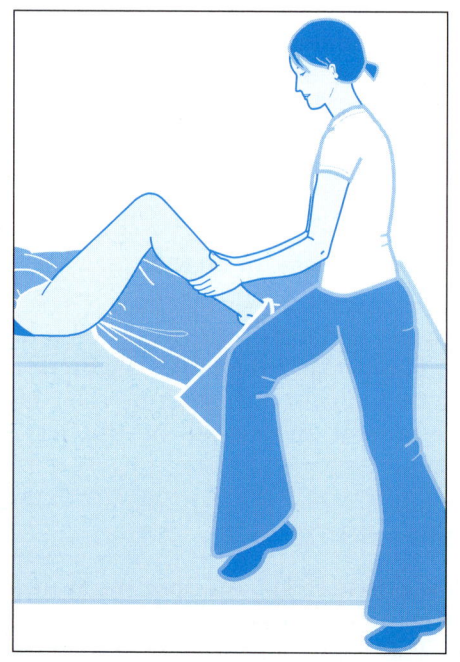

Figure 18.87c Drape and limb positions to manage bent knee

remain relaxed throughout the movement to allow the forearm flexors to remain soft in its contact with the calf muscle.

Movement: Slide the forearm up the calf with pressure on the outside of the muscle and return in a sweeping action down the calf with pressure on the inside of the muscle. Repeat this rolling action several times (Figure 18.88).

77. Split the calf

Therapist posture: The therapist sits at the edge of the massage table (Figure 18.87c).
Hands: Wrap both hands around the base of the calf muscle with the fingertips meeting at the midline.
Movement: The fingertips split the calf by pulling the muscle away from the centre and gliding to the edge of the muscle. Reposition higher up the leg and repeat the technique along the length of the leg (Figure 18.89).

78. Alternating circular thumb kneading around the knee joint

Therapist posture: The therapist sits at the edge of the massage table (Figure 18.87c).

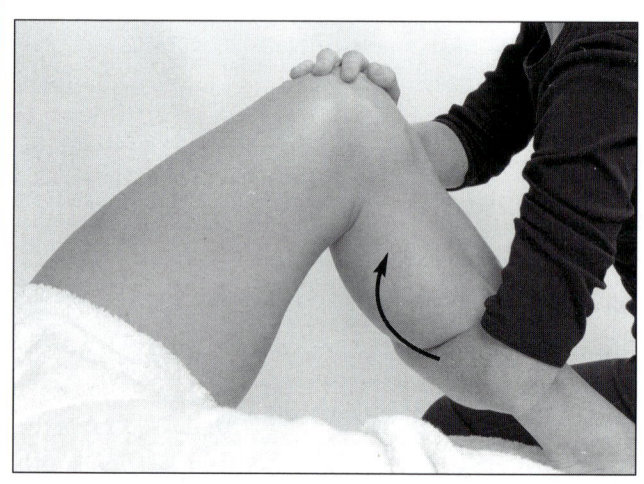

Figure 18.88 Rolling the calf

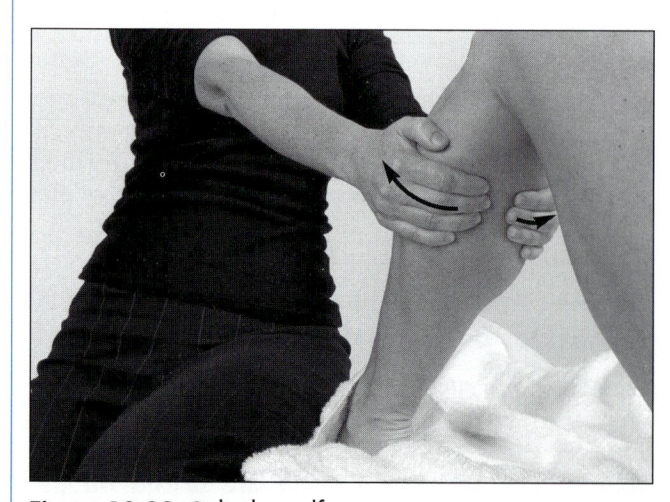

Figure 18.89 Split the calf

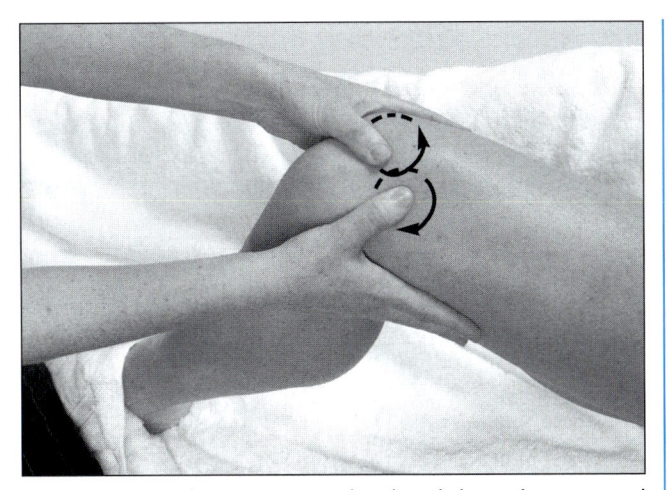

Figure 18.90 Alternating circular thumb kneading around the knee joint

Hands: Wrap both hands around the knee, with fingers spread on the underside and thumbs resting above the kneecap.
Movement: The thumbs perform small alternating circular movements with the thumb pads. One thumb will circle in a clockwise direction and the other anticlockwise. This movement is performed around the knee joint (Figure 18.90).

28, 53 and 54. Pummelling, hacking and plucking to the thigh

Therapist posture: The therapist stands at the side of the massage table at the level of the client's thigh. With wide stance, knees bent and facing the side of the table, the legs lunge from side to side as the stroke moves up and down the thigh (Figure 18.45).

Hands

Pummelling: With both hands, form loose fists and place them close together on the thigh (little finger side down) (Figure 18.65a).
Hacking: Both hands are open and fingers relaxed and spread on the thigh (see hacking in Figure 18.33).
Plucking: The superficial tissues of the thigh are picked up between the thumb and first two fingers (Figure 18.65b).
Movement: Using an even rhythm, alternately raise the hands up and down to contact the thigh and spring back off. The contact with the thigh and leg should be firm and quick.

79. Mobilise the ankle

Therapist posture: Wide stance at the base of the table (Figure 18.66).
Hands: Place the heel of the hands firmly on the sides of the foot below the ankle bones. The fingers point up the leg.
Movement: Keeping a firm contact with the side of the foot, the hands alternately and rapidly move back and forth, which shakes the client's foot from side to side (Figure 18.91).

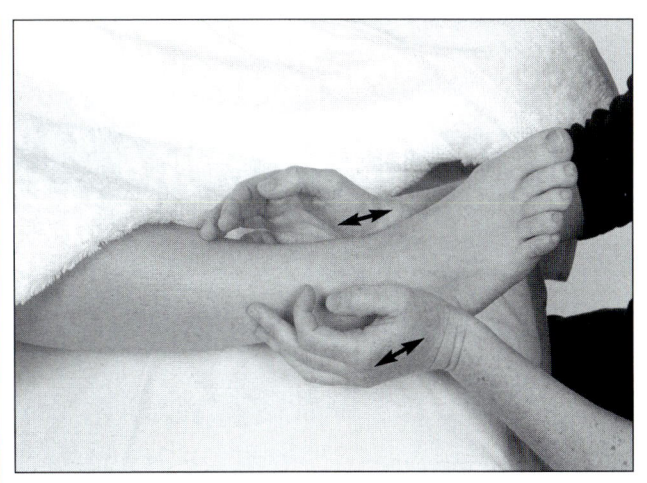

Figure 18.91 Mobilise the ankle

80. Broad compression of the foot

Therapist posture: Wide stance at the foot of the table (Figure 18.66).
Hands: Wrap the outside hand around the top of the foot. The hand should rest just below the base of the toes. The other hand forms a fist; the flat of the fist is held against the sole of the client's foot.
Movement: Compress the client's foot with the flat of the fist, hold and release and repeat. During the compression slightly relax the other hand allowing the client's foot to move backwards (Figure 18.92).

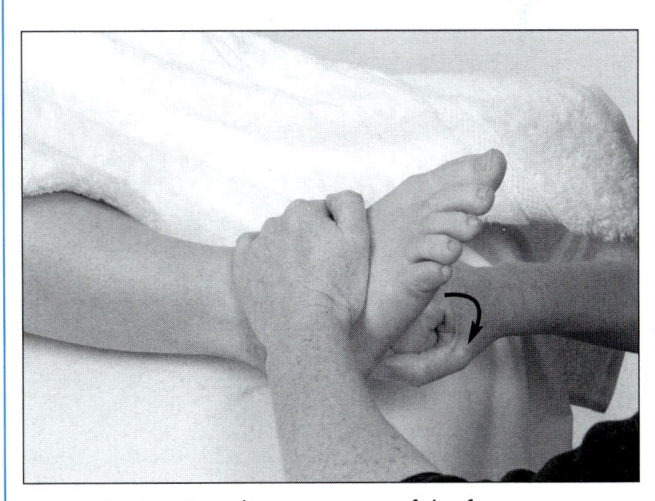

Figure 18.92 Broad compression of the foot

81. Thumb stripping between the metatarsals

Therapist posture: Wide stance at the foot of the table (Figure 18.66).
Hands: Place the thumb at the base of the toes, between the rays of the first and second toe.
Movement: Gently and slowly slide the thumb along each groove from the base of the toes as far along until bone is reached. Repeat between each ray (Figure 18.93).

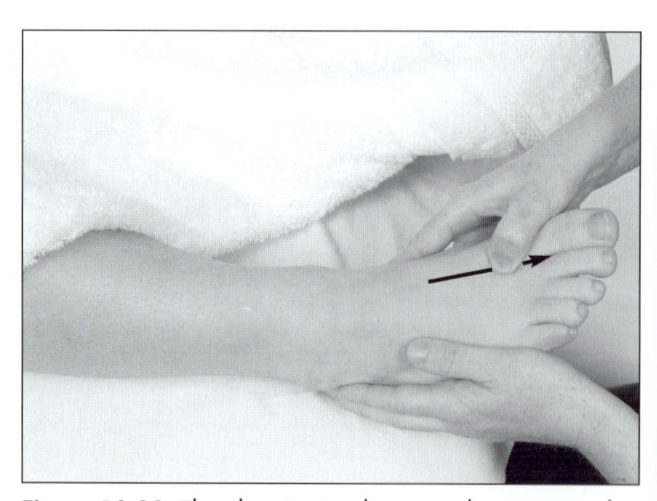

Figure 18.93 Thumb stripping between the metatarsals

82. Knead the toes

Therapist posture: Wide stance at the foot of the table (Figure 18.66).
Hands: Wrap the thumb and the first two digits around the base of a toe.
Movement: Knead around the circumference of each toe from the base to the tip. Repeat for each toe (Figure 18.94).

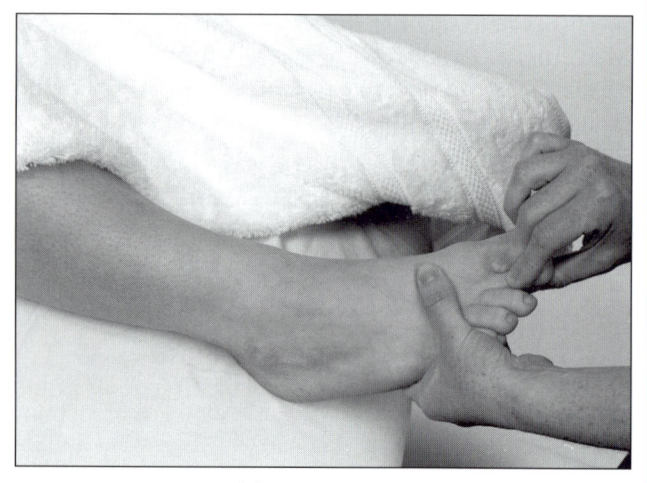

Figure 18.94 Knead the toes

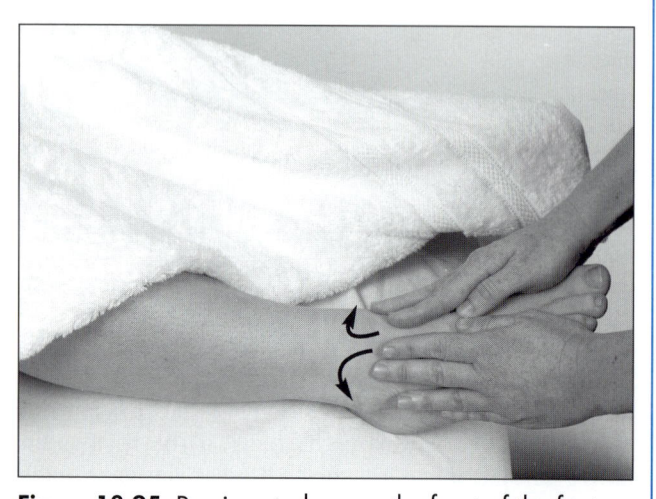

Figure 18.95 Rowing stroke over the front of the foot

83. Rowing stroke over the front of the foot

Therapist posture: Wide stance at the foot of the table (Figure 18.66).
Hands: Place your hands over the front of the foot.
Movement: Glide over the front of the foot, around the ankles and down the outside of the foot to the starting point (Figure 18.95).

Abdomen

Client positioning: The client is lying in supine position with a pillow at the head and under the knees for support and comfort.

84. Rest one hand on the abdomen and the other on the chest

Therapist posture: Wide stance facing the table at the level of the abdomen (Figure 18.96).
Hands: Place one hand on the abdomen and one on the top of the chest (Figure 18.97).
Movement: Hold the hands in this position and ask the client to take a few deep breaths.
Draping: A hand towel covers the chest and the main drape is folded back to expose the abdomen (refer to Chapter 15, Figures 15.5 and 15.6, for draping procedures).

85. Sun and moon stroke over the abdomen

Therapist posture: Wide stance facing the table at the level of the abdomen (Figure 18.96).
Hands: Place the hands on the abdomen on either side of the umbilicus with fingers facing away from the therapist.

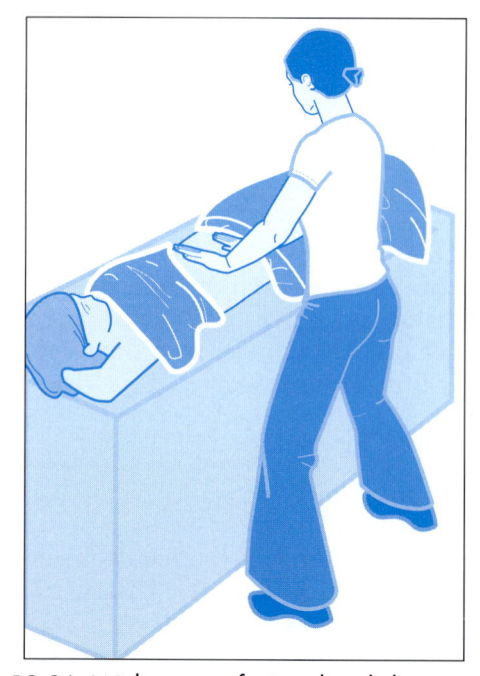

Figure 18.96 Wide stance facing the abdomen

CHAPTER 18 THE MASSAGE SEQUENCE   263

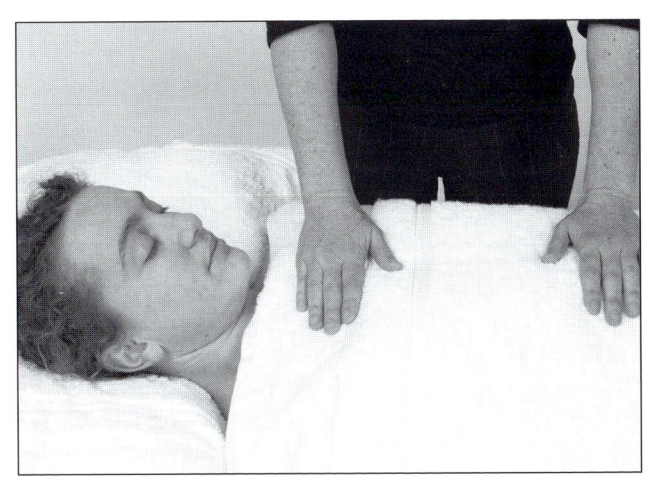

Figure 18.97 Rest one hand on the abdomen and the other on the chest

Movement: One hand performs a large continuous circular stroke in a clockwise direction below the ribs and above the pubic bone (sun). The other hand performs a half circular stroke when the hands are at opposite sides of the circle (half moon) and lifts off when it reaches the other side of the abdomen to allow the sun stroke to continue around the abdomen (Figures 18.98a and b).

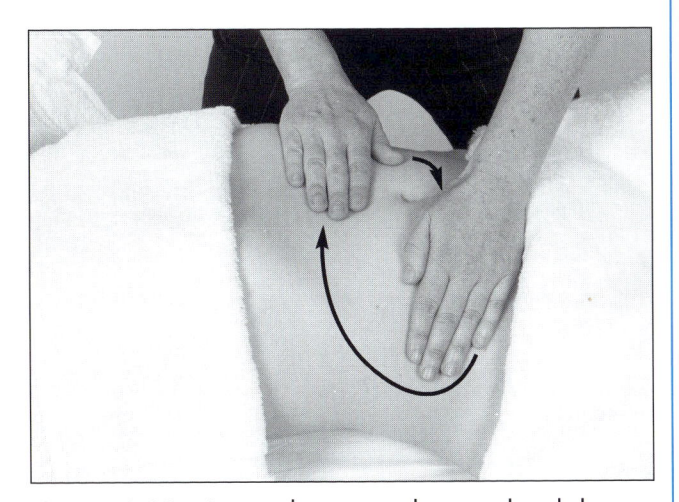

Figure 18.98a Sun and moon stroke over the abdomen

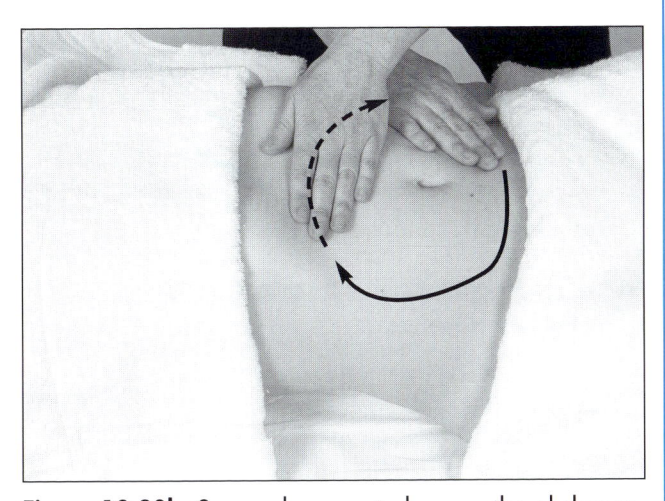

Figure 18.98b Sun and moon stroke over the abdomen

86. Hand after hand over the abdomen

Therapist posture: Stride stance standing at the level of the client's pelvis facing the client's opposite shoulder (Figure 18.99a). This stance changes during the movement to face the client's opposite hip (Figure 18.99b).

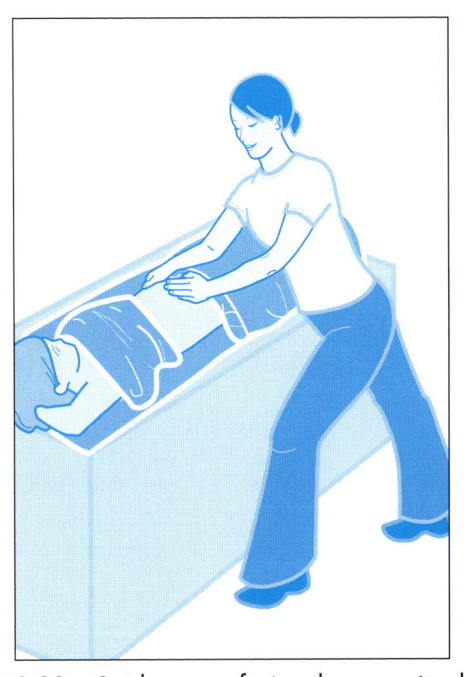

Figure 18.99a Stride stance facing the opposite shoulder

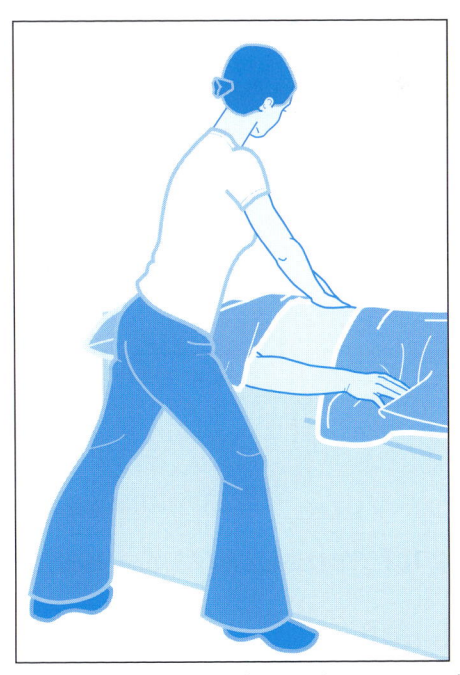

Figure 18.99b Stride stance facing the opposite hip

Hands: Place one hand on the client's waist (above the pelvis) on the opposite side.
Movement: Apply alternating palmer effleurage, in a clockwise direction in a diamond pattern using the ribs and pelvis as borders (Figure 18.100). The movement will vary between pulling toward the

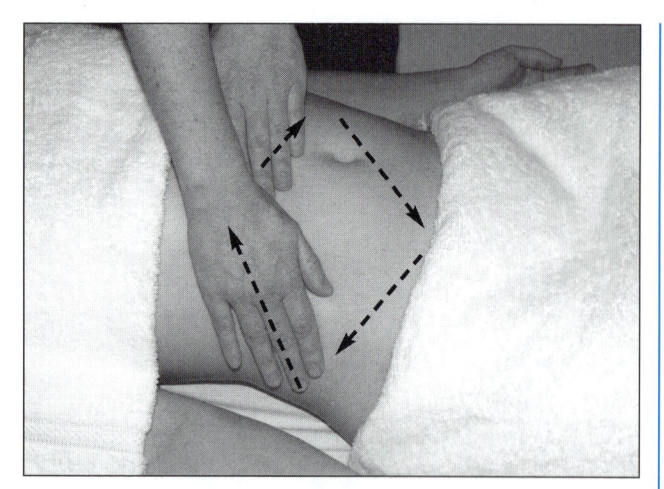

Figure 18.100 Hand after hand over the abdomen

therapist and pushing away from the therapist to maintain the movement in a clockwise direction.

87. Side pulls over the abdomen

Therapist posture: Wide stance facing the table at the level of the abdomen (Figure 18.96).
Hands: Place one hand on the client's waist (above the pelvis) on the opposite side.
Movement: Glide the hand across to the midline of the waist; as this hand reaches the midline the other hand follows the same path to create a continuous flowing stroke. Repeat this movement along the sides of the torso (Figure 18.101).

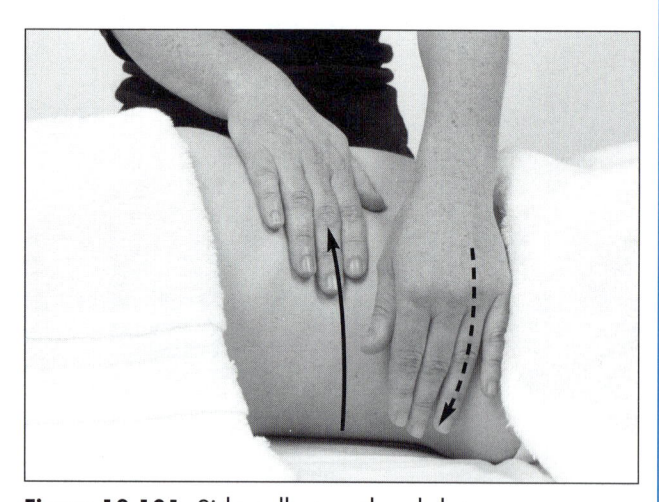

Figure 18.101 Side pulls over the abdomen

88. Rib raking

Therapist posture: Stand facing the table at the level of the hip on a slight angle facing the opposite shoulder (Figure 18.102).
Hands: Place the finger pads of one hand in the intercostal spaces of the lower ribs.
Movement: Gently stroke the finger pads between the rib spaces from the lateral aspect toward the midline (Figure 18.103).

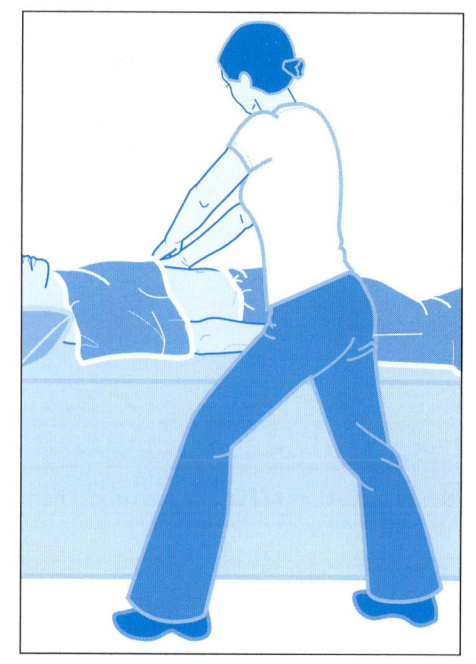

Figure 18.102 Short stride stance on an angle

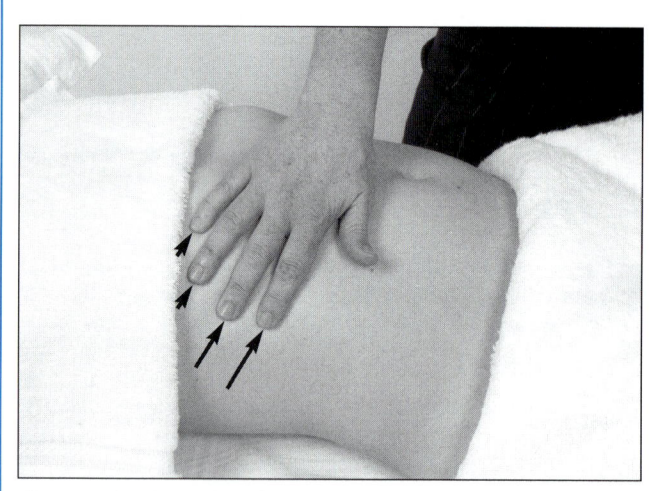

Figure 18.103 Rib raking

89. Broad circles over the ribs

Therapist posture: Stand facing the table at the level of the hip on a slight angle facing the opposite shoulder (Figure 18.102).
Hands: Place one hand over the lower ribs on the opposite side and the other hand sits on top to reinforce the stroke.
Movement: Apply broad circular strokes to cover the lower ribs; the circles should move from the midline laterally (Figure 18.104).

90. C-scoop opposite and lateral side of the abdomen

Therapist posture: Wide stance facing the table at the level of the abdomen (Figure 18.96).
Hands: The hands are placed on the side of torso facing each other with the thumbs and fingers separated creating a 'C' shape.

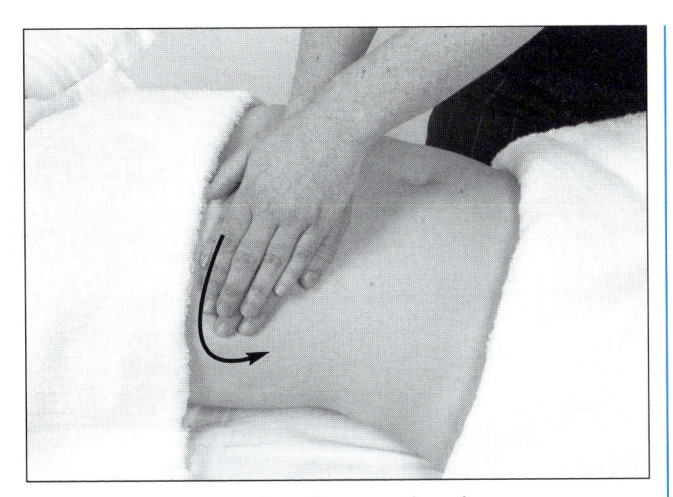

Figure 18.104 Broad circles over the ribs

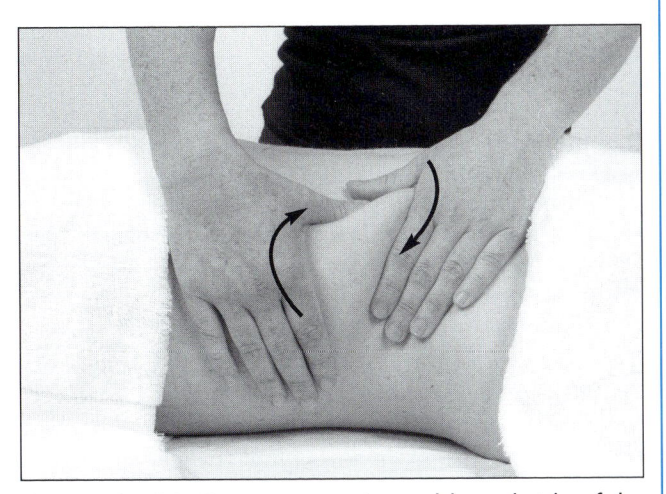

Figure 18.105 C-scoop opposite and lateral side of the abdomen

Movement: The hands alternately glide back and forth grasping and picking up the muscle between the fingers and thumbs. This stroke is performed covering the lateral side of the abdomen (Figure 18.105). Make the stroke broad and soft to prevent discomfort over the ribs.

91. Reinforced circular finger kneading over the large intestine

Therapist posture: Wide stance facing the table at the level of the abdomen (Figure 18.96).
Hands: Place a reinforced hand on the abdomen below the ribs.
Movement: Perform small circular movements with the finger pads around the abdomen in a clockwise direction (Figure 18.106).

92. Vibrations over the transverse colon

Therapist posture: Wide stance facing the table at the level of the abdomen (Figure 18.96).
Hands: The hands are placed on the abdomen below the ribs in the upper right quadrant. If the therapist is standing on the right-hand side of the body the fingers are facing toward the left side of the body. If the therapist is standing on the left-hand side of the body the fingers are pointing toward the right side of the body.
Movement: The movement travels along the transverse colon from right to left. The hands gently push into the abdomen and vibrate as they travel from one side to the other. The vibration action is achieved by contracting the forearm flexors and extensors (Figure 18.107).

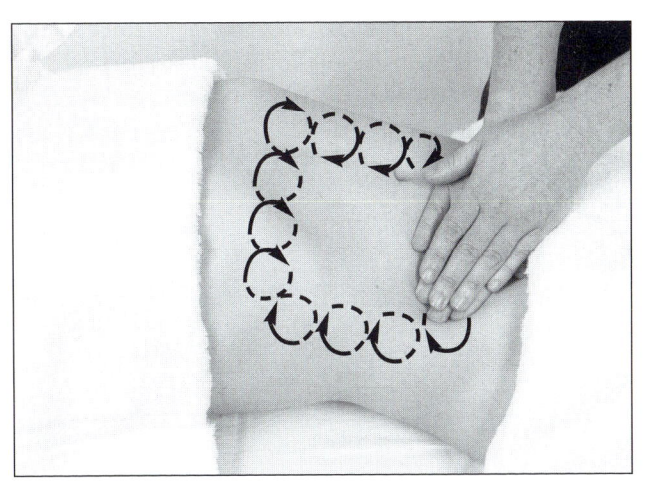

Figure 18.106 Reinforced circular finger kneading over the large intestine

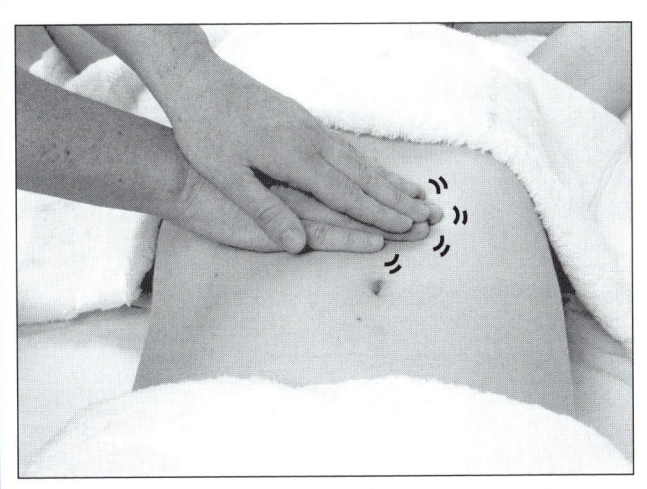

Figure 18.107 Vibrations over the transverse colon

93. Short rowing stroke lifting the low back

Therapist posture: Stride stance at the level of the client's pelvis facing the head of the table (Figure 18.3).
Hands: Place the palms on the abdomen close to the pelvis on either side of the navel with the fingers facing the head of the table.
Movement: Perform a rowing stroke over the abdomen to the lower ribs (Figure 18.108a). The hands glide outwards following the borders of the rib cage (Figure 18.108b). The fingers meet at the spine of the low back (Figure 18.108c). The hands

then lift and glide around the side of the abdomen to meet at the starting position (Figure 18.108d). The therapist should avoid their hands pinching the client's skin as they slide in under the lower back. This stroke can be repeated several times.

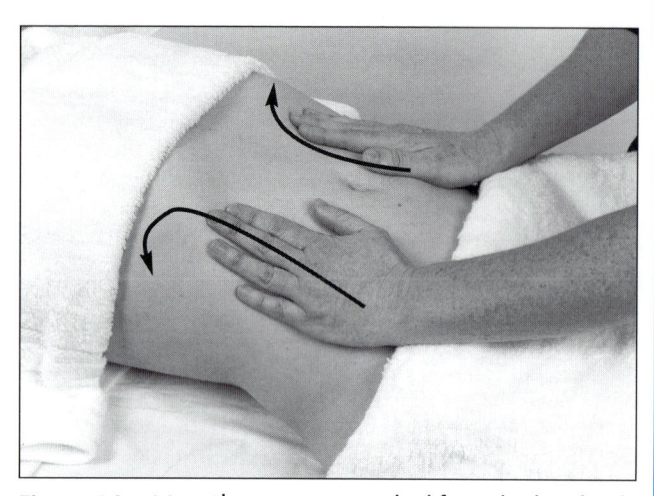

Figure 18.108a Short rowing stroke lifting the low back

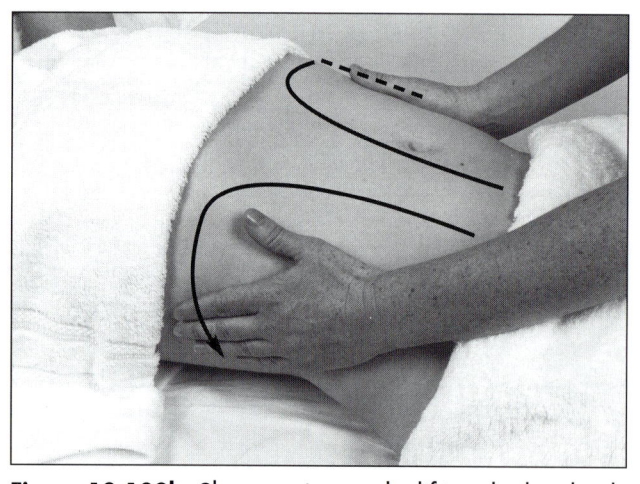

Figure 18.108b Short rowing stroke lifting the low back

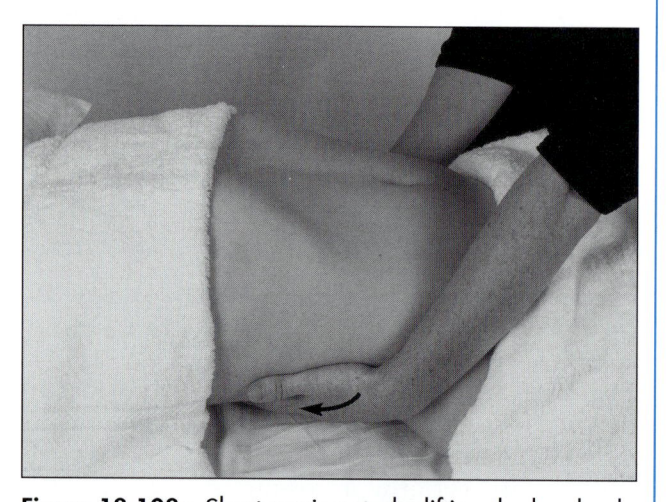

Figure 18.108c Short rowing stroke lifting the low back

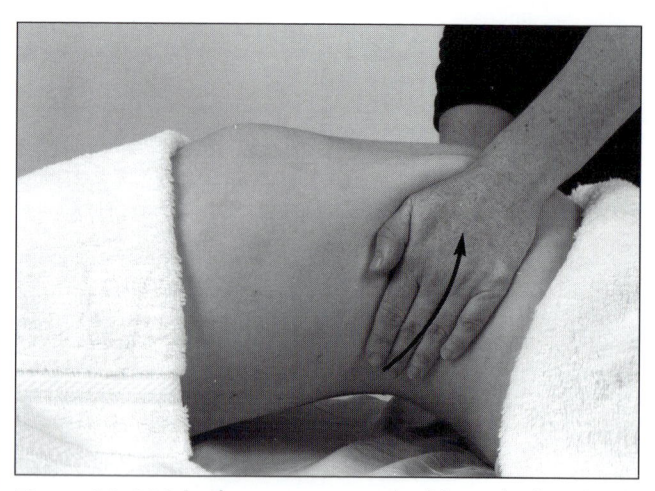

Figure 18.108d Short rowing stroke lifting the low back

Chest

Client positioning: The client is lying in supine position with a pillow at the head and under the knees for support and comfort.

Draping: The draping is folded back from the top of the chest to the axilla and anchored in under the arms (refer to Chapter 15 for draping procedures).

Therapist posture: Short stride stance facing the table at the level of the client's elbow (Figure 18.109).

Note: The therapist needs to stand on an angle facing the client's opposite shoulder to prevent their hands and arms from knocking the client on the chin. Massage is applied to the opposite side from where the therapist stands. The therapist should be aware that this area on a female is generally awkward to access. Therefore it is important that the therapist have relaxed hands that can mould

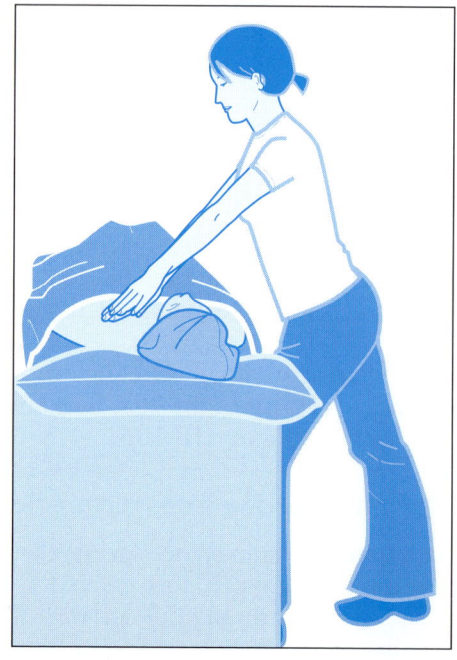

Figure 18.109 Short stride stance facing chest

easily into the area between the clavicles and the draping line.

94. Broad palmer stroke across the chest

Therapist posture: Short stride stance facing the client at the level of the client's elbow (Figure 18.109).
Hands: The hands are placed between the draping line and the clavicles on the muscles of the chest.
Movement: The aim of this stroke is to apply the oil across the top of the chest on both sides. Glide the hands across the chest in broad sweeping movements to cover the area that is about to be massaged (Figure 18.110).

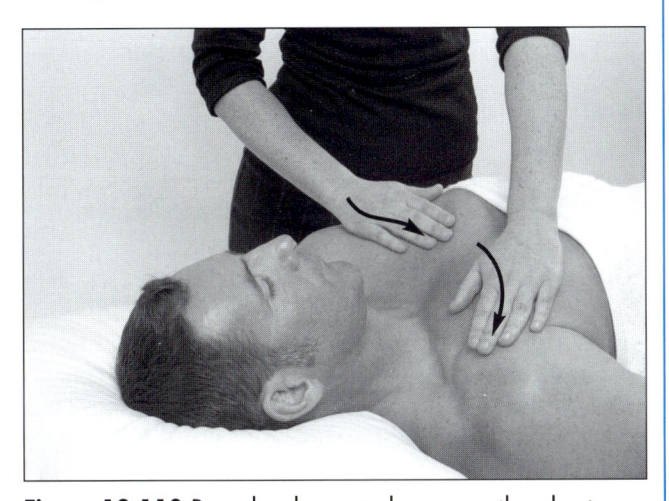

Figure 18.110 Broad palmer stroke across the chest

95. Hand after hand to the chest

Therapist posture: Short stride stance facing the client at the level of the client's elbow (Figure 18.109).
Hands: Place the palm below the clavicle on the pectoral muscle close to the sternum on the opposite side of the body.
Movement: Apply alternating gliding full palm strokes from the sternum to the shoulder. Repeat several times (Figure 18.111).

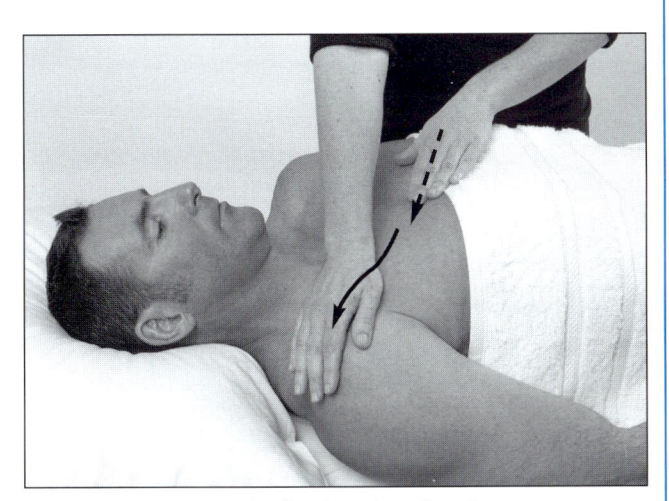

Figure 18.111 Hand after hand to the chest

96. One-handed reinforced effleurage to the chest

Therapist posture: Short stride stance facing the client at the level of the client's elbow (Figure 18.109).
Hands: Place the reinforced hands on the chest muscles of the opposite side.
Movement: With the hand glide across the pectorals, around the shoulder and behind the neck, lightly over the clavicle and then back to the pectorals (Figure 18.112). Repeat several times.

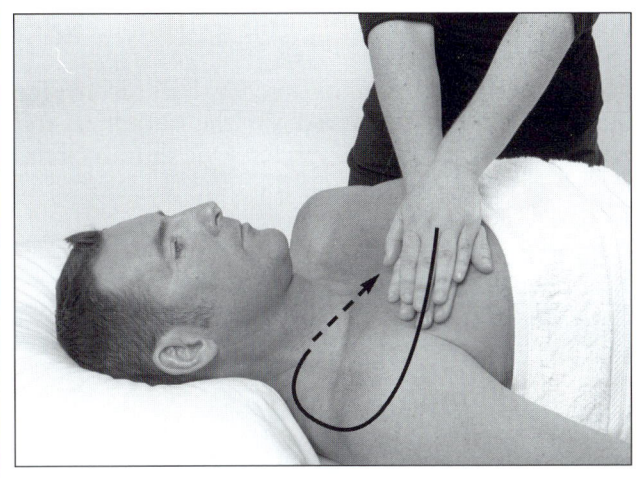

Figure 18.112 One-handed reinforced effleurage to the chest

97. Reinforced circular finger pad kneading to the chest

Therapist posture: Short stride stance facing the client at the level of the client's elbow (Figure 18.109).
Hands: Place the reinforced finger pads on the chest muscles of the opposite side. The palm of the hand needs to be lifted whilst performing this technique to prevent the hand resting on the chest of a female client.

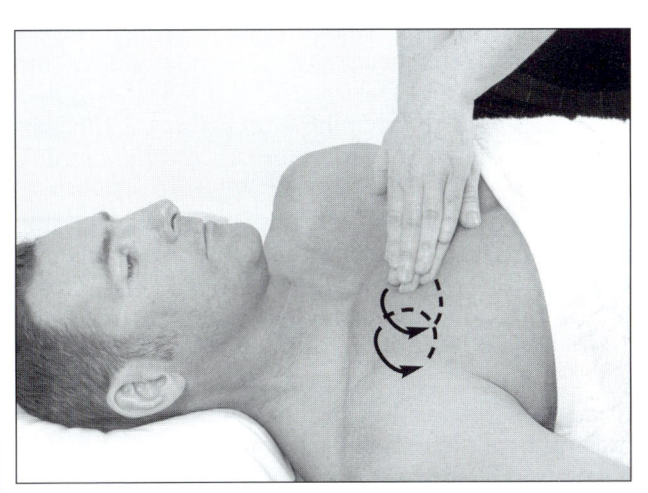

Figure 18.113 Reinforced circular finger pad kneading to the chest

Movement: Apply small circular finger pad strokes below the clavicle from the sternum to the shoulder in a clockwise direction (Figure 18.113). Repeat several times.

98. Alternating circular thumb kneading to the chest

Therapist posture: Short stride stance facing the client at the level of the client's elbow (Figure 18.109).
Hands: Place the thumbs over the chest muscle close to the shoulder on the opposite side of the body and rest the fingers on the top of the client's shoulder.
Movement: The thumbs stretch back from the hands which are anchored on the shoulder and perform small alternating circles. One thumb circles in a clockwise direction and the other anticlockwise to cover the undraped portion of the chest muscle (Figure 18.114).

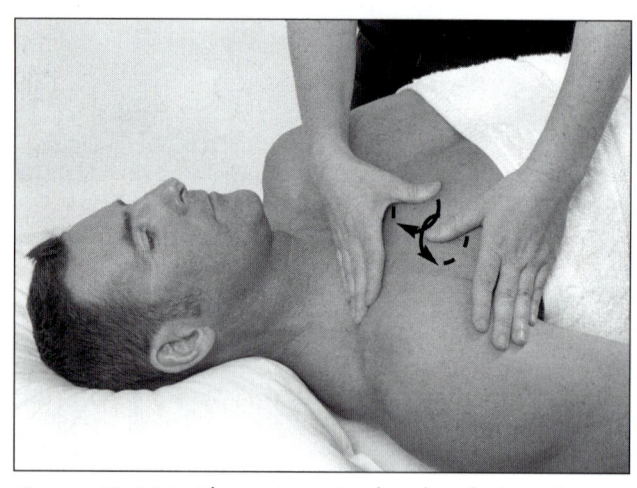

Figure 18.114 Alternating circular thumb kneading to the chest

Arm, forearm and hand

Client position: Client lies supine (face up), with a pillow under the head and a support under the knees.
Draping: Fold the draping back to reveal the arm (refer to Chapter 15, Figure 15.4, for draping procedures).
Therapist position: The therapist stands at the side of the massage table at the level of the client's elbow, facing the head of the table. The leg closer to the massage table extends behind the therapist and the outside leg is out in front. The width of this stance should be wide enough to allow the therapist's torso to be upright and not leaning over the arm being massaged. The knees are slightly bent to allow for easier movement and stability on the feet. This position is known as the stride stance (Figure 18.115).

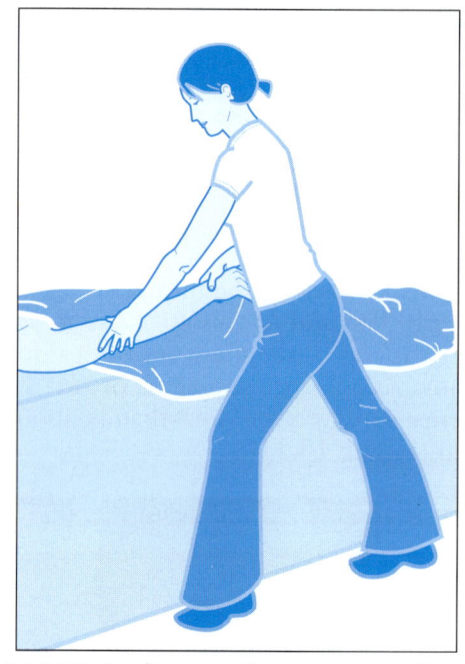

Figure 18.115 Stride stance for massaging the arm

Note: The most important aspect of the arm massage is learning to feel comfortable with supporting the client's arm securely. If the therapist has any apprehension, the client will attempt to assist by holding the arm up, thereby not allowing it to relax. The client's arm should also be supported away from the therapist's body rather than wrapped around their waist or resting on their torso.

99. Gently shake the arm with the arm bent

Therapist posture: Stride stance at the level of the client's abdomen, facing the head of the table (Figure 18.115).
Hands: Pick the client's arm up by the palm by interlocking the fingers around the client's thumb.
Movement: The therapist lifts the arm off the massage table and allows it to be bent at the elbow. The therapist shakes the arm back and forth

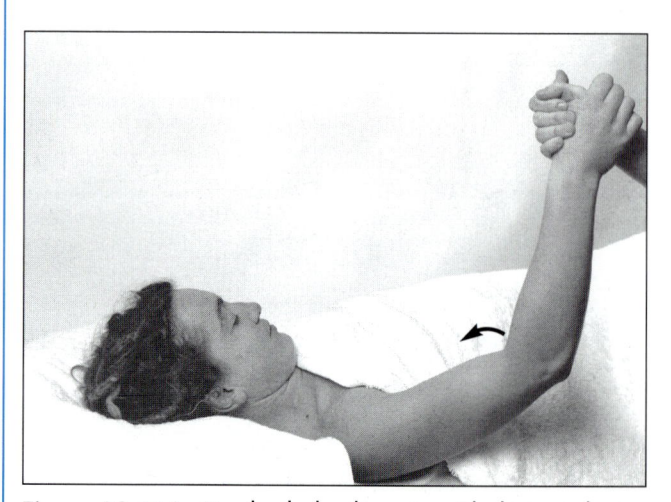

Figure 18.116 Gently shake the arm with the arm bent

allowing it to swing loosely at the elbow (Figure 18.116).

100. Alternating one-handed rowing stroke

Therapist posture: Stride stance at the level of the client's abdomen, facing the head of the table (Figure 18.115).
Hands: One hand holds the wrist and picks up the arm. The other hand is placed on the forearm, moulding to its contours.
Movement: Apply long gliding strokes on the upper surface of the upper limb from the wrist to the shoulder. The hand glides over the shoulder then to the under surface of the arm and glides down to the wrist (Figure 18.117a). Alternate the hands holding the wrist and repeat the stroke with the other hand to massage the inside of the upper limb (Figure 18.117b). Repeat several times.

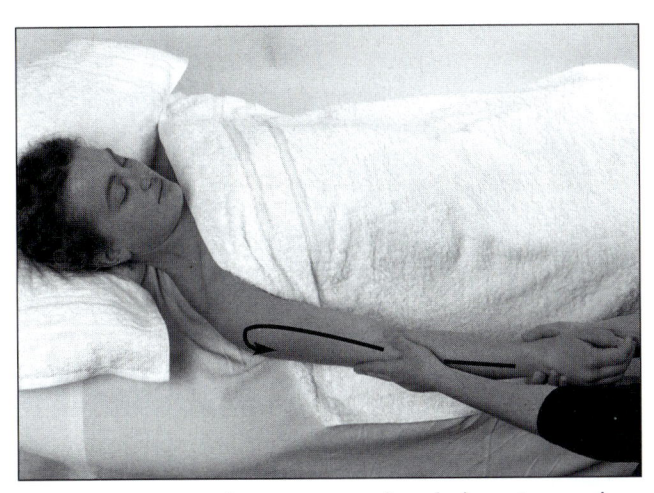

Figure 18.117a Alternating one-handed rowing stroke

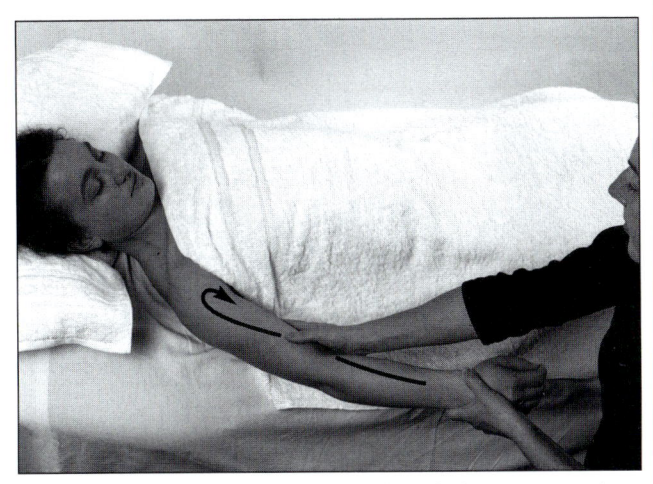

Figure 18.117b Alternating one-handed rowing stroke

101. One handed kneading to the front of the upper arm

Therapist posture: Stride stance at the level of the client's abdomen, facing the head of the table (Figure 18.115).

Hands: The therapist's outside hand picks up the client's wrist. The therapist's inside hand wraps around the client's elbow with the thumb across the elbow crease (Figure 18.118a). Bend the client's arm inward and have their forearm resting over the

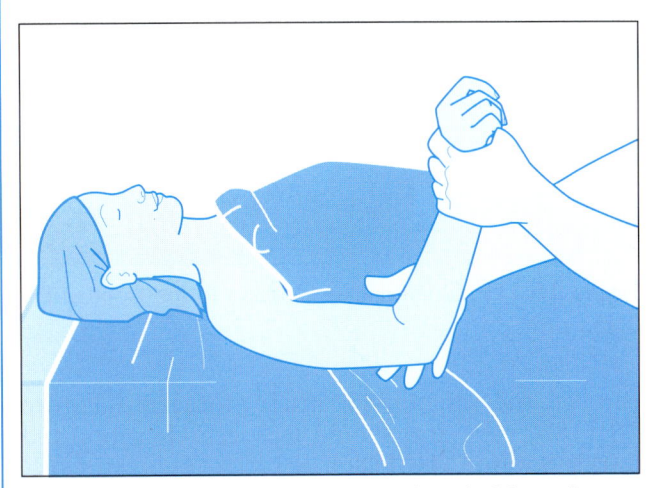

Figure 18.118a Arm hold for one-handed kneading to the front of the upper arm

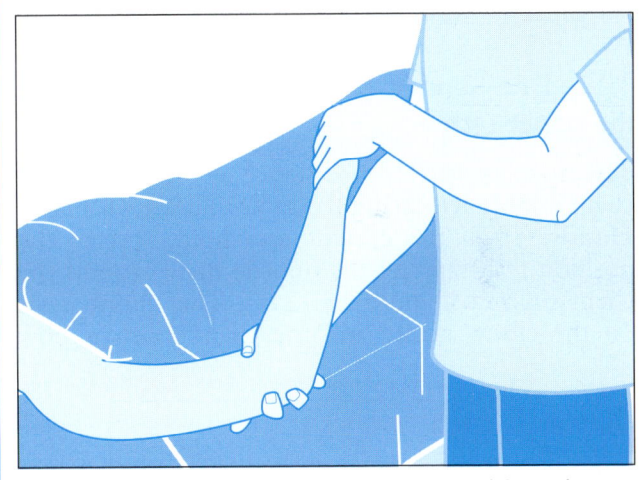

Figure 18.118b Arm hold for one-handed kneading to the front of the upper arm

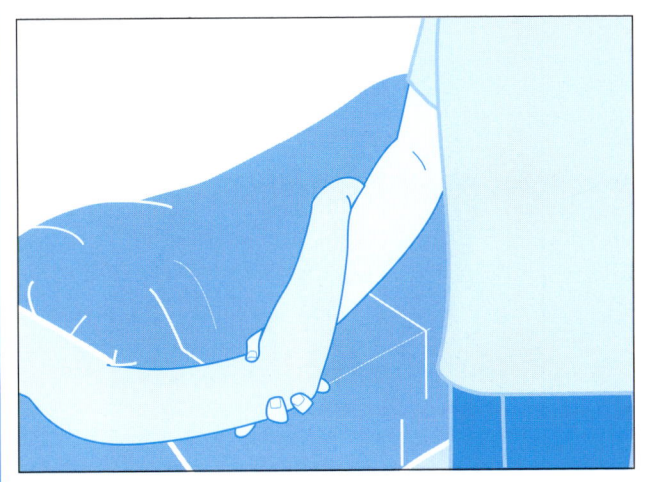

Figure 18.118c Arm hold for one-handed kneading to the front of the upper arm

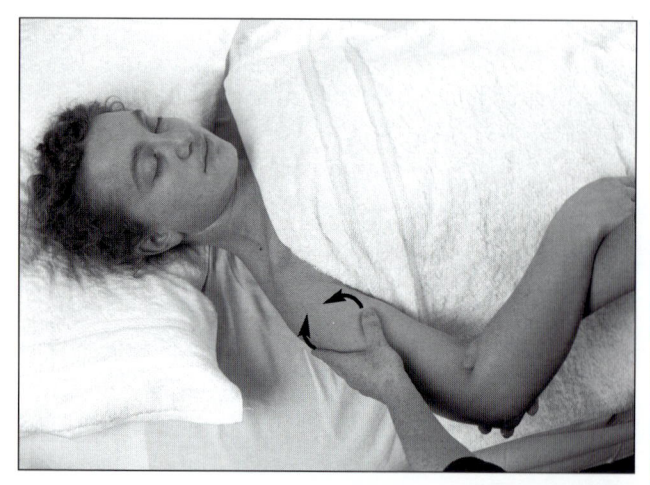

Figure 18.119 One-handed C-scoop to the front of the upper arm

top of the therapist's inside forearm (Figure 18.118b). The arm should feel securely supported in this position (17.118c).
Movement: With the outside hand use a one-handed C-scoop stroke to the upper arm. The pressure and direction of the stroke is from the elbow to the shoulder (Figure 18.119).

102. One-handed kneading to the back of the upper arm

Therapist posture: Wide stance at the level of the client's shoulder, facing the table (Figure 18.120).
Hands: From the current arm hold, reverse the position by wrapping the outside hand around the client's elbow (Figure 18.121a). The thumb rests on the elbow crease and the client's arm is now

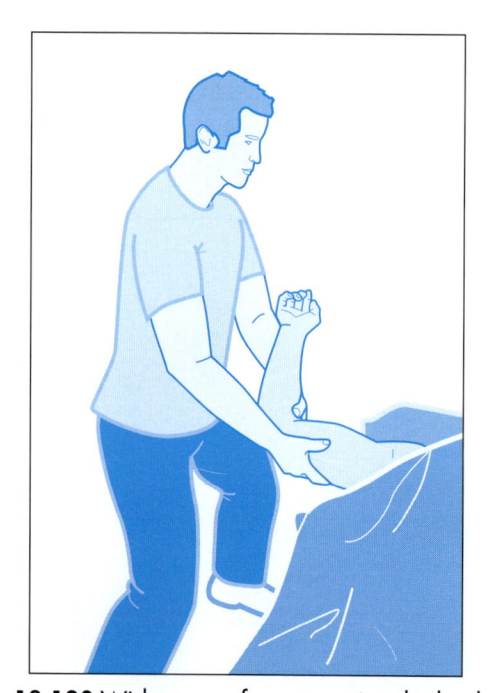

Figure 18.120 Wide stance for massaging the back of the upper arm

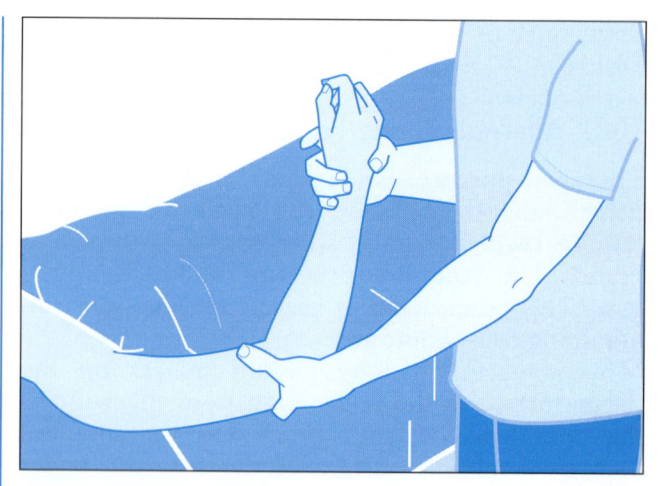

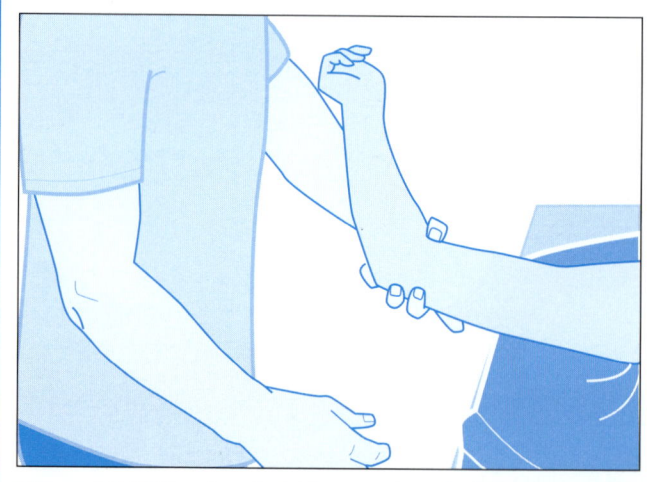

Figure 18.121a Arm hold for one-handed C-scoop to the back of the upper arm

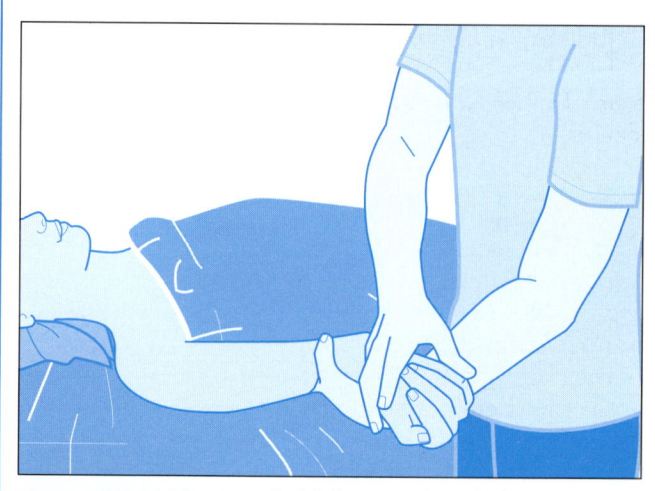

Figure 18.121b Arm hold for one-handed C-scoop to the back of the upper arm

Figure 18.121c Arm hold for one-handed C-scoop to the back of the upper arm

turned out to rest on the therapist's forearm (Figure 18.121b). The therapist moves to face the side of the table at the level of the client's shoulder; at the same time the client's arm will move outward. The back of the client's arm is now accessible for massage (Figure 18.121c).

Movement: With the inside hand, perform a one-handed C-scoop stroke to the back of the arm, covering the surface from the elbow to the armpit (Figure 18.122).

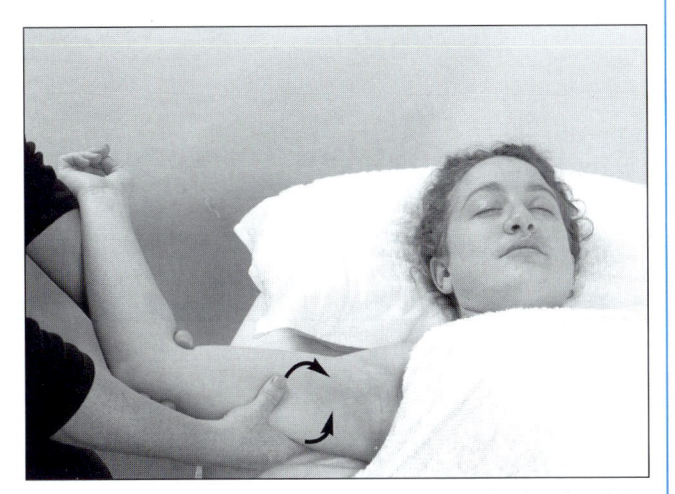

Figure 18.122 One-handed C-scoop to the back of the upper arm

103. One-handed C-scoop to the forearm

Therapist posture: Stride stance at the level of the client's abdomen, facing the head of the table (Figure 18.115).
Hands: From the previous position, return the arm to the table with the client's palm facing down. Grasp the client's wrist and lift the forearm slightly off the table whilst the upper arm remains resting on the table (Figure 18.123).
Movement: With the free hand, a one-handed C-scoop stroke is applied to the top surface of the forearm (Figure 18.124a). Alternate the supporting hand, so that the free hand now holds the client's wrist. The therapist turns the client's palm over so that the palm is now face up, allowing access to the inside of the forearm. Use a one-handed C-scoop stroke to the inside of the forearm (Figure 18.124b).

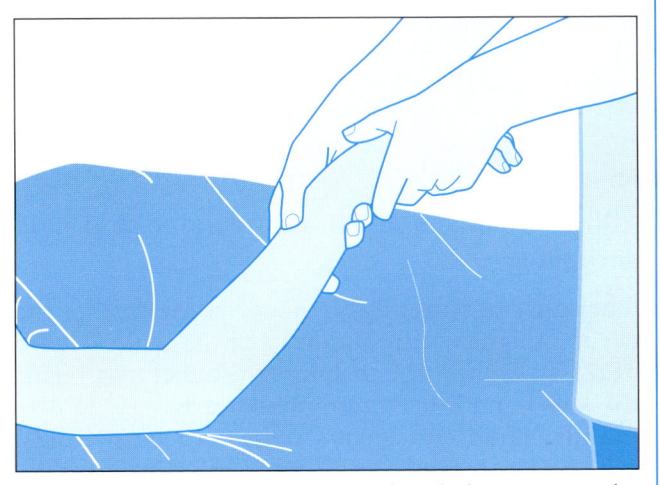

Figure 18.123 Arm hold for one-handed C-scoop to the forearm

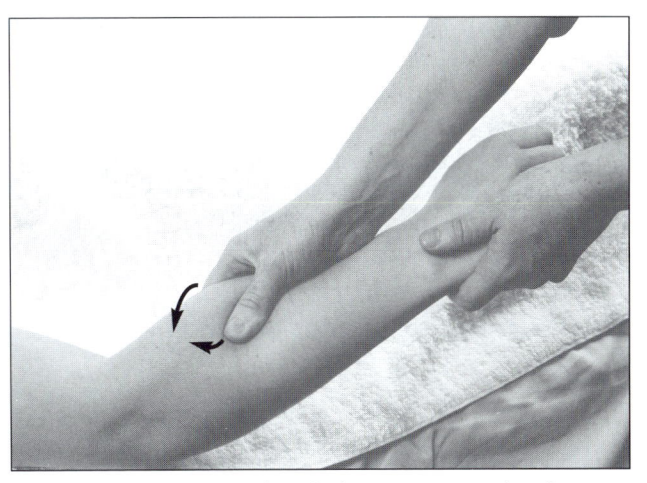

Figure 18.124a One-handed C-scoop to the forearm extensors

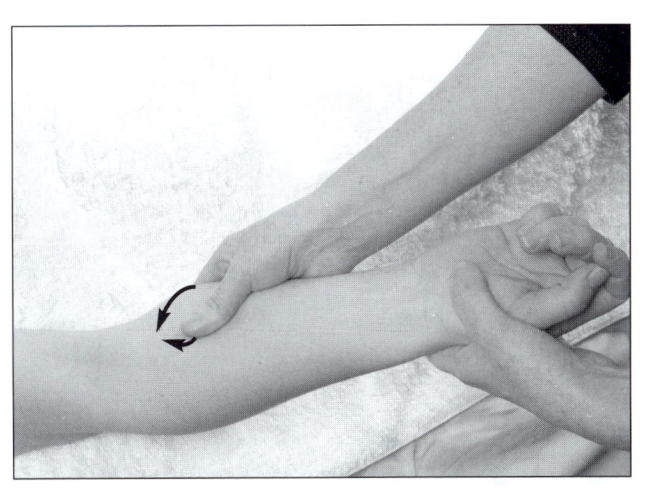

Figure 18.124b One-handed C-scoop to the forearm flexors

104. Alternating circular thumb kneading to the wrist

Therapist posture: Stride stance at the level of the client's abdomen, facing the head of the table (Figure 18.115).

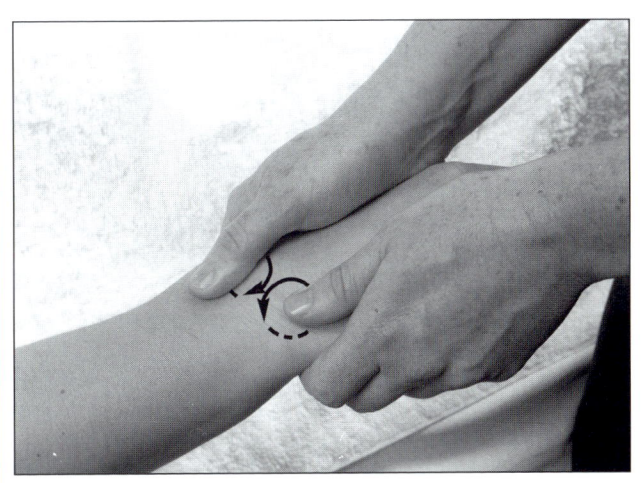

Figure 18.125 Alternating circular thumb kneading to the wrist

Hands: With the palm facing down, place both hands on either side of the wrist, supported loosely by the therapist's fingers below the palm. The thumbs come together over the top of the wrist.
Movement: Perform alternating circular thumb kneading to the top of the wrist with palm facing downward and then to the inside of the wrist with the palm facing upward (Figure 18.125).

105. Alternating circular thumb kneading to the palm

Therapist posture: Stride stance at the level of the client's abdomen, facing the head of the table (Figure 18.115).
Hands: From the previous stroke bend the elbow so the forearm is at right angles to the table. Support this position by placing the therapist's fingers on the back of the hand. The thumbs come together at the palm.
Movement: Perform alternating circular thumb kneading to cover the surface of the palm (Figure 18.126).

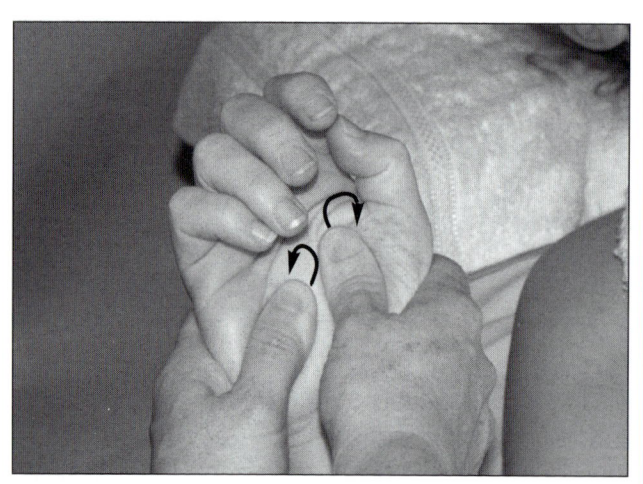

Figure 18.126 Alternating circular thumb kneading to the palm

106. Thumb stripping between the rays of the hand

Therapist posture: Stride stance at the level of the client's abdomen, facing the head of the table (Figure 18.115).
Hands: From the previous stroke the therapist turns the palm face down and supports the client's hand. On the dorsal surface (the back of the hand) use a thumb to find a space between the rays of the hand.
Movement: Gently and slowly slide the thumb along each grove, from the knuckles to the wrist (Figure 18.127).

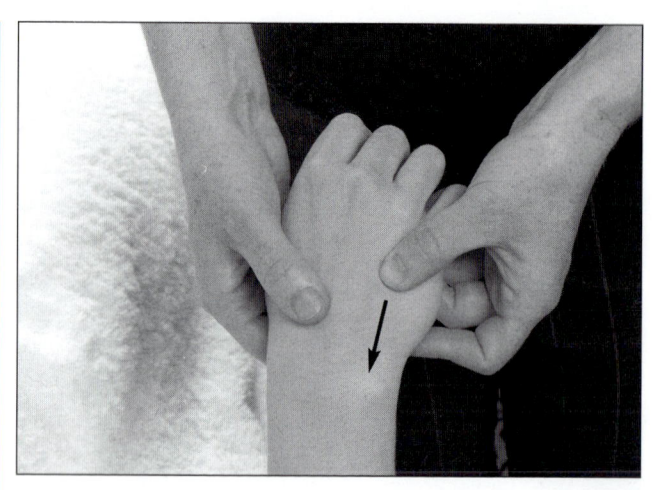

Figure 18.127 Thumb stripping between the rays of the hand

107. Kneading to each finger

Therapist posture: Stride stance at the level of the client's abdomen, facing the head of the table (Figure 18.115).
Hands: The client's palm faces down and the wrist is supported with the therapist's hand. Use the thumb, first and second digits to wrap around the base of a finger.
Movement: Knead around the circumference of each finger from the base to the tip (Figure 18.128). Repeat for each finger.

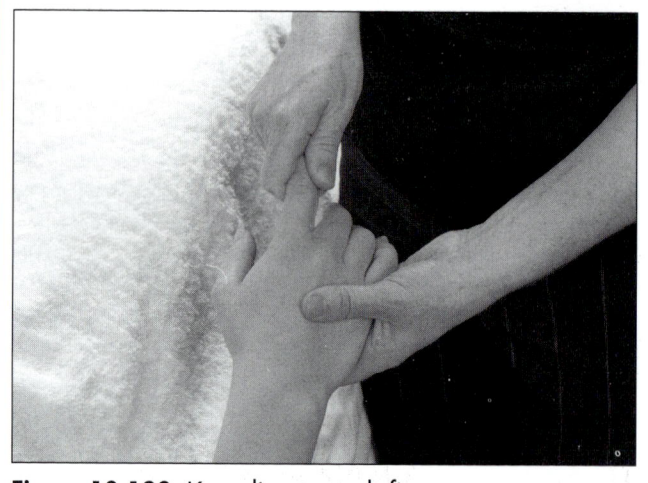

Figure 18.128 Kneading to each finger

108. Gently shake the arm with the arm straight

Therapist posture: Stride stance at the level of the client's thighs, facing the head of the table (Figure 18.115). During the technique the therapist bends the knees and leans slightly backwards.
Hands: Hold the client's wrist with both hands, hold it close to the client's torso and raise it off the massage table only slightly.

CHAPTER 18 THE MASSAGE SEQUENCE 273

Movement: Gently pull the arm allowing a small amount of traction to occur at the client's shoulder joint. Lightly shake the limb up and down ensuring the movement occurs at the shoulder rather than the elbow or wrist (Figure 18.129).

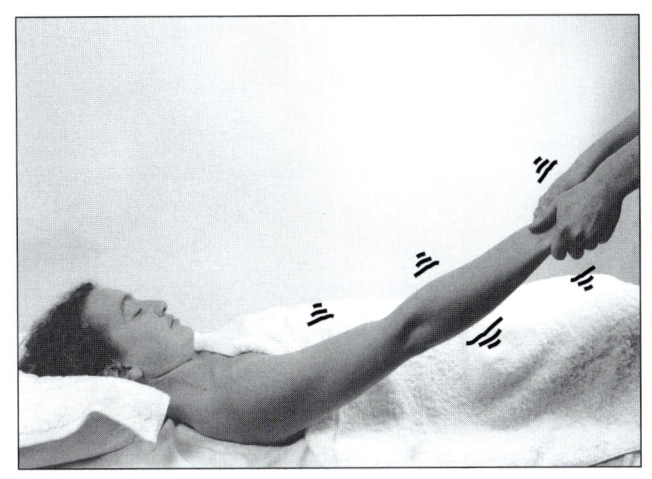

Figure 18.129 Gently shake the arm with the arm straight

Neck and shoulders

Client position: The client lies supine (face up) with their head at the end of the table. A pillow under the head may be used for comfort and support.
Draping: The client is completely draped. The drape is folded back at the chest to rest below the clavicles. (Refer to Chapter 15 for draping procedures.)

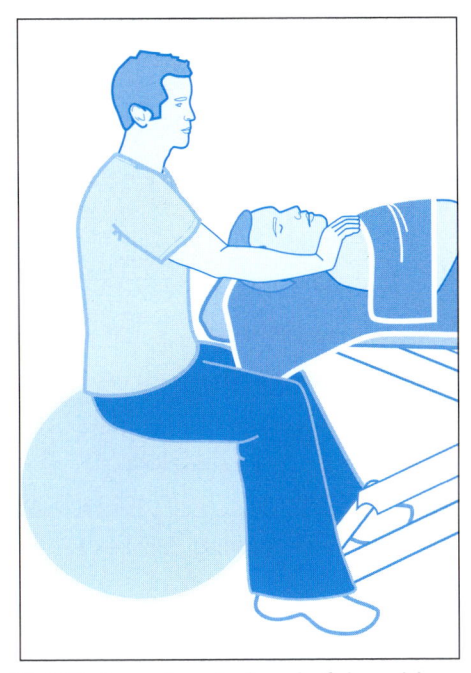

Figure 18.130 Seated at the head of the table

Therapist position: The therapist is seated at the head of the massage table (Figure 18.130).

Neck and Shoulders — Supine

109. Rowing stroke to the chest, shoulders and neck

Therapist posture: The therapist is seated at the head of the table (Figure 18.130).
Hands: Position the finger pads on the pectoral muscles near the sternum, the fingers face the feet (Figure 18.131a).
Movement: Apply oil to the hands and glide the finger pads outward over the chest (Figure 18.131b), around the shoulders and up the back of the neck (Figure 18.131c). Return the hands to the original position by sliding them over the sides of the neck back to the chest. Repeat this stroke several times ending at the base of the neck.

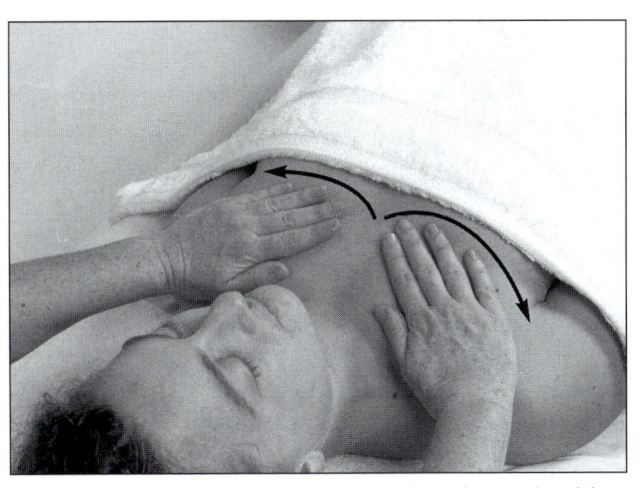

Figure 18.131a Rowing stroke to the chest, shoulders and neck

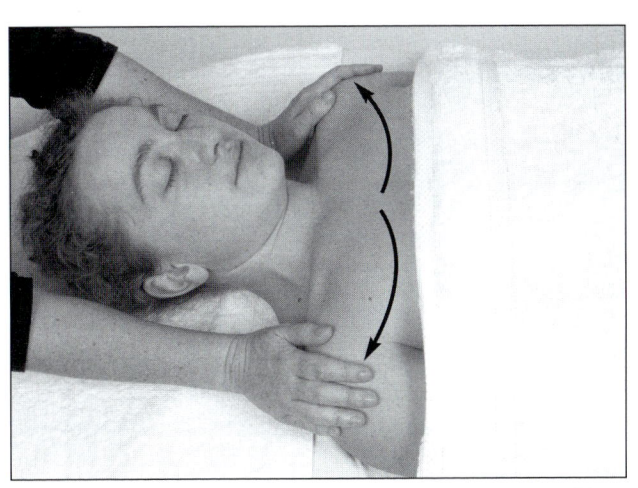

Figure 18.131b Rowing stroke to the chest, shoulders and neck

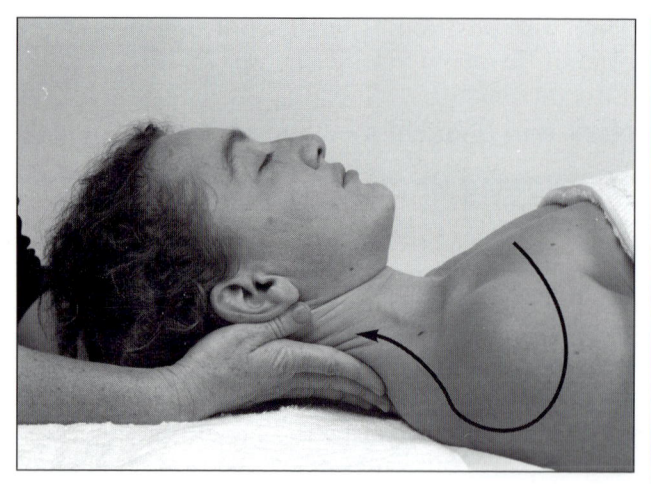

Figure 18.131c Rowing stroke to the chest, shoulders and neck

110. Knuckle kneading to the top of the chest

Therapist posture: The therapist is seated at the head of the table (Figure 18.130).
Hands: Position the knuckles below the clavicles on either side of the sternum on the pectoral muscles.
Movement: Perform circular kneading strokes using the knuckles along the top portion of the pectoral muscles. The direction of the circular kneading is away from the midline (Figure 18.132).

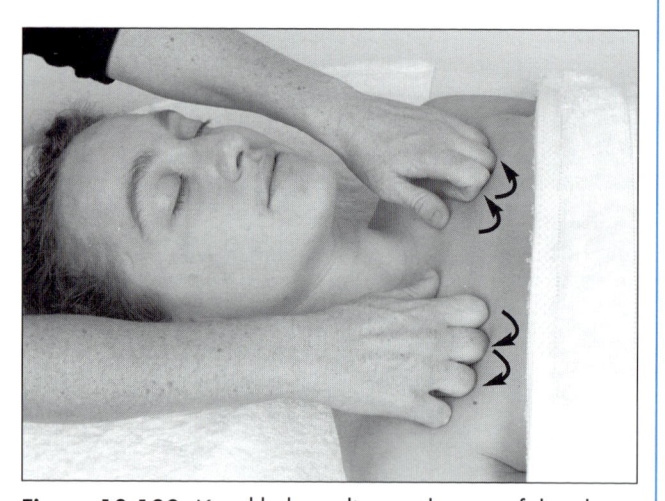

Figure 18.132 Knuckle kneading to the top of the chest

111. Trapezius alternating pinch knead

Therapist posture: The therapist is seated at the head of the table (Figure 18.130).
Hands: Place the head in a neutral position and position the fingertips of both hands on the shoulders under the trapezius muscle at the corner of the neck. The thumbs rest on top of the trapezius.
Movement: Apply an alternating pinch kneading stroke to the trapezius muscle by grasping the muscle between the thumbs and fingers. Grasp then

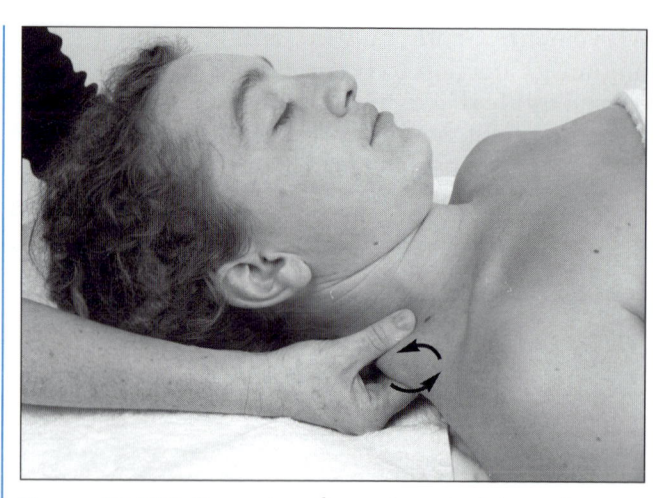

Figure 18.133 Trapezius alternating pinch knead

release to create a rhythmical effect (Figure 18.133).

112. Half rowing stroke to the chest, shoulders and neck

Therapist posture: The therapist is seated at the head of the table (Figure 18.130).
Hands: The hands are placed at the base of the neck. From this position rotate the head slightly to one side and support the head with the fingertips wrapped around the base of the skull and the thumb above the ear. With the other hand, position the finger pads on the pectoral muscles near the sternum, with the fingers facing the feet.
Movement: Glide the finger pads outward over the chest (Figure 18.134a), around the shoulders (Figure 18.134b) and up the back of the neck (Figure 18.134c). Repeat this stroke several times.

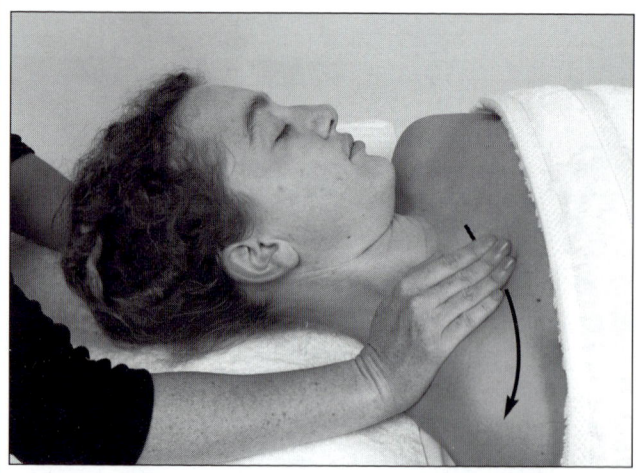

Figure 18.134a Half rowing stroke to the chest, shoulders and neck

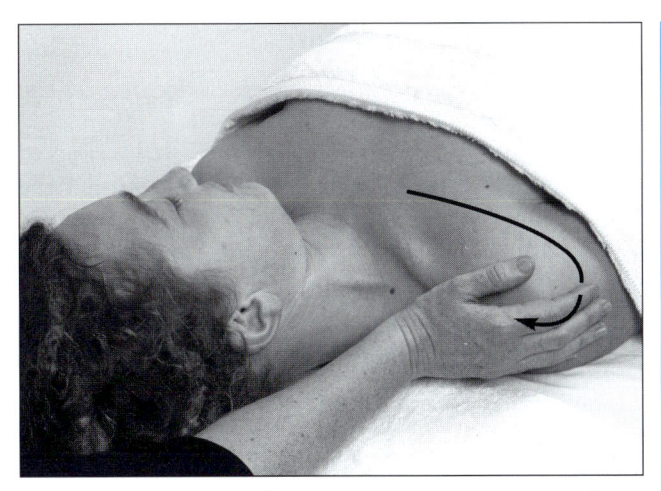

Figure 18.134b Half rowing stroke to the chest, shoulders and neck

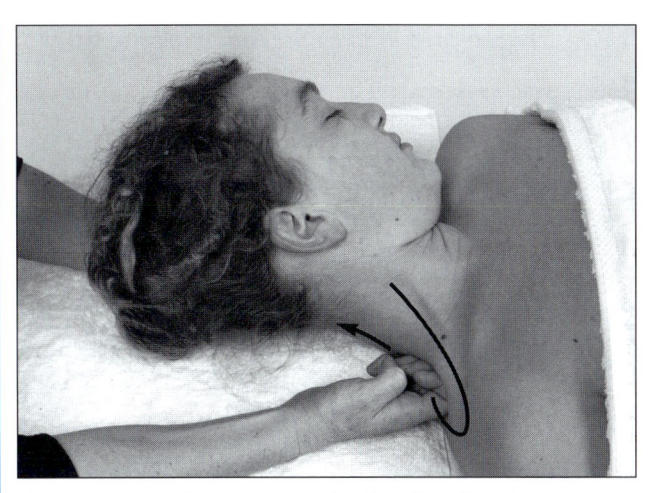

Figure 18.135b Return stroke for flat fist down upper trapezius

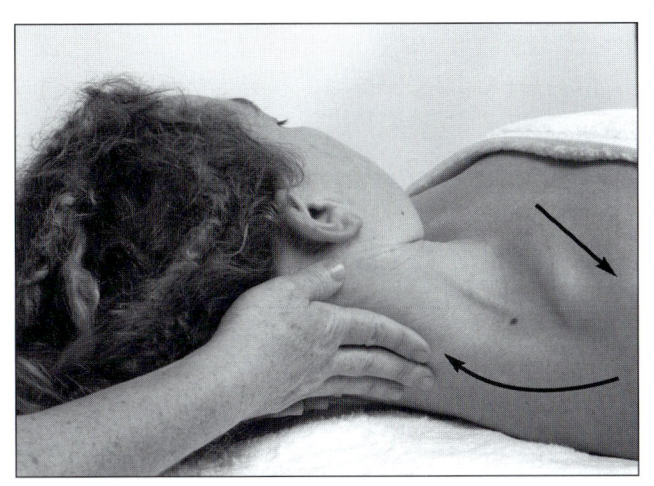

Figure 18.134c Half rowing stroke to the chest, shoulders and neck

113. Flat of fist down upper trapezius

Therapist posture: The therapist is seated at the head of the table (Figure 18.130).
Hands: The head is rotated and supported by one of the therapist's hands. Place the back of the fingers of the other hand on the side of the neck close to the skull. The fingertips face the skull.
Movement: Using the back of the fingers, glide down the trapezius muscle from the base of the skull to the shoulder (Figure 18.135a). At the shoulder turn the palm up, curl the fingers and use the flat knuckles to glide up the back of the neck (Figure 18.135b). Repeat several times.

114. Circular thumb kneading to the posterior triangle of neck

Therapist posture: The therapist is seated at the head of the table (Figure 18.130).
Hands: Place the thumb over the muscles on the side of the neck just beneath the scull. The fingers wrap around the back of the neck.
Movement: Perform circular thumb kneading to the side of the neck from the skull to the clavicle (Figure 18.136).
Note: the therapist must be aware of the endangerment site of posterior triangle (see Chapter 12).

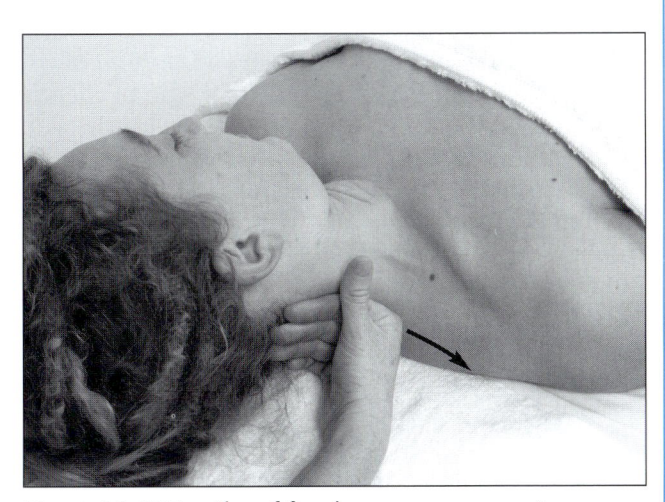

Figure 18.135a Flat of fist down upper trapezius

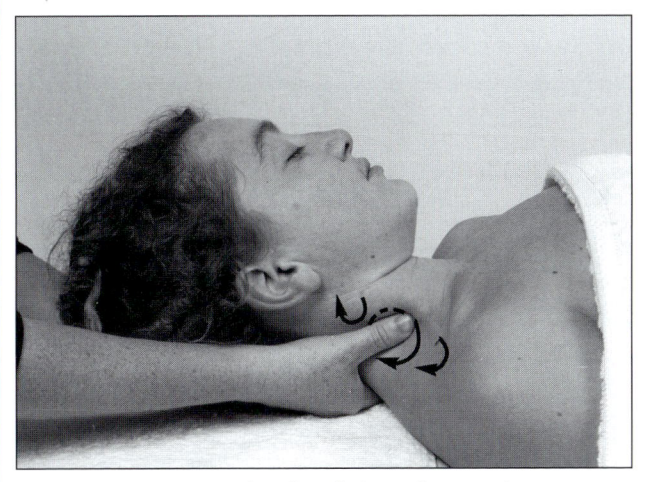

Figure 18.136 Circular thumb kneading to the posterior triangle of neck

115. Finger pad rub to sternocleidomastoid

Therapist posture: The therapist is seated at the head of the table (Figure 18.130).
Hands: Return the head to neutral position with one hand still supporting the head from beneath. With the other hand, gently place the finger pads over the sternocleidomastoid close to its bony attachment from the mastoid process.
Movement: Gently rub over the length of the muscle back and forth from origin to insertion. Repeat this movement along the muscle several times (Figure 18.137).

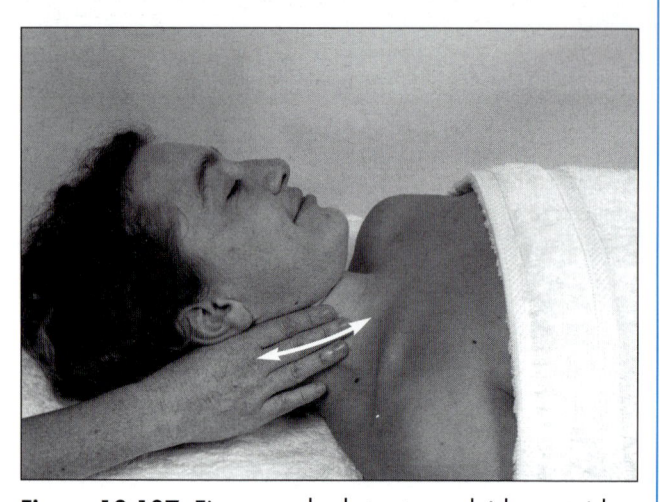

Figure 18.137 Finger pad rub to sternocleidomastoid

116. Circular fingertip kneading to the base of the skull

Therapist posture: The therapist is seated at the head of the table (Figure 18.130).
Hands: Rotate the head and support with one hand. Place the fingertips of the other hand on the muscles at the base of the skull close to the spine.
Movement: Perform small circular movements with the fingertips along the base of the skull, moving from the midline toward the ear (Figure 18.138).

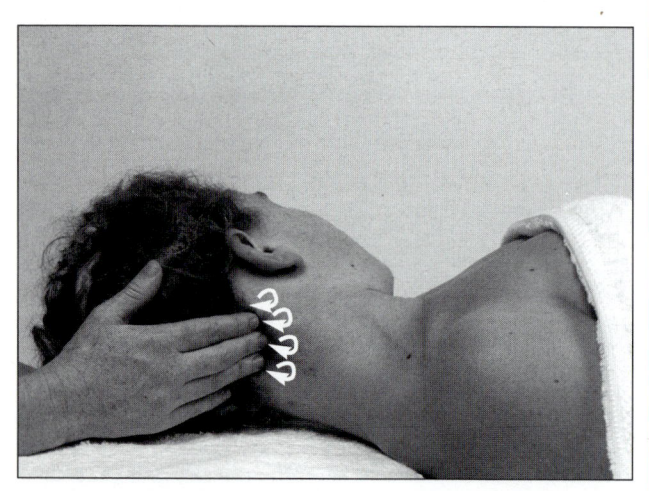

Figure 18.138 Circular fingertip kneading to the base of the skull

117. Sub-occipital release

Therapist posture: The therapist is seated at the head of the table (Figure 18.130).
Hands: The therapist's forearms rest by the sides of the client's head with the palms facing up under the back of the head. The tips of the fingers contact the sub-occipital muscles just beneath the base of the skull.
Movement: The therapist applies pressure up and in towards the crown (Figure 18.139).

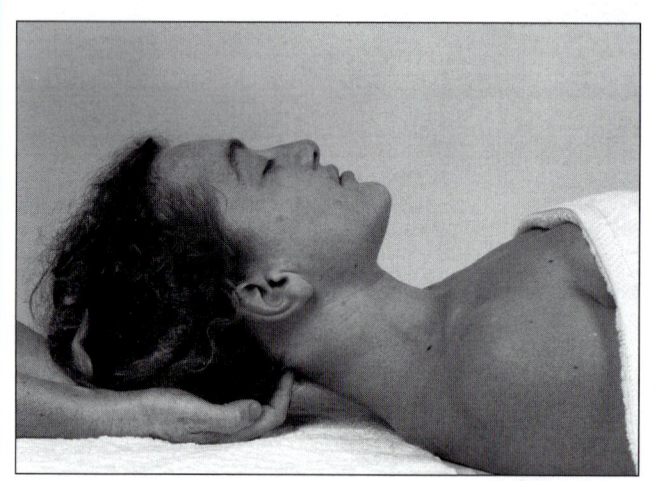

Figure 18.139 Sub-occipital release

Scalp and face massage

Client position: The client lays supine (face up) with their head at the end of the table. A pillow for support may be used if necessary.
Draping: The client is completely draped.
Therapist positioning: The therapist is seated at the head of the table. To reduce the distance between the therapist and the client's head, place the feet on either side of the massage table legs (Figure 18.130).

118. Fingertip kneading to the scalp

Therapist posture: The therapist is seated at the head of the table (Figure 18.130).
Hands: Position the hands on either side of client's head, spread the fingers and place them on the side of the skull above the ears.
Movement: Bend the fingertips and apply small circular movements with both hands simultaneously. Continue the stroke for a few moments then repeat the technique on another area of the scalp (Figure 18.140).

119. Palmer flat kneading to the sides of the scalp

Therapist posture: The therapist is seated at the head of the table (Figure 18.130).

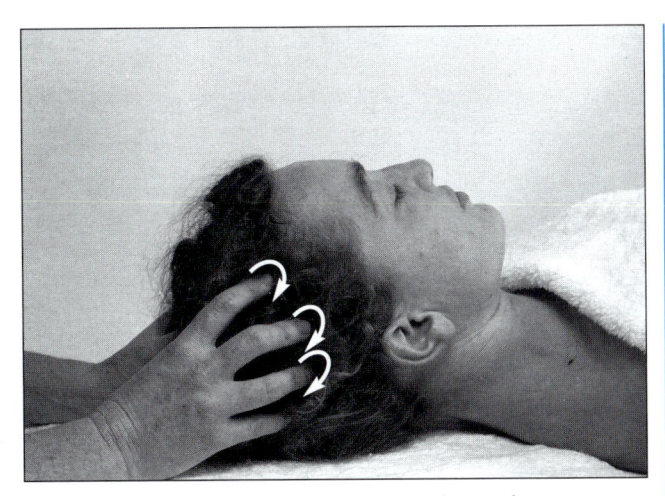

Figure 18.140 Fingertip kneading to the scalp

Hands: Position the hands on either side of client's head with the heel of the hand applying firm pressure above the ears with the palms and fingers loosely cupping the ears.
Movement: Apply circular compressions using the heel of the hand for several moments. The heels then slide closer towards the crown or top of the head and the technique is applied again. This can be repeated until the heel reaches the crown of the head (Figure 18.141).

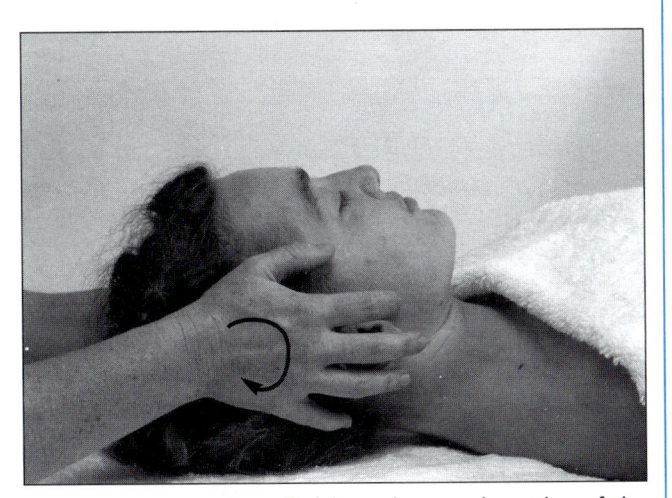

Figure 18.141 Palmer flat kneading to the sides of the scalp

120. Fingertip kneading around the hairline

Therapist posture: The therapist is seated at the head of the table (Figure 18.130).
Hands: Position the fingertips at the hairline of the temples.
Movement: The fingertips apply small circular movements. Repeat this technique as you follow the hairline toward the midline (Figure 18.142).

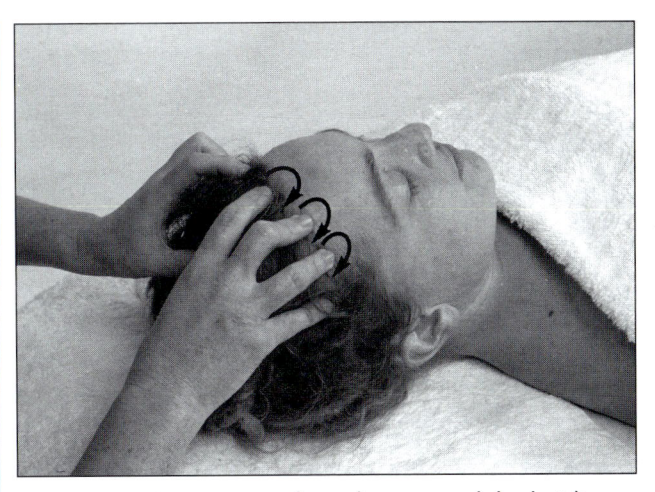

Figure 18.142 Fingertip kneading around the hairline

121. Circular thumb kneading along the midline of the head

Therapist posture: The therapist is seated at the head of the table (Figure 18.130).
Hands: Position the hands and fingers at the side of the head with the thumbs meeting at the junction of the forehead and hairline.
Movement: Apply stationary circular thumb kneading. Repeat as you move down along the midline across the top of the head (Figure 18.143).

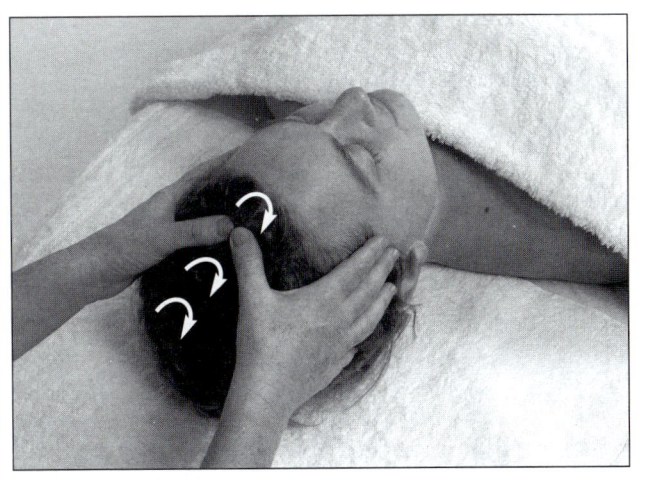

Figure 18.143 Circular thumb kneading along the midline of the head

122. Finger pad kneading across the forehead

Therapist posture: The therapist is seated at the head of the table (Figure 18.130).
Hands: The finger pads rest high on the forehead close to the midline.
Movement: Using the pads of the fingers perform circular movements in an outward direction. Repeat this technique several times, each time moving lower on the forehead (Figure 18.144).

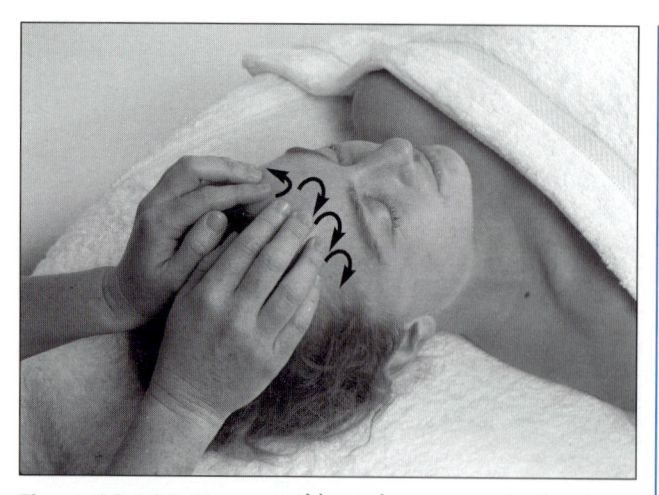

Figure 18.144 Finger pad kneading across the forehead

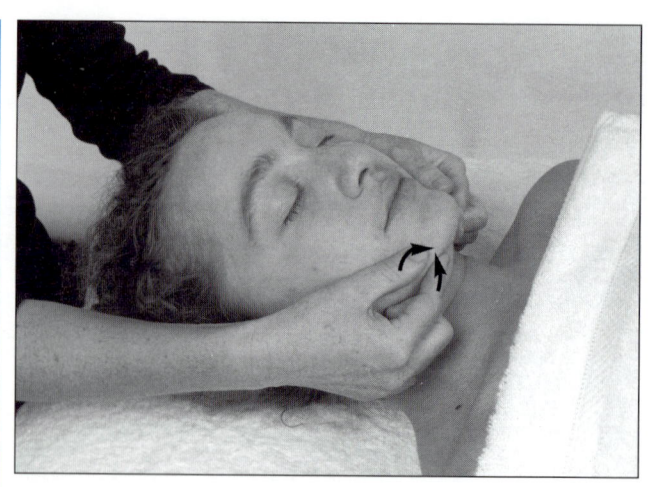

Figure 18.146 Jawline pinch kneading

123. Finger pad kneading to the temples and jawline

Therapist posture: The therapist is seated at the head of the table (Figure 18.130).
Hands: Place the finger pads on the temples.
Movement: Apply circular movements with the finger pads in an outward direction, travelling from the temples to the jaw (Figure 18.145).

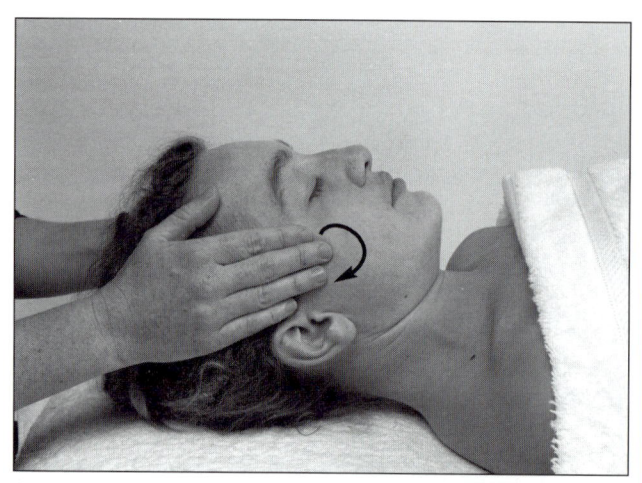

Figure 18.145 Finger pad kneading to the temples and jawline

124. Jawline pinch kneading

Therapist posture: The therapist is seated at the head of the table (Figure 18.130).
Hands: Gently place the thumb and index finger in a pinching position on the chin.
Movement: Slide the index finger and thumb away from each other. Repeat this stroke along the jawline from the midline toward the ears (Figure 18.146).

125. Alternate thumb stroking from the nose to the hairline

Therapist posture: The therapist is seated at the head of the table (Figure 18.130).
Hands: Place the thumbs between the eyebrows and rest the hand and fingers on the side of the head for support throughout the technique.
Movement: Apply alternating long strokes with the thumbs from the nose to the hairline (Figure 18.147).

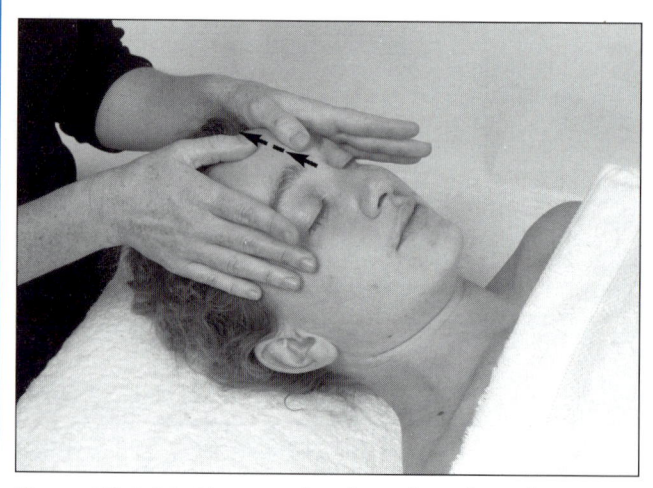

Figure 18.147 Alternate thumb stroking from the nose to the hairline

126. Index finger compression around the rim of the upper eye socket

Therapist posture: The therapist is seated at the head of the table (Figure 18.130).
Hands: Place the pad of the index finger at the bridge of the nose.
Movement: Apply static pressure moving outwards along the rim of the upper eye socket (Figure 18.148). Repeat on the other side.

CHAPTER 18 THE MASSAGE SEQUENCE 279

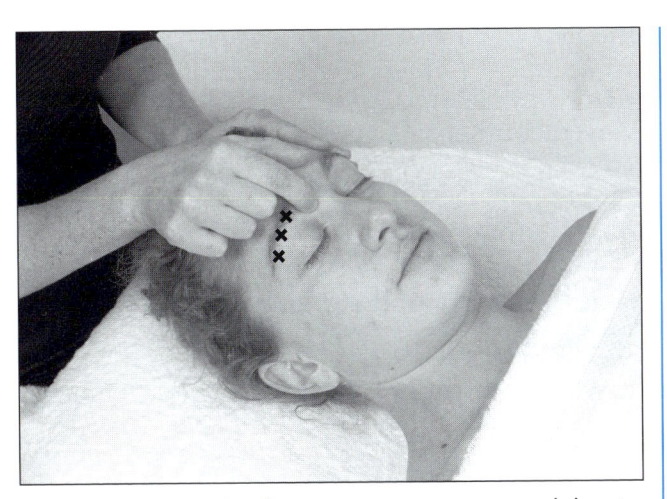

Figure 18.148 Index finger compression around the rim of the upper eye socket

127. Downwards thumb compressions on the eye socket

Therapist posture: The therapist is seated at the head of the table (Figure 18.130).
Hands: Place the pad of the thumb on the cheekbones beside the nose. Loosely place fingers and palm around the jawline to support the hand throughout the stroke.
Movement: Apply static pressure with the pad of the thumb along the upper side of the cheekbone, moving outwards (Figure 18.149). Repeat on the other side.

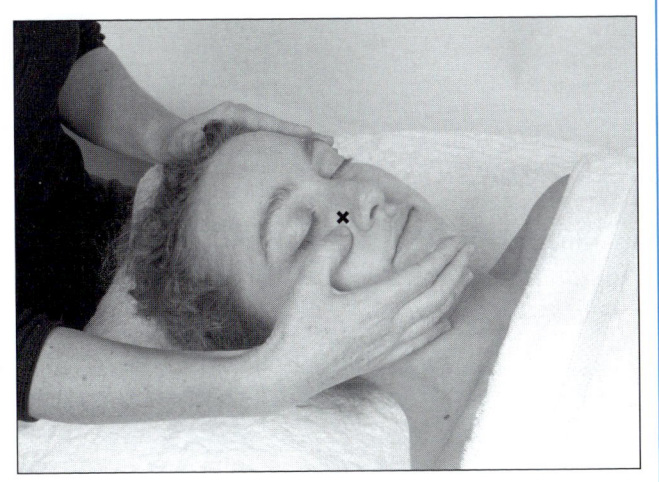

Figure 18.149 Downwards thumb compressions on the eye socket

128. Upwards index finger compressions on the cheekbone

Therapist posture: The therapist is seated at the head of the table (Figure 18.130).
Hands: Place the pad of the index finger on the cheekbone beside the nose. Loosely place the fingers and palm around jawline to support the hand throughout the stroke.
Movement: Apply static pressure with the pad of the index finger along the underside of the cheekbone, moving outwards (Figure 18.150). Repeat on the other side.

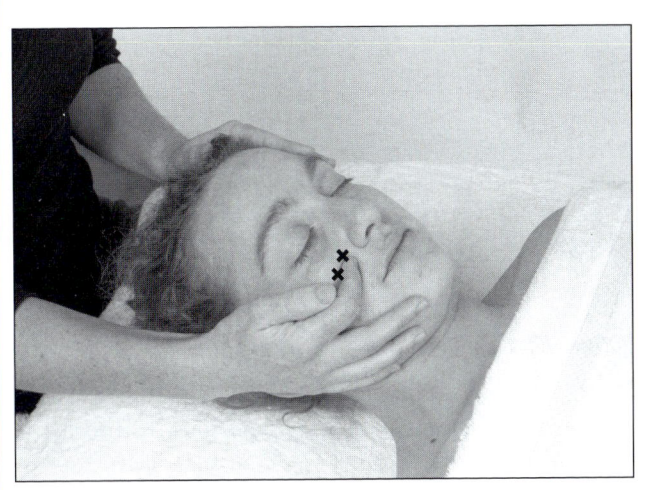

Figure 18.150 Upwards index finger compression on the cheekbone

129. Thumb stroking outward across the cheekbone

Therapist posture: The therapist is seated at the head of the table (Figure 18.130).
Hands: Place the pads of the thumb on either cheekbone close to the nose. Loosely place fingers and palm around the jawline to support the hands throughout the stroke.
Movement: Apply sliding outward strokes across both cheeks using the pads of the thumbs (Figure 18.151). Repeat several times.

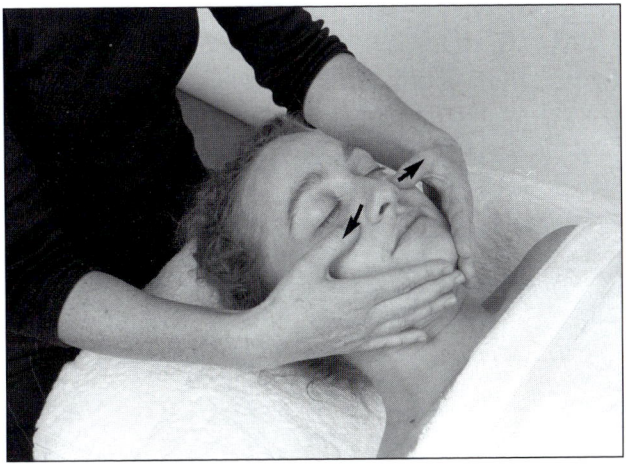

Figure 18.151 Thumb stroking outwards across the cheekbone

130. Pinch kneading the ear

Therapist posture: The therapist is seated at the head of the table (Figure 18.130).
Hands: Place the thumb and index finger in a pinching position on both ear lobes.

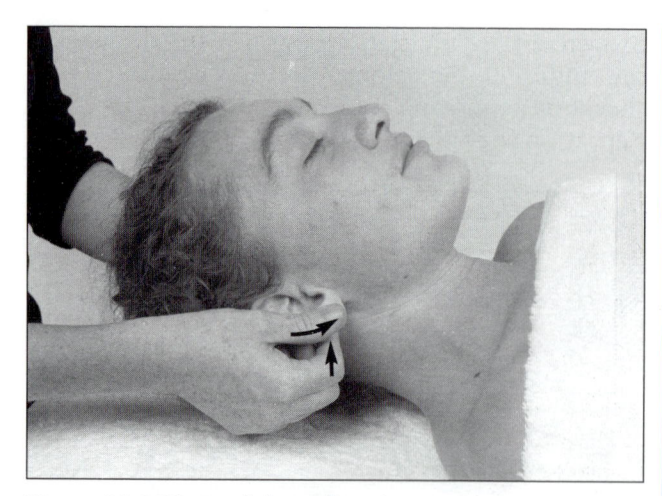

Figure 18.152 Pinch kneading the ear

Movement: Slide the index finger and thumb away from each other in a pinching action around the rim of the ear (Figure 18.152).

131. Long prayer stroke

Therapist posture: The therapist is seated at the head of the table (Figure 18.130).

Hands: The forearms cup the jawline with the hands together in a prayer position under the chin (Figure 18.153a).

Movement: Keeping in contact with the side of the face, slide the forearms, palms and fingers in a smooth motion along the side of the face and scalp through to the ends of the hair (Figure 18.153b).

132. Heels of hand stroking across the forehead

Therapist posture: The therapist is seated at the head of the table (Figure 18.130).

Hands: Place the heel of the hands on the forehead. The fingers face the chin and do not make contact with the face.

Movement: Compress and glide the heel of the hands from the centre of the forehead to the temples (Figure 18.154). Repeat this several times.

133. Tapping over the forehead

Therapist posture: The therapist is seated at the head of the table (Figure 18.130).

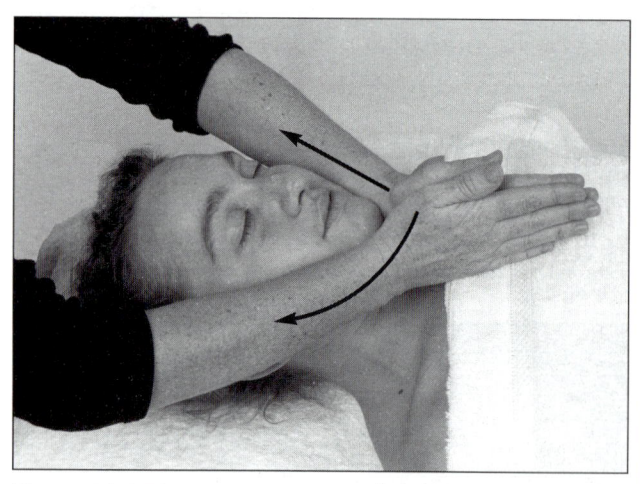

Figure 18.153a Long prayer stroke

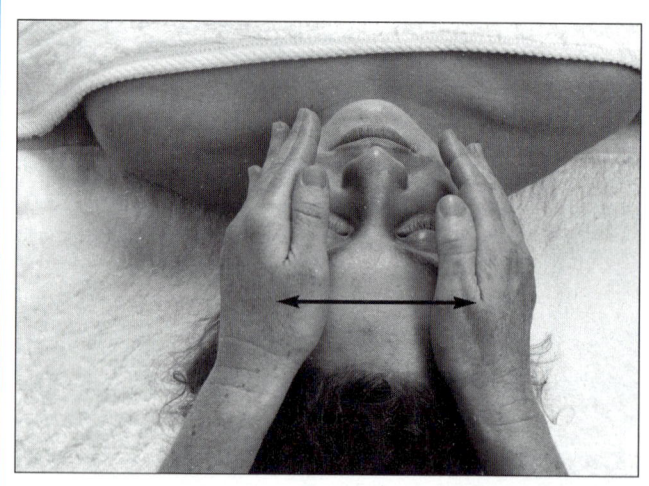

Figure 18.154 Heels of hand stroking across the forehead

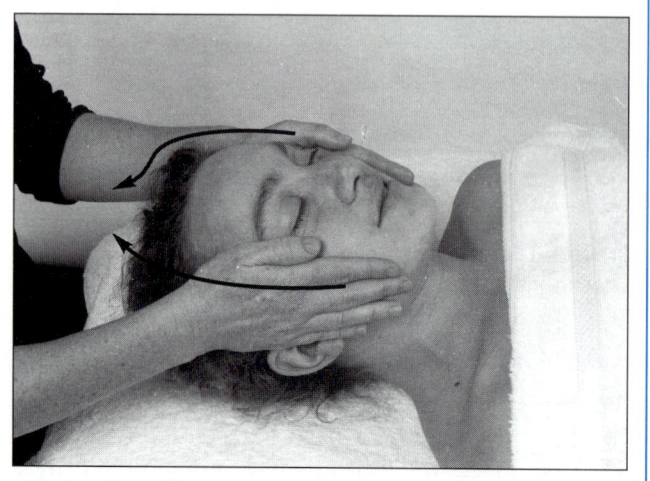

Figure 18.153b Long prayer stroke

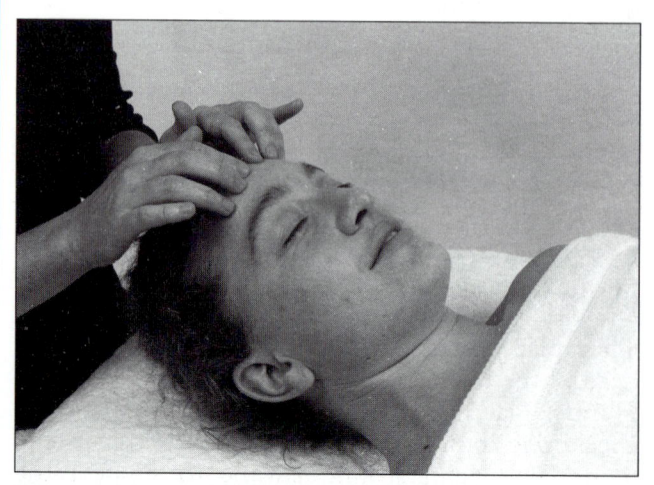

Figure 18.155 Tapping over the forehead

Hands: The finger pads of both hands are placed on the forehead.
Movement: The finger pads gently drum over the surface of the forehead (Figure 18.155).

134. Hot hand compressions over the eyes

Therapist posture: The therapist is seated at the head of the table (Figure 18.130).
Hands: Gently cup hands over eyes.
Movement: Rub hands together vigorously to warm the hands and then gently cup the hands over the client's eyes. There is no direct compression over the eyes (Figure 18.156).

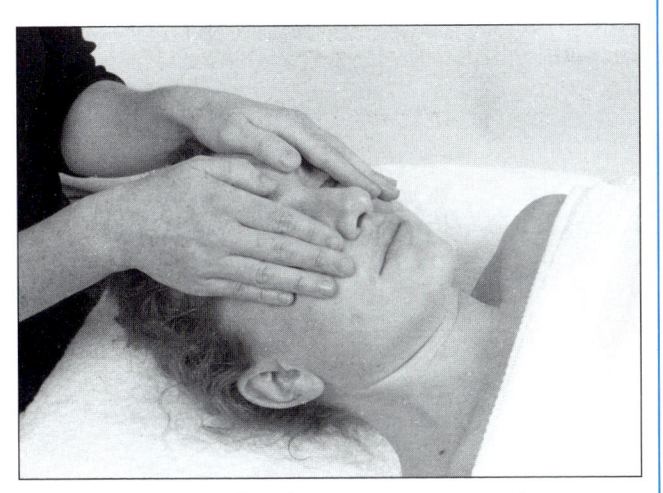

Figure 18.156 Hot hand compressions over the eyes

135. Hold the crown

Therapist posture: The therapist is seated at the head of the table (Figure 18.130).
Hands: Hold the thumbs together over the crown and the fingertips along the sides of the head (Figure 18.157).
Movement: Hold this position for 10–20 seconds.

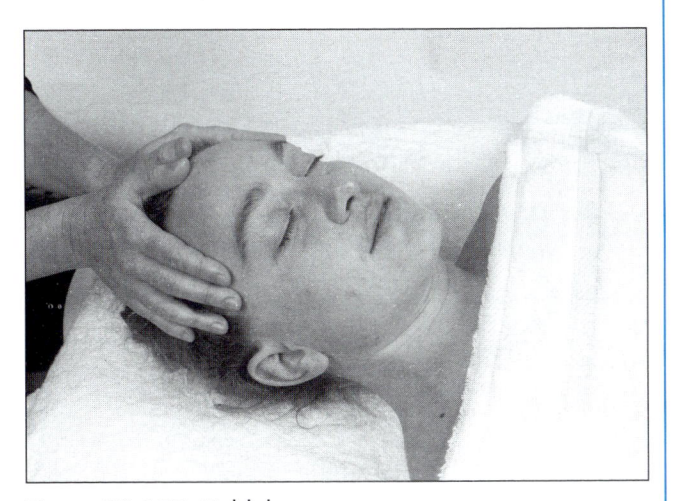

Figure 18.157 Hold the crown

136. Stroke fingers through the scalp and hair pulling

Therapist posture: The therapist is seated at the head of the table (Figure 18.130).
Hands: The therapist gently grips the hair between their fingers.
Movement: Using the fingers as a comb, stroke through the hair. Gently grip the hair between the fingers and slide through its length (Figure 18.158).

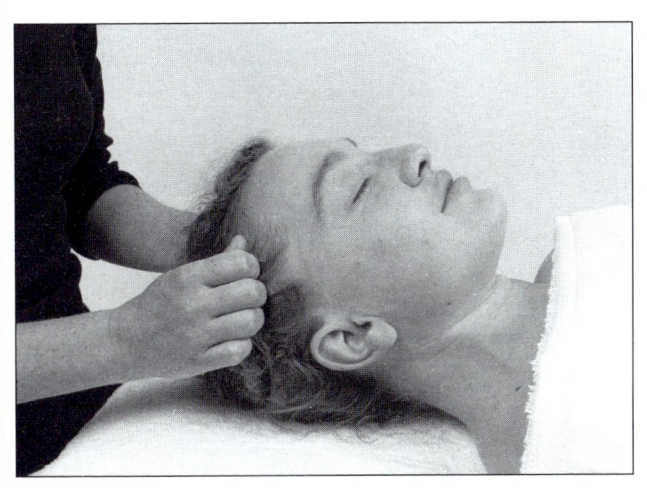

Figure 18.158 Stroke fingers through the scalp and hair pulling

Additional techniques

The sequence above introduces basic massage manipulations. As the massage student develops these skills, more advanced techniques can be integrated within the sequence. Chapter 17 introduces further massage manipulations, which the student may wish to add to their collection of techniques, such as using various deep effleurage manipulations and deep transverse frictions.

SEATED MASSAGE

The seated massage described is suitable for a clothed 10–15 minute massage. There are several variations for positioning the client when giving a seated massage and these include:

- using an adjustable desktop positioner (Figure 18.159);
- using a massage chair (Figure 18.160);
- using a stool and leaning forward onto a support (Figure 18.161);
- sitting upright in a chair (Figure 18.162).

The sequence below has been designed for the use of an adjustable desktop positioner or a massage chair. The therapist's stance and holding positions will need to be altered to accommodate the massage for other client positioning variations.

282   SECTION 6   THE MASSAGE TREATMENT

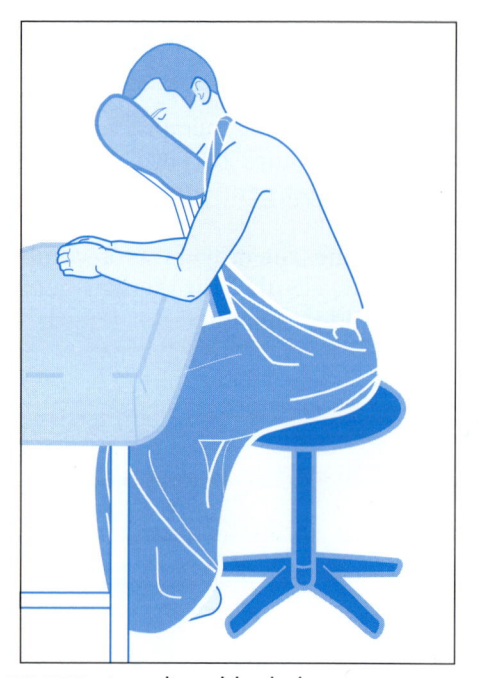

Figure 18.159 An adjustable desktop positioner

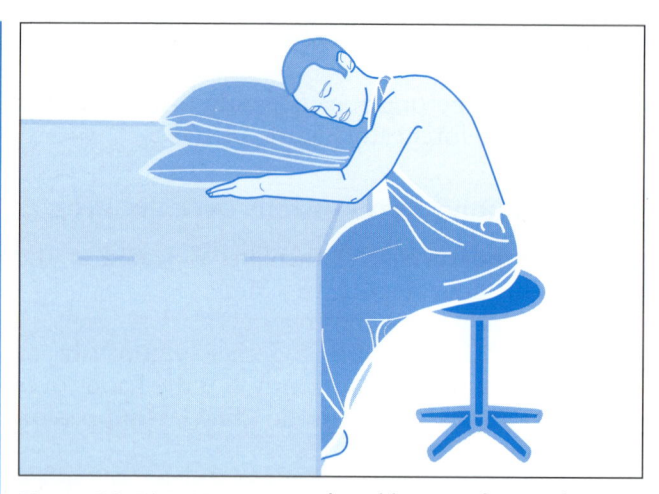

Figure 18.161 Using a stool and leaning forward onto a support

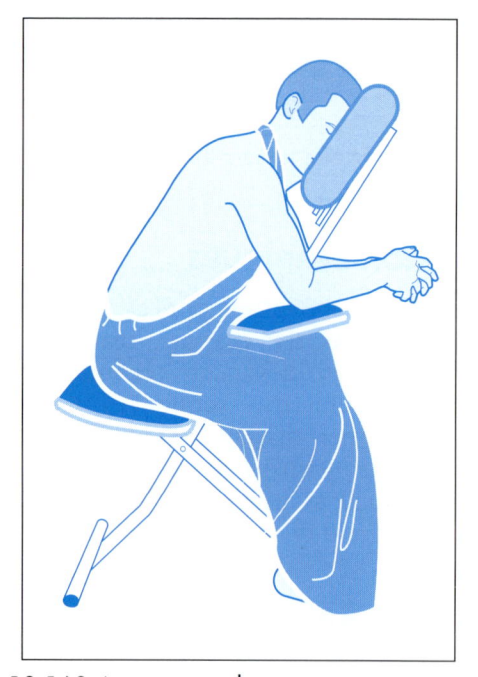

Figure 18.160 A massage chair

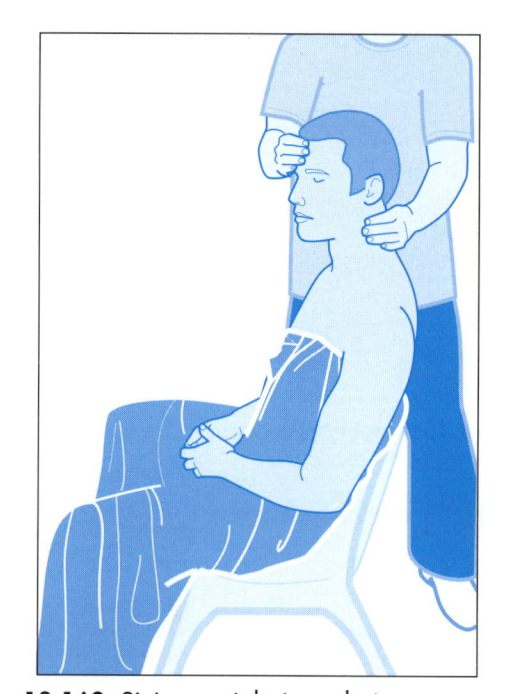

Figure 18.162 Sitting upright in a chair

BACK

Stance	Sequence reference	Description
Front stance	1	Kneading the upper trapezius
Wide stance at 45 degrees	2	Circular palm kneading
Stride stance	3	Loose fist compressions
Wide stance at 45 degrees	4	Heel frictions to the paraspinal muscles
Wide stance at 45 degrees	5	Forearm compressions on the trapezius
Stride stance	6	Specific compressions

CHAPTER 18 THE MASSAGE SEQUENCE   283

ARMS AND HANDS

Front stance	1	Kneading the upper trapezius
Front stance	7	Squeezing both upper arms
Kneel on one knee at side	8	Squeezing one arm
Kneel on one knee at side	9	Alternative circular thumb kneading to the wrist
Kneel on one knee at side	10	Alternative circular thumb kneading to the palm
Kneel on one knee at side	11	Thumb stripping between the rays of the hand
Kneel on one knee at side	12	Kneading to each finger
		Repeat arm and hand routine to other side 7–12

NECK AND SCALP

Front stance	1	Kneading the upper trapezius
Wide stance at side	13	Alternative knuckle kneading to the side of the neck
Stride stance behind client	14	Kneading the back of the neck
Front stance	15	Sub-occipital compressions
Front stance	16	Specific compression to the back of the neck
Front stance	17	Fingertip kneading of the scalp
Front stance	18	Finger pad kneading to the side of the head
Front stance	19	Stroking the hair

COMPLETING THE SEQUENCE

Front stance	1	Kneading the upper trapezius
Wide stance	20	Hacking the trapezius and muscles of the back
Front stance	21	Nerve stroke

Overview of the seated massage sequence

This section summarises the seated massage sequence. Once each stroke is mastered this overview will allow easy recall during practice. The column on the left indicates positional cues and the therapist's or the client's limb position. For easy reference the numbers in the centre column match the detailed description of each stroke given in the seated 'massage sequence in depth' section of this chapter.

The massage sequence in depth

This section breaks down the seated massage sequence and outlines each manipulation. Each stroke is fully explained in written form and supported with illustration. The therapist's posture is also described with each stroke.

1. Kneading the upper trapezius

Therapist posture: Front stance facing the client (Figure 18.163).

Hands: Place each hand on each upper trapezius muscle. The thumbs sit on the posterior aspect of the muscle and the fingers sit on the anterior aspect

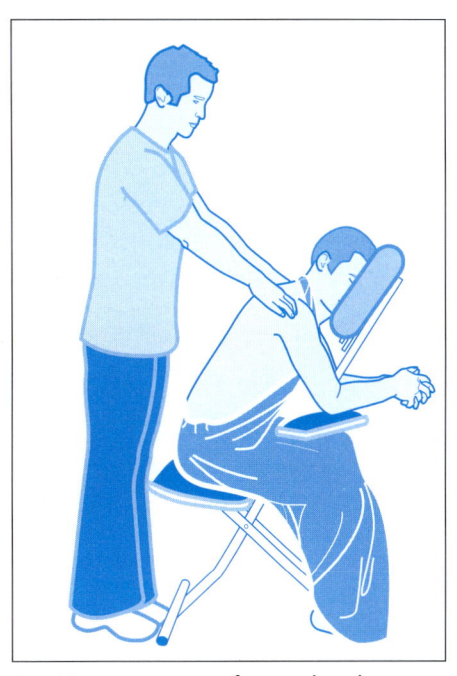

Figure 18.163 Front stance facing the client

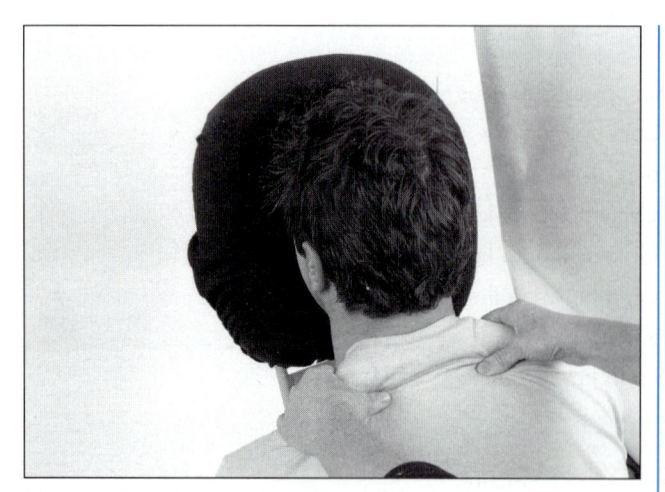

Figure 18.164 Kneading the upper trapezius

of the muscle with the fingers facing downwards and medially towards the sternum.
Movement: The thumb and fingers of one hand come together to grasp, lift and squeeze the muscle. The fingers then relax and glide to another position on the muscle and the stroke is repeated. Continue the stroke until the shoulders drop and move freely (Figure 18.164).

2. Circular palm kneading

Therapist posture: Wide stance standing at a 45 degree angle to the rear of the client (Figure 18.165).
Hands: Place the left hand on the client's left shoulder for support. Place the right hand on the paraspinal muscles of the upper back on the right side of the body.

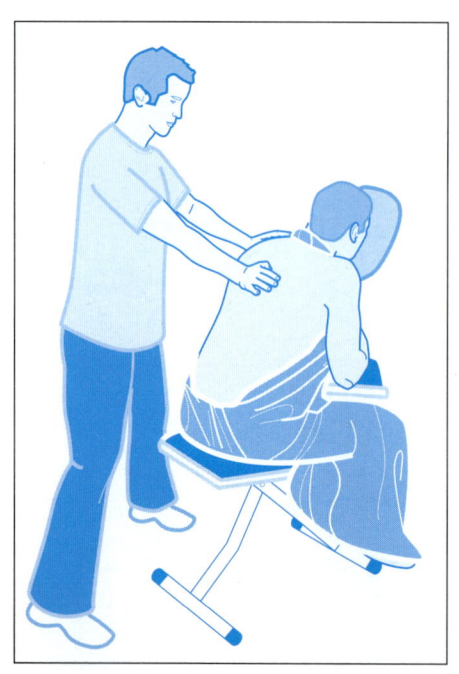

Figure 18.165 Wide stance standing at a 45 degree angle to the rear of the client

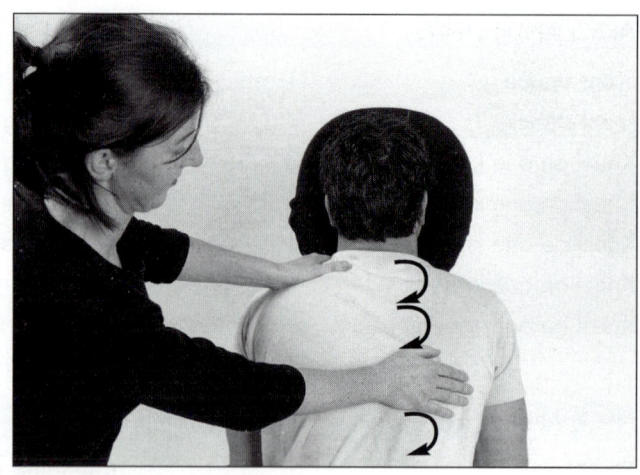

Figure 18.166 Circular palm kneading

Movement: Using the palm, perform gentle circular palm movements over the paraspinal muscle from the upper back to the low back (Figure 18.166).

3. Loose fist compressions

Therapist posture: Stride stance standing behind the client (Figure 18.167).
Hands: With a loose fist, place the knuckles of both hands on the paraspinal muscles of the low back.
Movement: Using the knuckles and posterior surface of the fingers, alternatively press into paraspinal muscles and push down, each compression moves towards the upper back (Figure 18.168).

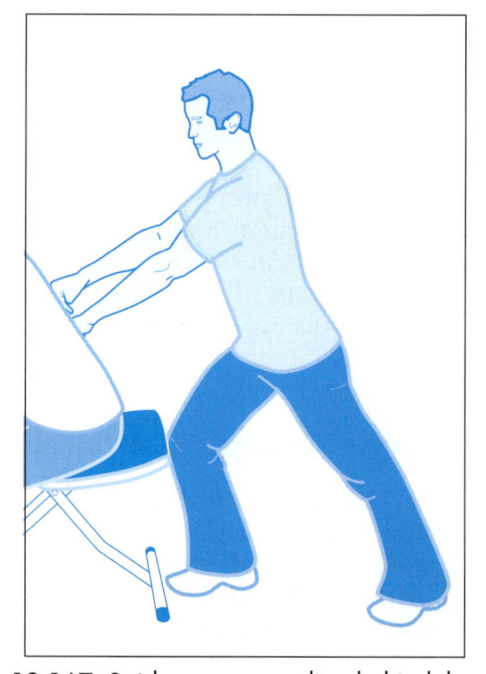

Figure 18.167 Stride stance standing behind the client

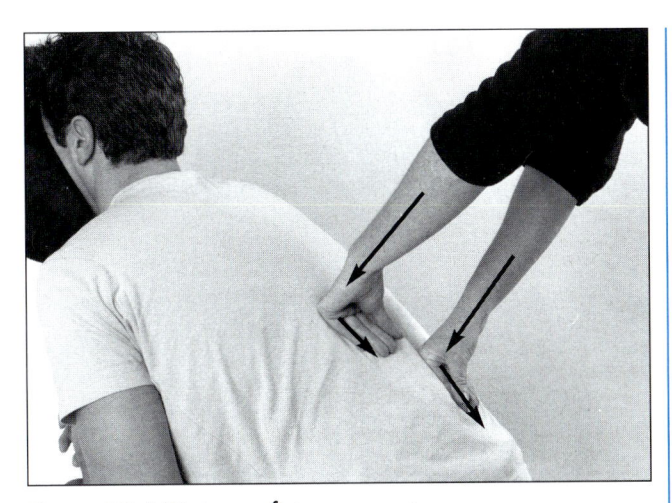

Figure 18.168 Loose fist compressions

4. Heel frictions to the paraspinal muscles

Therapist posture: Wide stance standing at a 45 degree angle to the rear of the client (Figure 18.165).
Hands: Place the left hand on the client's left shoulder for support. Place the right palm on the paraspinal muscle of the upper back. Ensure the fingers are relaxed and face the client's right shoulder.
Movement: Using the heel of the hand press into the paraspinal muscles and moves across the muscle fibres away from the spine. Glide the hands back towards the spine, moving further along the length of the paraspinal muscles, continuing the same movement. Repeat to cover the length of the spine from the upper back to the low back. Repeat on the other side (Figure 18.169).

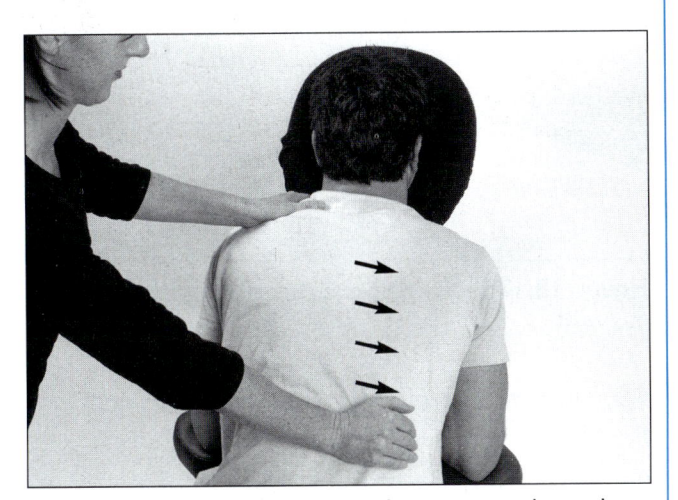

Figure 18.169 Heel frictions to the paraspinal muscles

5. Forearm compressions on the trapezius

Therapist posture: Wide stance standing at a 45 degree angle to the rear of the client (Figure 18.165).
Hands: Place the left hand on the client's left shoulder for support. Place the right forearm on the trapezius close to the angle of the neck.
Movement: Using the forearm, lean into the client and compress the trapezius muscles, hold for a short duration and release, move further laterally and repeat. Repeat the compression to cover the length of the trapezius muscle. Repeat on the other side (Figure 18.170).

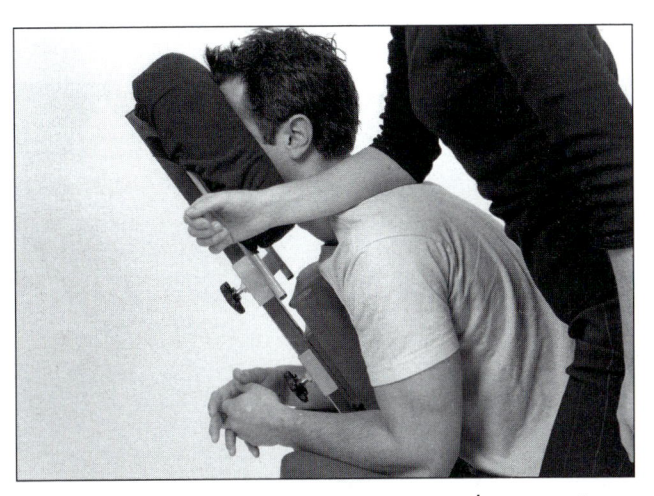

Figure 18.170 Forearm compressions on the trapezius

6. Specific compressions

Therapist posture: Stride stance standing behind client (Figure 18.167).
Hands: Place each thumb on the medial paraspinal muscles either side of the spine at the level of the angle of the neck.
Movement: Using the thumbs, working downwards, press into the paraspinal muscle and release. Repeat the technique to the base of the ribs. Repeat the technique several times; each time the thumb placement should be placed further away from the spine. Repeat on the other side (Figure 18.171).

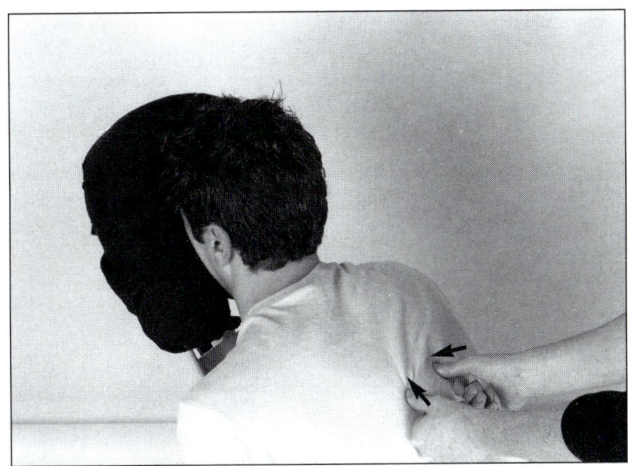

Figure 18.171 Specific compressions

7. Squeezing both upper arms

Therapist posture: Front stance (Figure 18.163).
Hands: From the previous position, move the hands so that they grasp the shoulders. The fingers should face forwards and the thumb should rest on the back of the muscle facing upwards.
Movement: Grasp, lift and squeeze the muscles between the palm of the hand and fingers. The hands then relax and glide to another position on the arm and the stroke is repeated (Figure 18.172).

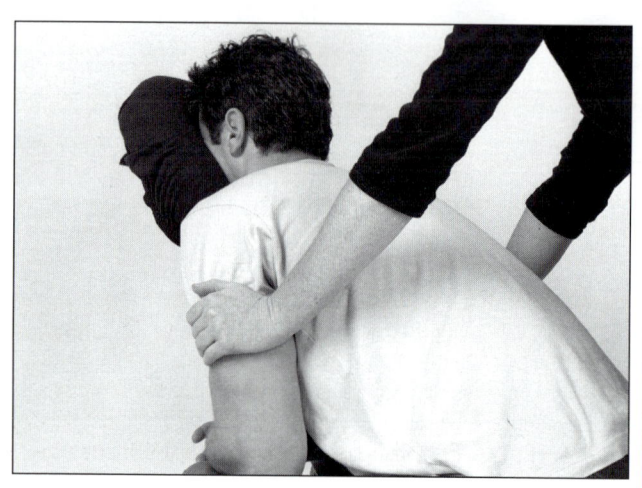

Figure 18.172 Squeezing both upper arms

8. Squeezing one arm

Therapist posture: Kneel on one knee, facing the client, at their side (Figure 18.173).
Hands: Place both hands on either side of the wrist supported loosely by your fingers around the palm. The thumbs come together over the top of the wrist.
Movement: Grasp, lift and squeeze the muscles in each hand and release. Repeat the technique at different positions as the hands slowly move down the entire length of the arm to the wrist (Figure 18.174).

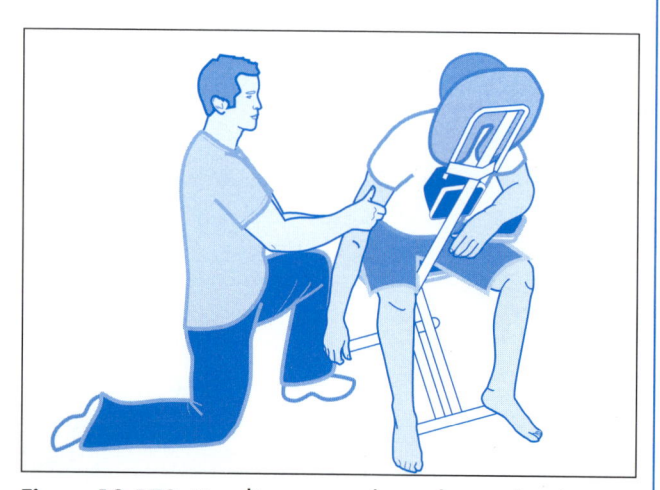

Figure 18.173 Kneeling on one knee, facing the client, at side

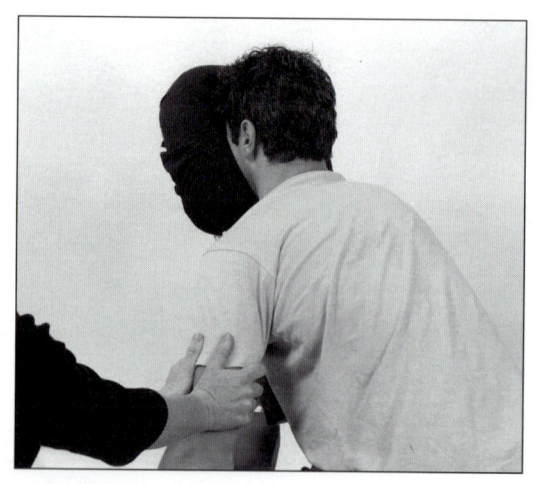

Figure 18.174 Squeezing one arm

9. Alternative circular thumb kneading to the wrist

Therapist posture: Kneel on one knee, facing the client, at their side (Figure 18.173).
Hands: Place both hands on either side of the wrist supported loosely by your fingers around the palm. The thumbs come together over the top of the wrist.
Movement: Perform alternating circular thumb kneading to the top of the wrist (Figure 18.175).

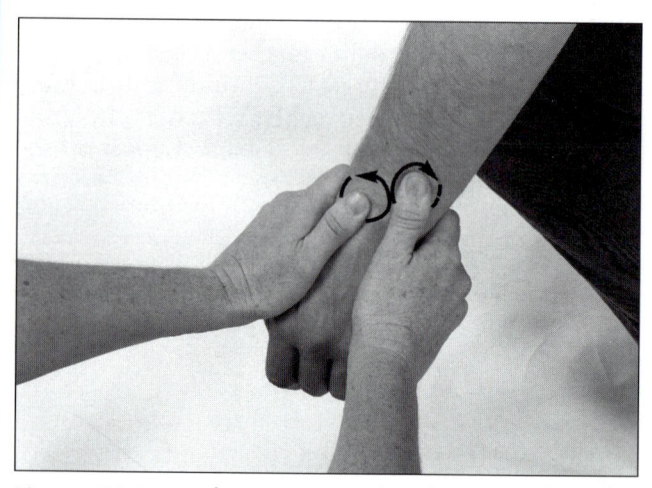

Figure 18.175 Alternative circular thumb kneading to the wrist

10. Alternative circular thumb kneading to the palm

Therapist posture: Kneel on one knee, facing the client, at their side (Figure 18.173).
Hands: Rotate the hand so that the palm faces towards the therapist.
Movement: Perform alternating circular thumb kneading to cover the surface of the palm (Figure 18.176).

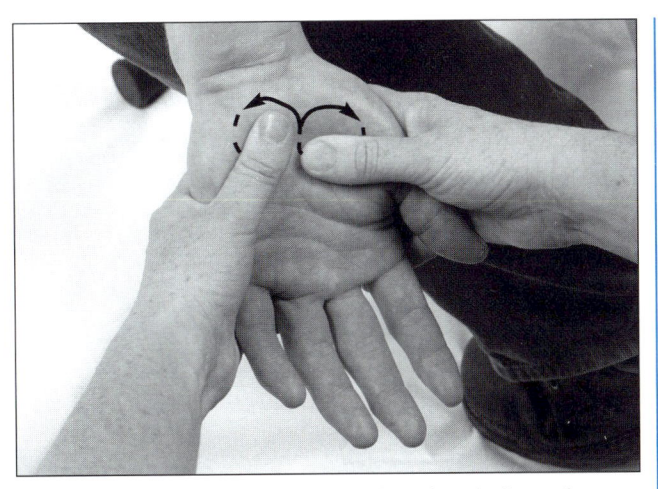

Figure 18.176 Alternative circular thumb kneading to the palm

11. Thumb stripping between the rays of the hand

Therapist posture: Kneel on one knee, facing the client, at their side (Figure 18.173).
Hands: On the dorsal surface (the back) of the hand use a thumb to find a space between the rays of the hand.
Movement: Gently and slowly slide the thumb along each grove, from the knuckles to the wrist (Figure 18.177).

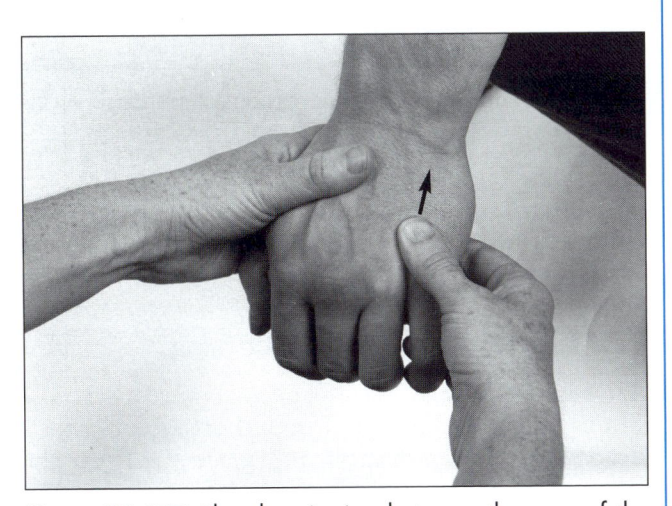

Figure 18.177 Thumb stripping between the rays of the hand

12. Kneading to each finger

Therapist posture: Kneel on one knee, facing the client, at their side (Figure 18.173).
Hands: Support the wrist with one hand. Using the thumb and first and second digits and wrap them around the base of a finger.
Movement: Knead around the circumference of each finger from the base to the tip. Repeat for each finger (Figure 18.178).

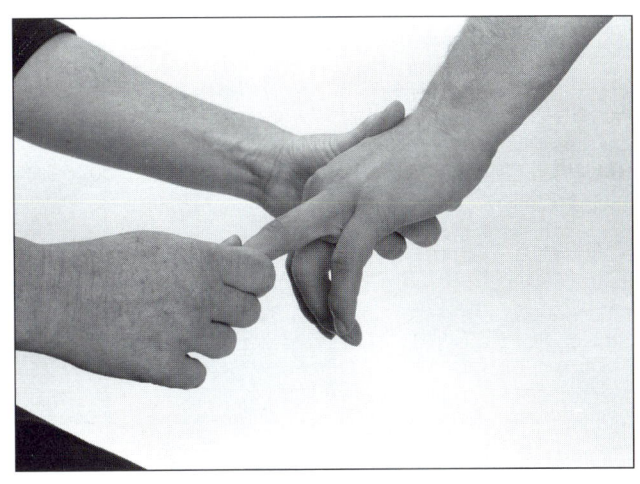

Figure 18.178 Kneading to each finger

13. Alternative knuckle kneading to the side of the neck

Therapist posture: Front stance (Figure 18.163).
Hands: Place one hand with loosely curled fingers on each side of the neck.
Movement: With loosely curled fingers, apply alternating circular movements, travelling up and down the sides of the neck (Figure 18.179).

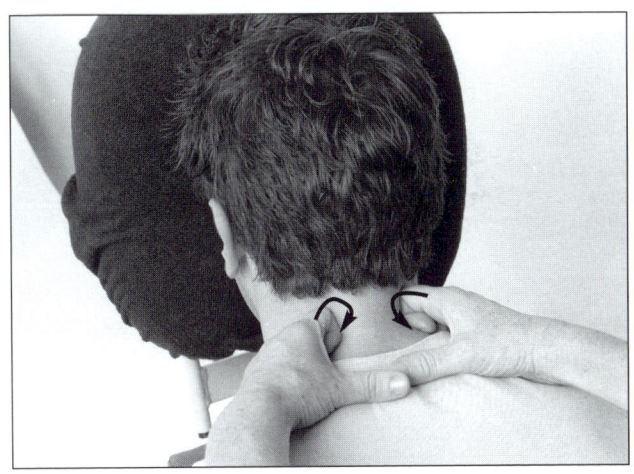

Figure 18.179 Alternative knuckle kneading to the side of the neck

14. Kneading the back of the neck

Therapist posture: Wide stance at the side of the client (Figure 18.180).
Hands: Place one hand around the back of the neck with the fingers on one side and the thumbs on the other side of the neck.
Movement: Grasp the back of the neck with thumbs and finger pads and gently pick up and knead the back and sides of the neck (Figure 18.181).

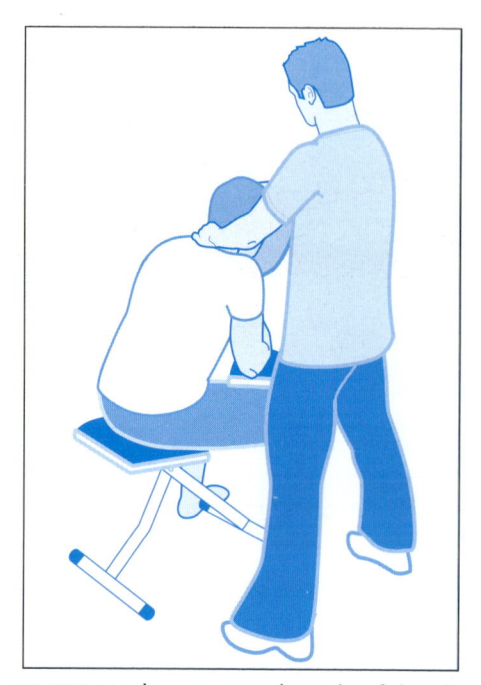

Figure 18.180 Wide stance at the side of the client

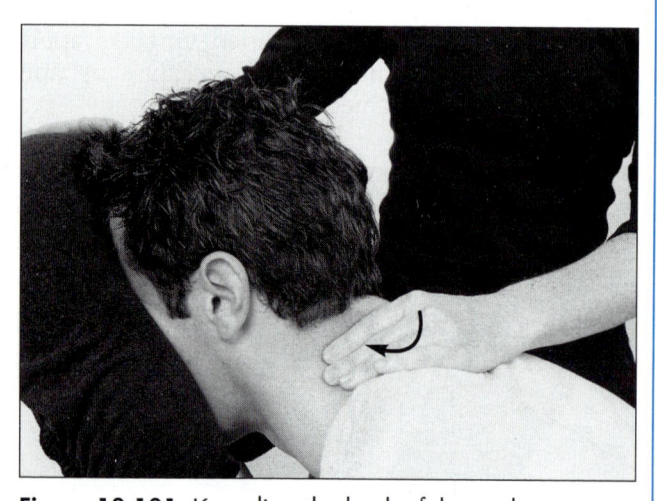

Figure 18.181 Kneading the back of the neck

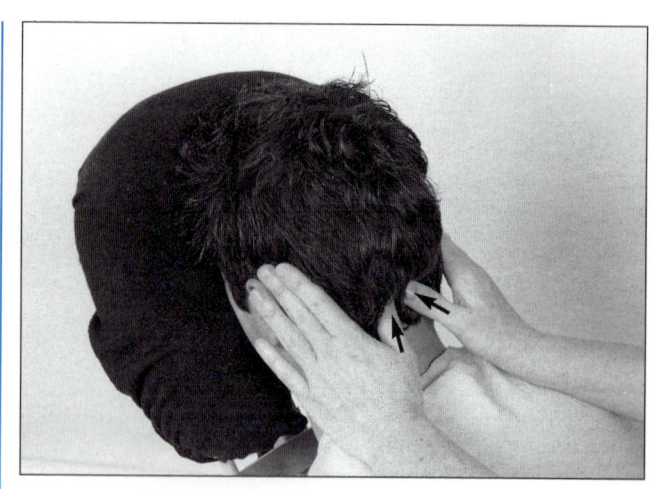

Figure 18.182 Sub-occipital compressions

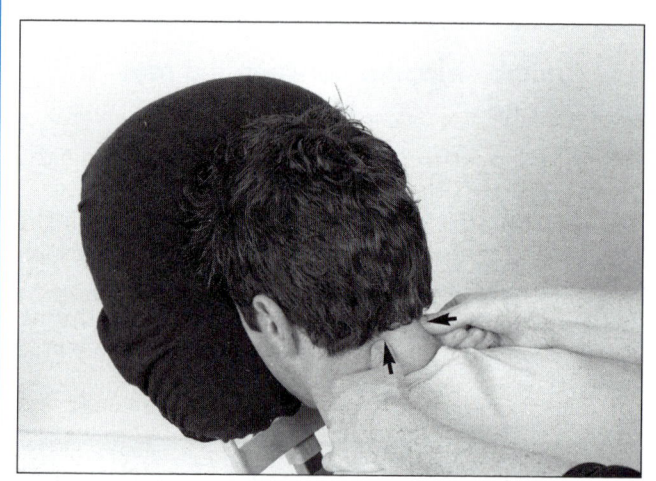

Figure 18.183 Specific compression to the back of the neck

15. Sub-occipital compressions

Therapist posture: Stride stance standing behind client (Figure 18.167).
Hands: Rest the fingers of each hand on the back of the client's head, place each thumb on either side of the spine, just beneath the occiput.
Movement: Using the thumbs press into the sub-occipital muscles and release. Repeat the technique moving laterally to the mastoid process of the occiput (Figure 18.182).

16. Specific compression to the back of the neck

Therapist posture: Stride stance standing behind the client (Figure 18.167).
Hands: Place the thumbs on muscles either side of the spine. Gently wrap the fingers around the side of the neck.
Movement: Apply gentle compressions as the thumbs travel down the length of the neck to the scapula (Figure 18.183).

17. Fingertip kneading of the scalp

Therapist posture: Front stance (Figure 18.163).
Hands: Position the hand on either side of client's head, spread your fingers and place them on the side of the skull above the ears.
Movement: Bend the fingertips and apply small circular movements with both hands simultaneously. Continue the stroke for a few moments then repeat the technique on another area of the scalp (Figure 18.184).

18. Finger pad kneading to the side of the head

Therapist posture: Front stance (Figure 18.163).
Hands: Place the finger pads on the temples.
Movement: Apply circular movements in a line from the temples to behind the ears (Figure 18.185).

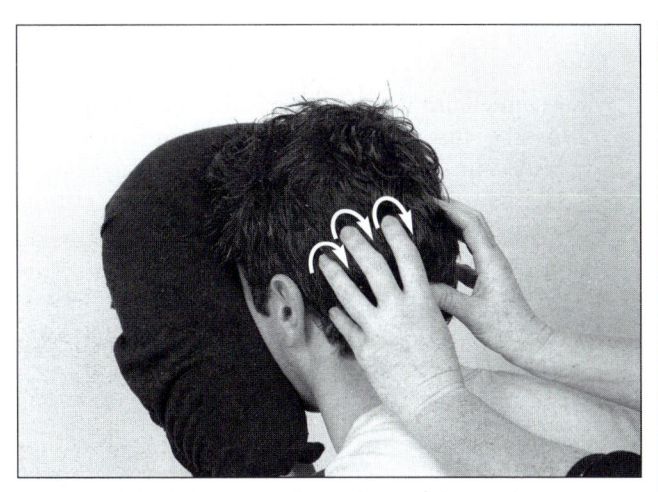

Figure 18.184 Fingertip kneading of the scalp

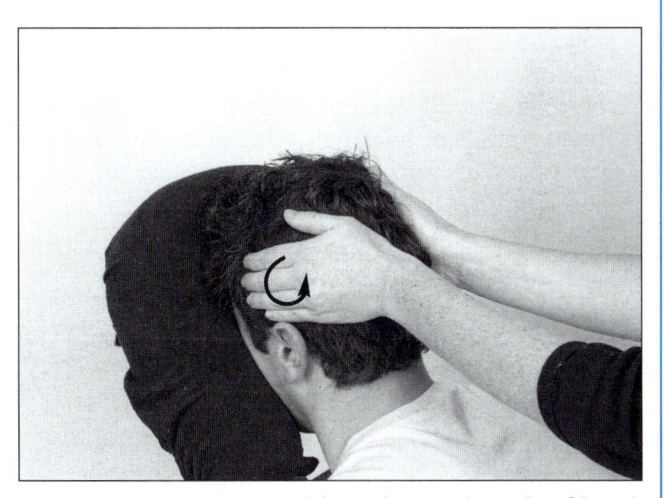

Figure 18.185 Finger pad kneading to the side of head

19. Stroking the hair

Therapist posture: Front stance (Figure 18.163).
Hands: Gently grip hair between the fingers.
Movement: Using the fingers as a comb, stroke through the hair. Gently grip the hair between the fingers as they pass through its length (Figure 18.186).

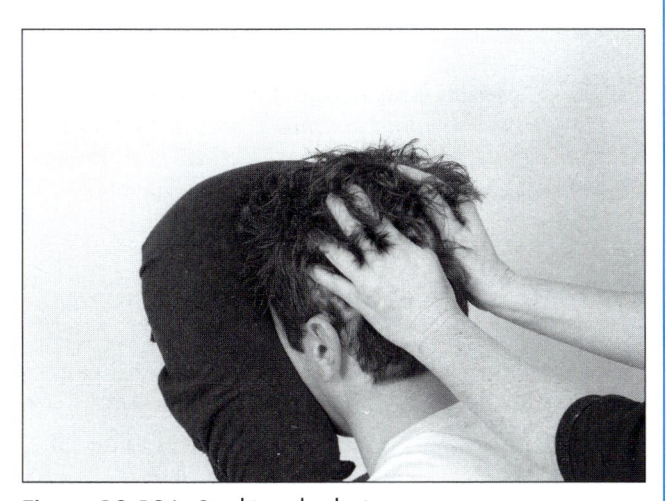

Figure 18.186 Stroking the hair

20. Hacking the trapezius and muscles of the back

Therapist posture: Wide stance facing the client (Figure 18.187).
Hands: Place the hands on the back with the little fingers in contact with the body and the palms parallel about five centimetres apart.
Movement: Flick the wrists back and forth alternately so that the little fingers come in contact with the trapezius and the back. The fingers are kept relaxed and the wrists are loose so that that the fingers spring up off the back rather than landing heavily in a chopping action (Figure 18.188).

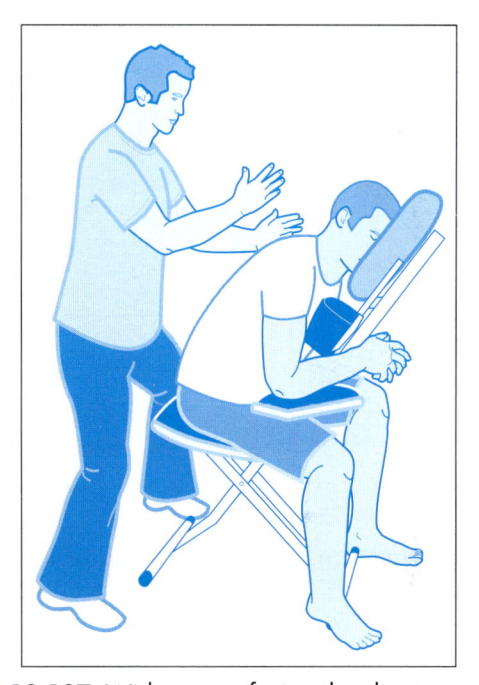

Figure 18.187 Wide stance facing the client

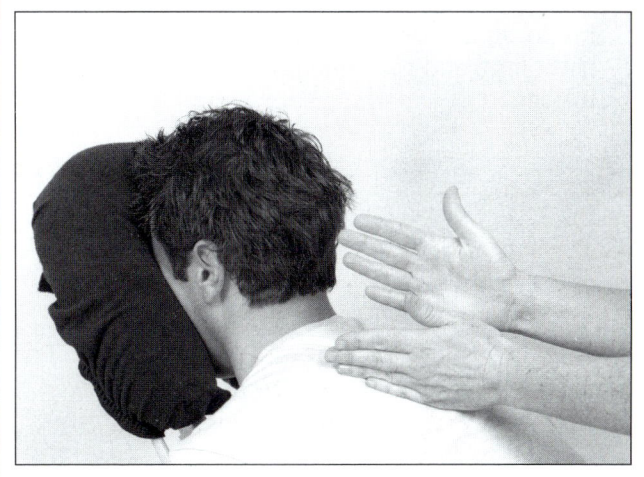

Figure 18.188 Hacking the trapezius and muscles of the back

21. Nerve stroke

Therapist posture: Stride stance standing behind the client (Figure 18.167).
Hands: The therapist places fingertips at the top of the head.
Movement: With the fingertips, stroke down the neck, shoulders and back with light and slow pressure (Figure 18.189).

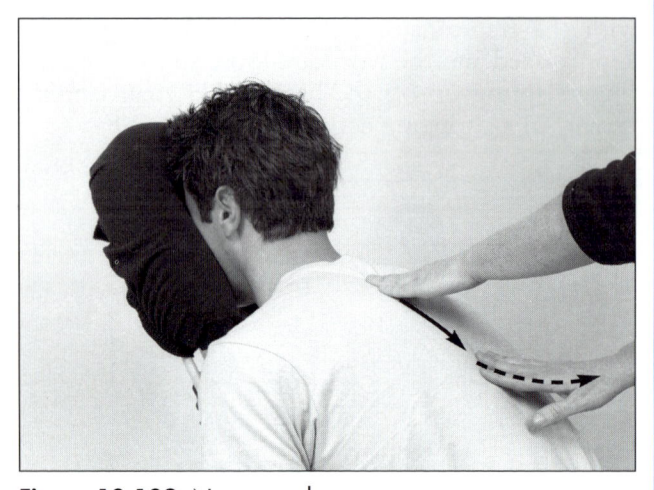

Figure 18.189 Nerve stroke

Questions and activities

1. Design your own one hour full body massage based on the principles of massage application.
2. Your client, Sam, is suffering from neck pain and shoulder pain. The pain experienced is a dull ache and is accompanied with restriction in movement. Headaches occur frequently for Sam and he attributes this to stress and tension caused by his senior managerial role where he is responsible for retrenching staff. Sam has visited his local doctor who has ruled out all serious pathology and recommend that he has a regular massage.
   (a) Sam is coming to you for massage for relief of tension in his neck and back. You are seeing him for the first time and wish to assess his needs thoroughly in this first meeting. What questions would you ask Sam to gain information about his presenting complaint?
   (b) Are there contraindications or precautions to this massage? If so, list them.
   (c) You have gathered all the appropriate information from your client. Design a massage sequence suitable to treat Sam's complaint.
   (d) How would you record all this information on an ASTER form?
3. Michael is a 21-year-old man who complains of low back and buttock pain. Michael visits his chiropractor who assures him that with a chiropractic adjustment and some massage therapy the muscles will relax and the pain will disappear. Design a half hour massage sequence suitable for Michael's condition.

Further reading

Andrale, C. and Clifford, P. (2001) *Outcome-based Massage*. Lippincott Williams & Wilkins, Philadelphia.

Cassar, M. (1999) *Handbook of Massage Therapy: A Complete Guide for the Student and Professional Massage Ttherapist*. Butterworth–Heinemann, Oxford.

De Domenico, G. and Wood, E. C. (1997) *Beard's Massage* (4th edn). W. B. Saunders, Philadelphia.

Holey, E. and Cook, E. (2003) *Evidence Based Massage*. Churchill Livingstone, London.

Loving, J. E. (1999) *Massage Therapy: Theory and Practice*. Appleton & Lange, Stamford, Connecticut.

REFERENCES

De Domenico, G. and Wood, E. C. (1997) *Beard's Massage* (4th edn). W. B. Saunders, Philadelphia.

Fritz, S. (2000) *Mosby's Fundamentals of Therapeutic Massage*. Mosby, St Louis.

Mennell, J. B. (1917) *Massage: Its Principles and Practice*. J. & A. Churchill, London.

Tappan, F. M. and Benjamin, P. J. (1998) *Tappan's Handbook of Healing Massage Techniques: Classic, Holistic and Emerging Methods* (3rd edn). Appleton & Lange, Stamford, Connecticut.

section 7

Pregnancy, the Infant and Massage

chapter 19

Massage during pregnancy and labour

Vicki Tuchtan

Learning outcomes

- Describe the benefits of massage therapy in pregnancy
- Describe the stages of pregnancy
- Discuss the considerations for massage and cautions for massage during the first trimester
- Discuss the considerations for massage and cautions for massage during the second trimester
- Discuss the considerations for massage and cautions for massage during the third trimester
- Describe the use of massage during labour

INTRODUCTION

The number of women seeking the services of a qualified massage therapist during their pregnancy and labour is increasing. Pregnancy is a natural occurrence for women, and is not considered a disease state or illness. During pregnancy, a woman undergoes significant physical and emotional changes; changes that can be assisted with massage therapy.

When working with the pregnant client, there are many considerations that must be taken into account. At every consultation, the women would have undergone change since their last visit to their massage therapist, and such changes need to be recognised and responded to appropriately. This chapter serves to outline the various stages of pregnancy, and describe the management of the client throughout the pregnancy. It also outlines the important role the massage therapist plays in the process of labour.

MASSAGE DURING PREGNANCY

Upon learning that she is pregnant, a woman embarks upon a unique journey that is a roller coaster of emotions and new experiences. The process of pregnancy is unique, as no two pregnancies are the same. A most joyous time for many women, the experience of pregnancy may also be extremely stressful. Fear, excitement, anticipation, uncertainty, sadness and exhilaration are all feelings that a woman may experience about the impending birth of her baby. At the same time she may feel anxious, bemused or overjoyed by the changes she notices physically to her body. Such changes include enlargement of the breasts, thickening of the waistline and changes in hair and nail growth. They may also notice other changes or conditions associated with pregnancy that may lead them to seek the services of a massage therapist. These conditions include low back pain, tiredness and fatigue, anxiety, headache, cramp, swelling of the hands and feet, insomnia and sciatic pain.

> **Box 19.1** Remember
>
> The process of pregnancy is a unique one, and each woman's experiences will be different.

Several authors describe the benefits of massage therapy during pregnancy (McPake and Shannon, 2002; Hicks and McPake, 2001; Stillerman, 2000; Osborne-Sheets, 1998). Some of the claimed benefits of pregnancy massage described by these authors include that it:

- encourages relaxation and reduce stress;
- improves blood and lymph circulation and reduce oedema;
- reduces pain;
- minimises varicose veins;
- reduces blood pressure;
- relieves muscular fatigue, cramping and contraction;
- improves energy levels;
- maintains skin elasticity, minimising stretch marks;
- relieves depression and anxiety; and
- stimulates glandular secretions that assist in balancing hormone levels.

Many of these claims are broad and generalised, and not supported by controlled and randomised clinical trials. Despite this fact, pregnant women are seeking out massage as a supportive and nurturing therapy during their pregnancy. Although the exact benefits of pregnancy massage are not known, anecdotal reports from pregnant women include improvements in mood and sleep and a reduction in pain.

When presented with a pregnant client, the massage therapist should have knowledge of the process of pregnancy. They should be aware of and expect the many changes that occur throughout the pregnancy, and be able to adapt their techniques accordingly. The skilled massage therapist must also be aware of the contraindications and precautions associated with massage during pregnancy. The way in which the massage therapist modifies their treatment for a pregnant client will depend on the stage of pregnancy that the woman is in.

THE STAGES OF PREGNANCY

The process of pregnancy is divided into three stages, referred to as trimesters. A trimester is a period of 13 weeks, or three months. Weeks 1–13 of the pregnancy are referred to as the first trimester. During this time the woman discovers that she has stopped menstruating and learns of the impending birth of her child. Many know this time as the trimester of nausea or morning sickness. The second trimester lasts from 14 to 26 weeks. During this stage the woman can no longer disguise her pregnancy, as the characteristic contour of pregnancy shows its form. By this stage of the pregnancy, the woman is usually comfortable with the idea of pregnancy and has adjusted her routine and lifestyle to accommodate her changing form, and nurture her unborn child. During the second trimester, at around 20 weeks, the mother would have felt the presence of the baby as it kicks and moves around in its cramped space. Depending on

> **Box 19.2** The stages of pregnancy
>
> First trimester — weeks: 1–13
> Second trimester — weeks: 14–26
> Third trimester — weeks: 27–39+

the onset of labour, the third trimester may run from the 27th to the 40th week of pregnancy or beyond.

As described above, each trimester is characterised by unique changes that mark the stages of pregnancy. Such changes occur not only in the mother but also in the unborn child. The therapist must be sensitive to the needs of the pregnant client, and be aware of the events that occur during each trimester. Such knowledge will equip them with the skills to manage the pregnant client and ensure the safety of both the mother and the unborn child during massage therapy.

The first trimester

When a woman becomes pregnant the body is subjected to a cascade of changing hormone levels. Throughout the first trimester, the mother-to-be must adjust to these changes in hormones, and in particular the higher levels of both oestrogen and progesterone hormones. The levels of both oestrogen and progesterone will continue to increase over the course of the pregnancy. In the first trimester these hormone levels are only slightly higher than the levels produced after ovulation each month in a non-pregnant woman. However, during pregnancy they are responsible for stimulating uterine growth; enhancing blood circulation to the uterus, placenta and baby; maintaining the balance of blood metabolites and glucose; promoting metabolism; and increasing the respiratory rate and cardiac output of the mother, to promote the healthy development of the foetus (Osborne-Sheets, 1998). Oestrogen increases uterine strength, whilst both hormones assist in preparing the mammary glands to produce milk. Progesterone also inhibits uterine contractions and maintains the lining of the uterus (Hicks and McPake, 2001; Osborne-Sheets, 1998).

Nausea is a symptom that is experienced by approximately 60 per cent of women during the first semester (Stillerman, 2000). It has been suggested that the release of human chorionic gonadotrophin — a hormone that conserves maternal use of glucose for the growing baby and prepares the mammary glands to produce milk (Hicks and McPake, 2001) — is responsible for the nausea commonly referred to as 'morning sickness' (Stillerman, 2000). Hormones are also partly responsible for the physical exhaustion and increased frequency of urination experienced throughout these first three months. Other symptoms that may be experienced during the first trimester include mood swings, breast tenderness, constipation, reduced appetite, and musculoskeletal problems. During the first trimester, the massage therapist must take care to devise a treatment plan that takes these maternal changes into consideration.

> **Box 19.3** Symptoms associated with the first trimester
>
> - Nausea or morning sickness
> - Mood swings
> - Breast tenderness
> - Constipation
> - Reduced appetite
> - Musculoskeletal aches and pains

Massage and the first trimester

At this early stage of the pregnancy the size of the baby is not so large that it would place undue pressure on internal structures, or produce pain and affect function by placing strain on utero-abdominal ligaments. As such, each of the following massage positions are considered safe for use during the first trimester, taking all other precautions and client comfort into consideration:

- supine position;
- prone position;
- side-lying position;
- semi-reclining position;
- seated position.

Most pregnant clients will not have difficulty lying supine (on their backs) for extended periods during the first trimester. When massaging a client in this position it is important to ensure the low back is supported. This can be done by placing bolsters or pillows under the knees, which will in turn reduce the curvature of the client's lumbar spine, thereby reducing strain on the lower back region. When lying prone, the growth of the breasts may produce pain and discomfort for some clients, thus position adjustments may be necessary. Another consideration when lying either supine or prone is the fact that towards the end of the trimester the

> **Box 19.4** Remember
>
> When the client is in the supine position, support the low back by placing pillows or bolsters under the knees.

baby may be getting close to the size of a grapefruit, and thus may place undue pressure on the bladder, increasing the frequency of urination.

When massaging a pregnant client during the first semester, the massage therapist should:

- allow the client to adjust their positioning if the breasts are uncomfortable;
- recommend the woman empty her bladder prior to the massage treatment;
- use pillows or bolsters under the knees when in the supine position to reduce strain on the low back; and
- encourage the client to attend appointments at times during the day when their energy levels are high and feelings of nausea are low.

Caution

The risk of miscarriage is highest during the first trimester. As such, the massage therapist must take additional care to ensure the comfort and safety of the client and her unborn child during this time. For clients with a history of difficult pregnancy, miscarriage or complications associated with pregnancy, it is advised that a medical clearance be sought prior to the application of massage therapy. When providing massage treatment during the first three months of pregnancy, the therapist should observe the following cautions:

- refrain from touching the abdomen of the pregnant client;
- seek medical clearance for any client who has a history of pregnancy-related complications prior to any treatment being administered; and
- avoid rhythmic rocking of the client if they are feeling nauseous.

The second trimester

Sometimes referred to as the 'quiet months', the second trimester is often a period of reduced symptomatology in contrast to the first trimester. For the majority of women the nausea and tiredness that characterised the first trimester will be replaced by a feeling of wellness. It is during this trimester that women often have that 'glowing' look associated with a healthy pregnancy. By the 14th week of pregnancy most women will have adjusted to the hormonal changes and will spend the second trimester grappling with the changes in their physical form. During the second trimester, most women take on the 'pregnant appearance' and exhibit an abdominal bulge or contour. Some women find this a glorious time, whilst others will seek to hide their changing shape.

The massage therapist needs to be empathetic towards the client at this time. They must respect the mother's feelings and be a supportive listener throughout the pregnancy as the women experiences changes in her body shape. The expectant mother will normally experience weight gain during the second trimester and the breasts will continue to enlarge. The additional weight gain may result in conditions associated with undue pressure, such as varicose veins, haemorrhoids and stretch marks or striae over the abdomen, and occasionally the buttocks and thighs. As the baby enlarges in the uterus it will encroach upon abdominal organs and may lead to abdominal pain and gastric reflux. The added weight may overload muscles and joints, especially of the legs, back and pelvis. Other complications associated with the second trimester include flatulence and constipation. When massaging a client during the second trimester, the massage therapist must take care to devise a treatment plan that takes these maternal changes into consideration.

> **Box 19.5** Symptoms associated with the second trimester
>
> - Differing emotional response to a changing body shape
> - Weight gain
> - Varicose veins
> - Haemorrhoids
> - Stretch marks
> - Abdominal pain
> - Gastric reflux
> - Musculoskeletal aches and pains
> - Flatulence
> - Constipation

Massage and the second trimester

The second trimester is an opportune time for the massage therapist to encourage the mother to massage her own abdomen (if she isn't doing so already) with an oil or cream that is emollient. This will assist in maintaining the suppleness of the skin and may serve to minimise the appearance of stretch marks.

This trimester is a time of rapid growth. During the second trimester the baby may grow to 36 cm in length and weigh up to 700 grams. As the size of the baby increases over this period, the postural alignment of the mother's body is altered, as her gravitational centre is shifted. This shift will place undue strain on areas such as the lower back and pelvis, and may produce great pain. Such growth of the baby also affects internal structures of the mother, as the uterus and baby now take up space equivalent to a rockmelon in the ventral body cavity (Osborne-Sheets, 1998). This growth encroaches on abdominal and pelvic organs, affecting functioning of structures such as the bladder, intestines and lungs.

In certain positions, the weight and size of the uterus places pressure on the major maternal veins, affecting the flow of blood returning to the heart. This in turn affects circulation to the placenta and the foetus. If a pregnant woman is required to lie supine for any extended period during this trimester, the weight of the uterus can impinge the inferior vena cava as it returns to the heart along the right side of the abdominal region. Such impingement will result in reduced maternal blood pressure and decreased blood circulation to the mother and baby. This condition is referred to as supine hypotensive syndrome (see Figure 19.1). It is recommended that, to avoid such a condition, supine positioning be limited to no more than five minutes after week 13 of pregnancy, and supported by a pillow or wedge placed under the client's right side at the level of the waistline (see Figure 19.2).

As the mother's body shape changes and the foetus grows in size during the second trimester, the mother will find it difficult to lie in the prone position. Due to the bulk of the uterus the prone position will be uncomfortable and should be avoided. To ensure that the massage experience is a safe and comfortable one during the second semester, it is advised to use the following positioning techniques:

- supported supine position — for no more than five minutes after week 13, and avoid after week 22 (Figure 19.2);
- supported semi-reclining position — recommended instead of supine position after week 22 (Figure 19.3);
- supported side-lying position (Figure 19.4); and
- seated position.

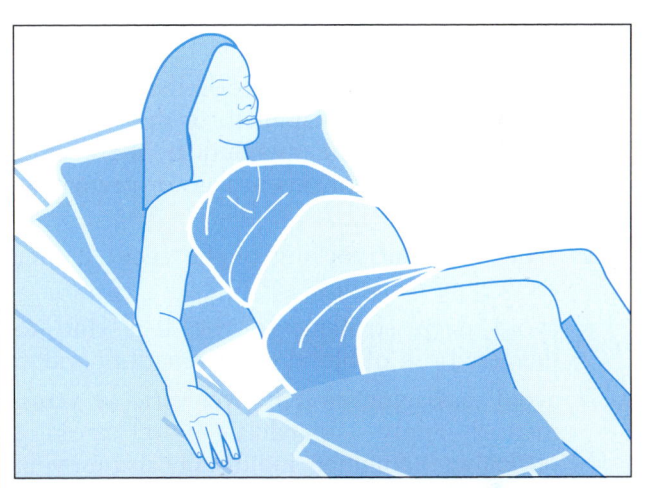

Figure 19.3 Supported semi-reclining position

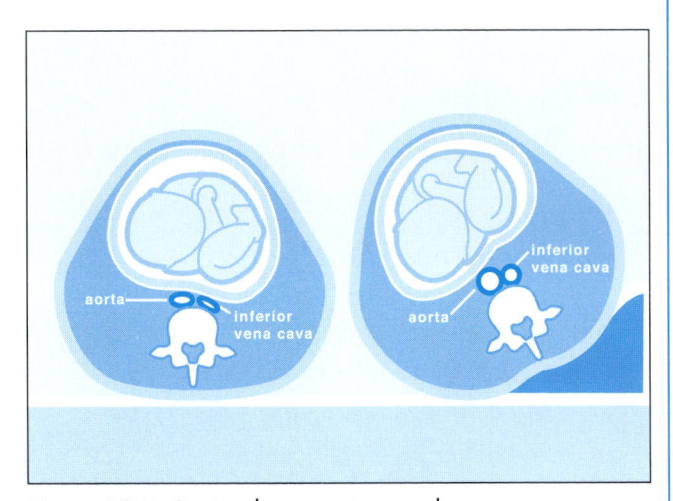

Figure 19.1 Supine hypotensive syndrome

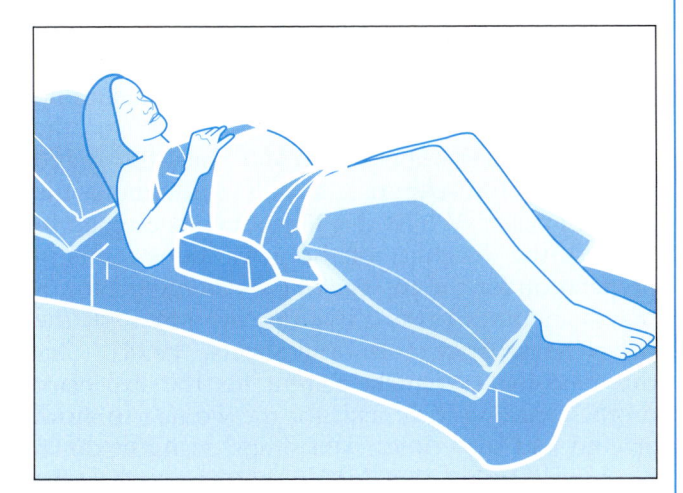

Figure 19.2 Supported supine position

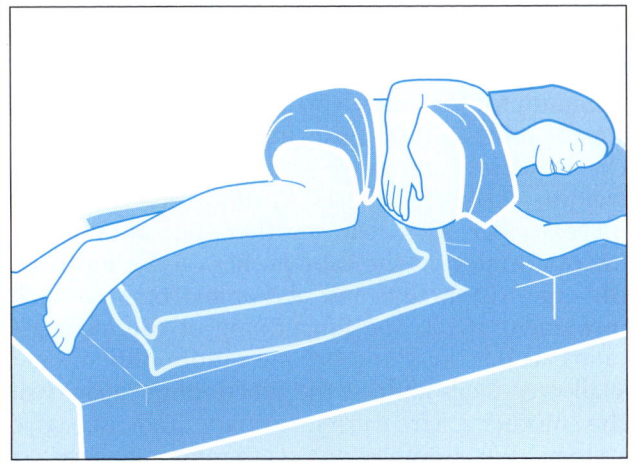

Figure 19.4 Supported side-lying position

Box 19.6 Remember

For the comfort and safety of both mother and baby, avoid placing the mother in a prone position for massage during the second or third trimesters.

Caution

The mother will feel for the first time the movements of the baby during this trimester, as it grows and enlarges in the ever-decreasing space of the abdomen. Some mothers will ask the massage therapist to feel or massage the abdomen at this stage, and the therapist must take care to use only light stroking if they choose to oblige. When massaging the legs during the second trimester, it is important that the therapist observe any varicose veins, as the mother may become more prone to blood clotting at this stage of the pregnancy. Due to the risk associated with varicose veins, it is best to avoid any deep stroking of the legs during the second trimester and beyond. Other precautions for the massage therapist to note during this stage are as follows:

- avoid all deep work over or around the abdominal region;
- application of light abdominal stroking (effleurage) may be applied for short periods though should be avoided if there is a previous history of miscarriage or premature birth;
- avoid rhythmic rocking of the client if they are feeling nauseous;
- avoid deep stroking of the legs due to increased risk of blood clot formation; and
- avoid massaging directly over varicose veins; instead apply superficial light stroking (effleurage) commencing distally and moving proximally.

The third trimester

In the last three months of pregnancy space is of a premium for the baby, who will more than triple its weight prior to birth, growing to an average of 50 cm in length and three and a half kilograms in weight (Osborne-Sheets, 1998). As the baby increases in size, the mother becomes more uncomfortable, as the baby pushes on the mother's rib cage, diaphragm and abdominal organs. Such movement affects the functioning of the mother's lungs, as her breathing becomes more difficult and shallower. It also affects the functioning capacity of the mother's circulatory, urinary and digestive systems. For example, due to the impingement on circulatory vessels by the size of the baby, the mother's reduced capacity to return fluid to the heart causes the amount of interstitial fluid to almost double, resulting in oedema and other pressure-related disorders, such as carpal tunnel syndrome (Osborne-Sheets, 1998).

In addition to the physical symptoms experienced during the second trimester, the mother will also experience breathing difficulties, fluid retention and increased urinary frequency during the final trimester. Fluid retention or oedema will often affect the peripheries of the body, the hands and the feet, and when severe will affect functioning and movement.

As the birth approaches, the mother prepares herself physically and emotionally for the arrival of the baby. During the third trimester the mother may again experience fluctuating moods, dependent on her feelings regarding the approaching labour and delivery. For a first-time mother, she may also be grappling with how her life will be after the birth, knowing it will be changed forever once the baby arrives. As such the expectant mother will exhibit different moods dependent on her emotions and her situation, ranging from frustration to eagerness, and anxiety to anticipation. At this time the therapist needs to be sensitive to the feelings of the mother and what she may be going through emotionally. When devising a treatment plan during the third trimester, the therapist must take care to ensure the treatment plan takes each of these physical and emotional changes into consideration.

> **Box 19.7** Symptoms associated with the third trimester
>
> - Weight gain
> - Varicose veins
> - Haemorrhoids
> - Stretch marks
> - Abdominal pain
> - Gastric reflux
> - Musculoskeletal aches and pains
> - Flatulence
> - Difficulty with breathing
> - Oedema or fluid retention
> - Increased frequency of urination

Massage and the third trimester

The hormone relaxin is released in the body during pregnancy to relax and ready the cervix for the birthing process (Hicks and McPake, 2001), and the levels of relaxin rise steadily throughout the third trimester. Whilst this hormone is designed to increase the flexibility of the pelvic bone joints in preparation for the passage of the emerging baby, it may sometimes cause the pubic symphysis of the pelvis to separate (Osborne-Sheets, 1998). This may become extremely painful for the expectant mother, making it difficult for the woman to move around and sometimes even simply walk, sit down or stand. During the third trimester the therapist must ensure they minimise the need to ask the pregnant client to make position changes throughout the treatment, and provide additional support to the expectant mother when she is getting on and off the massage table. Due to the continued body changes throughout the third trimester, the following positions are indicated for massage treatment:

- supported semi-reclining position (Figure 19.3);
- supported side-lying position (Figure 19.4);
- seated position.

These positions can be used right up until the birth of the baby. In this last trimester the pregnant woman will find it increasingly difficult to move and get comfortable during a massage. The therapist should be guided by the comfort needs of the expectant mother and use additional pillows for support as required. It may be prudent to use extra pillows under the knees and arms as the abdomen grows, to prevent strain on lumbar and utero-abdominal ligaments when the client is in the side-lying position.

> **Box 19.8** Remember
>
> Avoid asking the pregnant client to unnecessarily change positions during the third trimester.

In addition to affecting the pubic symphysis, the hormone relaxin may also affect other musculoskeletal structures. The therapist should take care during the third trimester not to apply any undue pressure over joints, ligamentous structures and musculature when applying massage. The pelvic girdle will be particularly mobile during this period, and the typical waddle of a late pregnancy is produced by the relaxation of the whole pelvic area. Late in the third trimester, the baby begins to move into a low position in the pelvic area, in preparation for delivery. The massage therapist may concentrate on relaxing and releasing musculature surrounding the pelvic girdle, and other structures that would be affected by the changed posture and gait.

Caution

The following guidelines should be considered when administering massage treatment to an expectant mother in the third trimester:

- avoid tapôtement strokes during the third trimester, as they may have an overstimulating effect;
- ensure clients affected by symphysis pubis are well supported when changing positions, and minimise the number of positional changes required; and
- employ only light stroking (effleurage), moving distal to proximal to relieve oedema associated with carpal tunnel syndrome.

> **Box 19.9** Positioning the pregnant client
>
> **First trimester**
> - Prone position
> - Side-lying position
> - Semi-reclining position
> - Seated position
>
> **Second trimester**
> - Supported supine position — for no more than five minutes after week 13, and avoid after week 22
> - Supported semi-reclining position — recommended instead of supine position after week 22
> - Supported side-lying position
> - Seated position
>
> **Third trimester**
> - Supported semi-reclining position
> - Supported side-lying position
> - Seated position

MASSAGE DURING LABOUR

As the benefits of massage therapy for pain relief are becoming more widely accepted, it is not uncommon for birthing units to offer massage services during the labour process. Although this service is a good idea, many women prefer to have their own support person trained in massage on hand for their birth. If they have been consulting with a massage therapist on a regular basis throughout their pregnancy and feel comfortable with this person, it is not uncommon for the pregnant woman to ask their massage therapist to attend their birth to provide massage during the labour.

For the professional massage therapist a request to provide massage during a labour may be greeted with confidence and humble acceptance or may leave the therapist feeling ill-equipped and unsure. For the therapist who falls into the latter group, a little bit of forward planning can increase their confidence in assisting a client.

The massage therapist is the ideal person to provide instruction to another who will act as the support person for the expectant mother during her labour. A woman may ask her partner, husband, mother or friend to act as their labour support person on the 'big day'. It is recommended that a labour support person be trained (close to the delivery date) to massage the expectant mother in preparation for the labour (Stillerman, 2000). The massage therapist can provide a service of simple instruction in the basic massage techniques used during labour.

Massage can be used during labour as an intervention that assists in relieving pain, encouraging relaxation and reducing anxiety. Although the pregnant woman may have thought about the process of labour and what interventions she would like to assist with the labour, one can never plan for this event. The process of labour can be most unpredictable, and may last for as little as one hour or may extend across days. A labour support person trained in massage may be asked to perform light strokes over the low back of the pregnant woman for hours, or may never have cause to test out their newly discovered skills. One thing that is certain is that the labour support person must be committed to last the distance of the labour.

CONCLUSION

As women become more aware of their health and the choices they have surrounding their care, they will increasingly seek out alternative options to complement their health care regime. This is evident with the increasing number of women adopting massage therapy as a form of adjunct treatment throughout their pregnancy and subsequent labour.

Massage therapy is an ideal treatment for the symptomatic relief of pregnancy-related disorders. The skilled massage therapist should be sensitive to the special needs of the pregnant woman, and have the skills to confidently adapt their techniques to accommodate the expectant mother. Massage therapy provides support for the changing emotions experienced by a woman during pregnancy, and has a role to paly in maintaining the healthy functioning of the musculoskeletal system. In addition, massage therapy improves a woman's acceptance of touch as a form of therapy. As such regular massage therapy on the part of the mother will only serve to encourage a healthy relationship based on touch between mother and child.

Questions and activities

1. A client of yours is in her second trimester of pregnancy, and claims she is 'hardly showing'. She believes she could receive a massage whilst lying prone for one hour.
   (a) As a therapist what concerns might you have for this positioning of the client?
   (b) What could you suggest to the client as an alternative?
2. Prepare a one-page information flier to give to clients, which details the benefits of receiving massage therapy during each of the stages of pregnancy.

Further reading

Osborne-Sheets, C. (1998) *Pre- and Perinatal Massage Therapy*. Body Therapy Associates, San Diego.

Stillerman, E. (1992) *Mother Massage — A Handbook for Relieving the Discomforts of Pregnancy*. Dell Publishing, New York.

REFERENCES

Hicks, S. and McPake, A. (2001) 'Pregnancy massage. Why it works — part 1', *Massage Australia*, 35, pp. 24–33.

McPake, A. and Shannon, P. (2002) 'Low back pain and the pregnant client', *Massage Australia*, 39, pp. 34–41.

Osborne-Sheets, C. (1998) *Pre- and perinatal massage therapy*. Body Therapy Associates, San Diego.

Stillerman, E. (2000) 'Partner labour-support massage', *Massage Magazine*, Nov–Dec, pp. 144–54.

BIBLIOGRAPHY

Beischer, N. A., Mackay, E. V. and Colditz, P. B. (1997) *Obstetrics and the Newborn — An Illustrated Textbook* (3rd edn). W. B. Saunders, London.

Kimber, L. (1998) 'How did it feel? An informal survey of massage techniques in labour', *The Practising Midwife*, 1(12), pp. 38–41.

O'Connor, L. J. and Gourley, R. J. (1990) *Obstetric and Gynaecologic Care in Physical Therapy*. SLACK Inc, Thorofare.

Stillerman, E. (1992) *Mother Massage — A Handbook for Relieving the Discomforts of Pregnancy*. Dell Publishing, New York.

—— (2000) 'Mother massage: touch for happier, healthier pregnancies', *Massage Magazine*, Sept–Oct, pp. 82–95.

chapter 20

Infant massage

Vicki Tuchtan

Learning outcomes

- Describe the benefits of infant massage
- Discuss the role of the International Association of Infant Massage in education and training
- Outline the research in the area of infant massage
- Discuss the role of the massage therapist in infant massage

INTRODUCTION

Researchers have documented the importance of touch for mother–infant interaction (Field, 1998; Onozawa et al., 2001). Touch is an instinctive response that has been around since the evolution of the human species. All animals use touch as a form of non-verbal communication, for inquisitive investigation, to communicate feelings and emotions and to comfort and soothe one another. The importance of touch can be profoundly observed at the birth of a baby, where the mother establishes a bond with the newborn through a loving, nurturing and caring touch.

Despite the fact that touch is an instinctive form of communication, many new parents feel awkward about handling their child, unsure of whether they are doing it correctly or fearful they may hurt the infant. The art of massage is increasingly being used as a tool to encourage parents to touch their infants, and many prenatal courses now include instruction in infant massage for parents (see Figure 20.1). This chapter serves to introduce the reader to the concept of infant massage, and describes the benefits of massage for parent and child. It also discusses the importance of massage therapy in the development of the child.

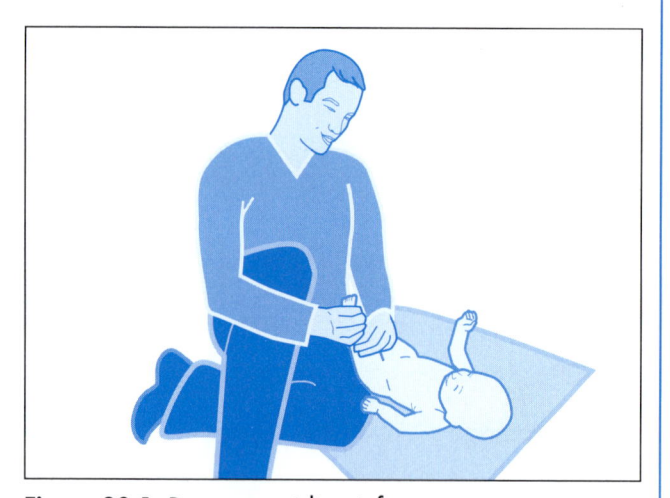

Figure 20.1 Parent providing infant massage

THE BENEFITS OF INFANT MASSAGE

Vimala Schneider McClure founded the International Association of Infant Massage (IAIM) in 1976. Prior to this time McClure observed the benefits to children of traditional Indian massage whilst travelling and studying in India. Upon her return to the United States McClure went on to study Swedish massage and later developed infant massage, writing the first book on the subject in 1977, entitled *Infant Massage: A Handbook For Loving Parents*, which has since been revised and updated (McClure, 2000).

Today the IAIM conducts specialised massage training courses. Such courses are designed to qualify professional massage therapists as certified infant massage instructors. These instructors then conduct instruction for parents in infant massage in hospital and community settings worldwide. In such classes, parents are instructed in the art of infant massage and are encouraged to maintain eye contact with their infant and to also use speech as a form of communication. Such positive interactions are used to enhance the baby's emotional and physical development, and cement the bonding between parent and child.

> **Box 20.1 Remember**
>
> The International Association of Infant Massage conducts training for professional massage therapists to become certified infant massage instructors.

The IAIM claims there are many benefits of infant massage (detailed in Box 20.2). According to Porter (1996) 'love expressed through touch affects both the baby and its parents and family ... it promotes bonding and well-being, gives pleasure and relaxation and inspires confidence' (p. 93). Unlike in pregnancy, the benefit of massage therapy for infants has been the subject of research. Although the quantity of research in this area is not

> **Box 20.2 Possible benefits of infant massage**
>
> - Improves communication between the parent and child.
> - Calms and soothes the baby's emotions.
> - Relieves stress and assists with sleep.
> - Helps babies to develop an awareness of their bodies.
> - Aids digestion and assists in relieving infant colic, wind and constipation.
> - Aids the development of muscle tone and coordination.
> - Strengthens the immune system.
> - Regulates breathing and relieves nasal congestion.
> - Improves skin texture.
> - Enhances the confidence and self-esteem of parents.
>
> (adapted from Simpson, 2001)

extensive, 'what little has been done has been quite equivocal' (Clarke et al., 2002, p. 121).

Research findings

It is widely accepted that touch in the form of massage positively affects the growth and development of infants born prematurely. Studies have reported pre-term infants who received massage gained more weight than infants who received no massage (Field, 2000).

Most of the studies conducted in this area employed the services of trained massage therapists to administer massage to pre-term infants, yet a recent controlled and randomised study aimed to ascertain whether massage performed by mothers had the same beneficial effect on infant growth and development (Ferber et al., 2002). The findings of this study suggest that massage performed by mothers achieved the same effect as that of trained professional massage therapists; in previous studies the infants experienced a significant gain in weight compared to the control group.

Massage not only improves the development of pre-term infants — according to the findings of Cigales et al. (1997) infants who receive massage have an enhanced recovery from habituation compared to infants that receive no massage. Field (1998) states that massage may prove useful in cases of maternal depression, as massage positively enhances the mother's mood and reduces arousal in the infant. Such factors promote positive interactions between the mother and infant and assist with bonding.

Another study investigated the effects of participation in a mother–infant massage class by mothers with postnatal depression (Onozawa et al., 2001). The findings from this study suggest that participation in infant massage classes assists with postnatal depression and facilitates improved mother–infant interaction.

> **Box 20.3** Remember
>
> Research investigating the benefits of infant massage suggests that it:
> - promotes growth and development as evidenced by increased weight gain;
> - enhances recovery from habituation;
> - may assist with postnatal depression; and
> - facilitates improved mother–infant interaction.

Porter (1996) describes the approach to care of the neonate over the past 50 years as having undergone significant change and outlines that in the past the focus was on establishing feeding routines, maintaining a constant temperature and minimising the risk of infection. Today the focus has shifted to include touch as a critical element in the care of the newborn.

> **Box 20.4** Remember
>
> Infant massage should always be a positive and pleasurable experience for the child.

CONSIDERATIONS FOR THE MASSAGE THERAPIST

When massage is provided to an infant, it should always be a pleasurable experience for the infant. If the infant is uncooperative or unsettled, the massage should not proceed. Massage of the infant is typically applied by the parent and consists of light and pleasurable stroking of the limbs and torso (Figures 20.2 and 20.3). The massage therapist would rarely massage an infant as a client, yet may treat a parent or grandparent of an infant. As such, they may be in a position to provide advice on the

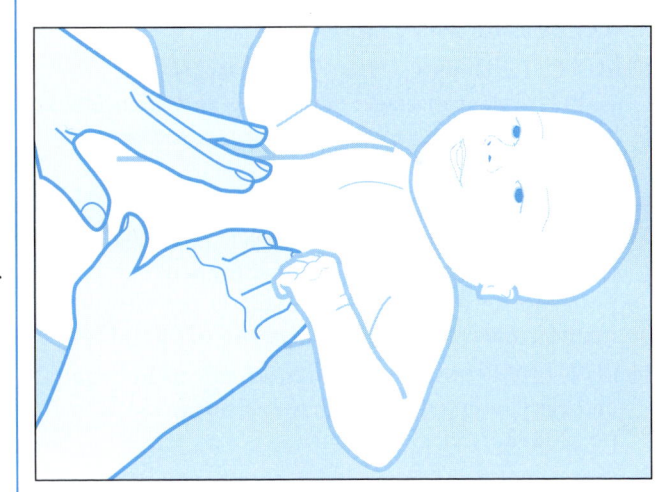

Figure 20.2 Light stroking used in infant massage

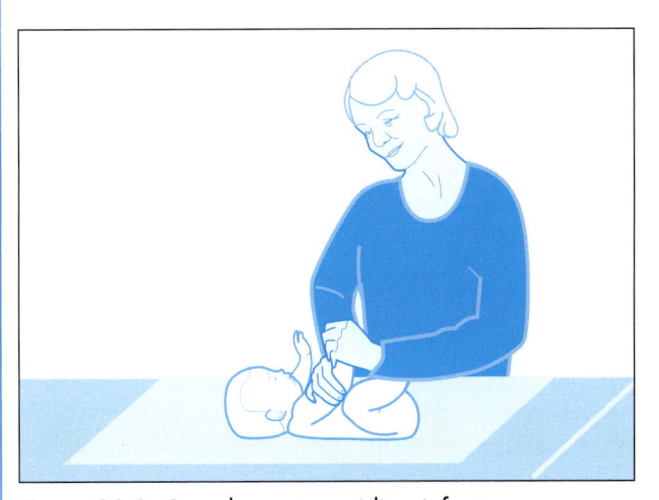

Figure 20.3 Grandparent providing infant massage

benefits of infant massage, and can refer the adult to suitable courses that provide instruction in infant massage.

CONCLUSION

There exist numerous and various benefits of infant massage for both the parent and child.

For infants, massage is more than just a pleasurable experience, it is a vital tool that promotes bonding and belonging, and enhances growth and development. For the parent it imparts feelings of confidence and connectedness with their child, and improves their mental wellbeing.

The IAIM provides certified training for instructors, who regularly conduct courses in infant massage at hospitals and community centres. The professional massage therapist should be aware of such courses, so they can refer their clients as required. By attending such sessions, parents and grandparents can learn simple techniques that can be used on a daily basis to massage their infant. Communicating and sharing through touch will reward those who adopt the practice of infant massage with a healthy and happy baby who benefits from and enjoys the intimacy of touch.

Questions and activities

As a professional massage therapist, you have a special interest in the benefits of massage for infants. You consult with many expectant mothers and have often thought of undertaking studies in infant massage, yet have a very busy clinical practice already.

Discuss how you could creatively expand your current practice into the area of infant massage.

REFERENCES

Cigales, M., Field, T. Lundy, B. Cuadra, A. and Hart, S. (1997) 'Massage enhances recovery from habituation in normal infants', *Infant Behaviour & Development*, 20(1), pp. 29–34.

Clarke, C. L., Gibb, C. Hart, J. and Davidson, A. (2002) 'Infant massage: developing an evidence base for health visiting practice', *Clinical Effectiveness in Nursing*, 6, pp. 121–8.

Ferber, S. G., Kuint, J. Weller, A., Feldman, R., Dollberg, S., Arbel, E. and Kohelet, D. (2002) 'Massage therapy by mothers and trained professionals enhances weight gain in pre-term infants', *Early Human Development*, 67, pp. 37–45.

Field, T. (1998) 'Maternal depression effects in infants and early interventions', *Preventive Medicine*, 27, pp. 200–3.

—— (2000) *Touch Therapy*. Churchill Livingstone, Edinburgh.

McClure, V. (2000) *Infant Massage: A Handbook For Loving Parents*. Barton Books, New York.

Onozawa, K., Glover, V., Adams, D., Modi, N. and Kumar, R. C. (2001) 'Infant massage improves mother–infant interaction for mothers with postnatal depression', *J of Affective Disorders*, 63, pp. 201–7.

Porter, S. J. (1996) 'The use of massage for neonates requiring special care', *Complementary Therapies in Nursing & Midwifery*, 2, pp. 93–6.

Simpson, R. (2001) 'Baby massage classes and the work of the International Association of Infant Massage', *Complementary Therapies in Nursing & Midwifery*, 7, pp. 25–33.

BIBLIOGRAPHY

Chapman, G. and Bond, C. (2002) 'Baby massage — a dialogue of touch', *Massage Australia*, 39, pp. 6–11.

Field, T., Grizzle, N., Scafidi, F., Abrams, S. and Richardson, S. (1996) 'Massage therapy for infants of depressed mothers', *Infant Behaviour & Development*, 19, p. 107–12.

Lynch, S. (1997) 'Baby massage — enhance the loving bond between you and your baby', *Massage Australia*, 1, pp. 6–10.

Miller, J. (1999) 'Baby massage — a touch of magic', *Australian Massage Magazine*, Oct–Nov, pp. 13–14.

Pelaez-Nogueras, M., Gewirtz, J. L., Field, T., Cigales, M., Malphurs, J., Clasky, S. and Sanchez, A. (1996) 'Infants' preference for touch stimulation in face-to-face interactions', *J Applied Developmental Psychology*, 17, pp. 199–213.

Walker, P. (1988) *The Book of Baby Massage*. Simon & Schuster Inc, New York.

appendix 1

Anatomical terminology

ANATOMICAL DIRECTIONAL TERMINOLOGY

TERM	DEFINITION
Superior (cephalic or cranial)	Towards the top of the body; above in relation to another structure
Inferior (caudal)	Towards the bottom of the body; below in relation to another structure
Anterior (ventral)	In front of; towards the front of the body
Posterior (dorsal)	Behind; towards the back of the body
Medial	Towards or at the midline of the body; relating to the middle or centre
Lateral	Towards the side; outside
Ipsilateral	On the same side
Contralateral	On the opposite side
Proximal	Towards the trunk; nearest to a point of origin
Distal	Away from the trunk; further from a point of origin
Supine	Lying face up
Prone	Lying face down

MOVEMENTS AT JOINTS

Common movements

Flexion

A bending motion where there is a decrease in the angle of a joint when two bones move towards each other.

Extension

A straightening movement where there is an increase in the angle of a joint when two bones move away from each other.

Internal rotation

The movement of a bone around its longitudinal axis towards the midline of the body; also known as medial rotation and inward rotation.

External rotation

The movement of a bone around its longitudinal axis away from the midline of the body; also known as lateral rotation and outward rotation.

Abduction

A movement of a body part away from the midline of the body.

Adduction

A movement of a body part towards the midline of the body.

Circumduction

A movement where the proximal end of the limb is stationary and the distal end moves in a circle forming a cone-like pattern. The movement results from a combination of flexion, extension, abduction and adduction.

Special movements

Elevation

Upwards movement.

Depression

Downwards movement.

Protraction

Forwards movement.

Retraction

Backwards movement.

Inversion

Turning the sole of the foot inwards or medially.

Eversion

Turning the sole of the foot outwards or laterally.

Dorsiflexion

Flexion movement of the ankle that results in the top of the foot moving towards the front of the leg.

Plantar flexion

Extension movement of the ankle that results in the foot and toes moving downwards; away from the front of the leg.

Supination

A movement where the forearm rotates laterally so that the radius lies parallel to the ulna, resulting in the palm facing upwards.

Pronation

A movement where the forearm rotates medially so that the radius lies diagonally across the ulna, resulting in the palm facing downwards.

Opposition

Diagonal movement of the thumb across the palmar surface of the hand to make contact with the fingers.

appendix 2

The human skeleton

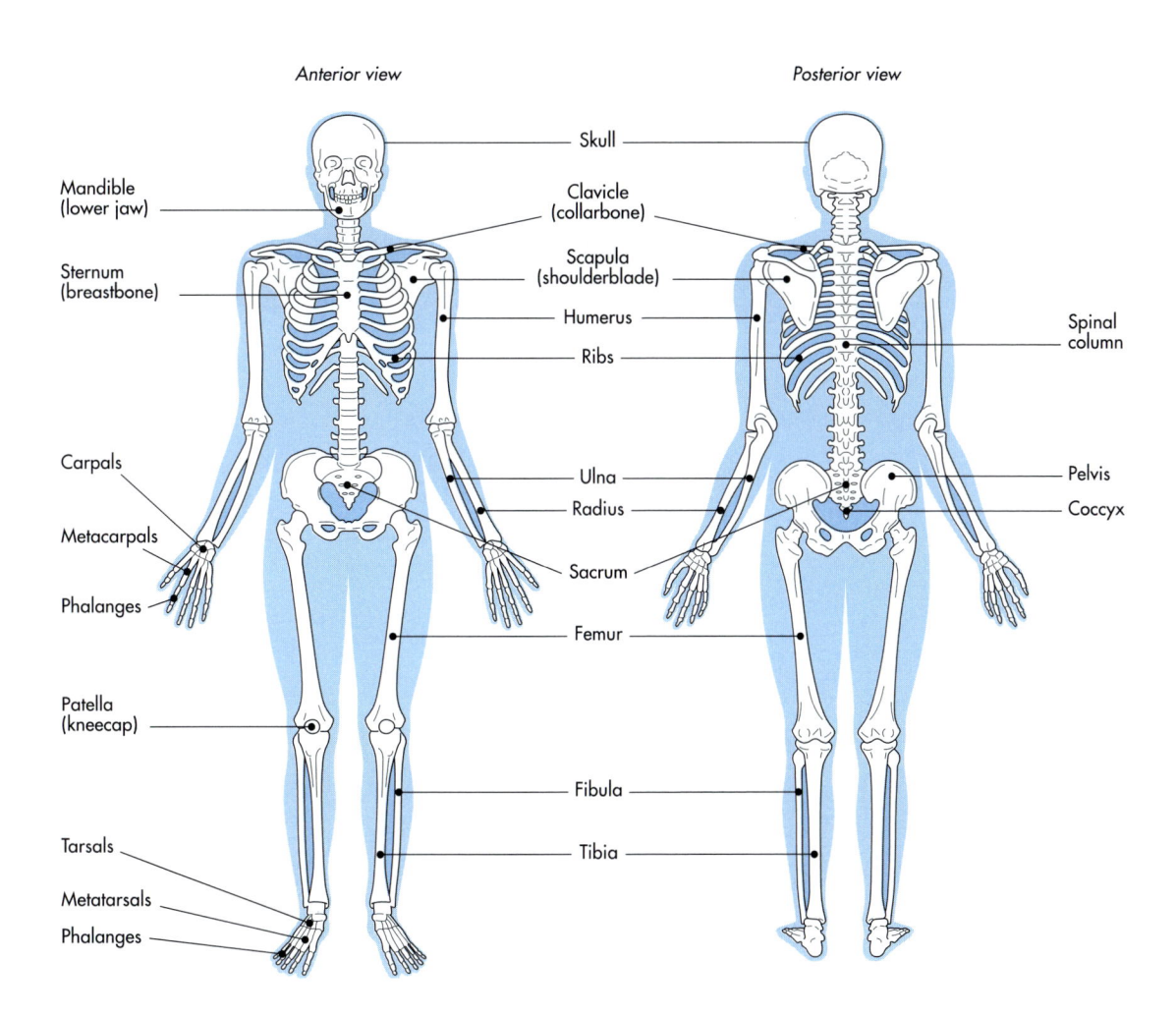

Anterior view

- Skull
- Mandible (lower jaw)
- Clavicle (collarbone)
- Sternum (breastbone)
- Scapula (shoulderblade)
- Humerus
- Ribs
- Carpals
- Ulna
- Metacarpals
- Radius
- Phalanges
- Sacrum
- Femur
- Patella (kneecap)
- Fibula
- Tarsals
- Tibia
- Metatarsals
- Phalanges

Posterior view

- Spinal column
- Pelvis
- Coccyx

appendix

appendix 3

Overview of the muscular system

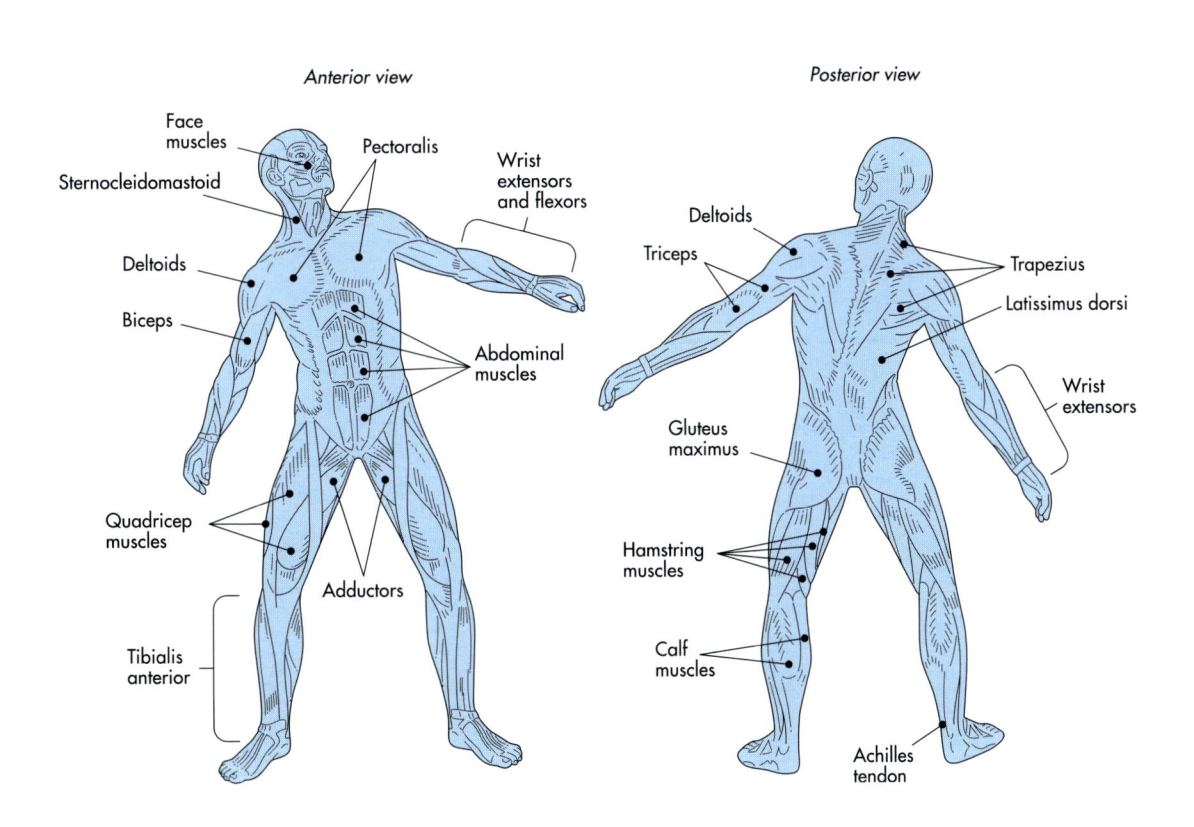

Glossary

Active listening is a communication skill that involves attentive listening followed by a response, which paraphrases what the listener heard. This technique assists with mutual understanding.

Adhesions see muscular adhesions.

Adrenalin is also known as epinephrine, and it is used by the body as a neurotransmitter for the sympathetic nervous system or as a hormone. As a hormone it mimics the effects of the sympathetic nervous system augmenting the flight or fight response; increasing respiration, blood pressure and heart rate; constricting blood vessels to the skin; and stimulating sweating.

Amputation is the removal of a limb or other appendage of the body.

Applied kinesiology (AK) is a system of assessment and treatment using muscle testing as a functional neurological evaluation, and corrective plans to align any imbalances.

Aromatherapy is the art and science of prescribing essential oils from aromatic plants to affect a psychological, physiological or spiritual change in the body.

Aura balancing is a technique that seeks to balance the electromagnetic field or aura, which surrounds all living organisms, via the use of light.

Autism is a neurological disorder affecting brain function. It is considered a developmental disability, and appears during the first three years of life.

Autonomy is the right of a person to make his or her own decisions and to act independently.

Blood pressure is the pressure of the blood measured in millimetres of mercury (mmHg).

Bowen technique is a therapeutic intervention that uses a series of gentle, rolling, connective tissue manipulations that encourage the body to realign and heal itself.

Brazelton scale or the Neonatal Behavioural Assessment Scale (NBAS) examines the behavioural portrait of newborns and infants (up to two months old). This scale identifies and describes the baby's strengths, adaptive responses and possible vulnerabilities. When shared with the parents, this data may serve to enhance the parent–baby relationship.

Breast augmentation is a surgical procedure to enlarge the breast.

Chakra balancing is a healing art that uses 17 vibrational frequencies to balance life-force energy. It can incorporate interventions such as holistic aromatherapy, guided meditation and releasing techniques to assist with the process.

Chronic refers to a condition or state that persists over an extended period of time.

Cortisol is a hormone that is secreted from the adrenal gland, which assists the metabolism of glucose, fats and proteins.

Cranio-sacral therapy is considered a gentle therapeutic intervention. This manual system of diagnosis and treatment involves the practitioner influencing the cranio-sacral motion by placing their hands on the cranium, sacrum or other body parts where this motion can be felt, and performing gentle movements to remove asymmetries or restrictions, thus restoring normal cranio-sacral motion.

Degenerate refers to the change of state or deterioration from a higher state or condition to a lower state or condition.

Diastole refers to the period of dilation of the heart.

Dilation refers to the stretching or increased hollowing of a blood vessel.

Dopamine is a neurotransmitter of the central nervous system.

Duty of care refers to the duty that exists when one person can reasonably foresee that their actions or omissions could cause harm to another person.

Eating disorder inventory (EDI) is a psychological assessment tool that evaluates several behavioural and psychological traits common in people who suffer from bulimia and anorexia nervosa.

Effleurage refers to a light stroking technique that is often used at the commencement and conclusion of a massage, and for transition between other types of massage techniques.

Electroencephalograph (EEG) is a medical tool that is used to record electrical signals from the brain.

Endorphin is a painkilling neuropeptide of the central nervous system.

Essential oils are highly concentrated and volatile plant essences, extracted from aromatic plant parts, which are used in aromatherapy.

Ethics refers to the moral principles by which our actions are guided.

Frictions are specific, localised massage techniques. Such massage strokes seek to produce movement between two surfaces or areas of tissue.

Hemiplegia refers to the paralysis of one side of the body.

Hippocampal region is a part of the limbic system of the brain. The limbic system is often referred to as the emotional brain, as it is responsible for such emotions as pain and affection.

Hypertonic muscle lesion refers is an area of abnormal muscle contraction within a muscle, characterised by bundles of muscle fibres in a state of excess tone.

Hypotonic muscle lesion refers to a muscle or part of a muscle that lacks muscle tone and is flaccid.

Informed consent refers to a client giving consent to any treatment protocol after first knowing all of the procedures and any risks associated with the treatment. As such, the client is able to decide whether they wish to proceed with the treatment protocol after being adequately 'informed' to make a judgment.

Jin Shin Do (The Way of the Compassionate Spirit) is a simple, gentle technique that addresses both physical and emotional tension and pain. Jin Shin Do combines traditional Japanese acupressure, classic Chinese acupressure theory, Reichian segmental theory, Taoist philosophy and Qigong exercises.

Joint mobility refers to the amount of movement or range of movement a joint can produce.

Justice refers to the maintenance of society's moral principles, as performed by governing bodies exercising their authority or power.

Lymphoedema is a condition characterised by chronic swelling affecting part(s) of the body. This condition results from damage to or blockage of the lymphatic system, thereby affecting its ability to restore interstitial fluid volume.

Manual lymphatic drainage is a specialised treatment technique that stimulates the lymphatic system to remove congestion and stagnation from within the body. This technique assists in promoting optimum lymphatic function, and commonly consists of specialised massage techniques, bandaging techniques and lymphatic exercises.

Muscle energy technique refers to manual techniques that require a contraction of a muscle or group of muscles against a counterforce. Such techniques are used to strengthen weak muscles, release hypertonicity, increase joint range of movement and improve lymphatic and vascular circulations.

Muscular adhesions occur when connective tissue abnormally adheres muscle fibres to each other, or adheres muscle fibres to another surrounding structure such as bone or fascia.

Myofascial release refers to specialised massage techniques, which are usually performed with sustained tensional force to increase the pliability and length of a muscle and its fascia.

Negligence is a term used to describe a lack of reasonable care and attention.

Neuromuscular techniques refer to a broad range of techniques, which positively affect the tone of a muscle. These techniques include deep effleurage, petrissage and compression techniques.

Non-maleficence refers to the intent to cause no harm.

Nutrient is a chemical substance obtained from a food source to provide energy to the body for development, growth and repair of tissue.

Oedema refers to the excessive or abnormal accumulation of interstitial fluid.

Ortho-bionomy is a gentle, non-invasive manual therapy. This technique involves the therapist moving the client on the treatment table in simple movement patterns and performing gentle compression-and-release techniques to encourage neuromuscular re-education of the body.

Oxytocin is a hormone secreted by the posterior pituitary gland, which stimulates uterine contractions to induce labour.

Paraplegia is the paralysis of the lower limbs and trunk.

Pétrissage refers to a group of massage techniques that involve lifting, squeezing, rolling, stretching and compressing the tissue under the hand.

Polarity therapy is a technique based on the theory that health is dependant on the uninterrupted flow of energy in the body between two polar opposites. This theory, developed by Randolf Stone, is not dissimilar to that of Ayerveda and traditional Chinese medicine (TCM).

Postural integration refers to a manual technique that combines gentle manipulations, bioenergetics, acupressure, breath-work, neo-Reichian techniques and Gestalt therapy.

Pranic healing refers to an energy-based healing technique that aims to balance and harmonise 'prana' or 'life-force'. This technique is based on the holistic principle that the body heals itself, and the treatment is performed on the body's electromagnetic field or aura.

Prosthesis refers to the artificial replacement for a missing body part, such as an artificial limb.

Psychiatrist refers to a medical practitioner who specialises in mental and emotional disorders.

Qigong is a system of self-healing, combining movement and meditation, to enhance the mind/body connection and promote wellbeing.

Reflexology refers to the therapeutic practice of applying pressure to reflex zones, primarily of the feet, hands and ears, to normalise body function.

Reiki is a form of Japanese spiritual healing that is based on the theory that vital life energy flows through all living creatures, and can be activated to promote healing. When performing a treatment, the Reiki practitioner channels life energy through their hands to the client, encouraging the body to heal itself.

Rolfing is a manual therapy that involves a series of deep massage treatments, which aim to re-establish the natural alignment and structural integration of the body.

Salivary cortisol is a glucocorticoid that may be found in saliva, that functions to regulate metabolism and the body's response to stress.

Scope of practice refers to the types of services that may be provided by a profession.

Sensory impairment refers to a loss of or altered sensory functioning.

Serum level refers to the quantity of blood plasma minus the clotting proteins.

Shiatsu is an ancient Japanese manual therapy that is based on the theory that vital energy flows through the body in a series of channels known as meridians. When performing a treatment, the Shiatsu practitioner aims to restore energy flow along the meridians using a variety of techniques that improve energy flow, including pressure work and dynamic stretches.

Sports massage involves the use of therapeutic massage strokes and related techniques to promote the health and wellbeing of an athlete.

Standard of care refers to a reasonably expected level of professional service.

Swedish massage is one of the most widely practised massage techniques in Western civilisation, and combines the seven major massage techniques; namely effleurage, pétrissage, tapôtement, frictions, vibrations, rocking and compressions.

Tapôtement refers to massage techniques that pat or tap the skin.

Therapeutic touch is an energetic technique that has been practised by health care workers since Dolores Krieger developed it in the 1970s. Therapeutic touch aims to promote wellness by a transfer of excess energy from the practitioner to the client, and it is often taught and practised by the nursing profession.

Trager therapy refers to a system of manual therapy that uses gentle, rhythmic movements to assist the release of physical or psychological stress patterns — either on a mental, emotional or physical level — and enhance the mind/body connection.

Tui Na (also known as traditional Chinese medicine remedial massage) is an ancient Chinese system of manual therapy that aims to restore energy flow within the body, and is used in conjunction with other forms of traditional Chinese medicine (TCM).

Urinary cortisol is a glucocorticoid that may be found in urine, and functions to regulate metabolism and the body's response to stress.

Vibrations are massage techniques that are rhythmic and trembling or oscillating in nature.

Visceral is a term used to describe that associated with an organ of the body.

Vitamin D is essential for the absorption of calcium by the body, and can be obtained from food sources such as fortified milk, fish-liver oils and egg yolk.

Zero balancing is a manual therapy developed by Dr Fritz Smith in the 1970s. Combining both Eastern and Western techniques, it aims to restore the flow of energy in the body and improve posture.

Index

abbreviations in record keeping 127–9
abdomen endangerment site 138
Aboriginal history of massage 19
absolute contraindications 136, 139
    see also contraindications
accessories for massage tables 89
ACT privacy legislation 130
acupuncture 7
    massage complementing 31
Additional Precautions 109
    see also infection control
ADHD *see* attention deficit hyperactivity disorder
aged care 176–7
alternative medicine *see* complementary and alternative medicine
Alzheimer's disease 216
ambience of the massage room 85
American history of massage 18, 23
amma massage writings in China 16
    see also traditional Chinese medicine 7
analgesics 40, 42
angina 156–7
ankylosing spondylitis 39
anorexia nervosa 52–3, 139–40
    drug therapy 158
anterior shoulder flexibility exercise 99
anxiety 140
    drug therapy 158
arm baths 103
arm endangerment sites 138
aroma of the massage room 84–5
aromatherapy 7
arthritis 41, 151–3, 163
aseptic techniques for infection control 109
    see also infection control
Asian therapies 8–9
assessing clients' needs 120–4
ASTER formula 120
    case study 132
    sample form 131
    see also consultation process
asthma 140
    drug therapy 158–9
atmosphere *see* massage settings
attention deficit hyperactivity disorder (ADHD) 140–1
    drug therapy 159
Austin and Repatriation Medical Centre 19
Australian National Training Authority (ANTA) 13, 63
Australian Physiotherapy Association 11, 20
Australian Traditional Medicine Society (ATMS) 63

autism 52
autonomy (ethical principle of) 64–5
Avicenna 18
axilla endangerment site 138
ayurveda 7

baby massage *see* infant massage; pregnancy and massage
back endangerment site 136
back loosening exercise 99–100
back pain research 41
bacteria 106–7
bathing culture in ancient Greece and Rome 17
Bell's palsy 141
beneficence 65
biomagnetic energy fields 54
biomedical health care model 32–3
biomedical practitioners 29
blood collection 114
    see also infection control
blood pressure 39
    see also hypertension
body fluid management 114
    see also infection control
body image 53
body language 55
body massage *see* full body massage
body mechanics 196
    leverage and 197–200
    principles for self-care 196–7
bodywork 8
bodywork qualifications 13
botanical medicine 7
boundaries 72, 78–9
    and the right to refuse 73–4
    cultural background affecting 65, 76–7
    dual roles and 74
    emotional 75
    guidelines for cultural 77–8
    intimacy and 75
    personal/professional 72–3
    physical 74
    self-disclosure 73
    sexual 75
breast massage 138
breast tissue endangerment site 138
British history of massage 18, 32
British Medical Association (BMA) inquiry into massage 18–19
broad compression 207–8

bulimia 52–3, 141
    drug therapy 158

CAM *see* complementary and alternative medicine
cancer 41, 43
case histories 54–5, 139
    including medication 156
case studies
    consultation process 132
    negligence 66
    standard of care breach 67
cellulitis 141
Celsus, Aulus 17–18
cerebrovascular accident 40, 141–2
CFS *see* chronic fatigue syndrome
charting 125
    see also record keeping
chemotherapy 43
chest endangerment site 138
Chinese massage history 16
    see also traditional Chinese medicine 7
chiropractic 10–11
    massage complementing 31
Chopra, Dr Deepak 7
Christianities influence on massage history 17
chronic fatigue syndrome (CFS) 121, 142
    drug therapy 158
chronically ill clients 177–8
circular friction 212
circular kneading 206
circulatory benefits of massage 30, 38–9
civil action in assault 69
civil law 65
    see also law of torts
Clancy, Jim 21
clean techniques for infection control 109
    see also infection control
Cleaver, Keith 21
client comfort 85
    special needs and 171–3
    see also massage settings
client interview 54–5, 122–4
    for homoeopathy 31
    see also consent to therapy
client needs assessment 120–1
client positioning 192–4
    for special needs 171–4
    prone to supine 191–2
    see also draping techniques
client questioning techniques 123
client referral 6, 62, 64, 67, 69
    multicultural considerations for 78
    with absolute contraindications 136, 139, 142
client–therapist relationship
    cultural considerations 65
    dual roles within 74
    importance of touch in the 30–1, 53
    trust 55, 76, 122
    see also boundaries; duty of care
clinic-based practice 87
clinic safety 67
    see also infection control
clinic set-up *see* massage settings
clinical nutrition 8

closed questions 123
clothing 112
codes of ethics 74
    see also ethics
codes of practice 63
colours for relaxation 85
common abbreviations 127–9
common law 65
communication
    draping as a form of 194
    regarding pain/discomfort 77
    through touch 52
    through touch therapy 55
    with special needs clients 171
complementary and alternative medicine
    (CAM) 6–7, 22
compression 207–9
confidentiality 67
consent to therapy 55, 62, 68, 77
    for special needs clients 171
    legal capacity to give 68–9
constipation 142
consultation process 85–6, 120, 134
    assess client needs 120–2
    ASTER chart sample 131
    client interview 122–4
    evaluation 125
    health history form 121–2
    recording 125–7, 130
    treatment 124–5
    see also treatment plan
contraindications 67, 123
    aged care 176–7
    effleurage 205
    friction 213
    pétrissage 209
    pre-natal massage 296, 298–9
    tapôtement 211
    vibrations 215
cramp 39–40
creams 92
criminal law 65
cross-fibre friction 212–13
C-scoop kneading 205–6
cubital fossa endangerment site 138
cultural boundaries 65
    guidelines for 77–8
cupping 210
Cyriax, James 19

Dark Ages (the) 17
DBE *see* deep breathing exercise
De Medicina 17–18
deep breathing exercise (DBE) 219
definition of
    a child for consent purposes 68
    boundaries 72
    complementary medicine 6–7
    effleurage 202
    friction 211
    holistic medicine 28
    infection 106
    infectious agents 106–7
    integrative medicine 28

manipulative therapy 9
massage therapy 4–5
pétrissage 205
tapôtement 209
vibrations 213–14
dementia 162, 177, 216
depression 43, 52, 142–3, 170
    drug therapy 159
desktop massager 90, 281–2
diabetes mellitus 143
    drug therapy 159–60
direct osteopathic technique 10
direction of massage 226
    see also full body massage
discrimination 65
disease in modern society 29
diseases see infection control; infectious agents
disinfecting the workplace 112–13
    see also infection control
dispensing lubricants 92
disrobing 74
    cultural boundaries and 76
doctor as teacher 6, 29, 32
Down syndrome 143–4
draping 184, 194
draping materials 184–5
draping techniques 185
    for anterior lower limb massage 255
    for arm, forearm and hand massage 268
    for back massage 234
    for chest massage 266
    for neck and shoulder massage 273
    for scalp and face massage 276
    for seated position 190–1
    fully draped client 185
    prone to supine 191–2
    side-lying position 188–9
    table preparation 185
    undraping abdomen and chest 187–8
    undraping lower limb 186–7
    undraping the arm 187
    undraping the back 185–6
    undraping the buttocks 189–90
    see also full body massage
drug abuse 160
drug therapy 166
    angina 156, 158
    anorexia nervosa 158
    anxiety 158
    asthma 158–9
    attention deficit hyperactivity disorder (ADHD) 159
    bulimia nervosa 158
    chronic fatigue syndrome 159
    depression 159
    diabetes 159–60
    dysmenorrhea 160
    endometriosis 160
    epilepsy 160
    fibromyalgia 161
    hay fever 161
    headache 161
    heart failure 161–2
    hypertension 162
    immunosuppressant therapy 162
    interacting with massage therapy 156
    menopause 162
    multiple sclerosis 162–3
    obesity 163
    osteoarthritis 163
    Paget's disease 163
    premenstrual syndrome 163
    rheumatoid arthritis 163
    schizophrenia 163–4
    topical steroid therapy 164
drug types 157–8, 164–6
dual roles in client–therapist relationship 74
duty of care 66–7
dynamic vibrations 214
dysmenorrhoea 144
    drug therapy 160

Eastern/Asian therapies 8–9
eating disorders 52–3
education see training
effleurage 202
    contraindications 205
    effects of 215–17
    techniques 203–4
Egyptian massage history 16
elderly clients 176–7
emotional boundaries 75
    see also boundaries
emotional state (massage benefits) 42–4
emotional trauma and touch therapy 53
endangerment sites 136–9
endometriosis 144
    drug therapy 160
endorphins 42, 51
    and drug therapy 156
energy healing through touch 54
environment see massage settings
epilepsy 145
    drug therapy 160
equipment 88
eyewear 109, 112
    face masks 109, 111–12
    for special needs clients 171–3
    gloves 109, 111
    handtowels 187–8
    lubricants 91–2
    maintenance 67
    massage chair 90
    massage table 88–90
    self-massage 103
    use for client positioning 192–4
errors in record keeping 127
Esalen Institute 21
ethics 62, 64
    codes of 74
    principles of 64–5
ethnic background affecting boundaries 76–7
ethnic stereotyping 78
evaluation 125
exercises for
    anterior shoulder flexibility 99
    back loosening 99–100
    finger flexibility 97
    finger strengthening 101

forearm flexibility 97
forearm strengthening 101
hand strengthening 101
latissimus dorsi flexibility 97–8
pectoralis major flexibility 97
rhomboid flexibility 98
rhomboid strengthening 101
rotator cuff strengthening 102
serratus anterior strengthening 101
thoracic spine flexibility 99
triceps brachii flexibility 99
upper trapezius flexibility 98
eyewear 109, 112
    see also protective equipment

face endangerment site 139
face masks 109, 111–12
    see also protective equipment
fatigue 196
Fay, Joseph 20
feet position for massage 199
femoral triangle endangerment site 138
FET see forced expiration technique
fibromyalgia 41, 145–6
    drug therapy 161
finger flexibility exercise 97
finger strengthening exercise 101
first trimester massage 295–6
    see also pregnancy and massage
fist effleurage 204
    see also effleurage
fitness therapy and massage 32
flow of manipulations 226–7
folliculitis 146
forced expiration technique (FET) 219
forearm
    endangerment sites 138
    flexibility exercises 97
    leverage for massage 199–200
    strengthening exercises 101
forearm effleurage 203–4
    see also effleurage
foreseeability (duty of care and) 67
fractures 146–7
free and voluntary consent 68
    see also consent to therapy
French history of massage 18, 32–3
friction 202, 211–12
    contraindications 213
    effects of 220
    techniques 212–13
full body massage 184, 228
    abdomen 262–6
    anterior lower limb 255–6
    arm, forearm and hand 268–73
    back routine 234–45
    chest 266–8
    foot 253–5
    front of leg 258–62
    front of thigh 256–8
    neck and shoulders 273–7
    posterior lower limb 245–53
    scalp and face 276–81
    sequence summary 228–34
    see also draping techniques; seated massage

fungi 107
future of massage 22–3

Galan, Claudius 17
gate-control theory of pain 40
gloves 109, 111
    see also protective equipment
government regulation 22
Graham, Douglas 4
Greek massage history 16–17
guardians 69
guidelines for
    cultural boundaries 77–8
    draping 184
    record keeping 126–7
    treating multicultural clients 77–8
Guillain-Barre syndrome 147

hacking 210
Hahnemann, Dr Samuel 7
half rowing stroke 203
Hall, Teepo 19
hand after hand effleurage 204
    see also effleurage
hand washing 110
hands
    care of 96–7
    healing power of 30, 54
    nerve receptor cells 50
    strengthening exercises for 101
hands-on healing 54
handtowels 187–8
hay fever 147
    drug therapy 161
headache 147–8
    drug therapy 161
healing environment 30
    see also massage settings
health (origin of the word) 28
health history form 121–2
health maintenance for therapists 103–4
Health Privacy Principles (HPP) 130
Health Training Package (Complementary
    and Alternative Health Care) 13
hearing impaired clients 175–6
heart failure drug therapy 161–2
hepatitis 148–9
herbal medicine 7
high blood pressure see hypertension
high velocity low amplitude (HVLA) adjustments 31
    chiropractic 11
    physiotherapy 12
    remedial massage 13
Hippocrates' theory 8
    of massage 17
history of infectious agents 106
history of massage 23
    3000 BC–AD 400 16–17
    Dark/Middle Ages 17–18
    in Australia 19–21
    in New Zealand 21–2
HIV 43–4
home-based practice 86–7
homoeopathy 7–8

holistic medicine 28–9
    massage complementing 31
hormone replacement therapy 162
HVLA adjustments *see* high velocity low
        amplitude adjustments
hydrotherapy to reduce therapist fatigue 103
hygiene 67, 106, 178
    personal 110
hygienic application of lubricants 92
hypertension 149
    drug therapy 162
    research into massage benefits for 39
    strokes and 40, 141–2
hypertonicity 39–40

ice (in treatment) 21
immune function improvement 43–4
immunosuppressant therapy 162
impaired mobility clients 174
indications for therapeutic massage 123, 139, 153
    anorexia nervosa 139–40
    anxiety 140
    asthma 140
    attention deficit hyperactivity disorder (ADHD) 140
    Bell's palsy 141
    bulimia 141
    cellulitis 141
    cerebral vascular accident 141–2
    chronic fatigue syndrome 142
    constipation 142
    depression 142–3
    diabetes mellitus 143
    Down syndrome 143–4
    dysmenorrhoea 144
    endometriosis 144
    epilepsy 145
    fibromyalgia 145–6
    folliculitis 146
    fractures 146–7
    Guillain-Barre syndrome 147
    hay fever 147
    headache 147–8
    hepatitis 148–9
    hypertension 149
    irritable bowel syndrome 149
    menopause 149–50
    multiple sclerosis 150
    obesity 150–1
    oedema 151
    osteoarthritis 151
    Paget's disease 151–2
    premenstrual syndrome 152
    psoriasis 152
    rheumatoid arthritis 152–3
    see also contraindications
indigenous culture and massage 19, 28
indirect benefits of massage 38
indirect osteopathic technique 10
infant development enhanced by touch 50–1
infant massage 302–4
infection control 106, 115–16
    cleaning equipment for 113
    cleaning the workplace for 112–13
    equipment 111–12
    managing waste for 113–14
    personal hygiene for 110
    risks 114
    Standard and Additional Precautions for 109
infectious agents 106–7
    entering/exiting the body 108–9
    location of 107–8
    transmission of 108
information for informed consent 68
information gathering 54–5, 77, 120–3
Information Privacy Principles (NZ) 132–3
informed consent 68, 124
    multicultural clients and 77
    see also consent to therapy
Institute of Touch 23
integrative health care 28–9
integrative health care model 29–33
intellectual disability 174–5
    and consent 69
    dementia 162, 177, 216
interview *see* client interview
intimacy 75
intimate distance 72
irritable bowel syndrome 149

jewellery 110
joint mobility 42, 146
justice (ethical principle of) 65

Kellogg, J. H. 16, 202
kidney region endangerment site 136
King, Harry and Arthur 21

labour and massage 299–300
    see also pregnancy and massage
large clients 171–2
lateral epicondyle endangerment site 138
latissimus dorsi flexibility exercise 97–8
laundering 85, 184–5
law of torts 66
    see also negligence action
Laws of Man 16
leg endangerment sites 138
legal action and record keeping 126
legal capacity for consent 68–9
legibility of records 127
legislation 22–3, 62, 65, 115
    privacy 73, 130, 132–3
    see also consent; negligence action
leverage in massage 197–200
lighting in the massage setting 85
    see also massage settings
limits of practice 64
linear friction 212
linen care 85, 184–5
linens for draping 184
Ling, Per Henrik 18, 202
literature on massage benefits 38
lotions and creams 92
lubricants 91–2
    application for back massage 234
Lucas-Championnière, Just Marie 18, 32
lymphatic drainage 19, 207, 216
lymphoedema relief 39

Maitland, Geoff 12
managing waste 113–14
    see also infection control
manipulations 226–7
    see also effleurage; friction; full body massage; pétrissage; tapôtement; vibration
manipulative therapies 9
    chiropractic 10–11
    osteopathy 9-10
    physiotherapy 11–12
    remedial massage therapy 12–13
manual lymph drainage (MLD) 216
Maori culture and massage 21
massage associations 62–3
massage chair 90, 172, 281–2
massage history see history of massage
Massage Institute of New Zealand Incorporated (MINZI) 22
massage parlours 19, 75
massage settings 84–5, 92–3
    clinic-based 87
    home-based 86–7
    mobile 87
    work-site 87–8
    see also special needs clients
massage table 88, 171
    accessories 89
    assisting clients on and off 192
    maintenance 89–90
    preparation 185, 192–3
    special needs clients and the 172–3
massage therapists'
    body mechanic principles 196–7
    flexibility/mobility exercises 96–100
    professional responsibility 84, 170
    resistance exercises 100–2
    self-care 96, 103–4
    self-massage 102–3
    use of leverage 197–200
massage therapy 13
    categories 4
    definition of 4–5
    Eastern/Asian 8–9
    integrative health care model for 29–32
    legislation for 22–3, 62, 65, 115
    qualifications 13, 23
    registration of 22
    right to refuse 73–4, 124
    scope of practice 7, 62–4, 69
    therapeutic 4–5
    training 13, 63
    within the biomedical health care model 32–3
    see also full body massage; indications for therapeutic massage
massage therapy benefits 30, 44–5
    during labour 300
    during pregnancy 294, 300
    for circulatory system 38–9
    for emotional state 42–4
    for infants 302–3
    for muscle tone 39–40
    for pain relief 40–2
    for sleep enhancement 44
    see also indications for therapeutic massage

medial epicondyle endangerment site 138
medical terminology in record keeping 127
medication history 156, 166
    see also drug therapy
Menell, Dr James 19, 202
menopause 149–50
    drug therapy 162
menstruation and massage therapy 77
Mercuriale, Girolamo 18
Mezger, Dr Johann 4, 18, 32, 202
micro-organisms 106–7
    see also infection control; infectious agents
Middle Ages (beliefs during) 9
migraines 161
mineral oils 92
Mitchell, Bill 21
MLD see manual lymph drainage
mobile massage practice 87
moxibustion 7
multicultural clients 76–8
multidisciplinary environment 64
multiple sclerosis 40, 150
    drug therapy 162–3
muscle tone 39–40
music 84
myofascial trigger points 209

nail care 110
National Privacy Principles (NPP) 130
natural medicine 4–5
    modalities 7
    philosophy/principles 5–6
    usage statistics 6
nature as healer 5
naturopathy 8
    massage complementing 29–31
neck endangerment sites 136
negligence action 66
    duty of care 66–7
    foreseeability 67–8
    standard of care 67
nerve receptor cells 50
nerve strokes 204
nervous system
    benefited by touch 51
    parasympathetic response to massage 75
neuromuscular excitability 39–40
New South Wales privacy legislation 130
New Zealand Association of Therapeutic Massage Practitioners (NZATMP) 22
New Zealand Qualifications Authority (NZQA) 64
New Zealand's
    history of massage 21–2
    legislative requirements 63
    privacy legislation 132–3
non-maleficence 65
Northern Territory privacy legislation 130
nutrition therapy 8

obesity 150–1
    drug therapy 163
objective assessments 73
objectivity in record keeping 126
oedema 39, 151

oil 67
oil application for back massage 234
open-ended questions 123
oriental bodywork 8–9
osteoarthritis 151
    drug therapy 163
osteopathy 9–10
    role of massage in 31
overuse injuries 96, 196

Paget's disease 151–2
    drug therapy 163
pain
    communicating about 77
    effect of massage on 40–2
    gate-control theory of 40
    medication 41
    threshold 227–8
Palmer, Bartlett Joshua, 10
Palmer, Daniel David 9–11
palpation assessment 124
parasites 107
parasympathetic nervous system 75
Paré, Ambrois 18
parent–child bond 51
pathogens 107–8
    see also infection control; infectious agents
PD see postural drainage
pectoralis major flexibility exercise 97
peripheral nervous system 75–6
person-centred health care 29
personal boundaries 72–3
personal space 54, 72
    see also physical boundaries
personal trainers using massage therapy 32
Peters, Alfred 19
pétrissage 202, 205
    compression and 207–9
    contraindications 209
    effects of 217–18
    for muscle tone 39–40
    techniques 205–7
physical boundaries 74
    see also boundaries
physical therapy 8
physicians 32
physiotherapy
    history of 11–12, 32
    role of massage in 31
    techniques 12
phytotherapy 7
pillowing 85, 171
plucking 210
popliteal fossa endangerment site 138
positioning 192–4
    for large clients 171–4
    see also draping; special needs clients
positive touch experience 54–5
post-natal massage 302–4
post-surgery massage benefits 39
postural drainage 219
pregnancy and massage 294
    during first trimester 295–6
    during labour 299–200

    during second trimester 296–8
    during third trimester 298–9
    see also infant massage
premenstrual syndrome 152
    drug therapy 163
prescription pain medication 41
prevention versus cure 6
principles
    body mechanics 96–7
    chiropractic 10–11
    natural medicine 5–6, 29
    of ethics 64–5
    osteopathy 9–10
    privacy 130, 132–3
privacy legislation 73, 130, 132–3
professional boundaries 72–3
professional negligence see negligence action
professional responsibility 84, 124, 170
    see also professional boundaries; negligence action
protective equipment
    eyewear 109, 112
    face masks 109, 111–12
    gloves 109, 111
psoriasis 152
psychological benefits of massage 42–4
psychological disorders and touch therapy 52–3
    see also intellectual disability
psychosocial development and touch 51–2
public distance 72
pummelling 210

Qi 7, 9
qualifications 13, 23, 63–4
questioning techniques 123

RA see rheumatoid arthritis
record keeping 125–6
    guidelines 126–7
    using ASTER 120, 130–2
referral of clients 6, 62, 64, 67, 69
    multicultural considerations for 78
    with absolute contraindications 136, 139, 142
registration 22, 62–3
relaxation massage 4–5
remedial massage 4–5, 12–13
research into biomagnetic energy fields 54
research into massage therapy benefits 44–6, 51–2
    for circulatory system 38–9
    for emotional state 42–4
    for infants 303
    for muscle tone 39–40
    for pain relief 40–2
    for psychological disorders 52–4
    for sleep enhancement 44
    of effleurage 215–17
    of friction 220
    of pétrissage 217–18
    of tapôtement 218
    of vibrations 220–1
resistance exercises 100–2
responsibility see professional responsibility
rheumatoid arthritis 41, 152–3
    drug therapy 163
rhomboid flexibility exercise 98

rhomboid strengthening exercise 101
right of refusal 73–4, 124
rocking vibration 214
Roman bathing culture 17
rotational movements of therapist's trunk 198
rotator cuff strengthening exercise 102
Roth, Mathias 18
rowing stroke 203
rubbish *see* infection control

Sandford, Jim 22
schizophrenia 163–4
Scientific Massage for Athletes 20
scope of practice 7, 62–3, 69
    guidelines 63–4
    limits 64
seated massage 171–3, 281
    sequence 283–90
    sequence summary 282–3
second trimester massage 296–8
    see also pregnancy and massage
self-care 96, 103–4
    arm baths 103
    flexibility/mobility exercises 96–100
    good body mechanics for 196–7
    resistance exercises 100–2
    self-massage 102–3
    using leverage for 197–200
self-concept 53
self-disclosure 73
self-healing, 10–11, 31
self-massage 102
sensory impaired clients 175
sequence 226, 228–34
    see also full body massage
serratus anterior strengthening exercise 101
sexual boundaries 75
    promoting clear 76
shaking vibration 214
shiatsu therapy 16
shock treated with touch therapy 53
side pulls 204
skin and tactile sense 50
skin rolling 207
sleep enhancement 44
slow manual chest percussion (SMCP) 219
slow-stroke back massage (SSBM) 215
SMCP *see* slow manual chest percussion
SOAP *see* Subjective Objective Assessment Plan
social distance 72
societal touch deprivation 52
society's contribution to disease 29
society's standard of behaviour 72
soft tissue injury 42
spasm 30–4
special needs clients 170, 178–9
    aged and frail 176–7
    chronic/terminal illness 177–8
    communicating with 171
    impaired mobility 174
    intellectually challenged 174–5
    massage positions for 171–3
    sensory impaired 175–6
    techniques for size and shape 171–2

specific compression 208–9
speech impaired clients 175
spinal chord injury 40
sports masseurs 32
squeezing 206–7
SSBM *see* slow-stroke back massage
standard of behaviour 72
standard of care 67
    see also negligence action
Standard Precautions 109
    see also infection control
static vibrations 214
Still, Andrew Taylor 9
stoicism 77
stress reduction 42, 52
stroke (cerebral vascular accident) 40, 141–2
    see also hypertension
subjective assessments 73
Subjective Objective Assessment Plan (SOAP) 120, 130
subluxation (chiropractic approach) 11
subtle energy practices 4
surgery 32, 42
Swedish massage 222
    history of 18, 202
    sequence 226, 228–34
    see also full body massage
symbols in record keeping 127
sympathetic nervous system 75–6

tactile sense 50
tactile therapies 8
    see also manipulative therapies
tactile-kinaesthetic stimulation 51
talcum powder 92
tapôtement 202, 209
    contraindications 211
    effects of 218–20
    techniques 209–11
tapping 210–11
TCM *see* traditional Chinese medicine
techniques
    chiropractic 11
    effleurage 203–4
    for adapting massage to client size and shape 171–2
    friction 212–13
    hand washing 110
    infection control 109
    osteopathic 10
    pétrissage 205–9
    physiotherapy 12
    questioning 123
    tapôtement 209–11
    vibrations 214
    see also draping techniques
technological advances affect on touch 52
TEE *see* thoracic expansion exercises
temperature assessment of clients 124
temperature in the massage setting 85
tenderness or pain 125
terminally ill clients 177–8
texture 124–5
The Yellow Emperor's Classic of Internal Medicine 16
therapeutic massage *see* massage therapy
Therapeutic Massage Association (TMA) 22

therapists'
    overuse injuries 96
    presentation 85, 103
    strategies for positive touch 54–5
    see also client–therapist relationship; self-care
thigh endangerment sites 138
third trimester massage 298–9
    see also pregnancy and massage
thoracic expansion exercises (TEE) 218
thoracic spine flexibility exercise 99
throat endangerment site 136
time for record keeping 126–7, 130
time management 84
tone 39–40, 124–5
topical steroid therapy 164
touch
    deprivation 51–2
    developing a sense of self 51
    enhancing infant development 50–1
    everyday role of 50
Touch Research Institute (TRI) 50–1
touch therapy 8
    approaches 55
    benefits for human development 50–1
    energy healing through 54
    for psychological disorders 52–3
    psychosocial development and 51–2
traditional Chinese medicine (TCM) 7
    tactile therapy within 31
training 13, 63
tranquillity 84
transmission of infectious agents 108–9, 115
    see also infection control
transverse friction massage 19
trauma 53
traverse friction 212–13
treatment plan 124, 153
    to avoid boundary violation 74
    evaluation 125
    see also record keeping
triceps brachii flexibility exercise 99
trigger-point therapy 5, 11–12, 208–9, 219
trust 55, 76, 122
tsubo points 16
tui na 31
turning client prone to supine 191–2

umbilicus area endangerment site 138
undraping see draping techniques
undressing see disrobing
upper trapezius flexibility exercise 98

valid consent 68
    see also consent to therapy
VAS see visual analogue scale
vector transmission of infectious agents 108
    see also infection control
vegetable oils 91–2
vibration 202, 213–14
    contraindications 215
    effects of 220–1
    techniques 214
Victorian privacy legislation 130
violence and negative touch 51
viruses 106–7
visual analogue scale (VAS) 40–1, 227–8
visually impaired clients 175
vital energy (Qi) 7, 9
Vocational Education and Training (VET) 13
Vodder, Emil 19

war's impact upon massage development 12, 20
Wareham, Bill 22
Warren, Anne 19
waste collection 113–14
    see also infection control
water soluble vegetable oils 92
Western biomedical health care model 29
    massage therapy within the 32–3
wheelchairs (massage in) 172, 174
WHO see World Health Organisation
whole person approach 5–6
World Health Organisation 6, 28
World War I 20
World War II 12, 20
work-site massage practice 87–8
wringing technique 207
wrist leverage for massage 199
written consent 124
    see also consent to therapy

yoga 16, 43